Psychopathology

Carter's *Psychopathology* is an accessible, engaging, and well-organized text covering the study, understanding, diagnosis, treatment, and prevention of psychological disorders. Fully integrating gender and culture in the presentation of mental disorders, and using sensitive and inclusive language to encourage an empathic approach to psychopathology, this introductory textbook offers students a strong foundation of the socio-cultural factors influencing how we treat mental disorders. Featuring boxes such as "the power of words," promoting the use of respectful, empathic language, and "the power of evidence," demonstrating that scientific evidence can answer questions about psychopathology treatments; real-world case studies and examples; "concept checks" questions to test the student's mastery of the material covered in each section; chapter summaries listing the "take-home" points discussed; and key terms and glossary highlighting terms that students will need to understand and become familiar with, this textbook provides a hands-on approach to the study of psychopathology.

KENNETH CARTER is Charles Howard Candler Professor of Psychology and interim Dean at Oxford College of Emory University, where he teaches introductory courses in psychopathology as well as advanced courses in clinical psychopharmacology, research methods, and personality. Before joining the Oxford College faculty in 1994, Carter served as a senior assistant research scientist in the Centers for Disease Control and Prevention's prestigious Epidemic Intelligence Service, with a research focus on smoking as a risk marker for suicidal behaviors in adolescents. He has published extensively in both academic and lay publications, actively engaging in the translation of research in psychology into everyday language. His articles have been published in magazines such as *Psychology Today* and *Women's Health*, and he has appeared on programs such as *CNN Tonight* and NBC's *Today* show and hosted NBC's *Mind of a Motorhead*. His most recent book is *Buzz! Inside the Minds of Thrill-Seekers, Daredevils, and Adrenaline Junkies* (Cambridge University Press, 2019).

T0370736

Psychopathology

Understanding Psychological Disorders

Kenneth Carter

Oxford College, Emory University

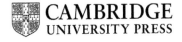
CAMBRIDGE
UNIVERSITY PRESS

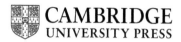

Shaftesbury Road, Cambridge CB2 8EA, United Kingdom

One Liberty Plaza, 20th Floor, New York, NY 10006, USA

477 Williamstown Road, Port Melbourne, VIC 3207, Australia

314–321, 3rd Floor, Plot 3, Splendor Forum, Jasola District Centre,
New Delhi – 110025, India

103 Penang Road, #05-06/07, Visioncrest Commercial, Singapore 238467

Cambridge University Press is part of Cambridge University Press & Assessment,
a department of the University of Cambridge.

We share the University's mission to contribute to society through the pursuit of
education, learning and research at the highest international levels of excellence.

www.cambridge.org
Information on this title: www.cambridge.org/highereducation/isbn/9781108437516

DOI: 10.1017/9781108525985

© Cambridge University Press & Assessment 2023

First published 2023

A catalogue record for this publication is available from the British Library.

A Cataloging-in-Publication data record for this book is available from the Library of Congress.

ISBN 978-1-108-43751-6 Paperback

Additional resources for this publication at www.cambridge.org/psychopathology

Cambridge University Press & Assessment has no responsibility for the persistence
or accuracy of URLs for external or third-party internet websites referred to in this
publication and does not guarantee that any content on such websites is, or will remain,
accurate or appropriate.

To my clinical supervisors and clients who helped me understand the world through the experiences of others.

Brief Contents

Contents

Figures

Tables

Boxes

Case Studies

The Power of Evidence

The Power of Words

Pulling it Together

Preface

Psychopathology, the science of psychological disorders, is one of the most popular courses in undergraduate psychology. Understanding psychological disorders and treatments not only informs us about people experiencing psychological conditions – it reveals truths about all of us.

I remember the first time I ever saw the *Diagnostic and Statistical Manual for Mental Disorders* (*DSM*). I was mesmerized. "It's the psychiatrist's Bible," I was told, "a clear and easy way to categorize psychological disorders." It was neither.

Fast-forward four years and I am a graduate student using the *DSM* in both clinical and research settings. Fast-forward another 20 years and I'm teaching *DSM-5* to mental health counselors all around the United States and to my students. I've come to know psychological diagnosis and treatment as a student, a clinician, a researcher, and a professor. And psychological diagnosis and treatment can be both complex and elegant at the same time. There are also some important gaps in the way we understand and categorize psychological disorders. Anyone who's taught psychopathology has bumped up against these gaps: How to balance the medical model with the challenge of avoiding stigma, how to encourage empathy, and how to avoid "othering" as we introduce these important concepts. This book is my attempt to help you accomplish these goals.

A textbook in psychopathology must strike a delicate balance. It must reflect the current science of disorders and treatments – both therapeutic and medical – while also folding in cultural and gender issues. A textbook that does this in an engaging, sensitive way is a rare find. Even more uncommon is one at an accessible price.

My goal in *Psychopathology: Understanding Psychological Disorders* is to provide students and instructors with a textbook offering modern pedagogical features, presenting the information in an easy-to-understand format that is engaging and scientifically sound.

Key Features

To help meet the challenge of teaching this enormous and complex field, I have made the following themes the keystones of my presentation:

Keeping the student in mind. The language is accessible and conversational, and the tough-to-understand concepts, such as the discussion of the difference between bipolar and depressive disorders in Chapter 6 and the explanation of patients' rights in Chapter 15, are highlighted in visuals as well as in the text. I take the time to thoroughly explain theories and models to help the student avoid common "sand traps," such as how medications for bipolar disorders can be different from medications for depressive disorders (Chapter 6), and how to tell the difference between disorders that sometimes look like each other, such as post-traumatic stress disorder (Chapter 5) and major depressive disorder (Chapter 5) and avoidant personality disorder and schizoid personality disorder (Chapter 12).

Keeping instructors in mind. Each chapter contains several numbered sections that each address a major topic or concept. Because these sections are largely self-contained, instructors can assign them independently.

Fully integrate culture and gender into the presentation. We know that psychological conditions are influenced by culture and gender, but previous editions of the *DSM* have largely ignored them. *DSM-5tr* has integrated research on both culture and gender and I've done the same. Culture and gender are incorporated throughout the chapters, not limited to special features and boxes. See, for example, the discussion of how gender stereotypes may influence the perception of symptoms of depression (Chapter 6), and the impact of implicit bias on the diagnosis of conduct disorder (Chapter 10). Research around culture and gender is not just worked into the narrative of the text but is also highlighted in the figures, charts, and photos. You'll also find some of the current prevalence data visualized in world maps throughout the book. I've taken the time to discuss differences in the cultural expression of disorders, too, and to point out where the research is lacking regarding inclusiveness.

Inclusive, cultural, and linguistic support. Words are important. When used incorrectly they can be harmful, but used carefully they can help to create an inclusive experience. In this book we worked hard to embrace and incorporate inclusive language throughout. To support our efforts, Dr. Leslie Berntsen, a teaching faculty member in the Department of Psychology at the University of Southern California, has reviewed the entire manuscript for inclusive language and research. We have also followed the American Psychological Association's (APA) guidelines for inclusive language. According to APA, "These guidelines aim to raise awareness, guide learning, and support the use of culturally sensitive terms and phrases that center the voices and perspectives of those who are often marginalized or stereotyped." For more information about APA's language guidelines for inclusive language, please take a look at www.apa.org/about/apa/equity-diversity-inclusion/language-guidelines.pdf.

Tackle the disorders in a consistent and structured way that also captures key details within *DSM-5tr*. The text is faithful to *DSM-5tr*, with a focus on clarity, application, and ease of understanding. In each chapter where we cover disorders, we discuss:

- *Symptoms and Diagnosis:* An introduction to the disorder, its functional consequences, and cultural and gender diagnostic issues.
- *Statistics and Trajectory:* The development of the disorder and its course over the life span, as well as prevalence, risk, and prognostic factors. Where available, current worldwide prevalence data is included.

- *Models and Treatment:* The underlying etiology and treatments from various perspectives are discussed (where the evidence supports), including biological, psychodynamic, cognitive and behavioral, sociocultural, and multiperspective approaches.

Employ an integrated approach. The inclusion of multiple perspectives and an integrative approach to evidence-based treatments provides for a deeper understanding of the field. To this end, I have proactively avoided presenting only the one-dimensional approaches, such as biological, behavioral, and social and cultural. Instead, I have used them as a base upon which perspectives such as the interaction of medication and culture, or the way behavioral interventions can influence the family system have been integrated.

Introduce *DSM* and *DSM-5tr* early in the text. Most texts present *DSM* later, often in the fifth chapter. We introduce *DSM* in Chapter 1, because an early introduction provides students with a more complete framework for the disorders, the course, and the field of psychopathology.

Pedagogical Features

This book is based on a modular format that provides a clear organization of the key topics in psychopathology. The format also offers professors more control over the way they teach the content. Every chapter in the book is organized with the following structure to help the students engage with the concepts as they read:

Chapter-Opening Vignette

The case studies at the beginning of each chapter focus on real people's stories, as often described in their published biographies or autobiographies. References to this literature have been provided so that students can dive deeper into these stories, if they so desire (which makes a great end-of-term project). Moreover, these cases introduce some of the challenges that we face in understanding a specific disorder covered in the chapter, with numerous call-outs throughout the text.

The Power of Words

This feature aims to help students develop empathy toward people with psychological disorders, and become aware of ongoing evolution in the way psychological disorders are discussed. To achieve this, I explain how the language we use can impact the way we view psychological disorders and those who experience symptoms of psychological disorders, as covered in "The Power of Words: Hysteria" in Chapter 5 and "The Power of Words: Misgendering" in Chapter 8.

The Power of Evidence

This feature aims to show students how scientific evidence can answer questions about psychopathology treatments, and encourages them to apply critical thinking and evidence-based approaches when evaluating the effectiveness of different treatments (for example, see "The Power of Evidence: Lavender for Anxiety" in Chapter 4).

Concept Checks

A list of application-style questions that tests the student's mastery of the material covered in each section, applying their knowledge to fresh examples and from different perspectives.

Key Terms

Key terms appear in bold throughout the text when they are first discussed, and are defined in an integral way that doesn't interrupt the main idea of the sentence. They are also reinforced in the margins, and gathered at the very end of the book into a glossary.

Pulling It Together

This feature appears at the end of each chapter, providing a visual presentation of one or several key concepts that have been discussed. It helps to tie the chapter and its segments into a cohesive whole.

Chapter Review

This section includes:

- Chapter summary, to recap the main ideas in each chapter using brief, bulleted sentences keyed to the chapter's main sections.
- Discussion questions, to give students the opportunity to use their critical thinking skills while reviewing important material in the chapters.
- Answers to concept checks, for effective self-study.

ONLINE RESOURCES FOR INSTRUCTORS

- Test bank
- PowerPoint lecture slides
- Jpeg and ppt figure files from the book

ONLINE RESOURCES FOR STUDENTS

- Link to the author's website, which includes additional cases, interviews, book reviews, and links to podcasts with discussion questions.

Coverage and Organization

Psychopathology: Understanding Psychological Disorders is for a first course in psychopathology sometimes named Abnormal Psychology or Adult Psychopathology. It reflects the current science of psychological disorders and treatments – both therapeutic and medical – while also folding in cultural and gender issues.

The first three chapters focus on the background and history of psychological disorders.

Chapter 1 introduces the ways in which psychologists define psychopathology both historically and today, as well as the key features of modern mental health care. The chapter also introduces the research methods psychologists use to study psychopathology. Chapter 2 surveys the various theories and treatments of psychopathology including the biological, psychodynamic, behavioral, cognitive, sociocultural and multiperspective approaches. Chapter 3 reviews research, assessment, diagnosis, and treatment. It includes discussions of clinical assessment, the components of intake reports, the purpose and limitations of diagnosis, and dives into how diagnostic manuals have changed over time. It also contains a summary of how psychologists evaluate the effectiveness of psychotherapy.

The next eight chapters cover current diagnostic categories and information about treatment (adhering to the chapter structure previously described). Chapter 4 reviews anxiety and obsessive-compulsive and related disorders as well as their treatments. It includes a discussion of the difference between adaptive and maladaptive anxiety, and discusses the key symptoms of the fight or flight response. Chapter 5 surveys both the trauma and stressor-related disorders and the dissociative disorders. Chapter 6 takes a look at depressive and bipolar mood disorders including the new *DSM-5tr* diagnosis of prolonged grief disorder. Chapter 7 addresses somatic symptom disorders, sleep disorders, and psychological factors affecting health. It contains a review of sleep architecture, as well as the techniques psychologists use in the treatment of various medical conditions. Chapter 8 discusses three separate topics: gender variation, sexual dysfunctions, and paraphilic disorders. The chapter includes a description of the differences between gender, sex, and sexual orientation. It addresses gender dysphoria and includes a separate discussion of sexual dysfunction as well as the paraphilic disorders. Chapter 9 focuses on eating disorders. It describes the symptoms and physical consequences of eating disorders. Chapter 10 surveys the disruptive impulse control and conduct disorders. Chapter 11 reviews the substance-related and addictive disorders. It describes the categories of psychoactive drugs as well as the effects of psychoactive drugs on the nervous system. Chapter 12 features personality disorders. It defines the main features of personality disorders and describes the three clusters of personality disorders. Chapter 13 examines schizophrenia and psychotic disorders. The chapter describes the symptoms associated with psychotic disorders and compares the positive and negative symptoms of psychosis. Chapter 14 surveys neurodevelopmental and neurocognitive disorders. It includes discussion of the difference between neurodevelopmental and neurocognitive disorders.

Finally, Chapter 15 introduces the legal and ethical issues in psychopathology. It discusses the process of civil commitment and competency to stand trial. It also reviews and compares the laws regarding the "insanity defense" and includes discussions of how mental health practitioners protect patients' rights.

Acknowledgments

There's a particular recipe for being helpful: heaps of encouragement, a dash of support, and even sometimes a pinch of constructive abuse. That's where it starts. Not everyone gets this right, but I'm fortunate to have people in my life who have mastered this tricky recipe and made this project possible. A sampling of the many deserved acknowledgments follows.

This book would have consisted entirely of blank pages had it not been for the guidance and assistance of the developmental editors Lisa Pinto and Elisa Adams. From mentor to editor, to advocate to cheerleader, it's hard to overstate how valuable their help has been. Their unflinching faith, artful strategies, and keen editing eye have made them powerful partners (Elisa is a literary alchemist).

A hat tip to all the people I interviewed, wrote about, or quoted, especially those featured in the case studies. There were many who weren't mentioned specifically in the book but who really helped me to think about mental health, and who transformed the tables, graphs, and statistics of research studies into the reality of how people live their lives every day. I hope I have conveyed their lived experience into the manuscript.

The team at Cambridge University Press is truly exceptional. Thanks go to managing editor Ilaria Tassistro, content manager Rachel Norridge, and especially to my commissioning editor David Repetto, whose patience is exceeded only by his encouragement and good nature.

I want to thank the many scientists whose work is described, cited, and synthesized in this book; also Tracy Darbeloff, Adam Stanaland, Jee Young Kim, and Haruka Notsu, who as my research assistants gave help in the research process; and in addition the patient and careful academic reviewers who worked so hard. A special thank-you goes to Dr. Leslie Berntsen, whose thoughtful review helped to make the text more inclusive and diverse. Her depth of knowledge, student-centered focus, and understanding of the importance of inclusion and diversity reveal that she is a teacher-scholar who is clearly a master teacher.

I'm grateful to Jack Hardy, Debra Woog, Jaquelyn LaVictoire, Teddy Ottaviano, Michael McGloin, Susan Ashmore, Sharon Lewis, Jennifer McGee, Molly McGehee, Shira Miller, and of course my parents, Bill and Eugenia Carter. Many other people and organizations have been important in this process. You can find their names on my gratitude website www.drkencarter.com/thanks. Thank you all for relentless support, encouragement, and reassurance. It absolutely made a difference.

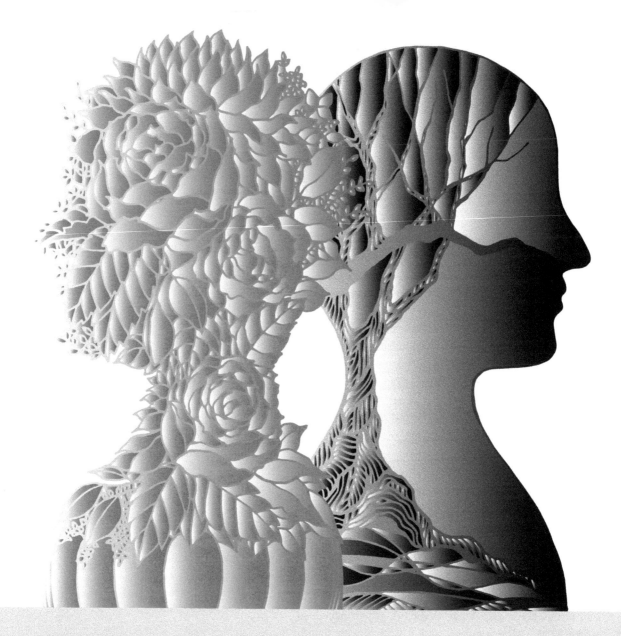

CHAPTER CONTENTS

Benjavisa/iStock/Getty Images Plus.

1

Overview of Psychopathology and Psychological Disorders

CASE STUDY: **The Madness of King George**

The nearly 60-year reign of Britain's King George III (Figure 1.1), from 1760 to 1820, was considered to be mostly a success, including as it did the start of the industrial revolution, the British agricultural revolution, and years of notable advances in the sciences. The king himself was fascinated by magnetism and electricity and even had his own collection of scientific instruments, including a gilded microscope. In 1781, a new planet was discovered and named Georgium Sidus or "George's Star" in his honor (it's now called Uranus). Yet despite his successes, King George is usually remembered for just two things: the loss of the North American colonies and his precarious mental state.

Although Great Britain was a dominant power in Europe, the American Revolutionary War (1775–1783) left some in Parliament saying that King George could have been more flexible in responding to the colonists' demands. Many blamed him for the war, which ended with the colonies gaining their independence from Britain.

As for his mental state, by late October 1788 something seemed off about the king. He had trouble sleeping, spoke incessantly for long periods, and was once caught shaking hands with a tree that he claimed was the King of Prussia. The first few times this happened people shrugged it off and said nothing (he was the king, after all), and by early winter, everything was back to normal. But only for a while. George had relapses over the next few years, and each time his condition got worse. During these times, George would race

Learning Objectives

- Summarize how psychologists decide which kinds of behaviors are abnormal and the role culture plays in this determination.

- Discuss the various ways that abnormality was viewed historically.

- Describe the key features of modern mental health care.

- Identify the various kinds of research methods that psychologists utilize.

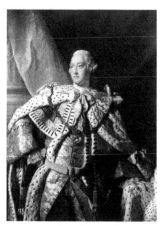

Figure 1.1 King George III.
Source: Tony Baggett/iStock/
Getty Images Plus.

around the grounds in his nightclothes, walking and talking at great speed, or he would get out of bed after only four hours of sleep and make sure everyone else was awake too. He'd forget the names of people he had known all his life. Even the king knew something wasn't right.

Officials halted all his public appearances, and the most famous doctors of the time hedged their bets on a diagnosis. They examined what they could – physical signs and symptoms including persistent abdominal pain and discolored urine. But because it violated convention to look the king in the eye, much less examine him closely, and because the king wasn't the best patient, a real physical exam wasn't possible. The king's emotional, behavioral, and physical symptoms provided the only clues to an underlying cause. Doctors treated him with state-of-the-art medicine, often against his will. Among other efforts, they heated glass cups with candles to sear his skin and create blisters, intended to increase blood circulation on his back and legs. Nothing helped.

The king's mental and physical health perplexed his doctors. Had he been poisoned? Was he possessed? Did he have a brain tumor? Were his mental faculties slipping under the stress he was facing in his old age? What was wrong with their king?

More information about King George's symptoms and treatment appears later in the chapter.

1.1   WHAT IS ABNORMAL PSYCHOLOGY?

Most people would likely consider behaviors like the ones King George III exhibited to be out of the ordinary, even unusual or unhealthy. Over the years, medical professionals and even laypeople have labeled such behaviors madness, lunacy, mental illness, abnormal, or psychopathology.

If you look up the word *abnormal*, you will find something like "deviating from what is normal, usual, or typical in a way that is undesirable or wrong." When something is abnormal, it's different from the usual. Psychology is the science of behavior and mental processes. **Abnormal psychology** is the scientific study of **psychological disorders**, meaning psychological conditions that depart from the norm, are usually maladaptive, and may cause personal distress. Often these psychological disorders are identified through the abnormal or unusual behaviors the person exhibits.

Abnormal behavior is conduct that differs from typical developmental, cultural, or societal norms and creates distress or impairment in functioning. When you tell people you are studying abnormal psychology, most of them probably think this means the psychology of the weird and strange people in the world (it's not). Crack open or launch any number of contemporary "Abnormal Psychology" textbooks and you'll see similar content in all: descriptions and listings of psychological disorders. Why? Abnormal psychology isn't the psychology of the strange.

Abnormal psychology: the scientific study of psychological disorders.

Psychological disorders: psychological conditions that depart from the norm, are usually maladaptive, and may cause personal distress.

Abnormal behavior: conduct that differs from typical developmental, cultural, or societal norms and creates distress or impairment in functioning.

More accurately, it is **psychopathology** – the science of diagnosing and under-standing all psychological disorders, including their causes, descriptions, and treatments.

Let's think back to one of King George's symptoms – abdominal pain. What might cause someone's stomach to hurt? A typical stomach has a certain shape and functions in a specific way, and it's usually not painful. An abnormal stomach, on the other hand, deviates in function or structure, such as by having difficulty digesting certain foods or maybe prompting unexpected pain. But stomachs don't deviate in an infinite number of ways. There are certain patterns to these differences. A physician might ask you to describe the kind of abdominal pain you are experiencing (dull, stabbing, throbbing) and what other types of symptoms accompany your stomach pain, such as discolored urine. Scientists will categorize and describe these differences, what might lead to them, and ultimately how to correct and help with those differences that could lead to problems.

The same process occurs in the behavioral and emotional world of psychology and psychological disorders. While some psychologists study typical processes in terms of how we think, feel, and behave, those who study psychopathology categorize other variations in behavior that can cause problems in the way people function at work and home and in how well they get along with others or even themselves.

Deviance, Distress, Dysfunction, and Danger

How do you set about deciding which kinds of behaviors are normal and which are abnormal? Mental health professionals train intensively to observe and record symptoms before they make a formal diagnosis (more on that in Chapter 3). In general, psychologists focus on a few constructs to guide their reasoning: *deviance*, *distress*, *dysfunction*, and *danger*. These four D's help them to establish whether the observed behaviors might be problematic. Most are present to some degree in all of us and can lie on a **continuum**, which means that abnormality can exist in mild everyday ways at one end of the continuum, or it can be disruptive and severe or even harmful at the other end. Abnormality is a *variation* of functional behaviors, thoughts, or feelings (Wakefield 2009). Thus *deviance*, *distress*, *dysfunction*, and *danger* are most helpfully examined on a scale, instead of being considered as either present or absent (Aftab & Rashed 2021).

DEVIANCE

To **deviate** means to depart from typical or accepted standards. Sometimes this departure can be helpful, as when we are thinking divergently and creatively, "outside the box." Other times deviance can impair someone's ability to live their best life, as when a person becomes terrified of going outside the home. Deviance can also be a departure from commonly accepted cultural standards.

Psychopathology: the science of diagnosing and understanding all psychological disorders, including their causes, descriptions, and treatments.

Continuum: a range of severity from mild to disruptive.

Deviate: a departure from typical or accepted standards.

For example, not wearing shoes is perfectly normal or even expected in many cultures (it might be strange to wear shoes to walk into the ocean). On the other hand, you will be expected to wear shoes next time you go to your chemistry laboratory. People's explanation of deviance can correlate with the way they see the world. For example, for cultures that emphasize individualism, going away to college and separating from your parents is an important aspect of development. If you decided to pick a college just because your sibling was also going there, some people might suggest you are deviating from the norm of going off on your own, but for cultures that prioritize family connections, going off on your own would be a deviation. Some deviations from norms might be easy to overlook, such as when King George III forgot the names of some of his subjects. But forgetting where you are when you are at home is a completely different matter. Deviations exist on a continuum; some are minor, others major.

By itself, the statistical frequency or infrequency of an unusual behavior isn't a foolproof way to establish whether it is a psychological disorder. Nonconformity in itself is not a disorder. Besides, sometimes we behave outside the norm on purpose, like when we order breakfast for dinner just to mix things up. But there are times when the deviations are beyond our control, such as when King George felt a pressure or compulsion to talk and talk and talk.

DISTRESS

Distress: a feeling of anxiety or pain.

Being unusual doesn't make a behavior or symptom problematic. It's important to consider whether the behavior is also causing the person **distress**, a feeling of anxiety or pain. Sometimes people behave in ways that cause them stress or even make them miserable. Or they take actions or focus on thoughts that make them feel unhappy, such as when someone consistently feels that others are out to harm them despite evidence to the contrary.

The world is full of distressing things like mass shootings, troubled relationships, and stressful work environments, and we do our best to avoid them. Sometimes even small matters like running out of coffee or being in an unfamiliar environment will cause overwhelming and debilitating distress. But that alone doesn't mean that a person has a psychological condition. In fact, many psychological disorders aren't associated with distress at all, like some of the personality disorders we'll discuss in Chapter 13.

DYSFUNCTION

Dysfunction: behaviors, emotions, or thoughts that are outside the ordinary and that result in a person's being impaired or distressed.

Dysfunction refers to behaviors, emotions, or thoughts that are outside the ordinary and that result in a person's being impaired or distressed. Such dysfunction can interfere with the way a person goes about their daily life (Bergner & Bunford 2017) at work, school, home, and social life.

King George experienced dysfunction in controlling his emotions. He saw and believed things that weren't objectively there, and this caused problems with his family and concerns about his ability to be king. Consequently, much of his power was eventually transferred to his son.

DANGER

Sometimes our thoughts, feelings, or behavior can be dangerous or be associated with discomfort to ourselves or others. This is the fourth D: **danger**, a tendency toward violence. Although danger is extremely rare (Honberg 2020), abnormal behavior will sometimes put a person at risk of harming themselves or others.

Danger: a tendency toward violence.

Cultural Norms and Cultural Relativism

It's not unusual to think that the way you or your family does something is the norm – the way everyone does it. Sometimes you don't realize you've made this assumption until you bump up against someone who does things completely differently. Imagine traveling out of the country for the first time. It's easy to be amazed by the differences in food, traditions, and clothing. What might be unusual for one person will be quite normal for others.

Sometimes norms are explicit, such as the way you order your lunch at a fast-casual restaurant (there's often a sign that will tell you what to do). At other times norms are much less explicit, such as the proper way to act during a religious ceremony. When you violate or deviate from norms, you stand out – and that is usually awkward for you and for others and draws attention to you. But norms aren't universal, especially when it comes to culture.

Culture refers to the shared customs, institutions, values, and habits that distinguish a group. **Cultural relativism** is the idea that our understanding of abnormality should be based on a person's culture rather than on one universal definition of the term. So whether it's common to eat with your fingers or use utensils, for instance, or whether an intersex person is considered deviant or holy, is a matter of culture rather than of rules and definitions. Cultural relativism suggests that the norms can vary by place or even time. How does this relate to abnormal psychology and psychopathology? Cultural norms help us to understand which behaviors are acceptable. We apply specific cultural expectations and norms to a behavior or emotional reaction that is culturally based.

Culture: the shared customs, institutions, values, and habits that distinguish a group.

Cultural relativism: the idea that our understanding of psychopathology should be based on a person's culture rather than on one universal definition of the term.

Take grief, for example. While grief is a perfectly normal reaction to the death of a loved one, the way people grieve can vary dramatically depending on religion or culture (Figure 1.2). In some cultures, it's perfectly acceptable to laugh and celebrate a deceased person's life, while in other cultures mourning is more somber and focuses on the family's loss. Wearing black clothes is typical in some cultures, while white was a traditional color of mourning for medieval European queens. In some times and places, a widow was expected to wear black for an entire year following her husband's death (Queen Victoria took this to an extreme, wearing black for the rest of her life – nearly 40 years – after her spouse, Prince Albert, died). In other times and places, most family members and friends at least wear black to the funeral.

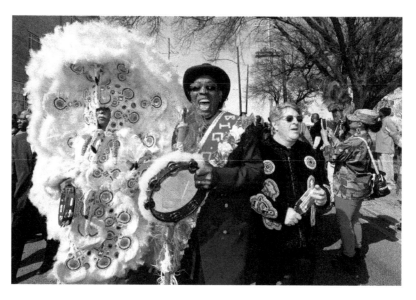

Because the expression of grief can be so variable, it would be harmful to try to establish a best (or conventional, or appropriate) way to grieve based on a single perspective. Cultural relativism reminds us there are multiple right ways in which to think, behave, or feel. Cultural relativism can also give us **empathy**, the willingness to understand another person's inner world.

Empathy: the willingness and ability to understand another person's inner world.

Culture can have a strong impact on the ways in which psychological conditions are expressed. In fact, some psychological disorders, called culture-bound syndromes, are specific to certain populations and recognized within those cultures. See Table 1.1 for a few examples.

Culture influences not only how abnormal behavior is expressed through symptoms but also how willing people are to admit or talk about their symptoms (Dow & Siniscarco 2021). For example, in cultures where anger isn't normally expressed, people might be reluctant even to talk about their feelings of anger.

Table 1.1 Some culture-bound syndromes

Name	Location/ Population	Description
Ataque de nervios	People of Latino descent	Loss of control and intense emotional upset. Often related to stressful family-related events.
Kufungisisa ("thinking too much")	Zimbabwe	Anxiety, depression, or bodily sensation. Complaints related to persistent and upsetting thoughts caused by social difficulties.
Maladi moun ("sent sickness")	Haiti	Illness caused by the hatred of others.
Uamairineq	Inuit people	An out-of-body experience and paralysis often described as spirit possession.
Pa-leng ("frigophobia")	Taiwan	Anxiety, fear, and fatigue related to being too cold.

Source: Richey et al. (2019).

Thomas Szasz (1920–2012) suggested that societies often label and marginalize people in order to control or silence them. In the American South, for example, enslaved people who attempted to escape were often diagnosed as having a mental disorder that caused them to desire to be free (Cartwright 1851; Szasz 1971). The treatment? Hard labor and beatings. This idea of using labels to control others might seem familiar even today. Until recently many who were sexual and gender minorities were thought to be somehow deviant, and it was wrongly believed they could be "converted." Szasz regarded mental illness as a myth and held the controversial view that mental health professionals like psychologists and psychiatrists were pathologizing and attempting to treat what was essentially everyday behavior. Szasz's impact on psychopathology has remained, and it's important to consider how some psychological conditions may not be disorders at all.

CONCEPT CHECK 1.1

Match each construct of abnormality with the appropriate example.
   A. Deviance
   B. Distress
   C. Dysfunction
   D. Danger

1. Kenzo is concerned about how his friends will judge him. Although they have tried to reassure him whenever he tells them this, he still worries so much that his stomach hurts.
2. Briar is a huge fan of vampire movies, so much so that she is considering filing her own teeth into points to resemble vampire fangs.
3. Layton prefers to be alone. Although he checks in with his parents occasionally, he has been missing class and failed to present his final project in chemistry because it meant he would have to stand in front of the entire class to speak. He received a zero on the assignment.
4. Chad often has trouble controlling his temper. He was frustrated about a flight delay of 45 minutes and as a result he threw his water bottle at the gate agent and slammed his fist on the counter. The other passengers were so nervous that the gate agent decided to call security.

1.2 HISTORICAL VIEWS OF ABNORMALITY

It's likely that humans have noticed variations in personality, emotions, or behavior ever since they noticed the behaviors themselves. In fact, the more deviant, distressing, dysfunctional, or dangerous the behavior, the more humans have generally tried to explain or attempt to change it. Their explanations often correlate with the way they see the world.

Several big ideas have influenced the way we think about problematic variations in behaviors. One big question (that we still have) is whether abnormal behavior is prompted by what is going on within or outside the person. In general, three types of theories are used to explain abnormal behavior: **biological theories** explain abnormal behavior as evidence of a disease or some kind of biological imbalance; **supernatural theories** explain it as caused by demons or sin; and **psychological theories** explain abnormal behavior as influenced by environmental factors such as stress, trauma, or family situations.

The treatments for abnormal behavior are linked to the **etiology** or presumed cause of the disorder. Biological treatments focus on changing the body, for example through medicine or diet. Supernatural treatments focus on boosting a person's morals, for example by using faith healers or herbs, or by expelling demons from the person (Exline et al. 2021). And psychological treatments focus on changing the environmental factors or their impact on the person, such as the way a person thinks or feels about their family life. The predominance of each of these three treatment types has shifted over the course of history.

Abnormality as Seen in Ancient Times

For early humans, it was probably easy to believe that supernatural forces were everywhere. Rain, sun, wind, lightning, and trees all seemed somehow magical (they still do to me), and people understood their appearance or disappearance to be influenced by unseen forces, whether Mother Nature, the god Thor, the Christian God, or the sun god Ra, for example. Perhaps they believed that helpful events were caused by powerful positive forces and harmful ones by powerful evil ones. It's likely that prehistoric humans thought abnormal behavior too was caused by supernatural forces like gods and demons.

Treatments attempted to reduce the influence of those supernatural forces or even cast them out. There was no lack of creative (and sometimes dreadful) ways in which to do this: coax the forces out through prayers, pleading, insults, or potions, or make them uncomfortable by starving or beating the person they afflicted. Another technique (which some religious groups use to this day) was **exorcism**, a religious ritual that treated abnormality by coaxing spirits such as demons from the body. If all else failed, the community might even kill the person, often in dramatic and public ways like burning at the stake or drowning.

From the Stone Age to the Middle Ages, another treatment for demon removal was **trephination** (Figure 1.3), which entailed drilling holes in the skull, presumably to release demons or evil spirits from within (Exline et al. 2021). However, other researchers have a different idea. They think the holes found in the skulls of Stone Age humans were made not to facilitate the release of demons but to treat blood clots (Newman et al. 2016).

Biological theories: an explanation of psychopathology that suggests that psychological disorders are caused by human physiology.

Supernatural theories: a theory that suggests that psychopathology is caused by demons or sin.

Psychological theories: theories of psychopathology that explain psychopathology as influenced by environmental factors such as stress, trauma, or family situations.

Etiology: the presumed cause of a disorder.

Exorcism: a religious ritual that treated abnormality by coaxing spirits such as demons from the body.

Trephination: a procedure which entailed drilling holes in the skull, presumably to release demons or evil spirits from within.

In ancient China, some people thought abnormality was caused by an imbalance between the forces of yin (negative) and yang (positive) (Tseng & Hsu 1970). Others believed that emotions were influenced by bodily organs. The heart was associated with joy, lungs sorrow, liver anger, spleen worry, kidneys fear. Later writings moved away from this biological interpretation to a more religious view of abnormality (we'll come back to this in a bit).

Abnormality as Seen in the Greek Era

The Greek physician Hippocrates of Kos lived from 460 to 377 BCE and is often described as the founder of Western medicine (hence, the Hippocratic oath). Like other ancient Greek and Roman physicians, Hippocrates suggested that psychological disorders should be treated just as physical diseases were (Wallace & Gach 2010).

Hippocrates considered the brain the organ that contained wisdom, intelligence, and emotion, so he thought psychological disorders might be a disease of the brain. This was in stark contrast to the ideas of others who thought of the heart as the center of consciousness. (As a vestige of such thinking, we sometimes still point to our chests as our "me" spot.) Hippocrates put abnormal behaviors into several categories: epilepsy, mania, melancholia, and brain fever.

Hippocrates thought normal brain function was connected to four bodily fluids or **humors** that influenced mental functioning: blood (from the heart), black bile (from the spleen), phlegm (from the brain), and choler or yellow bile (from the liver). Too much or too little of one of these fluids would throw the whole system out of balance. For example, too much black bile could lead to melancholia. The four humors were also linked to the Greek concepts of the Four Basic Qualities. These qualities (or aspects) described the nature of the things around us. Was something hot or dry, wet or cold? Aspects of these four humors were linked to personality traits as well (Maher & Maher 1994).

Humors: bodily fluids that were thought to influence mental functioning.

Since Hippocrates believed that abnormal behavior was due to imbalances in the four humors, the solution was clear – balance them. Too much of any humor was treated by increasing heat, prescribing rest, changing the climate or the diet, or applying moisture or cold, depending on which humor was off-kilter. Bloodletting, for example, removes excess blood through cuts or leeches, while blowing your nose was a great way to reduce excess phlegm. These remedies endured for a long time. In King George's case, the deliberate heat blistering on his back and legs was an attempt to move blood to different parts of his body and balance the amount of blood in his system. Environment was also important. Hippocrates acknowledged that removing a person from a stressful or difficult family could restore mental health.

Figure 1.3 Although undoubtedly painful, the ancient treatment of drilling holes in the skull (trephination) was not fatal.
Source: C. M. Dixon/Print Collector/Getty Images.

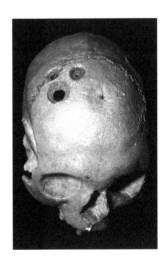

Abnormality as Seen in Europe in the Middle Ages and the Renaissance

The Middle Ages are the time from the fall of the Roman Empire in the fourth century to the beginning of the Renaissance in the fourteenth century. As Roman society started to decline, there was an uptick in beliefs about supernatural forces as the cause of psychological disorders. Although in the Middle Ages most people believed supernatural forces to be real, physicians and scientists generally regarded the supernatural not as an actual force in everyday life, but rather as the preoccupation of overly superstitious people (Neugebauer 1979). Typically, most doctors believed that abnormality was caused by emotional shock or physical illness.

THE POWER OF WORDS

LUNATIC

Paracelsus was a Swiss physician who lived from 1493 to 1541 and who thought the movement of celestial objects like planets and the moon affected our personalities (Figure 1.4). It is from the Latin word for moon (*luna*) that we get the word *lunatic* to describe those with psychological conditions.

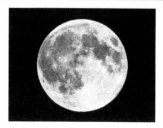

Figure 1.4 The word *lunatic* is linked to the idea that the moon affects our personality.
Source: Smartshots International/Moment/Getty Images.

The Catholic Inquisition was a major force in Europe in the later Middle Ages. The Church's questioning (or inquisition) of assumed heretics and non-believers typically resulted in their death or banishment to other countries. Prompted by the Church's pursuit of deviance from its strictures, this period saw a marked (and often forced) return to the belief that deviant behavior was the work of the devil (Kroll 1973). This led to an increased focus on the supernatural, including the influence of the planets, as an explanation for psychological disorders.

Today the word *lunatic* conjures the idea of wild and unpredictable behavior in a dehumanizing way that isn't descriptive of the specific behaviors a person with a psychological disorder might exhibit. It's easy to think that terms like *idiot* and *lunatic* are embedded only in everyday language, but they can actually be found in laws that describe people with psychological conditions, which can influence the way not only everyday people but also judges and juries understand mental conditions, with a consequent effect on legal decisions (LaFortune 2018). Fortunately, some lawmakers have started to remove such language from laws. For example, California has enacted a *Strategic Plan on Reducing Mental Health Stigma and Discrimination* that evaluates laws and attempts to correct problematic language.

Sources: Kroll (1973); LaFortune (2018).

Abnormality as Seen in the Age of Discovery

The rapid growth of cultural and scientific curiosity and activity that began in the Renaissance continued in the Age of Discovery (the fifteenth to seventeenth

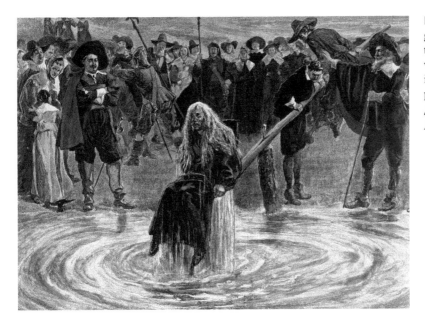

Figure 1.5 An accused witch going through the judgment trial, where she is dunked in water to prove her guilt or innocence of practicing witchcraft.
Source: Bettmann/Getty Images.

centuries), and progress extended to the views of mental health. For example, the sixteenth-century Spanish nun Teresa of Avila suggested that some psychological disorders nuns experienced could be the result of a physical illness (Sarbin & Juhasz 1967). German physician Johan Weyer (1515–1588) suspected that the mind could have illnesses in the same way the body could. Some historians see Weyer as the founder of modern psychopathology. The Catholic Church, however, banned writings that linked physical illness and psychological disorders, most likely to emphasize the role of individual behavior and beliefs in the conditions rather than biological ones.

Eventually, earlier treatments for psychological disorders returned, hand in hand with the return of belief in demonic possession. Evil needed to be rooted out and destroyed. Witch hunts reached their height during this time (Mora 2008), including in the North American colonies, and those found guilty of being witches suffered consequences including confinement, beatings, dunking in cold water, other tortures, and death (Figure 1.5).

It's quite possible that some people who were accused of witchcraft would have been diagnosed with psychological disorders today. Many confessed to engaging in unusual thoughts and beliefs, suggesting that they may have been hallucinating or having delusions (false beliefs), all signs of schizophrenia (Zilboorg & Henry 1941). Some researchers believe those accused of witchcraft were depressed and suffering from dementia. And some confessions of witchcraft came after hours or days of torture and may have been made to prevent execution.

As cities started to grow and consolidate their political power, governments became responsible for some new functions, including caring for those with psychological concerns. The Church's influence on the identification and treatment of these conditions began to diminish, and medical explanations and treatments grew in popularity and use once again, although remnants of supernatural beliefs remained until well into the seventeenth century. (Even today, studies reveal that a surprising number of people believe psychological disorders are due in part to "immoral" behavior (Witte et al. 2019).)

With the eventual spread of the idea that mental disorders were not caused by evil within the person or the environment, treatments eventually improved, becoming more humane and appropriate. Many were beginning to suspect that psychological disorders were caused by external factors such as stress (Maher & Maher 1994), which meant they could be treated by altering the environment as well. At the time, the state-of-the-art treatments were rest, baths, ointments, and a healthy environment. But these treatments were expensive, and improvements didn't last long.

In the twelfth century the trend in Europe had been to take family members with mental disorders into the home, rather than having them fend for themselves or live on the streets (Kroll 1973). Later, in the mid-1700s, hospitals began to set up special rooms and wings devoted to people experiencing symptoms of psychological disorders. Eventually entire hospitals began to be devoted to these patients.

Asylums: inpatient institutions created to provide care for people with psychological disorders.

Known as **asylums** (meaning refuge or sanctuary), these were inpatient institutions created to provide care for people with psychological disorders. Unfortunately, many patients were poorly treated, for example by being chained to a wall or locked in boxes. In some locations, for a fee you could gawk at them. At the time, laws protected only the public and relatives, not the patients themselves.

Before too long the asylums became overcrowded and devolved into storehouses for those with disorders. Patients received few if any treatments at best and were treated inhumanely at worst. Some patients, for example those in the Bethlehem (or Bedlam) Hospital in London, were bound in chains (Figure 1.6). Given the conditions there, the word "bedlam" came to mean a chaotic uproar (Harris 2017).

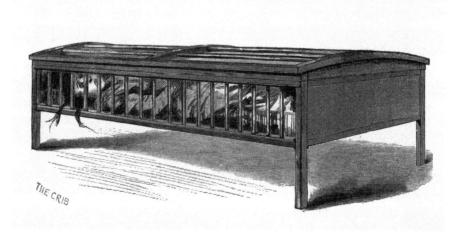

Figure 1.6 Restraint bed used in early mental hospitals. *Source: Stock Montage/ Getty Images.*

Abnormality as Seen in the Eighteenth and Nineteenth Centuries

The chaotic conditions of the asylums were noticed. Clifford Beers, for example, an 1897 Yale graduate who experienced depression, was one of five children in his family, all of whom spent time in mental institutions. Beers both witnessed and suffered maltreatment by the staff, and in 1908 he published a book chronicling his experiences that is still in print (*A mind that found itself*). This work and that of others started the movement toward more humane treatment of those in mental hospitals.

A few years earlier, in 1887, the journalist Elizabeth Cochrane (writing as Nellie Bly) had spent 10 days undercover at a New York City asylum. She pretended to be from Cuba and said she was looking for "missing trunks," and in her ground-breaking two-part series for the *New York World*, later published as a book called *Ten Days in a Mad-House*, she chronicled the conditions at the asylum. They included ice-cold baths in dirty water, towels shared among 45 other patients, beatings, and forced and excessive medication. After the publication of her story, which paved the way for the modern practice of investigative journalism and made her famous, more than $1 million (about $28 million in today's dollars) was added to the budget for the hospital (Noyes 2016).

MORAL TREATMENT

One theory that became popular during the **mental hygiene movement** (Kritsotaki 2019), in the early twentieth century in the United States, proposed that psychological disorders were a result of people's being separated from nature (Freis 2019). Treatment, also known as **moral treatment**, emphasized moral discipline and humane care and included prayers, rest, and a serene, beautiful environment. The idea was simple: treat hospitalized patients as normally as you can. The use of moral treatment led to asylum reform.

Asylum reform began at La Bicêtre, a French facility for men where Philippe Pinel (1745–1826) served as chief doctor (Figure 1.7). Pinel insisted that patients be treated with dignity, tranquility, and humanity (Yakushev & Sidorov 2013). Rather than being beaten and chained, the patients had clean, sunny, air-filled rooms and appetizing food and were able to move about the hospital grounds. The staff received special training to be sure that patients had plenty of social engagement and serene surroundings. The reforms were so successful that Pinel applied the same principles to La Salpêtrière, a hospital in Paris for women.

Similar reforms were instituted in Northern England by William Tuke (1732–1822) at The York Retreat in England, which opened in 1796. Patients were treated with rest, talk, prayer, and manual labor (Kibria & Metcalfe 2016). Some seemed calmer after treatment, and some who had been locked away for years were subsequently released from the hospital.

By the mid-nineteenth century, there were many state-funded mental hospitals in the United States. Thanks to retired Boston school teacher Dorothea Lynde Dix

Mental hygiene movement: a theory of psychopathology that proposed that psychological disorders were a result of people's being separated from nature.

Moral treatment: a treatment that emphasized moral discipline and humane care and included prayers, rest, and a serene, beautiful environment.

Figure 1.7 La Bicêtre, a French facility for men that undertook reforms in treatment of psychological disorders in the early 1800s.

Source: Gabriel Cloquemin, La prison de Bicêtre à Gentilly (1832/1833); http:// parismuseescollections.paris. fr/fr/20eha-carnavalet/ oeuvres/la-prison-de-bicetre- a-gentilly-la-toilette-des- forcats-avant-le-depart- de#infos-principales. Work in public domain.

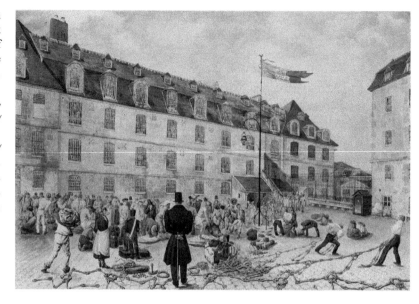

Figure 1.8 US reformer Dorothea Lynde Dix (1802–1887) advocated for moral treatment of patients in receiving psychiatric care.

Source: Samuel Bell Waugh (1814–1885), Oil painting of Dorothea Lynde Dix, 1868; https://upload.wikimedia.org/ 4ehave4li/commons/6/65/ Samuel_Bell_Waugh_-_ Dorothea_Lynde_Dix_-_ Google_Art_Project.jpg. Work in public domain.

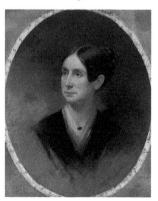

(1802–1887) (Figure 1.8) and others, legislative solutions for asylum reform led to increased government funding and regulations (Dvoskin et al. 2020) and laws to improve conditions and train professionals dedicated to the philosophy of moral treatment. Over a period of 40 years, Dix established more than 30 institutions in the United States, Canada, and Scotland based on the ideas of Pinel and others, and many more were inspired by her efforts.

Despite the successes of moral therapy, a few factors led to the reduction of its use (Bowrey & Smark 2010). First, although treating patients humanely is important, many patients required more than humane treatment, and some patients didn't improve using the moral treatment approach. It's also possible that the moral treatment movement grew too fast and created problems in acquiring proper funding and staff. This led to overcrowding, and individual care couldn't occur. Another factor was prejudice. During the time of the moral therapy movement, a new current of prejudice against people with psychological disorders emerged. One possible cause was a wave of immigration that brought in people who needed care and overburdened the system (Bowrey & Smark 2010). Because of the large influx of patients, a shift occurred from traditional moral therapy to custodial care. Treatment returned to the warehouse approach, and public mental hospitals once again became little more than long-term human storage facilities – with all the stress that induces (Figure 1.9).

By the mid-1950s, large state facilities in the United States had fallen into disrepair because of lack of funding, leading to too many patients and too few well-trained staff members. Mental hospitals again became notorious for poor treatment. Many patients were discharged before receiving sufficient treatments, and a community-based system was established for those experiencing psychological conditions. Community mental health services including hosting, with oversight by either full- or part-time mental health professions, in assisted-living facilities or halfway houses.

BIOLOGICAL TREATMENTS

In the twentieth century, two dominant perspectives began to emerge to explain and treat psychological disorders. One focused on biological causes and treatments, and the other suggested that the main causes of psychological disorders were psychological.

Interest in the biological causes of psychological disorders increased our understanding that symptoms could arise biologically. Many biological treatments were stumbled upon by chance or by improvements in medications originally used for other purposes. For example, insulin was sometimes administered to stimulate patients' appetites, and some doctors found that in patients with hallucinations and other symptoms of psychosis, it also seemed to calm them down.

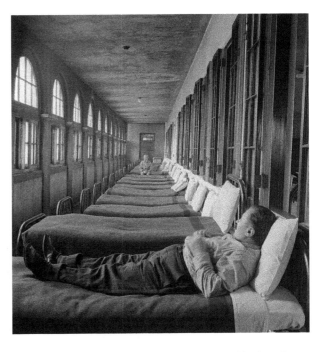

Figure 1.9 Psychiatric patients in an asylum sleeping area, *circa* 1900.
Source: Jerry Cooke/Corbis via Getty Images.

In 1929 Manfred Sakel started using ever higher doses of insulin, which caused some patients to convulse and led to a surprising reduction of their symptoms (Conseglieri & Villasante 2021).

Emil Kraepelin (1856–1926) suggested that biological factors are central causes of psychological disorders. In addition, he classified abnormal behaviors and described and listed their causes (Alda 2021). Kraepelin proposed that biology and genetics were the most influential factors for psychological conditions. He rejected the psychological ideas of Sigmund Freud and suggested that classification of disorders should be based on patterns of common symptoms. He would observe his patients, formulate common outcomes, try to ascertain the cause of the condition, and do his best to predict the best course of action. Kraepelin's method laid the foundation of the modern diagnostic system for mental disorders.

PSYCHOANALYTIC THEORY

Austrian physician Franz Anton Mesmer (1734–1815) (from whose name the term "mesmerize" comes) had an idea about why psychological problems arose in humans. He believed that an invisible fluid universal to all living things, which he called animal magnetism, could become blocked and cause havoc in humans (Gravitz & Page 2019). The solution? Unblock the fluids. Mesmer set up a clinic in Paris to treat what were known then as histrionic disorders. Vats of chemicals were set up with rods coming out from them that might be used to tap on various parts of the body where the animal magnetism was allegedly blocked. Mesmer often performed this treatment in darkness, while wearing elaborate robes and with music playing in the background. Few medical professionals agreed with Mesmer's ideas, but they show the creative lengths to which people went to try to address psychological problems.

And some of Mesmer's patients improved, intriguing a few professionals like Jean-Martin Charcot (1825–1893), who showed that some of Mesmer's techniques could be useful. For example, hypnosis (developed from Mesmer's techniques) not only could be helpful at reducing the symptoms of what was then called hysteria (a condition often marked by numbness or blindness); it could also be used to create symptoms like paralysis in the arm or loss of feeling. Charcot made hypnosis more mainstream as a treatment, which appealed to a new student of his eager to learn these techniques. His name? Sigmund Freud.

Freud became intrigued with the idea that much of what influences our personality is beyond our awareness. After training with Charcot, he returned to his hometown of Vienna and in the 1890s started to work with Josef Breuer (1842–1925), who had discovered that some patients were cured of hysteria after describing their problems under hypnosis. It was during these patients' trances that Freud and Breuer discovered the power of the unconscious mind and its influence on personality and psychological disorders, thus developing the foundations of psychoanalysis including the work of the Neo-Freudians (more on this in Chapter 2).

CONCEPT CHECK 1.2

For each case, indicate the proposed cause of psychopathology (either supernatural, psychological, or biological).
1. Thiago has been taught that depression is a curse passed down from prior generations.
2. Kay suspects her symptoms of depression are due to the stressors she experiences on a daily basis.
3. Patrick believes his symptoms of depression are due to a chemical imbalance.

1.3   MODERN MENTAL HEALTH CARE

Though still similar in certain respects, modern mental health care is fortunately markedly different from the treatment King George experienced. It has been influenced by advances in medications and treatment philosophies, as well as by changes in the way we pay for and deliver treatments.

Deinstitutionalization

The 1950s saw the invention of new psychotropic medications. Imipramine, for example, was one of the first medications marketed as an antidepressant (López-Muñoz & Alamo 2009). Over the next 68 years, more than 25 medications for mental health symptoms were developed for depression alone (Preston et al. 2021).

On the positive side, many people who started to take these medications saw dramatic improvement in their symptoms and were often able to be discharged from psychiatric hospitals. However, this **deinstitutionalization**, meant to replace inpatient psychiatric care with community outpatient services, also released many patients with severe conditions, few work skills, and limited access to the level of care they required.

Between 1955 and 1998, a 90 percent reduction in inpatient population occurred in the United States (Lamb & Weinberger 2020) (Figure 1.10). Where did these patients go? Halfway houses, day treatment centers, and nursing homes took some, but others became homeless and many ended up in prison. Four of five long-term homeless adults in the United States have a major mental disorder or substance abuse condition (Toro 2007). According to the Pew Charitable Trusts, some states such as Hawai'i are working hard to identify homeless people in need of mental health services to get them treatment (Pew Charitable Trusts 2019). Clearly, much more is needed.

Today, outpatient care is the mainstay of treatment for patients with psychological disorders, especially those with mild to moderate symptoms. Outpatient therapy is offered in the form of private psychotherapy or in community mental health centers and other social service agencies. One of six US adults receives outpatient treatment such as weekly therapy sessions for psychological disorders in any given year (NIMH 2019). Twenty percent are there because of milder problems to do with marriage, family, job, friends, or school issues, for example (Ten Have et al. 2013). Outpatient psychotherapy can also be beneficial for severe psychological disorders such as anxiety or depression, or even as an add-on treatment for managing health conditions such as diabetes. Even when symptoms do become so severe that inpatient treatment is needed, it typically occurs only for a short period of time, often just a few days. After that, some people are moved into community programs.

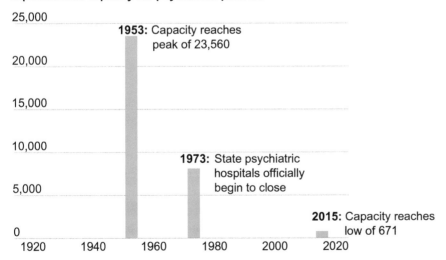

Inpatient bed capacity for psychiatric patients

Figure 1.10 Massachusetts' experience is an example of the dramatic decline in inpatient beds. Since 1953 the number of available beds for psychiatric patients has decreased by over 97%.

Source: Data from Massachusetts Department of Mental Health.

TREATMENT CENTERS AND MANAGED CARE

Managed care: a health care system in which the insurance companies control and coordinate medical and psychological services.

The second half of the twentieth century saw the start of a new approach to health care called **managed care**. Managed care is a health care system in which the insurance companies essentially control and coordinate medical and psychological services – because they make the decision whether to pay for the treatment or not. Insurance administrators assign practitioners, set the cost of and number of sessions, and even decide under what conditions the treatment is no longer needed. The benefit of managed care is that it's a one-stop system, often orchestrated by a primary care physician, nurse practitioner, or physician's assistant, which makes it easier for the insurance company to coordinate client care among various providers since they use the same systems. Providers can share information, help book appointments, and even assist in preventive treatments. Costs are reduced because therapists typically agree to accept lower fees from the insurance companies in exchange for being listed as preferred providers. In the United States, three of four privately insured people are enrolled in a managed-care program (Stewart et al. 2021).

Some therapists and clients feel the quest to reduce costs has affected the quality of care in some cases. For example, the insurance company, not a qualified doctor, therapist, or psychiatrist, may decide someone does not require treatment despite the fact that the person clearly doesn't feel well, or perhaps the type of treatment the person needs isn't covered by the insurance company. In the United States, only 50–60 percent of those with serious psychological disorders receive treatment, often due to the lack of low-lost treatment options, and sometimes due to the stigma of seeking treatment in the first place. The numbers of those in need who are not getting help are even higher in many other countries (NIMH 2019).

Mental Health Professions

Several professions are engaged in the research and treatment of psychological disorders including psychiatrists, psychiatric doctors of nursing practice, counseling and clinical psychologists, and master's level therapists (see Figures 1.12–1.14).

PSYCHIATRISTS

Psychiatry: a branch of medicine that treats mental and behavioral conditions.

Psychiatry is a branch of medicine that treats mental and behavioral conditions. The first two years of medical training in this field focus on the biomedical clinical sciences. After that, students receive training in clinical specialties such as primary care, cardiology, or pediatrics. Depending on the school, students earn professional doctoral degrees such as Doctor of Medicine (MD) or Doctor of Osteopathic Medicine (DO). After medical school, those interested in psychiatry practice serve as psychiatric residents for four years of in-depth training. Psychiatrists spend the bulk of their time treating severe psychological conditions and may prescribe psychotropic medications and order and interpret laboratory tests.

Practitioner-Scholar Model:	Scientist-Practitioner Model:	Clinical-Researcher Model:
More clinical work	Balance of clinical work and research	More research

Figure 1.11 Types of psychological training programs in the United States.

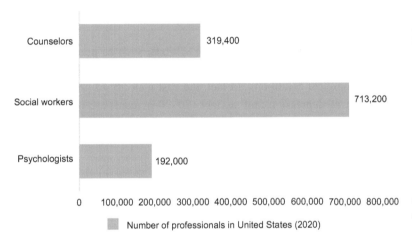

Figure 1.12 A number of professionals, including hundreds of thousands of psychologists, social workers, and counselors, provide treatment for psychological conditions in the United States. The chart shows the number of people in each category as of 2020.

Source: Based on data from www.bls.gov/ooh/life-physical-and-social-science/psychologists.htm.

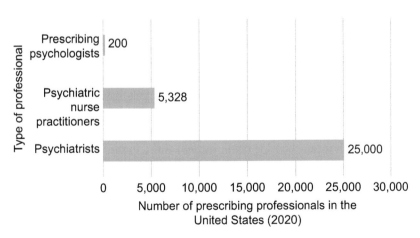

Figure 1.13 Specialists including psychiatrists, psychiatric nurse practitioners, and prescribing psychologists may prescribe medication for psychological conditions in the United States. The numbers in each profession shown here are from 2020.

Source: Based on data from www.aanp.org/about/all-about-nps/np-fact-sheet and Bureau of Labor Statistics, U.S. Department of Labor, Occupational Outlook Handbook, Physicians and Surgeons, at www.bls.gov/oes/current/oes291223.htm.

Figure 1.14 Primary care professionals in the United States including physicians, nurse practitioners, and physician assistants often prescribe medication for psychological conditions. These data on their numbers are from 2020.

Source: Based on data from Bureau of Labor Statistics, U.S. Department of Labor, Occupational Outlook Handbook, Physicians and Surgeons, at www.bls.gov/ooh/healthcare/physicians-and-surgeons.htm; Bureau of Labor Statistics, U.S. Department of Labor, Occupational Outlook Handbook, Physician Assistants, at www.bls.gov/ooh/healthcare/physician-assistants.htm; Bureau of Labor Statistics, U.S. Department of Labor, Occupational Outlook Nurse Practitioners, at www.bls.gov/ooh/healthcare/physician-assistants.htm; www.bls.gov/oes/current/oes291171.htm.

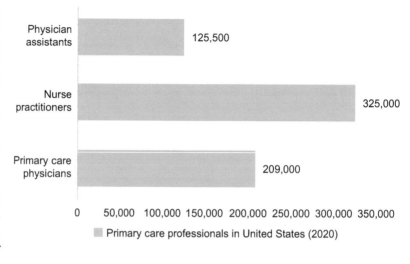

Many practitioners in primary care settings, such as primary care physicians, physicians in family medicine, and physician assistants, also prescribe medication for psychological conditions. In fact, the vast majority of prescriptions for conditions such as depression and anxiety (70–90 percent) are prescribed outside the practice of psychiatry (Preston et al. 2021).

PSYCHIATRIC DOCTORS OF NURSING PRACTICE

Psychiatric Doctors of Nursing Practice, or Psychiatric DNPs, are advanced practice nurses trained to provide mental health services. Psychiatric DNPs diagnose psychological disorders and prescribe and manage medications but may also conduct therapy and provide assessments. As of 2020, DNPs can practice without the involvement of a physician in 25 states. In other states they are required to have a collaborative agreement with a physician.

COUNSELING AND CLINICAL PSYCHOLOGISTS

Counseling psychologist: a mental health professional who helps those with difficulty adjusting to life stressors to achieve greater wellbeing.

A **counseling psychologist** is a mental health professional who helps those with difficulty adjusting to life stressors to achieve greater wellbeing. The verb "to counsel" comes from the Latin *consulere*, which means to consult or seek advice. Counseling psychologists originally delivered occupational advice to help people choose careers best suited to their abilities and interests. Since then, counseling psychologists have broadened their role by providing psychotherapy.

Clinical psychologists: mental health professionals who research, evaluate, and treat psychological conditions.

Clinical psychologists are mental health professionals who research, evaluate, and treat psychological conditions. The word "clinical" derives from the Greek *klinike*, which means bedside (as in re*cline*), since in the early days most medical clinical work was done at the patient's bedside. Clinical psychologists began by providing testing services and have added psychotherapy (previously practiced only by psychiatrists) to their portfolio of professional activities.

Clinical psychology training programs vary in their emphasis on the different roles of clinical psychologists, whether the scientist-practitioner model, the practitioner-scholar model, or the clinical researcher model (see Figure 1.11).

The **scientist-practitioner model** (also called the Boulder model because it was developed at a conference held in Boulder, Colorado) is a balanced program in which students learn both clinical skills and research skills. Having clinical research skills can help clinicians to keep up with new treatments, evaluate the treatments they offer, and even conduct research that informs others of new effective treatments. However, not everyone interested in clinical psychology wants to have a career that includes doing any scholarly research at all.

Scientist-practitioner model: a balanced clinical psychology program in which students learn both clinical skills and research skills.

The **practitioner-scholar model**, also known as the Vail model (because it was developed at a conference in Vail, Colorado), along with a professional doctorate in psychology (Doctor of Psychology, or PsyD), is well suited for individuals who wish to focus on treatment (Maree 2020). It emphasizes understanding, synthesizing, and applying existing research. Still others who are interested in psychology prefer to generate new research. Research is the basis of the **clinical research model**, a training program that emphasizes clinical psychology research over direct work with clients. In fact, some clinical researchers aren't licensed and never do direct work with clients.

Practitioner-scholar model: a clinical psychology program that emphasizes clinical practice.

Clinical research model: a clinical psychology training program that emphasizes clinical psychology research over direct work with clients.

In addition to coursework, doctoral students in psychology undertake two to three years of supervised training and complete scholarly work, typically a dissertation (in PhD programs) and an extensive literature review (in PsyD programs). Recently, some psychologists with advanced training in **psychopharmacology**, or the treatment of psychological conditions using medication, have been licensed to prescribe medicine. New Mexico granted properly trained psychologists prescriptive authority in 2002, and Louisiana, Illinois, and Idaho also now have prescribing psychologists.

Psychopharmacology: the treatment of psychological conditions using medication.

MASTER'S LEVEL THERAPISTS

So far, we've discussed mental health practitioners at the doctoral level. However, there are also many mental health practitioners who are trained at the master's level. These include social workers, pastoral counselors, licensed professional counselors, and marriage and family therapists. While practice laws can vary from state to state, those with master's degrees may be limited to performing certain actions (such as administering and interpreting neurological tests), or they may have hospital privileges or perform certain actions only under the supervision of a doctoral level practitioner.

CONCEPT CHECK 1.3

Match the professional with the description.
1. Dr. Ballard is a medical doctor who has in-depth training to treat psychological conditions. She prescribes psychotropic medication as well as orders and interprets laboratory tests.
2. Dr. Welch has an advanced degree in nursing and prescribes and manages medications.
3. Dr. Day works in a college mental health center. In addition to helping students adjust to life stressors, he also conducts both group and individual therapy sessions. His field originally provided occupational services.
4. Dr. Rios works in a hospital and provides testing and psychotherapy services for people with severe depression.

1.4   THE SCIENCE OF PSYCHOPATHOLOGY RESEARCH

Moods, motivations, and behaviors can be difficult to define in ways we can measure; fold in cultural differences and different expectations of gender, and measurement or assessment becomes even more difficult. Luckily clinical researchers have several tools in their arsenal to describe and predict psychological disorder as well as test the results of treatments. These include case studies, correlational techniques, and experimental research methods along with epidemiological studies.

Case Studies

Case study: an extensive examination of the experience of a single individual or group that allows researchers a deep look at the subject.

A **case study** is an extensive examination of the experience of a single individual or group that allows researchers a deep look at the subject. Case studies can be helpful vehicles for presenting discoveries about rare psychological disorders, for supporting a new theory to challenge an established theory, and for describing new therapeutic techniques.

You'll see many case studies throughout this book. But while they are helpful in describing one person very well, applying to other situations what you've learned in a case study can be challenging. Early in my career as a clinical psychologist I attended a workshop that featured a case study of a person with obsessive-compulsive disorder and a particular treatment that made a huge difference in the client. I tried the technique on my own client with no success at all. That doesn't mean the case study was flawed or that the treatment didn't work, but rather that I probably needed to adapt the treatment to my client's unique situation.

Correlational Research

Variables: the characteristics of behavior or experiences.

Some descriptive studies aim to establish the correlational relationship between two types of observations or variables, for example what kinds of factors are associated with insomnia. **Variables** are the characteristics of behavior or experiences, such as exposure to trauma, that can be described and measured. In psychopathology, these variables are often the symptoms of psychological disorders, or environmental or biological factors that could influence the presence or severity of the symptoms. The variable can be measured, and in some cases manipulated and assessed, to discover what might lead to the disorders or what treatments can be helpful in relieving the symptoms.

Correlational method: a research design that explains how two or more conditions vary in relation to each other.

Sometimes it's important to know what kinds of symptoms occur together, or what kinds of events are associated with a particular symptom – panic attacks, for example. To uncover this information, some psychological researchers employ the **correlational method**, a research design that explains how two or more conditions vary in relation to each other, such as how the number and types of toppings on a

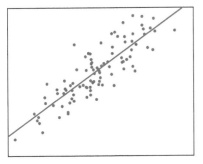

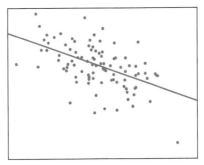

Positive correlation → r > 0

Negative correlation → r < 0

Figure 1.15 Correlation coefficients show the relationship between variables such as a positive correlation (on the left) and negative correlation (on the right).

pizza affects the number of calories in the pizza. A **correlation coefficient** describes the direction and strength of this relationship.

To show the pattern of relationship between variables, a scatterplot includes a line representing the average trend across the points. Do the points fall close to this average (along the line), and are they close together or scattered in a very diffuse pattern? Figure 1.15 shows a few possible patterns of scatterplots.

Correlations can be positive or negative (see Figure 1.15). A **positive correlation** occurs when both variables move in the same direction (the quantity of cheese and meat on the pizza heavily increase the calorie count; both quantities go up together). A **negative correlation** occurs when increasing scores on one variable are matched with decreasing scores on the other (as when extra vegetables rather than extra cheese on the pizza result in a proportionately negative price increase in a store that charges by the topping). When two variables are unrelated, their correlation is close to zero and there is no pattern to the spread of points on the distribution.

But knowing the relative strength and direction of a correlation raises other questions we might want to answer, such as whether one of the two measured variables causes changes in the other. For example, if there is a correlation between low self-esteem and depression, it's hard to say whether low self-esteem leads to depression or the symptoms of depression lead to self-esteem problems. A third possibility is that another factor such as biological predisposition or distressing events could lead to both low self-esteem and depression and there's really no link between the two at all, in which case the correlation merely describes the statistical relationship of the variables and not the causal relationship.

Experimental Method

Suppose you want to find out how high bread dough will rise at a given temperature. The best way to find out is to conduct a test or **experiment**, a method that helps us understand the relationship between two types of variables (Figure 1.16). The variables we manipulate, such as the temperature in the kitchen, are **independent variables**,

Correlation coefficient: a numerical description of the direction and strength of relationship between two variables.

Positive correlation: an association between two variables where both variables move in the same direction.

Negative correlation: occurs where increasing scores on one variable are matched with decreasing scores on the other.

Experiment: a method by which one or more independent variables is manipulated by researchers and the result is measured through one or more dependent variables.

Independent variables: the factor that an experimenter manipulates to create different experiences for participants.

Figure 1.16 Experiments can be carried out to understand the link between variables such as self-esteem and depression.

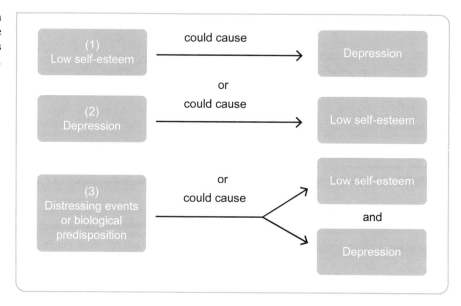

Dependent variables: in an experiment, the measurement collected to determine if there was any effect of the independent variable.

Experimental group: in an experiment, the group that receives some treatment or experience.

Control group: in an experiment, the participants who do not receive a treatment or experience.

Confounding variables: outside factors that might account for differences in the dependent variable.

Random assignment: assigning participants to the experimental group and the control group entirely by chance, so that each person has an equal likelihood of appearing in each group.

Experimenter bias: inaccurate measurements due to the researcher's expectations.

and those that change as a result of that manipulation, such as the amount by which the dough rises, are **dependent variables**.

In the simplest studies of human behavior, an **experimental group** of participants receives some treatment or experience – via the independent variable – and a **control group** of participants does not. Control groups are important because they allow us to compare those who receive the treatment to those who do not receive it, allowing us to conclude that the treatment has an effect – the dependent variable.

In a true experiment we conclude that the independent variable has *causality*; that is, it *causes* the difference in the dependent variable. How can we be sure? We must rule out **confounding variables**, or outside factors that might account for differences in the dependent variable. The important feature of experiments that allows us to draw solid conclusions about causality is the effort we take to be sure every participant in the study has an equal chance of being assigned to the experimental group, minimizing the occurrence of confounding variables. This method is called **random assignment**; it means assigning participants to the experimental group and the control group entirely by chance, so that each person has an equal likelihood of appearing in each group. Without random assignment, we are not able to say which factors might be responsible for causing the outcomes. But if we know the two groups differ *only* in the experience they had, then the outcome must be due to the independent variable. You can flip a coin or use a computer program to randomly assign participants to groups.

Careful controls are also needed to avoid inaccurate measurements due to the researcher's expectations, called **experimenter bias**. For example, an experimenter who knows which participants have received a particular treatment might form expectations about how they will react. Participants may also alter their behavior in a study to be more socially desirable and perhaps fail to answer honestly. For example, knowing they received a medication during the study, they may believe it has an effect and change their behavior as a result. For this reason, researchers sometimes administer **placebos**, or medications without active ingredients, to one group of subjects so they can separate the *placebo effect* from the effect of the medication. When subject or experimenter bias is expected to be a problem, a **double-blind** procedure is followed in which neither the subject nor the experimenter knows which experimental conditions that subject is assigned. In a **meta-analysis**, dozens (and sometimes hundreds) of studies on a single topic are considered together and conclusions drawn about our current knowledge.

The keys to good psychological research include a clear hypothesis, well-defined variables, and as much care as possible to control for confounding variables as well as experimenter bias. If well done, experiments can be useful for evaluating the effectiveness of treatments.

Placebos: medications without active ingredients.

Double-blind: an experimental procedure in which neither the subject nor the experimenter knows to which experimental conditions that subject is assigned.

Meta-analysis: a research technique in which many studies on a single topic are considered together and conclusions drawn about our current knowledge.

Epidemiological Studies

Epidemiology is the study of the frequency and distribution of health conditions. Epidemiological studies help us to discover the number of people in a certain population who may have a condition and how this carries over time and within specific populations such as certain countries and groups of people (such as people of different incomes, or different ethnicities). Epidemiological techniques can also be applied to mental health conditions (Das-Munshi et al. 2020). Among other pieces of data, epidemiology examines the incidence, recovery, mortality, and prevalence of health conditions.

Incidence refers to the number of individuals who develop a specific disease or experience a specific health-related event during a particular time period (such as a month or year). Incidence focuses on the number of new cases during that time. *Recovery* refers to the number of people who had a health condition but who no longer have the symptoms. Recovery may be due to treatment, or the symptoms getting better by themselves over time. Unfortunately, some people have symptoms that will lead to their death. *Mortality* refers to the number of people who die as a result of their health condition. **Prevalence** is the proportion of a population who have a disease or health condition at a specific period of time. Prevalence is typically expressed as a percentage of the population. Many researchers report the proportion of people who will have the condition at some point in their lives (lifetime prevalence), or the proportion who will have the condition in a population in the last year (12-month prevalence). Prevalence takes into consideration several factors including the number

Prevalence: the proportion of a population who have a disease or health condition at a specific period of time.

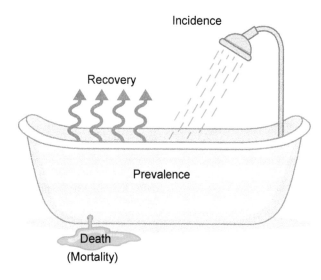

Incidence

Recovery

Prevalence

Death
(Mortality)

Figure 1.17 The prevalence of a condition is influenced by incidence, recovery, and mortality, as depicted here in the "epidemiologist's bathtub."

of new cases (incidence) and taking out the number who have recovered or died from their condition (see Figure 1.17).

Over the last decade several large-scale epidemiological studies have been done to estimate the prevalence of psychological conditions, including the Epidemic Catchment Area Study and the World Mental Health Surveys that you'll see cited in many graphs in this book. The Epidemic Catchment Area Study interviewed more than 20,000 people in five specific cities in the United States to estimate the prevalence of psychological disorders. The World Health Organization (WHO) conducted the World Mental Health Surveys by interviewing more than 150,000 individuals in 26 countries on 6 continents. Epidemiological data helps us to examine cross-national consistencies and variations in mental health, which we'll examine in the chapters to come.

CONCEPT CHECK 1.4

For each of the following, identify the type of psychopathology research study that is used.

> Case study
> Correlational research
> Experimental method
> Genetics research

1. A researcher examines sets of twins in order to help explain whether the environment or inherited biological factors are more important in developing public speaking phobias.
2. A therapist develops a new procedure to treat clients with eating disorders. She creates a detailed account of a client who is successfully treated using this procedure.
3. Researchers randomly assign study participants who agree to receive a new virtual-reality treatment for social anxiety disorder. One group receives the treatment: the other watches an interactive game.
4. Researchers survey 100 college students. They find that those who report having strict parents are more likely to report higher scores on a scale of thrill- and adventure-seeking as adults.

1.5 CHAPTER REVIEW

SUMMARY

What is Abnormal Psychology?

- Abnormal psychology is the scientific study of psychological disorders.
- For most behaviors to be abnormal they must be deviant, create distress or dysfunction, or be dangerous.
- Psychopathology must be seen through the lens of culture.

Historical Views of Abnormality

- Explanations of abnormality correlate with the way people see the world.
- The ways in which people have viewed abnormality have changed over time.
- Treatments for psychopathology are linked with the cause of the disorder.

Modern Mental Health Care

- Modern mental health care has been influenced by advances in treatment philosophies and medications.
- The development of medications led to a reduction to the inpatient population and to deinstitutionalization.
- There are several mental health practitioners with various approaches to mental health concerns.
- Psychiatrists are medical doctors with a clinical specialty in treating psychological conditions.
- Psychiatric nurse practitioners also treat mental health conditions with medications.
- Clinical and counseling psychologists both study and treat individuals with psychological concerns.
- In some states prescribing psychologists can treat psychological conditions with medications.

- Master's level therapists such as licensed professional counselors also treat individuals with psychological conditions.

The Science of Psychopathology Research

- Clinical researchers use various tools to describe and predict psychological disorders.
- A case study is an examination of the experience of a single individual or a group that allows researchers a deep look at the subject.
- Correlational research aims to examine the relationship between two types of variables.
- An experiment is a method that allows researchers to understand the relationship between two types of variables.

DISCUSSION QUESTIONS

1. Why is it important for us to understand the perspectives researchers have used to explain psychological disorders?
2. Explain how the study of abnormality has changed from its beginnings to its current status as a scientific discipline.
3. Are there times when deviance, distress, dysfunction, and danger might be inadequate in explaining a behavior? Why or why not?
4. What role do you think etiology might play in assigning a stigma to certain psychological disorders? What are some ways stigma could be reduced?
5. What are some of the advantages and disadvantages of having some clinical psychologists who focus on direct clinical treatment but not on research, and others who focus on research but not on direct clinical treatment?

ANSWERS TO CONCEPT CHECKS

Concept Check 1.1

1. B
2. A
3. C
4. D

Concept Check 1.2

1. Supernatural
2. Psychological
3. Biological

Concept Check 1.3

1. Psychiatrist
2. Doctor of nursing practice
3. Counseling psychologist
4. Clinical psychologist

Concept Check 1.4

1. Genetics research
2. Case study
3. Experimental method
4. Correlational study

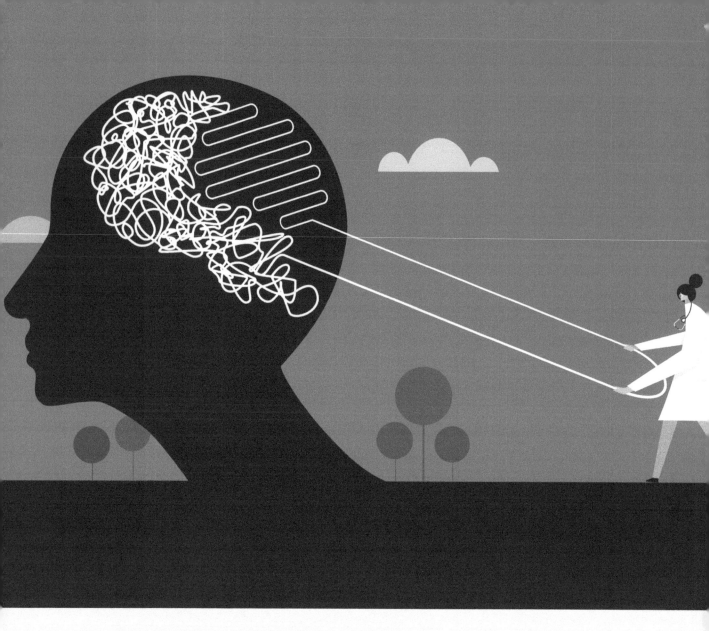

CHAPTER CONTENTS

2

Psychopathology Perspectives: Theories and Treatments

CASE STUDY: **Gloria Szymanski**

Gloria Szymanski is recently single and thinking of dating again for the first time since her divorce some six years ago. But Gloria is in a quandary. Dating has been difficult for her. She realizes that she doesn't present herself well and seeks out men who bring out the "worst in her." What's more, her daughter Pammy recently asked Gloria whether she has had sex since her divorce and she doesn't know what to do. Should she tell the truth, or would a lie hurt her relationship with her daughter?

Many of us might reach out to friends and family for advice, but Gloria has done something unique. She's presented her questions to not one but three different psychologists, Carl Rogers, Fritz Perls, and Albert Ellis. Each represents a different perspective in psychopathology and treatment, and we'll see in this chapter that two will give her different ways to solve her problem, while the third will give her no answers whatsoever. But their perspectives are just some of the many ways to conceptualize what's going on with Gloria and her daughter.

Why so many perspectives? Why so many treatments? The reason is that personality is complex, and various theories of personality take various positions on why people behave the way they do. Psychopathology describes problematic variations from these personality theories. Different models outline assumptions about personality and psychopathology and are often in conflict with each other. After introducing them in this chapter, we'll revisit these perspectives (and a few more) in each chapter as we discuss the various psychological disorders and their treatments.

More discussion of Gloria Szymanski's case appears later in the chapter.

Learning Objectives

- Explain the physiological processes and the medical treatments behind the biological perspective of psychopathology.
- Define the psychodynamic perspective and the techniques used in psychodynamic therapy.
- Describe the humanistic perspective and the techniques used in humanistic psychotherapy.
- Describe the behavioral perspective and related techniques.
- Contrast the cognitive theories of Beck, Ellis, and the Third Wave approaches of ACT and DBT.
- Describe the sociocultural perspective and how systems and group therapy utilize this approach.
- Analyze how multiperspective approaches to psychopathology integrate various approaches.

2.1   THE BIOLOGICAL PERSPECTIVE

The biological perspective suggests that our body and its physiology (or functioning) are the essential components of both our personality and psychopathology. To understand how biology influences psychological disorders, we need to understand the typical biological functioning of the brain and nervous system. We'll start with the basics, and by the end of this section, you'll understand some of the molecules, cells, organs, and systems that underlie the biology of psychopathology. What you'll notice is that variations in anatomy, neurotransmitters, and genetics are often involved in the connection between psychopathology and biology.

The Nervous System

Biologists study the body by looking at its various organ systems. We have a circulatory system that moves blood to and from our organs, a digestive system that breaks down and processes the food we eat, and a muscular system that helps us move. The *nervous system* is the network of organs, nerves, and supportive systems that send and receive signals to and from various parts of the body. Those signals consist of both electrical and chemical activity.

Biological psychology: also known as *neuropsychology*, is the branch of psychology that examines the connection between bodily systems and behavior.

Biological psychology, also known as *neuropsychology*, is the branch of psychology that examines the connection between bodily systems and behavior. Understanding *neuroscience*, the study of the nervous system, can also be helpful in connecting the body and behavior. Neuroscience can tell us how the nervous system is involved in psychopathology and its symptoms, and even the connection between the nervous system and some of the side effects of medications. Most of the communication within the nervous system occurs through messages that flow between neurons (nerve cells) to activate or deactivate various parts of the nervous system. Communication can also occur over long distances through the bloodstream via hormones.

Central nervous system: a division of the nervous system that comprises the brain and spinal cord.

Peripheral nervous system: a division of the nervous system that joins the rest of the body to the central nervous system.

The nervous system has two main branches (Figure 2.1). The **central nervous system** (CNS) connects and controls the body, while the **peripheral nervous system** (PNS) joins the rest of the body to the central nervous system. These two parts work together to operate the body's actions and reactions and in the following sections we will briefly cover their anatomy and the roles they play in our everyday life.

The Central Nervous System

The central nervous system consists of the brain and the spinal cord. The brain is protected by the skull, and the spinal cord by the spinal column. In addition, the central nervous system is protected by cerebrospinal fluid (CSF), a clear liquid that is created in the brain's ventricular system. The brain sits in CSF, which allows it to float and reduces the net weight of the brain from 3 pounds (on average) to

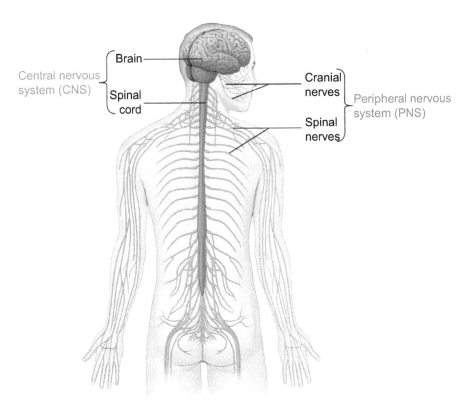

Central nervous system (CNS)
- Brain
- Spinal cord

Peripheral nervous system (PNS)
- Cranial nerves
- Spinal nerves

Figure 2.1 The nervous system is organized into the central and the peripheral nervous systems. Neurons in the CNS (orange) reside entirely within the brain and spinal cord. Nerves that extend from the CNS to the PNS (or vice versa) are part of the PNS (green).

less than 0.2 of a pound. Having a lighter brain is handy because it is much easier for our neck to carry it around. CSF also transports hormones around the brain and helps to wash away the waste products from the cells.

ANATOMY OF THE BRAIN

Housing more than 87 billion neurons and trillions of support cells such as glial cells, the brain is the chief of the nervous system. It's a hungry machine, using over 20 percent of all the oxygen you breathe in every day. What does the brain do with all that power? What *doesn't* it do? It controls muscles and organs and integrates, stores, and retrieves all that you know.

A good way to understand how the brain works is to highlight the location and functions of some of its main structures, like the forebrain, the cerebrum, and the cerebral cortex.

FOREBRAIN

The largest part of the brain is the *forebrain* (Figure 2.2). It consists of the thalamus, the hypothalamus, the limbic system, and the cerebrum. The *thalamus* acts as a relay point for most sensory information. It sorts and distributes information to other areas of the brain, and also helps us notice and react to the stimuli around us.

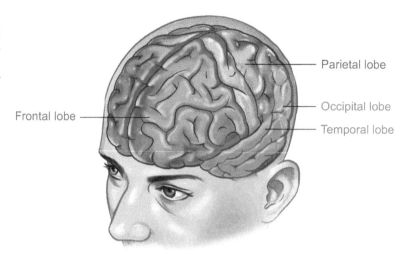

Figure 2.2 The occipital, frontal, temporal, and parietal lobes are important brain areas in psychopathology.
Source: Mark Garlick/Science Photo Library/Getty Images.

The *hypothalamus* detects drives and need states, such as the fight or flight response to a stressful/frightening event and hunger. It also controls the autonomic nervous system, which manages our involuntary responses, and the production of the pituitary hormone, which is largely responsible for the actions of metabolism like hunger.

The *limbic system* is a collection of brain structures that governs emotions (e.g. anger, happiness, and fear), memory, motivations, unconscious drives, and olfaction. There are many structures in the limbic system, but in this section we will look at three central structures in the limbic system: the amygdala, the hippocampus, and the nucleus accumbens. The *amygdala* is an area in the temporal lobe that has been implicated in our emotional responses, such as fear and anger (Dębiec et al. 2010). The amygdala helps to guide our responses to emotions, and a recent study by Bonnet et al. (2015) has reinforced its role in the perception of emotional intensity and positive emotions. The *hippocampus* is deeply embedded into the temporal lobe, right below the cerebral cortex. It plays an important role in learning and memory, making things easier to recall. The *nucleus accumbens* is a limbic system structure of the basal ganglia and integrates information from cortical and limbic structures to mediate goal-directed behavior. It is key in mediating emotions related to motivation, reward, and pleasure.

CEREBRUM

The *cerebrum* is the largest part of the forebrain, located superiorly and anteriorly in relation to the brainstem. It contains nearly 90 percent of the brain's overall volume and is the source of intellectual activities. Not only does it hold your memories, it also makes you plan, enables you to imagine and think, and allows you to recognize friends, read books, and play games. Only about a quarter-inch thick, it has hills (*gyra*) and valleys (*sulci*) that make it compact; otherwise it would be about 3 feet wide and 3 feet long. The cerebrum has two hemispheres, one on the left and one on the right, each containing four lobes. The two hemispheres communicate with each other through a dense network of nerve fibers called the *corpus callosum*. Curiously, although these two hemispheres seem identical, they have different abilities; for instance, the left is where our ability to form words lies, whereas the right one controls many abstract reasoning skills.

CEREBRAL CORTEX

What most people envision when they think of the brain is the *cerebral cortex*, the outside layer of the cerebrum just under the skull. Each of its four lobes has been associated with a range of tasks. The *occipital lobes* are an area in the back of the cerebral cortex. At the rear area of the occipital lobes is the visual cortex, which processes image information. The *temporal lobes* are near the temples and contain the primary auditory cortex, which helps us process the sounds we hear. The *frontal lobes* are at the front of the cerebral cortex and play an important role in planning and organization. The frontal lobes also contain the motor cortex, which functions in planning, controlling, and executing movements. The *parietal lobes* are located behind the frontal lobe, at the top of your head. These contain the somatosensory cortex, which processes body-sensation information, such as the way things feel, including texture, warmth, and weight.

NEURAL COMMUNICATION

Like the rest of your body, your nervous system is composed of millions upon millions of highly specialized cells. In general, the cells in the nervous system fall into two major categories: glia and neurons. In this section we'll focus on neurons.

The standard cell of the nervous system is the **neuron** (Figure 2.3). Also known as nerve cells, neurons are abundant. By some estimates your brain consists of around 87 billion neurons, each with thousands of connections to sensory or motor systems. Most of the neurons in our body are interneurons, which are neurons that communicate only with other neurons.

There are thousands of specialized types of neurons, but most have a few structures in common: dendrites, soma, and axons. *Dendrites* are neuron cell structures that receive messages from other neurons and funnel them to the cell body or soma of the neuron. The *soma* is the core part of the neuron and keeps the cell functioning. It contains the genetic material for the cell. The *axon* is a long, tube-like structure that extends from the soma and is used to carry messages away from the soma to another neuron's dendrite. At the end of the axon is the axon terminal.

The area between two neurons is called the *synapse* and consists of three structures: the *axon terminal* of the neuron that's sending the message, the *synaptic gap* (sometimes called the synaptic cleft) which is the space between one neuron and the next, and the *dendrite* of the neuron that's receiving the message (Figure 2.4).

Neuron: a standard cell of the nervous system.

Figure 2.3 A typical human brain cell (a neuron).

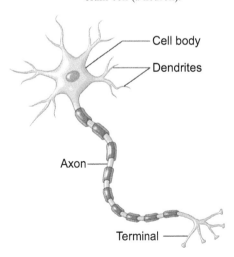

Cell body

Dendrites

Axon

Terminal

Figure 2.4 The synapse consists of three structures: the axon terminal, the synaptic gap, and the dendrite.

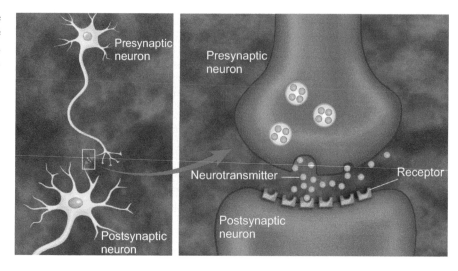

The billions of neurons in your brain are in constant communication with each other, but they don't actually touch. How do they exchange information without touching? They use chemicals called neurotransmitters to bridge the tiny space between them. **Neurotransmitters** are molecules that communicate, or transmit, messages from one neuron to the next, including neurons in particular areas of the brain. Neurotransmitters can therefore affect behavior.

Neurotransmitters: molecules that communicate, or transmit, messages from one neuron to the next, including neurons in particular areas of the brain.

Neural communication takes place across extremely tiny spaces and is incredibly fast; messages travel at speeds up to 268 miles an hour. These messages tell the neuron either "Fire!" (meaning the next neuron will pass along the message of the neural impulse) or "Don't fire!" (meaning the next neuron will stop the neural impulse from continuing).

Since neurotransmitters can send only two kinds of messages, you might think we need only two types of neurotransmitters. Actually, however, more than 100 different types of substances play the role of neurotransmitter at least some of the time (Greengard 2001). A single neurotransmitter can also be active in many different functions and thus have overlapping responsibilities in the nervous system. Serotonin, for example, is involved in both mood and anxiety. Table 2.1 describes neurotransmitters with some of their functions.

Drugs can cause neurons to fire or not fire, and some drugs can also influence the effects of neurotransmitters. An *agonist*, for example, is a substance that mimics or increases the effect of a neurotransmitter. Gamma-aminobutyric acid (GABA) is the nervous system's primary inhibitory ("Don't fire") neurotransmitter. GABA agonists like valium can slow down the nervous system and relax us. *Antagonists*, on the other hand, are substances that can block the action of a neurotransmitter. Botulinum toxins act as an antagonist and block the release of acetylcholine, causing paralysis

Table 2.1 Common neurotransmitters and selected functions

Neurotransmitter	Selected functions
Acetylcholine	Memory and muscle functions
Dopamine	Movement and reward system
GABA	Inhibition of action
Norepinephrine	Learning and memory
Serotonin	Sleep, mood, anxiety, and appetite

of muscles and the illness known as botulism. Agonists and antagonists each can act directly by binding to or blocking neurotransmitters at receptor sites, or by affecting the release neurotransmitters, or destroying neurotransmitters in the synaptic gap.

The Peripheral Nervous System

The peripheral nervous system consists of all the parts of the nervous system residing outside the brain and spinal cord. What's left? A lot. The peripheral nervous system includes 37 miles of nerves, or bundles of neurons, connecting the muscles, glands, and organs of your body. It has two parts: the *somatic nervous system*, which controls the voluntary movement of your muscles, and the *autonomic nervous system*, which controls internal organs such as the heart, glands, etc.

The autonomic nervous system, in turn, has two components: the *sympathetic nervous system*, which is involved in preparing the body for emergencies or stress (for example in response to stress, by activating the organs and the glands in the endocrine system), and the *parasympathetic nervous system*, which slows your heart rate and breathing, and conserves your bodily functions.

The Endocrine System

One of the main functions of the sympathetic and parasympathetic nervous systems entails interacting with the endocrine system. The endocrine system is formed by glands, which are groups of cells whose function is to secrete chemicals called hormones (Figure 2.5). Hormones, in turn, circulate in our body with the goal of regulating emotions and behavior. The adrenal glands, for instance, have a broad influence over many organs in the body. For example, in times of stress, they will secrete stress hormones like epinephrine that increase blood pressure, heart rate, and the other parts of the fight, flee, or freeze response of the sympathetic nervous system. One gland can affect your heart, blood vessels, and pupils all at once.

So far we have discussed how areas of the body and even cells can affect our behavior. In the next section we look at how even structures as small as molecules can influence our behavior. These molecules, small clusters of atoms, can have an impact on your behavior as well.

Genetic Influences and Psychopathology

Are you familiar with the nature-nurture debate? Although common sense would suggest that we are certainly born with specific traits but that we acquire others as we navigate life, this is still one of the most controversial questions in the history of psychology. Also, common sense often doesn't agree with science.

Figure 2.5 Major endocrine glands include the adrenal glands. The endocrine system can communicate over long distances in the body.

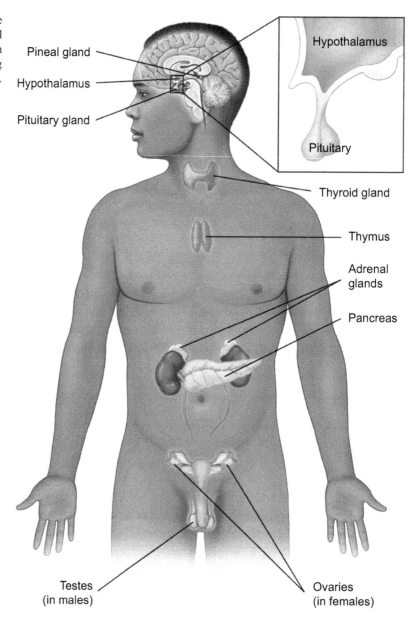

So, if you wonder how genetic some particular behavior is, the answer isn't straightforward.

We know that deoxyribonucleic acid, or DNA, is a complex molecule that contains the directions to make each and every structure and substance in your body, and it's tucked away in nearly every cell in your body. There are nearly 6.5 feet of tightly bundled DNA per cell that contain the specific recipe to make you. All the parts of your body are created from this instruction manual.

Chromosomes are the parts of the cell that contain segments of DNA called *genes*. You got half your chromosomes from your biological mother and the other half from your biological father back when you were a zygote, or a fertilized egg. Our genes' ability to make copies of themselves allows our parents to give us certain characteristics like dark hair or brown eyes. Genes can also pass along the likelihood for acquiring some psychological conditions, as we learned in Chapter 1. But with half our genes from mom and half from dad, what influences which traits and tendencies get expressed? Once again, the answer isn't straightforward.

Most traits are polygenic, meaning that multiple genes are probably needed for them to appear, not just one. For example, it's unlikely that there is only one gene for shyness. Second, the way traits are expressed also depends on the characteristics of the genes that are linked to them. We receive two versions of the same gene (known as alleles) from each parent. If the alleles of a gene (e.g. eye color) are different, one allele will be expressed, meaning that it is the *dominant* gene, and the other one will be masked, meaning that it is the *recessive* gene. So, say that your dad has brown eyes, your mother has blue eyes, and you have brown eyes, we can conclude that brown is the dominant gene (as it has overpowered blue) and blue is the recessive gene. A recessive gene's influence, such as the appearance of blue eyes, will be seen only when that gene teams up with an identical recessive gene (one from each parent).

At the same time, the environment plays a very important role as well. Some combinations of DNA cause the parents' offspring to remain healthier in a particular environment, meaning that, given that environment, those genes are more likely to appear in future generations. For example, over time, mutations in genes resulted in humans' ability to detect greater spectrums of light, allowing us to see more colors. Being able to spot ripe, colorful fruit became an advantage over other species. In such cases, the offspring's mutated DNA is an adaption, a new characteristic that gradually increases in a population to make reproduction or survival more likely. Such adaptations can accumulate over generations in both individuals and populations, giving them a distinct advantage.

Some researchers believe the genes involved in abnormal functioning may simply be triggers for responses that were once critical to survival (Sipahi et al. 2014). For example, fear was an evolutionary advantage that may be problematic today because so many things may set off the adaptable fear response even when it's not necessary. The triggering of this fear response might in turn be associated with high blood pressure, stress, and depression (Brefczynski-Lewis 2020).

The Research Methods of Genetics

Most research into genetics attempts to describe the relative influence of our genes and the environmental factors we encounter, including family, friends, work, home, and even specific experiences from everyday life, such as what we eat and environmental influences to which we are exposed, like diseases or toxins.

Family studies, for example, allow researchers to test hypotheses about the respective weights of genetic and environmental factors by examining a group of biological relatives. Just looking at families won't reveal everything. It's possible that one family is more likely to have depression, for example, because the family lives in an atmosphere charged with unexpressed rage. Certainly some environmental factors also increase the chance that a person might become depressed, such as lack of resources, chronic stress, or lack of personal control. This is where adoption studies can be beneficial. In an *adoption study*, researchers examine traits of children that are expressed in both their biological and their adoptive parents. This technique allows researchers to estimate the differences between environmental and biological influences.

Even family and adoption studies tell only a small part of the story, however. While biological family members share a genetic history, they aren't identical. Each has a unique combination of genes from both parents. *Twin studies*, however, can give us a better idea of the contribution of environment and biology. First let's take a look at the two types of twins.

Monozygotic or MZ twins are identical; they form when a single zygote divides, so they share 100 percent of their genetic material. The incidence of MZ twins is rare, accounting for only 1 in 259 births (Van Baak et al. 2018). *Dizygotic or DZ twins* are fraternal. They form from two eggs and two sperm (Figure 2.6) and are no more genetically similar than two non-twin siblings from the same parents. Since MZ twins share 100 percent of their genes, and those raised together also share 100 percent of their environment, researchers use MZ twins raised in different families as a means to research the strength of the environment versus the strength of genetic factors. For example, researchers have investigated MZ twins whose biological parents were diagnosed with schizophrenia. Although the twins were adopted separately and raised by different parents with no family history of schizophrenia, the studies discovered a genetic influence for the disorder, providing evidence that schizophrenia has a strong genetic component (Henriksen et al. 2017). Twin studies are the gold standard of genetics research.

Figure 2.6 MZ twins come from one egg and one sperm cell, while DZ twins come from two eggs and two sperm. *Source: ttsz/iStock/Getty Images Plus.*

From twin studies we can also make a *heritability estimate*, which describes the influence of heredity and how much of the variation in a specific trait might be due to genes as opposed to the environment. It helps us to determine the part (or proportion) of the variance in a population that can be attributed to genetics. *Behavioral genetics* is a field of research that works to discover how much of the variation is due to biology (genetics) and how much is due to environmental influences. Heritability estimates range from 0, meaning genes have no influence, to 1.0, meaning genes determine everything about the trait being studied.

The Minnesota Study of Twins Reared Apart, or MISTRA, is a longitudinal study (that is, a study over a given time period) of twin pairs who were separated in infancy, reared in different homes during their formative years, and reunited as adults. In 1979, these twins went through some 50 hours of medical and psychological assessments over a six-day span at the University of Minnesota Psychology

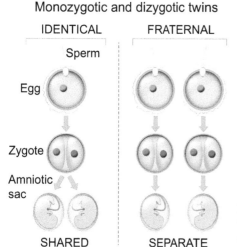

Monozygotic and dizygotic twins

IDENTICAL   FRATERNAL

Sperm

Egg

Zygote

Amniotic sac

SHARED   SEPARATE
PLACENTA   PLACENTA

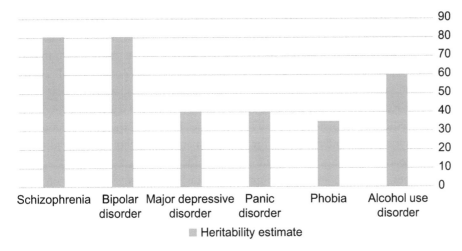

Figure 2.7 Thanks to twin studies, we know that many psychological conditions show evidence of heritability.
Source: Data from Owen et al. (2000).

Department and medical school. Follow-up studies were also conducted. Twin studies can inform us about the connection between genetics and the environment. For example, another twin study shows some of the evidence of the link between genes and certain psychological disorders (Figure 2.7).

Family, twin, and adoption studies can all be helpful, but they do have limitations (Hoffman 1991; Palma-Gudiel et al. 2020). Birth order, gender, and experiences with teachers, friends, sports, interests, and parents and siblings all conspire to make children's individual experiences living in the same family as different as if they came from completely different families. Even identical twins don't have identical environments. On the other hand, some researchers have suggested that there is a "twin effect," meaning that living as a twin is a unique experience because twins are raised a little differently than non-twin children. This, researchers note, makes it difficult to compare twins to non-twins (Plomin et al. 2001). After all, many twins are treated differently from other people simply because they are twins, especially if they are identical. How many other members of the same family are routinely mistaken for one another or dress in identical clothes?

If psychological disorders are caused at least in part by biology, what kind of treatments might be beneficial? Let's take a look at the variety of biological treatments we have in our toolbox.

Biological Treatments

The biological perspective has its own set of expectations about how psychopathology develops and how it should be treated. If psychopathology is caused at least in part by biology, as this perspective proposes, then the treatment should also be biological. For example, trauma and stressor-related disorders, which we will discuss in Chapter 5, by their very nature include an environmental element (a trauma). However, not every person who experiences a trauma ends up with one of these conditions. The biological model suggests that there might be a biological vulnerability in those who develop trauma and stressor-related disorders. For example, in 2020 Lori Zoellner and her colleagues suggested that specific brain regions connected with fear and the way people responded to threats were correlated with post-traumatic stress disorder (PTSD) (Zoellner et al. 2020). Those individuals who were most likely to develop PTSD had areas of their brain that over-responded to fear and avoided activities that might lead to fear.

Biomedical therapies: a family of therapies that use surgery, medication, or other physiological interventions for the treatment of psychological conditions.

Biomedical therapies are a family of therapies that use surgery, medication, or other physiological interventions for the treatment of psychological conditions. While most biomedical therapies are pharmaceutical or drug treatments, there are other types, and more are in development. In this section, we will focus on drug treatment as well as on more invasive medical procedures such as electroconvulsive therapy, transcranial magnetic stimulation, and deep brain stimulation.

PSYCHOTROPIC MEDICATIONS

Psychopharmacologists: researchers and practitioners who study and often prescribe medications for psychological disorders.

Psychopharmacologists are researchers and practitioners who study and often prescribe medications for psychological disorders. They include physicians, nurse practitioners, doctors of nursing practice, pharmacists, medical psychologists, and prescribing psychologists. All these practitioners have extensive knowledge of medicines that treat psychological conditions. As psychopharmacologists, they assume that psychological conditions are in part the result of biological problems including neurotransmitter abnormalities.

In the United States, prescription medications undergo extended review by the Food and Drug Administration (FDA). For a medication to be approved for use, its developers have to provide evidence that it is both safe and effective. "Safe" does not mean it has no risk. In general, a medication is considered "safe" if its benefits outweigh its risks. For example, some medications have significant or even dangerous side effects, such as nausea or seizures. Similarly, "effective" does not mean the medication cures or removes all symptoms of a condition. A medication is considered "effective" if its treatment effects outperform those of a placebo, a substance without an active ingredient. In fact, many placebos can have treatment effects as well as side effects. When a placebo helps a condition, the result is called a *placebo effect*, a treatment response to a physiologically ineffective treatment. People have reported side effects such as nausea, sweating, rash, and fever while using placebos (Hróbjartsson & Norup 2003).

After the FDA has approved a medication for a particular use, the developer of the drug is granted a patent for it. Medicines normally have both a generic name (often related to the molecule or how it works) and a brand name used for marketing the medication. Brand names are usually written with the first letter capitalized, while the generic name is lowercase. For example, if you have been to the supermarket in search for something to help your headache, you may have chosen Tylenol ® (a brand name) or a supermarket version of acetaminophen (the generic name).

Once the patent for the medication has run out, other companies can produce generic versions of it. While generic medications are usually less expensive

Table 2.2 Major categories of psychotropic medications

Category	Example of brand and generic equivalent	Indication (used to treat)
Antianxiety drugs	Xanax, *alprazolam*	Reduce the symptoms of agitation and nervousness
Antidepressant drugs	Paxil, *paroxetine*	Reduce the symptoms of depressive mood disorders as well as some anxiety symptoms
Anticonvulsants	Lamictal, *lamotrigine*	Reduce the symptoms of bipolar disorder
Antipsychotic drugs	Geodon, *ziprasidone*	Reduce the symptoms of psychosis

because their manufacturers do not have to recoup any development costs, they contain the same active ingredients as the brand-name medication. Some brand-name medications also contain inactive ingredients that might make them work better, but in general, generic medications are quite similar to brand-name medications (Alderfer et al. 2021). See Table 2.2 for some typical psychotropic medications and their uses.

NON-MEDICATION TECHNIQUES

Other medical procedures can help alleviate some psychological conditions. *Psychosurgery,* or treatment of mental and behavioral conditions using an invasive biological procedure, has come a long way since early treatments mentioned in the last chapter. One example of a newer medical procedure is *transcranial magnetic stimulation* (TMS) (Figure 2.8). This treatment uses magnetic fields generated by electromagnetic coils to stimulate or deactivate neurons in specific areas of the

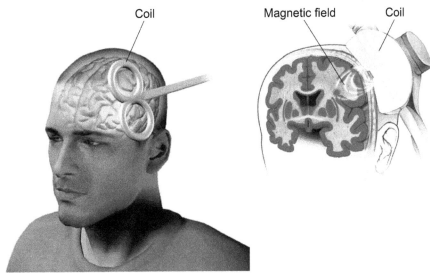

Figure 2.8 Transcranial magnetic stimulation (TMS) uses magnetic fields to treat psychological conditions.
Source: Images used with permission of Mayo Foundation for Medical Education and Research (all rights reserved).

brain. Depressed moods seem to improve when TMS is applied. About 50 percent of those who have received TMS show an improvement in their symptoms (Fitzgerald 2020).

Another procedure is *deep brain stimulation* (DBS), in which a small electrode connected to a generator stimulates the overexcited junction between the limbic system and the frontal lobe in order to regulate abnormally activated electrical impulses. In addition, some patients with chronic depression have found relief through a chest implant that stimulates the vagus nerve, which sends signals to the brain's mood-related limbic system (Bhat & Kennedy 2018). You'll learn more about these and other non-medication procedures in the chapters that follow.

Assessing the Biological Perspective

Biological theories of psychopathology are compelling and can be combined with other theories of psychopathology that we'll discuss next. Given what we know about the brain, it is hard to ignore that biological processes are at the root of who we are. Another strength of the biological approach is its emphasis on a scientific explanation of psychopathology.

Despite their strengths, though, biological approaches tend to ignore hard-to-evaluate concepts like thoughts or motivations, and thus they often overlook the multiple influences that culture and society have on our personalities. It is easy to oversimplify personality as brain and hormonal functioning alone. But can this be all it means to be human? Some suggest that because of their limited focus, biological theories are not complete theories of personality.

We know that life is an interplay between biology and environment, but many biological theories ignore the role of environmental influences. Also, many medications have undesirable side effects because they circulate throughout the body; for example, fluoxetine (Prozac) prescribed for depression can also affect the digestive system and cause nausea. And while medication can be beneficial, it can't solve everything. As we'll discuss in Chapter 10, for example, methylphenidate can benefit people who have attention deficit hyperactivity disorder because it can help them focus, but it can't make them want to study.

Looking at the chapter opening story from the biological perspective, Gloria's anxiety and indecision regarding her relationship might have been due, at least in part, to the areas of her brain that are involved in decision making and the fear response, such as the amygdala. Treatment to help temper this response in the biological perspective might be prescribed medication.

CONCEPT CHECK 2.1

Match the term with the correct definition
   A. Sympathetic nervous system
   B. Parasympathetic nervous system

C. GABA

D. Serotonin

E. Psychotropic medications

F. Antianxiety medications

1. An inhibitory neurotransmitter.

2. A part of the autonomic nervous system involved in the fight, flee, or freeze response.

3. A part of the autonomic nervous system that calms and slows the body down.

4. A neurotransmitter involved in sleep, mood, and appetite.

5. Medications that reduce the symptoms of agitation and nervousness.

6. A general class of medications to treat psychological disorders.

2.2   THE PSYCHODYNAMIC PERSPECTIVE

The **psychodynamic theories** (sometimes referred to as dynamic, psychoanalytic, or Freudian theories) are a family of personality theories that emerged from the work of Austrian neurologist Sigmund Freud (1856–1939) and that focus on unconscious motivation. The idea was that the psyche, or personality, moves what was known as psychic energy, the source of all thoughts and emotions, around the body to where it is needed. This movement of energy is the reason the theory is called dynamic.

Freud is often thought of as the founder of one of the first well-organized grand theories of personality. His early work used hypnosis to help bring about catharsis, or a release of emotions, in many of his patients. Inspired by that work, Freud shifted to examining the *unconscious*, or the thoughts, memories, feelings, and wishes that reside outside our awareness.

Freud's theory didn't suggest that we have access to all our motivations. Instead he described the mind as having several realms, some in awareness and some beyond it. The conscious mind included current thoughts and feelings. The majority of our mind, however, is in the vast and mysterious unconscious, containing thoughts, memories, feelings, wishes and instincts, drives, and memories that may have been repressed or forgotten. As you can see in Figure 2.9, most of our personality also resides outside our awareness in the unconscious mind. Many Freudian theorists compare the massiveness of the unconscious to an iceberg: you might see or be aware of only the tip, but much lurks beneath.

Freud described three structures within our personality: the id, ego, and the superego. The *id* is the part of the personality that functions on the *pleasure principle*, which means it seeks to reduce basic physiological tension, which then leads to the production of pleasure. The id is laser-focused on what it

Psychodynamic theories: a family of theories that focus on unconscious motivation.

Figure 2.9 Iceberg metaphor of Freud's theory of personality. *Source: Shutterstock.*

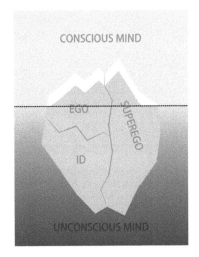

likes, and what it likes is reduction of tension. What kind of tension? All kinds. As a human, you have all sorts of physiological needs and drives. When these are unmet, tension builds up. Being thirsty creates tension; sipping a glass of iced water will reduce that tension. Being hungry creates tension; crunching on a yummy salad will reduce that tension. When the tension is reduced, the id feels satisfied, which brings a sense of gratification.

The physical and physiological needs that motivate the id keep us alive, causing us to eat, drink, and perpetuate the species by having sex. Freud grouped these drives into a cluster of instincts called *eros*, or the life instinct. Eros is the id instinct that reduces tension associated with basic biological drives. Freud also suggested that the id has a death instinct, an unconscious desire to be dead – the ultimate state of tension reduction called *Thanatos*. According to Freud, Thanatos is a way in which we reduce tensions that are aggressive and destructive.

What stops you from satisfying your id instincts in inappropriate ways all the time? According to Freud, good behavior is due, in part, to the ego and the reality principle. The *ego* is the part of your personality responsible for interacting with conscious reality. Rather than the pleasure principle, the ego operates according to the *reality principle*, which guides the ego to defer pleasure until a reasonable way to satisfy id instincts is available.

But the ego has another limitation, the superego. While not fully developed until age 2 or 3, the *superego* is the internalization of society's values. It is governed by the *perfection principle*, which provides an image of the perfect person. The superego can make us feel proud when we do well, but it can also cause us to feel shame and guilt when we don't measure up to its expectations. While the id's demands are generated from biological needs, the superego's demands come from societal pressures. As you can imagine, sometimes these demands can clash, forcing the ego to compromise.

Personality Development

Freud realized that the pleasure principle was dynamic, and that over the course of several developmental stages (which he called psychosexual stages), tension reduction was focused in different parts of the body for which he named the stages. The first area of the body where Freud believed tension reduction centered was the mouth. In the psychodynamic perspective, biting, sucking, chewing, and crying are all ways tension is reduced.

But tension reduction does not stay in the mouth forever. The oral stage, which begins at birth, gives way to the anal stage at around 18 months. This lasts until about age 3, when tension reduction shifts during the phallic stage. The following are Freud's psychosexual stages of development and the relevant ages:

- Oral, 0–18 months.
- Anal, 18–36 months.
- Phallic, 3–6 years.

- Latency, 6 years – puberty.
- Genital, puberty – adulthood.

Freud suggested that too much or too little tension reduction at a certain stage can lead to *fixation* at that stage even as the child grows older. For example, a child who always gets a bottle during the oral stage may become fixated at that stage and seek oral tension reduction when under stress as an adult. If you talk a lot, eat, or chew your pencil when you are stressed, a Freudian might say you may have an oral fixation. Fixation isn't bad; it just describes where you go to seek a reduction of tension – it is a way of explaining one aspect of your personality. Fixation can occur at any stage. For example, too much tension reduction during the anal stage can lead to an anal-retentive personality. Those who are perfectionistic or exceptionally clean are attempting to control their world in the same way they receive pleasure from the tension reduction of controlling their bowels.

Defense Mechanisms

Remember, the ego has some limitations: it must meet the demands of the id and the prohibitions of the superego. Often, to satisfy the id, the superego, and the realities of life, the ego has to compromise. One way it does this is through **defense mechanisms**, which are unconscious arrangements that the ego uses to satisfy id instincts indirectly. This is a list of some Freudian defense mechanisms:

Defense mechanisms: these are unconscious arrangements that the ego uses to satisfy id instincts indirectly.

- Denial: A psychoanalytic defense mechanism in which a person fails to accept reality.
- Sublimation: A psychoanalytic defense mechanism in which a person unconsciously redirects an id instinct in a more socially acceptable way.
- Repression: A psychoanalytic defense mechanism in which a person forces a threatening memory out of awareness.
- Projection: A psychoanalytic defense mechanism in which a person unconsciously attributes their own impulses to another person.
- Regression: A psychoanalytic defense mechanism in which a person reverts to an earlier stage of functioning.

Not all defense mechanisms are problematic. For example, in *sublimation*, a person unconsciously redirects an id instinct in a socially acceptable fashion, basically performing an id instinct in a superego way. According to Freud, a person who has an id instinct to beat up another person may unconsciously transform that into a desire to be a boxer, or a person with a hostile unconscious impulse to cut other people may long to be a surgeon. All positive activities, according to Freud, are sublimations of negative id impulses.

Psychodynamic Therapies

Like many personality theories, the psychoanalytic tradition was developed alongside a psychotherapy technique. **Psychodynamic therapies** are a family of

Psychodynamic therapies: a family of treatments that have at their core the exploration of unconscious internal conflict.

treatments that have at their core the exploration of unconscious internal conflict. They use insight about this conflict to bring about therapeutic change.

According to Freud, unresolved unconscious conflict from childhood can cause difficulties in adulthood. These difficulties include psychological disorders that are manifested as unhealthy defense mechanisms, anxiety, and problematic ways of guarding against the wishes of the id. Unhealthy defense mechanisms need to be dismantled because they are not successful at reducing anxiety and cause problems in everyday life. For example, a person might sabotage healthy relationships because they feel unlovable, but they may not be aware of this feeling.

According to psychodynamic therapists, in order to be healthy, people should come to understand their unconscious conflicts and gain the ability to make informed, mature decisions about fears and desires created in the formative childhood years. Insight into these internal workings of the psyche requires emotional understanding. After all, someone can intellectually understand an unconscious conflict but not really appreciate its potentially overwhelming emotional force.

Psychodynamic therapists employ many techniques to help clients bring unconscious conflicts into awareness, including free association and working through. *Free association* is a psychodynamic therapy technique that reveals unconscious conflicts by interpreting the client's spontaneous responses to given words. Awareness allows the client to *work through* unresolved conflicts in an adaptive way. The therapist can see patterns in the evidence or material revealed by the client and make carefully timed interpretations of the client's unconscious motivations.

But the therapist's work is more complex than simply revealing the interpretation. If it is revealed too quickly or in the wrong way, the client may reject it. *Resistance* is a client's employment of a defense mechanism during therapy. Resistance blocks the therapeutic process and can show up in subtle ways, such as coming late to a session or revealing important information so late that there is little time to address it.

There are dozens of types of psychodynamic therapies. However, in this section we'll outline just two: classical psychoanalysis and short-term psychodynamic therapy.

Psychoanalysis: a psychodynamic treatment rooted in Freud's approach to psychotherapy.

When most people imagine what therapy might be like, they conjure up the image of classical **psychoanalysis**, in which the client lies on a comfortable couch while the therapist sits out of view and encourages free association. Psychoanalysis is intense, with hour-long sessions taking place three to five times a week for years. Though based on Freud's traditional approach to psychotherapy, it is not actually practiced very broadly. It is much too expensive and time consuming for most people, though it does have a track record of helping those with complex psychological conditions (Leichsenring & Klein 2020).

Short-term psychodynamic therapy is rooted in Freud's classical psychoanalysis but is solution-focused, taking place within a much less formal client–therapist relationship in which the two people sit face to face on chairs for 12 to 50 weekly sessions. This therapy is more active and direct than psychoanalysis, with the goal of figuring out the client's current problems rather than restructuring their personality. Because of its brief duration, short-term psychodynamic therapy is more affordable than psychoanalysis but not necessarily appropriate for in-depth personality change, which might be required for personality disorders, for example (Knekt et al. 2008).

Assessing the Psychodynamic Perspective

Though both Freud and his work have been criticized over the years and many of Freud's specific ideas do not hold up against the scientific method, they have nevertheless provided a general foundation that informs the way that psychologists think to this day. It is hard to go even a week without stumbling over one of Freud's terms: repression, denial, unconscious. Freud has become part of our culture. In fact, psychodynamic therapists are fairly common. Almost one in five therapists identifies as a psychodynamic practitioner (see Figure 2.14) (Prochaska & Norcross 2018).

However, there are shortcomings to the psychodynamic approaches. Freud is understandably criticized for his views of women, which reflect the ideas and norms of society during the time he lived; every personality theory does so to some degree. Some of Freud's first work was published in 1895 – only two years before the first European country allowed women to vote, and some 25 years before women were allowed to vote in the United States. But his views are manifested in his work. For example, Freud believed that women may not develop the same superego strength as men. Values always seep into science, despite how objective we hope to be. Culture is also dynamic, however, and changes over time.

Another criticism leveled at Freud is that many of his theories were derived solely from case studies of his patients. This makes the evidence difficult to generalize to everyone and hardly objective. Many of Freud's theories are not scientifically sound, in fact, because they defy the *principle of falsifiability* (Prochaska & Norcross 2018). In order to be scientific, a theory must be testable and able to be disproved. It is difficult to disprove the existence of the ego and superego since, by definition, they are outside our awareness. In fact, many psychodynamic theories may be impossible to study scientifically, but there have been some attempts (Pretsky 2020; Western 1998).

Despite this, Freud's theories have been tested by modern psychodynamic researchers, and many have withstood the challenge. For example, evidence supports Freud's core theories suggesting that early experience affects later behavior, and his theory of unconscious motivation. While psychoanalytic theory has its critics, no one person or theory has had as much influence on psychology as have Sigmund Freud and his work. Today his ideas have morphed into contemporary psychodynamic approaches including object relations theory, self-psychology, and ego psychology.

Referring back to the chapter opening story, a psychodynamic therapist might focus on Gloria's unconscious motivations, such as her defense mechanisms.

For example, in one interview she explains that when she meets someone she really likes, she acts "flip" and tries to sabotage the relationship. A psychodynamic therapist might help Gloria explore her motivations for doing so.

CONCEPT CHECK 2.2

Fill in the term that best completes the statement.
1. After the car accident Austin had no memory of the details, though his physician said there was no physical reason he should have forgotten. Austin's psychodynamic therapist felt his forgetting was a defense mechanism known as _____.
2. Although she really wanted to leave class, Clara decided to stay because it was the right thing to do. The Freudian perspective would say her choice reflected a strong _____.
3. Miguel's Freudian therapist insists that his desire to become a therapist is due to a need to cut that, due to his superego, has transformed into something more socially desirable. This transformation is the defense mechanism known as _____.

2.3   THE HUMANISTIC PERSPECTIVE

While Freud and many adherents of the psychoanalytic perspective saw people as basically selfish and needing to be tamed by society's influence on the superego, humanists see people as inherently good. They believe that all humans, indeed all living things, have an *actualizing tendency*, an innate drive to be the best possible version of themselves. It is just in our nature. *Humanism*, or the phenomenological approach, is a family of personality theories that emphasizes growth and potential.

The Humanistic Approach

According to the humanist perspective, your actualizing tendency allows you to know – internally and maybe even unconsciously – what is best for you. You have an *internal wise mind* that points you in the correct direction for your best growth. Thus, if you are in touch with yourself, you will make the best choices. Because a person's way of being the best version of themselves is unique, humanists believe it is important to examine each person as a unique individual and understand the world from their perspective (think of the saying that you need to "walk a mile in someone else's shoes").

Where does this innate tendency come from? Psychologist Carl Rogers (Rogers 1989) suggested that besides food, water, and shelter, humans have a need for *positive regard*, a sense of being loved and respected. At some point, we also develop positive *self-regard*, which is a kind of grow-your-own version of positive regard developed through the positive regard you get from others, like parents, siblings, friends, and teachers. The ideal way to obtain positive regard that grows into positive self-regard is through *unconditional positive regard* – that is, a sense of others' respect and love that is not linked to your specific behaviors. People love you no matter what you do. Unconditional positive regard allows you to love and respect yourself and get in touch with the internal sense of what is best for you.

If you feel like you must act a certain way in order to be loved and respected, however, you are receiving *conditional positive regard*, or love and respect earned only when you act in ways that others want. Parents, teachers, and friends often deliver conditional regard unintentionally, and not usually out of some desire to control you. But what starts off as an easy way to prod someone to do something ("If you were really my friend, you'd ditch your family vacation and go to the beach with me instead") or a way to shame someone into doing something ("No daughter of mine is going to take a gap year – you're going to get a job once school is over!") can instead be heard as, "I'm loved only if I behave in a specific way."

Conditional regard becomes a problem if it causes you to act for an external reason (in order to get that respect and love), as a result of which you are no longer listening to your own internal wise mind. Rogers suggested that the internal wise mind that directs you by means of the actualizing tendency is your real self. Through conditional regard, however, you develop an idea of what you "should" be in order to get maximum feelings of worth from others. You develop an internal idea of an ideal self, which tries to meet all the conditions of worthiness you discern from others. The difference between your real self and this artificial ideal self creates incongruence. The more incongruence you have, the more miserable you are.

Rogers believed that a fully functioning person is open to experience, accurately perceives the world, and correctly reads their own feelings and motives. The person lives in the here and now, trusts themselves to do what is right, feels free to make independent choices, and contributes to the actualization of others. In order for them to help people regain connection with their internal wise mind, Rogers felt therapists should be genuine and honest and have empathy and genuine respect for clients.

Humanistic Therapy

Carl Rogers established **client-centered therapy** based on humanistic personality theory; this treatment method takes place in a nondirective and accepting environment and leads the client toward personality change. The therapist's major role is to clarify the client's experience and establish the proper therapeutic setting for change by providing feedback with minimal advice giving, instruction, or interpretation. An important part of client-centered therapy is thus *active listening*, a communication method in which the listener responds in ways that demonstrate understanding of what another person says. Using these techniques, the therapist helps clients deeply explore their emotions and approaches to life.

Client-centered therapy: a psychotherapy based on humanistic personality theory that works to create a nondirective and accepting environment and leads the client toward personality change.

Client-centered approaches are powered by the active ingredients of genuineness, acceptance, and empathy (Rogers 1989). *Genuineness* refers to authenticity and transparency in the relationship, meaning the therapist is encouraged to behave according to feelings, revealing their inner experiences to the client and focusing on the here and now rather than the past. As clients sense genuineness in the therapist, they will offer more genuineness themselves, becoming more aware of their experiences and better able to know and express what is going on in the moment.

Acceptance, or communication of respect, is also important for client-centered therapy. Rogers suggests that the client is more likely to be able to change if the therapist grants them the respect all humans should receive, communicated as unconditional positive regard. Respect from the therapist will increase self-respect and self-acceptance in the client and, according to Rogers, will lead to greater self-understanding.

Empathy refers to the therapist's attempt to understand the client's inner world. The client-centered approach is rooted in the idea of *phenomenology*, which emphasizes each individual's unique perspective and the need to understand what it feels like to be that person and see the world from their perspective.

By exposing clients to an atmosphere of genuineness, acceptance, and empathy, the therapeutic environment helps clients to understand hidden aspects of themselves, relate more directly to themselves, better tolerate the nuances of situations, and emphasize conscious over unconscious processes. The relationship encourages clients to focus on growth and to appreciate and be accountable for their own behavior.

Assessing the Humanistic Perspective

Despite the positive view that the humanistic theory holds of humans, not all psychologists hold humanistic theory in such high regard. As with Freudian theory, it is difficult to muster scientific evidence for humanist theory. Much of it comes from case studies of the healthiest of people. And many believe the humanistic approach to be so overly confident about the positive nature of personality as to be impractical.

Still, humanistic ideas have found their way into our everyday language: "living authentically" and "awareness" are part of our understanding of ourselves and others. In addition, humanist influences have informed our understanding of therapy and influenced other research trends, such as positive psychology, which helps clients recognize and relish positive experiences (Joseph & Linley 2006). Humanistic interventions have had mixed results when used alone, however, and may not be appropriate for those with the most serious psychological concerns (Elliott et al. 2020).

In the chapter opener we mentioned that one theorist had no answers for Gloria. In particular, Gloria struggled because her young daughter had recently asked whether she had had sex since her divorce. Gloria had always been honest with her daughter and didn't know whether she should be honest now or lie and protect her. She really wanted to know what Carl Rogers, a humanist therapist, thought she should do. Rogers' response? Many pauses and looks of empathy and active listening. From the client-centered view, the answer has to come from the client, as opposed to advice coming directly from the therapist.

> Gloria: "And I . . . I . . . I . . . have a feeling that you are just going to sit there and let me stew in it (laughs) and I – I want more. I want you to help me get rid of my guilt feeling. If I can get rid of my guilt feeling about lying or going to bed with a single man, any of that, just so I can feel more comfortable."

> Rogers: "And I guess I'd like to say, No, I don't want to let you stew in your feelings, but on the other hand, I, I also feel that this is the kind of very private thing that I couldn't possibly answer for you. But I sure as anything will try to help you work toward your own answer. I don't know whether that makes any sense to you, but I mean it." (Shostrom 1965)

CONCEPT CHECK 2.3

Indicate whether each example demonstrates genuineness, empathy, or acceptance.
  A. Genuineness
  B. Empathy
  C. Acceptance
  1. When Max's therapist Jill found that Max had suddenly quit his job, Max could tell she wasn't pleased, yet he still felt she respected his decision.
  2. Coral disliked the way the cake looked when she picked it up from the bakery, so she decided she would express her displeasure rather than pretend she liked the design.
  3. Although he was really enjoying the day, when Blake found that his friend Devon had recently broken up with his boyfriend, he stopped what he was doing so he could listen to the story and try to understand what Devon was going through.

2.4 THE BEHAVIORAL PERSPECTIVE

In the 1950s some psychologists wanted a model more concrete and measurable than the psychodynamic perspective offered. They felt that psychological disorders are rooted in behaviors, and that psychology should therefore study objective behavior rather than subjective experience. These psychologists applied the tenets of the behavioral model to explain and treat psychological disorders. The **behavioral perspective** assumes that psychological disorders are the result of

Behavioral perspective: a theory of psychopathology that uses learning theory to understand problematic behaviors and change them to more constructive ones.

maladaptive behavior patterns, so it uses learning theory to understand those behaviors and change them to more constructive ones.

Behavioral Theory

According to behavioral therapists, behavioral symptoms are not a sign of the problem – they *are* the problem. While insight into the motivation for your behavior is essential for psychodynamic therapies, behaviorists argue that knowing why you do something doesn't necessarily stop you from doing it. And sometimes that insight isn't necessary to change the behavior at all.

Some behavior therapists will treat a specific set of symptoms related to the client's complaint. Behaviorists, for example, believe that lack of social skills can lead to nervousness and in extreme cases to social isolation. Since according to behaviorists social skills are attained through learning, behavior therapy uses social skills training to increase social ease and improve interaction with others. It has been used to treat many issues, including social anxiety (Horigome et al. 2020) and autism spectrum disorder (Wood et al. 2020).

More often, however, behavioral therapies are applied to change the connections between certain behaviors. Behavioral therapists use classical conditioning and operant conditioning to achieve therapeutic change. Let's look at each of these techniques in turn.

Behavioral Therapies

Behavioral therapies assume that all behaviors, even problematic ones, are learned. Behavioral therapies use the principles of the behavioral approach such as classical and operant conditioning to treat psychological disorders.

CLASSICAL CONDITIONING

Classical conditioning: a type of learning in which a response typically associated with one stimulus becomes associated with a new stimulus.

Classical conditioning is a type of learning in which a response typically associated with one stimulus becomes associated with a new stimulus. Learning begins when an *unconditioned stimulus*, an unlearned signal that leads to a reflexive response, is associated with a *neutral stimulus*, an event that contains no reflexive response. After we experience learning, the neutral stimulus will become a *conditioned stimulus*, which will activate the behavior associated with the original stimulus. Sometimes people make accidental associations with a stimulus that leads to problematic behaviors or reactions. For example, loud noises naturally induce fear. Lightning is associated with the boom of thunder, so some people will become frightened and flinch when they see any quick flash of bright light, even outside the context of a thunderstorm. Behavioral therapists attempt to decouple these associations by using *counter-conditioning*, a behavioral technique in which a response to a stimulus is replaced by a new response. Classical conditioning techniques attempt to extinguish behaviors in various ways (Figure 2.10).

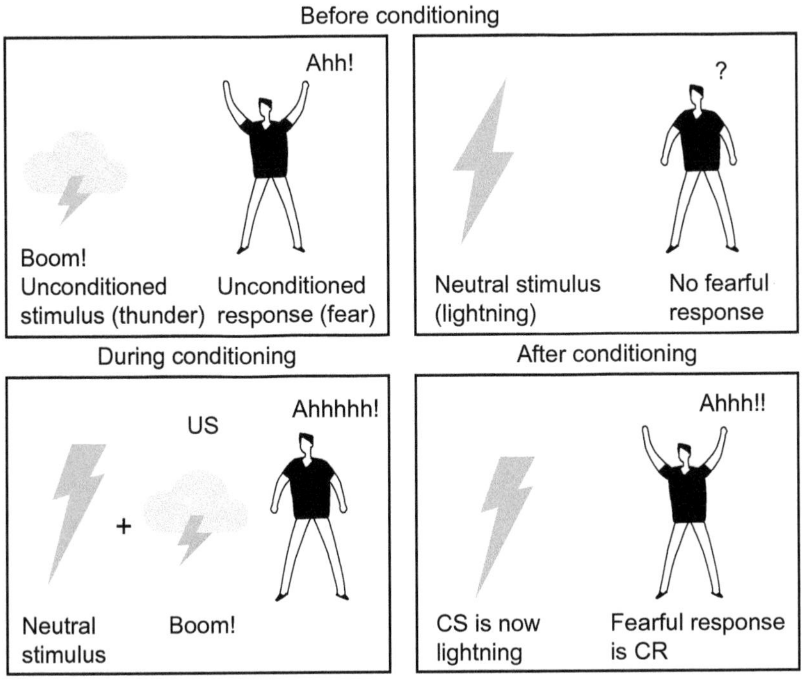

Before conditioning

Ahh!

Boom!
Unconditioned   Unconditioned
stimulus (thunder) response (fear)

Neutral stimulus   No fearful
(lightning)   response

During conditioning

US   Ahhhhh!

+

Neutral   Boom!
stimulus

After conditioning

Ahhh!!

CS is now   Fearful response
lightning   is CR

Figure 2.10 Classical conditioning might be able to explain why some people flinch when there is lightning. Notice how in the first panel the unconditioned stimulus (thunder) is associated with an unconditioned response (fear), and through classical conditioning the conditioned stimulus (lightning) becomes associated with fear (the conditioned response).

For example, anxiety can be countered by using relaxation as a substitute. Since anxiety is produced by the sympathetic nervous system, which as we learned earlier prepares the body to fight, flee, or freeze, and relaxation is produced by the parasympathetic nervous system, which conserves bodily functions and energy, these two states cannot exist at the same time. Mary Cover Jones (1924) developed **exposure therapy**, which repeatedly presents the client with a distressing object to reduce associated anxiety and the fear response over time (Deacon & Abramowitz 2004). A common type of exposure therapy is *systematic desensitization*, in which a client practices relaxation while facing progressively more fear-inducing stimuli. Systematic desensitization has three steps:

Exposure therapy: a therapeutic approach which repeatedly presents the client with a distressing object to reduce associated anxiety and the fear response over time.

1. Constructing a hierarchy of fears such as the one in Table 2.3.
2. Training the client in progressive relaxation.
3. Alternately exposing the client to succeeding levels of the fear hierarchy and then to relaxation until the fear response is extinguished and fear no longer occurs.

Exposure therapies including systematic desensitization can be done *in vivo*, meaning actual exposure to the thing that causes the anxiety; using imagination, in which the person will create a mental image of the feared object; and using computers, as in virtual reality

Table 2.3 Example of a fear hierarchy

Level of distress	Situation
40	Look at a cartoon drawing of a spider
50	Look at a photo of a real spider
60	Hold a spider in a box
70	See a spider on a desk
80	See a spider on my pants
95	See a spider on my sleeve
100	See a spider on my arm

Figure 2.11 Virtual reality therapy can help some clients overcome their fears, such as fear of heights, in a simulated environment.
Source: Kobus Louw/E+/ Getty Images.

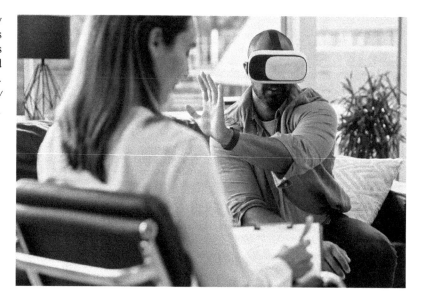

exposure therapy. Virtual reality therapy has been used to treat postpartum stress disorder, flight anxiety, and public-speaking anxiety, among other disorders (Kaussner 2020; Kim 2021; Krijn et al. 2004) (Figure 2.11).

Aversive conditioning pairs an unpleasant stimulus with an undesired behavior in order to reduce that behavior. Painting an unpleasant-tasting liquid on the fingernails of people who bite their nails is one example (Vargas & Adesso 1976). Although aversive conditioning has been shown to be beneficial in the short run, its use has been limited because of the availability of more effective treatment such as operant conditioning techniques.

OPERANT CONDITIONING

Operant conditioning: a type of learning that uses training to make desirable behaviors more likely to occur again and reduce the occurrence of others.

First described by psychologist B. F. Skinner, **operant conditioning** uses training to make desirable behaviors more likely to occur again and to reduce the occurrence of others. Operant techniques include *positive reinforcement*, which sets a consequence of desired behaviors that creates a pleasant state, making the behavior more likely to occur again, and non-reinforcement and sometimes punishment of behaviors that are undesired. Often, desired or adaptive behaviors are encouraged through *shaping*, in which a part of a behavior is reinforced first, and over time more of the behavior is reinforced. We use techniques like positive reinforcement all the time. For instance, not only is it polite to thank a friend for taking you to the airport, it also makes it more likely that they will take you to the airport again in the future.

Assessing the Behavioral Perspective

One advantage of the behavioral theories is that they lend themselves much more easily to the scientific method than do the psychoanalytic theories, because they are more observable and easier to measure. Therefore, we have more scientific evidence about the effectiveness of behavioral therapies.

Behavioral intervention can be particularly helpful in treating anxiety disorders through behavioral conditioning, as we saw above (Antony 2014). But it has some limitations. Some therapists think behavioral interventions are too simplistic to address complex human conditions such as schizophrenia, and that the improvements in behavior don't always translate to real life or persist over the long term. However, making their results easier to measure might also make the behavioral theories less like actual life, because actual life may have many uncontrolled variables that are difficult to predict accurately.

Applying a behavioral perspective to the chapter opener, we can say that Gloria's ordeal about what to do centered on balancing the potential reinforcement of telling her daughter Pammy about her dating life and the potential punishment of how Pammy might respond to the truth. Not knowing whether her action will cause a reinforcement or a punishment is what causes the anxiety Gloria experiences.

CONCEPT CHECK 2.4

Indicate whether the example illustrates classical conditioning, operant conditioning, or observational learning.

1. Belen snaps a rubber band to punish herself whenever she thinks about spending time on social media.
2. Sam always feels slightly sick to his stomach whenever he even thinks about eating at The Chicken Salad Sandwich Shop after he got food poisoning there three weeks ago.
3. Even though she didn't get punished by the teacher, Darla makes an extra effort to get to class on time after her friend was embarrassed for being a few minutes late last week.

2.5   THE COGNITIVE PERSPECTIVE

The behavioral perspective offered something new that the psychoanalytic perspective didn't have – a way to test, measure, predict, and shape behavior that was more scientific than relying on the unseen forces predicted by Freud. But it also left out something: the idea that our thoughts, feelings, and attitudes contribute to the human condition.

Cognitive Theory

The **cognitive perspective** in psychology emphasizes the internal processes of thought, or cognition, that help us make sense of the world. Cognition encompasses all aspects of thinking including knowing, remembering, reasoning, deciding, and communicating. In addition, the cognitive perspective studies our thinking

Cognitive perspective: a theory in psychology that emphasizes the internal processes of thought, or cognition, that help us make sense of the world.

shortcuts and the biases and errors that can come from them, leading to the symptoms of psychological disorders.

Some psychologists found the explanations of the behaviorists to be unsatisfying. They wanted to know more about the motivations behind the behaviors humans performed. One investigation into the cognitive approach started with a conditioning study using dogs. Seligman and Maier (1967) studied operant conditioning using an escape-learning procedure. They placed dogs in a box with two compartments and used a mild electrical current, like static electricity, to teach the dogs to jump over the partition to escape the shock. A second group of dogs were placed in a different situation in which they could neither control nor escape the shock. After this initial training, the second group was placed in the partitioned box and shown that they could easily avoid the shock. However, these dogs failed to learn to escape, even though escape was easy and was readily learned by the dogs without the initial training.

Seligman called the phenomenon demonstrated by the second group of dogs *learned helplessness*. The dogs seemed to have generalized their learning to feel they no longer had any control of consequences. As a result, they were unable to learn to respond when the consequences changed. Seligman extended this concept to human behavior in people suffering from depression. When you feel your efforts at controlling events in your life repeatedly fail, you may give up even trying to succeed. Later, you may be in situations in which you *can* control the consequences and may still fail to act because you believe you aren't able to control the outcome.

Peterson and Seligman reformulated the helplessness approach by examining *explanatory style*. Our explanatory style reflects what we think causes or explains an event, such as getting a crack on your cell phone screen or misplacing your keys. By nature, we tend to accept positive things that occur in our lives. A negative event, on the other hand, requires an explanation so we can prevent it from happening again. Humans tend to be more consistent about the ways we explain negative events than positive events (Peterson et al. 1982). Peterson and colleagues (1982) have suggested that our response to the negative events we experience – our explanatory style – is demonstrated by our answers to three questions about the events and how we perceive them:

1. Is the event's cause internal or external? Was it your fault or did someone else cause the event to occur? If you have an *internal locus of control*, you believe that any good or bad things that happen to you are the result of your own actions. An *external locus of control* leads you to feel that both good and bad things are outside your control.
2. Is the event stable or unstable? In other words, is the cause there to stay, or does it come and go?
3. Is the event global or specific? That is, does it affect other aspects of your life, or does it have a relatively localized impact?

Those whose answers reflect internal, stable, and global explanations will have a pessimistic explanatory style and be more prone to helplessness in the face of negative events. If you've lost your keys, you are likely to see the event as internally caused ("It's my fault that I lost my keys"), stable ("I'm always doing things like this"), and global ("This is exactly why I shouldn't get an expensive cell phone – I'd lose that too").

However, a person with an optimistic explanatory style will often attribute the negative event to an outside or external factor ("I was distracted") and believe it is a temporary or unstable occurrence ("because my phone was ringing"), whose impact has a limited or specific effect ("It will likely never happen again"). See Table 2.4 for a summary of these explanatory styles.

Table 2.4 Explanatory styles for negative events

Explanatory style	Internality	Stability	Globality
Optimism	External	Unstable	Specific
Pessimism	Internal	Stable	Global

Source: Adapted from Peterson et al. (1982).

Cognitive Therapies

Cognitive psychotherapy emphasizes the link between thoughts and emotions and suggests that thoughts are the cause of psychological disorders. The goal of cognitive therapy is to help clients understand their thinking patterns, which may be maladaptive, and develop healthier ways of thinking in order to change the way they feel. Therapists use specific techniques to help clients recognize patterns of maladaptive thoughts and to apply intervention strategies to reshape their ways of thinking. The two most common types of cognitive therapy are Beck's cognitive behavior therapy and Ellis' rational emotive therapy.

COGNITIVE BEHAVIOR THERAPY

As a psychoanalyst, Aaron Beck noticed that his clients' language underwent a shift over the course of therapy (Beck et al. 1987). Some of his depressed patients experienced negative thoughts about themselves, their world, and their future that seemed to occur automatically. Beck tried to evaluate these thoughts and wondered whether a therapist could change them more directly using the therapeutic process. The basis of the model he developed is that psychological conditions, like depression, result from maladaptive thoughts. Specifically, people who are depressed tend to have a pessimistic explanatory style, and when bad things occur, they tend to blame themselves. In addition, they are also more likely to discount positive events (Beck et al. 1987).

In **cognitive behavior therapy (CBT)**, the goal is to identify any negative self-talk and examine it fully. Rather than just advocating positive thinking, the therapist encourages clients to notice and test their maladaptive or distorted beliefs through questioning techniques and homework. The treatment emphasizes the link between thoughts, emotions, and behavior. A cognitive therapist will give clients tools that can help them address distortions in their thinking. Here are some examples of common cognitive distortions:

Cognitive behavior therapy (CBT): a psychotherapeutic technique where the goal is to identify any negative self-talk and examine it fully.

- *All-or-nothing thinking*: Seeing things in inflexible extremes such as good or bad.
- *Overgeneralization*: Seeing one negative event as an ongoing pattern.

- *Jumping to conclusions*: Assuming something is negative without enough evidence.
- *Emotional reasoning*: Assuming that feeling negative emotions means negative things are really happening.

RATIONAL EMOTIVE THERAPY

Like Aaron Beck, Albert Ellis was also trained as a psychoanalyst, but Ellis' active, directive, *rational emotive* approach emphasizes the link between thoughts and emotions. Ellis rejected the notion that the past is important to a person's current condition. In fact, he believed you affect your future more than the past affects you. Your current problems are based on the idea that we teach ourselves false notions about ourselves, the world, or other people over and over again (Ellis 1980).

How do we do this? Ellis says we use self-talk to focus on irrational or unrealistic expectations, leading to unwanted feelings. Statements like "I am worthless" are illogical overgeneralizations associated with anxiety and depression. Ellis also emphasizes the importance of action. Like cognitive therapy, rational emotive therapy includes homework in which clients practice their new ways of thinking.

THIRD WAVE COGNITIVE APPROACHES

New leaders in cognitive-behavioral therapy started to challenge the traditional way of explaining their clients' relationships with their thoughts and emotions. They proposed that perhaps eliminating the symptoms was only part of the treatment, and that some of the strategies to treat the symptoms might be useful in and of themselves. *Third wave cognitive approaches* fold together behavioral and cognitive (the first two waves) and other traditions such as mindfulness meditation and Buddhism.

Particularly helpful for mood, substance use, and personality disorders (Campbell-Sills & Barlow 2007; Kring & Sloan 2009), third wave therapies help clients understand, accept, and regulate their emotions. Avoiding emotions can often cause problems (such as when people avoid thoughts, memories, feelings), so third wave approaches include acceptance and commitment therapy and dialectical behavioral therapy. *Acceptance and commitment therapy* (ACT) helps clients accept problematic thoughts as opposed to changing them (Hayes 2019). *Dialectical behavioral therapy* (DBT) was developed for treatment of borderline personality disorder (Linehan 1999). It helps clients deal with conflicting emotions, focus on managing negative emotions and controlling impulses, and learn mindfulness techniques to increase problem-solving skills and tolerance of negative emotions. It has been helpful not only with borderline personality disorder and eating disorders (Fogelkvist et al. 2020) but also in reducing suicidal thoughts (Lyng et al. 2020) and self-harm, and increasing interpersonal skills (Bernal-Manrique et al. 2020).

Assessing the Cognitive Perspective

Cognitive approaches are popular among therapists, with up to a third identifying with this approach (see Figure 2.14) (Prochaska & Norcross 2018). It's no surprise, since cognitive approaches are particularly helpful for mood, anxiety, and substance use conditions.

But cognitive approaches do have their limitations. Some therapists and clients find them too cold and impersonal. The highly structured nature of CBT isn't for everyone. In fact, sometimes the symptoms of a condition may make it difficult for clients to do the work of CBT (for example, if they have learning difficulties or problems with thought processes). Some people critical of CBT think it doesn't focus on the insight and depth of problems and changes things only on the surface. Despite these challenges, cognitive techniques remain some of our most effective tools.

Gloria, from the chapter-opening story, worried excessively about not being able to find people to date. According to the cognitive approach, this behavior would be due not to the way Gloria was reinforced or punished (as the behavioral perspective suggested), but rather to her perceptions of herself, others, or the world. The therapeutic intervention would focus on helping her to change the way she thought about herself in order to change the way she feels.

CONCEPT CHECK 2.5

Identify each technique with the correct cognitive approach.
Cognitive-Behavioral Therapy (CBT)
Acceptance and Commitment Therapy (ACT)
Dialectical and Behavioral Therapy (DBT)

1. Rather than working to change Ivy's thoughts about losing her dream job, her therapist is helping her to accept that she no longer has the job.
2. In his therapy group for borderline personality disorder, Devin is working on discovering what kinds of events trigger his anger and what to do when he feels that way.
3. When she feels sad, Liana's therapist encourages her to stop and analyze her thoughts.

2.6 THE SOCIOCULTURAL PERSPECTIVE

The perspectives in psychopathology we've looked at so far have emphasized parts of the individual: our biology, our unconscious, our human striving for perfection, and even our thoughts. The **sociocultural perspective** emphasizes the way social and cultural elements in the environment might interact with the person. *Social psychology* and *cultural psychology*, for example, examine the ways in which

Sociocultural perspective: a theoretical perspective that emphasizes the way social and cultural elements in the environment might interact with the person.

people affect one another and differences in cultural values and norms, respectively (Kashima 2019).

The sociocultural perspective suggests that you can't understand abnormal behavior (or really any behavior) without understanding a person's cultural and social context. For example, socioeconomic disadvantages can be a risk factor for psychopathology, and members of some cultural groups are more likely to witness trauma and violence than others (Gustafson et al. 2009). For example, social norms can stigmatize some groups, and marginalized people in the United States have increased rates of anxiety, depression, and substance use (W. L. Huang et al. 2021). These problems are often due to the impact of their treatment in society. For this reason, some types of therapy that focus on the individual might not be comprehensive enough to make an impact on the causes of distress (such as poverty or racism). The sociocultural perspective focuses on prevention and community interventions that can address the root causes of inequality. These will improve individuals' mental health outcomes because people are no longer treated poorly by society.

The sociocultural perspective has grown in the United States as the field of psychology – and the country – have become more diverse. By 2050, ethnic and racial minorities will represent nearly half the US population (US Census Bureau 2016). While some psychotherapies focus only on the individual in treatment, sociocultural perspectives consider the relationships in clients' lives. For example, the systems and group therapy approaches both recognize the influence of other people in an individual's life.

Systems Approaches

According to the *systems approach*, psychopathology is an indication of a dysfunctional system, which could be a family, a couple, or even a group of friends. In the belief that therapists cannot change the individual without also changing their system, systems therapies examine the interdependence of people in the system as a means of improving their relationships.

Families, for example, often interact by following certain rules and norms (Goldenberg et al. 2014). These structures and patterns teach the members to behave in ways that might seem unusual to outsiders but are quite functional in that particular family system. Sometimes, however, the system is dysfunctional, and therapy will examine intergenerational patterns, using genograms or family trees to understand the roles people play. *Family therapy* and *couples therapy* (Figure 2.12) both aim to identify and change dysfunctional ways individuals in a family or a couple relate to each other. They have been used to help clients with eating disorders (Fisher 2019) as well as bipolar disorders (MacPherson 2020). The goal is to get the entire family to change. *Structural family therapy* works to change the power structure within families (Goldenberg et al. 2014), while *conjoint family therapy* seeks to change dysfunctional communication patterns (Sharf 2015).

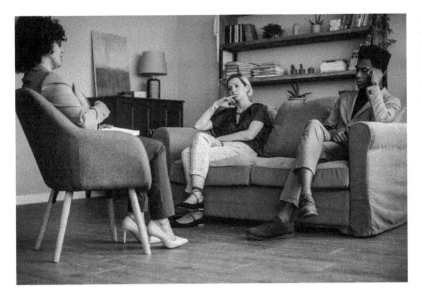

Figure 2.12 Couples therapy is a systems approach that can help to change ways that couples relate to each other.
Source: svetikd/E+/Getty Images.

THE POWER OF EVIDENCE

Understanding culture can benefit treatment

Despite the progress that has been made in psychotherapy in general, marginalized populations show less improvement in psychotherapy than others, stop treatment sooner, and use it less often (Cook et al. 2014). Among the many factors responsible for the disparity are the interactions between clients and their therapists, including poor communication and microaggressions. There is evidence to suggest that these factors can lead to misdiagnosis, shorter client visits, less empathy, and increased anxiety in clients (Kanter et al. 2020; Montgomery et al. 2020).

What can help? Researchers have found that greater therapist sensitivity and the inclusion of cultural mores in treatment (Comas-Díaz 2014), including culturally sensitive approaches (Wyatt & Parham 2007) in graduate training, can help therapists to be aware of their own values and the values of others whose cultures may be different from their own. It can make them aware of the hardships faced by their clients and understand the stress that comes from negative prejudices and stereotypes (including their own). What's more, cultural competency training can assist therapists in helping clients understand the impact that culture can have on their own self-view, and to identify and express anger and pain and increase self-esteem that may have been damaged by negative messages from society. Many states now require some evidence of cultural competency training to obtain or maintain a license to practice.

Group Therapy

Group therapy: a psychotherapy treatment technique that treats multiple clients in a collective setting.

Many therapists devote some portion of their practice to working with groups (Norcross & Goldfried, 2005). **Group therapy** can be as effective as individual therapy for many kinds of conditions (Grier et al. 2010). It treats multiple clients in a collective setting, often under the direction of one or several therapists (or even on their own), and relies on some of the same intervention techniques as systems approaches, except that clients in a group setting share similar concerns rather than a family relationship. One type of group therapy is the *support group*, in which members meet without a therapist to provide social and emotional support for each other.

Group therapy has both strengths and weaknesses. It is much less expensive than individual therapy since the members share the cost of the therapist. In addition, the group experience can reveal patterns of problematic relationships that may not show themselves in individual settings. For example, a client may work well with an individual therapist but have difficulty balancing a situation in which they have to control their own anxiety and impulse and wait while another person in the group takes a turn to speak. Members of the group may compete for the therapist's time, however, and confidentiality is harder to control in group settings. Groups are also helpful for some concerns but not all, especially when a client may require more attention from a therapist due to such concerns as severe depression, impulsivity, or symptoms such as hallucinations. However, group therapy can be useful to many clients because of its affordability and the increased motivation that clients often receive from the other group members.

Assessing the Sociocultural Perspective

One benefit of the sociocultural perspective is that it acknowledges the obvious impact of society and culture on the individual. In fact, some states now require culture competency as a continuing-education requirement for some mental health professionals (see The Power of Evidence). And family systems approaches have been particularly helpful in treating children.

However, among the challenges to the sociocultural approach is that sometimes the findings of the research in this area are difficult to interpret and implement. Associations between behavior and culture don't necessarily mean there is a causal link between culture and certain ways of being in the world. Members of any given cultural group aren't all alike, and the way one person interacts with their culture or family can be as individual as the way that person interacts with their thoughts. Nevertheless, the sociocultural perspective is an essential perspective in psychopathology.

CONCEPT CHECK 2.6

Indicate whether the statement is true or false.
1. The sociocultural perspective focuses only on society.
2. Family therapy is primarily useful only when working with small children.

3. Because of the importance of the sociocultural perspective, some states require cultural competency as part of continuing education for mental health professionals.
4. Being part of a cultural or social group could be a risk factor for some mental health conditions.

2.7 PULLING IT TOGETHER: A MULTIPERSPECTIVE APPROACH

People often wonder whether depression might be biological or environmental in origin. Or they wonder whether they are afraid of storms because of a childhood experience or should take a genetic test to find out whether they have a biological fear of storms.

Because the experiences we have in the moment are the result of biological, environmental, and cultural factors, a **multiperspective approach** is most appropriate. The psychological symptoms we develop (or fail to develop) are likely the result of multiple factors, and multiperspective models take this into account. Psychological risk factors can be biological (such as a genetic predisposition for increased amygdala reactivity, which could heighten anxiety), sociocultural (such as a family of origin that freely expresses anger), or environmental (such as exposure to a dangerous neighborhood in childhood) (see Figure 2.13).

Risk factors alone might not be enough to lead to a psychological disorder, however. It's more likely that a certain triggering event, called a *diathesis*, is also needed. The **diathesis-stress model** implicates stressors such as a move to a new city, the death of a close friend, or a change in hormone levels in the development of psychological symptoms.

Another multiperspective theory picks up where the diathesis-stress model leaves off. The **reciprocal-gene environment model** suggests that while there might be biological predispositions for certain conditions, patients themselves can increase the stress that makes symptoms worse. For example, if you have a biological predisposition to become depressed during times of stress, and if during times of stress you tend to withdraw from friends and family, this response might make it less likely you will reach out to people who might be able to help you when you are overwhelmed and stressed.

Because of the multiple factors that can lead to psychological disorders, many mental health care practitioners take multiple approaches to treatment. While many practitioners claim a primary theoretical orientation (Figure 2.14), 22 percent of clinical psychologists, 34 percent of counseling psychologists, and 26 percent of social workers describe themselves as *eclectic*, meaning they take their treatments from a diverse range of therapies.

Multiperspective approach: a perspective that assumes the psychological symptoms we develop (or fail to develop) are likely the result of multiple factors.

Diathesis-stress model: a multiperspective approach that implicates stressors are involved in the development of psychological symptoms.

Reciprocal-gene environment model: a multiperspective approach that suggests that with biological predispositions for certain conditions, patients themselves can increase the stress that makes symptoms worse.

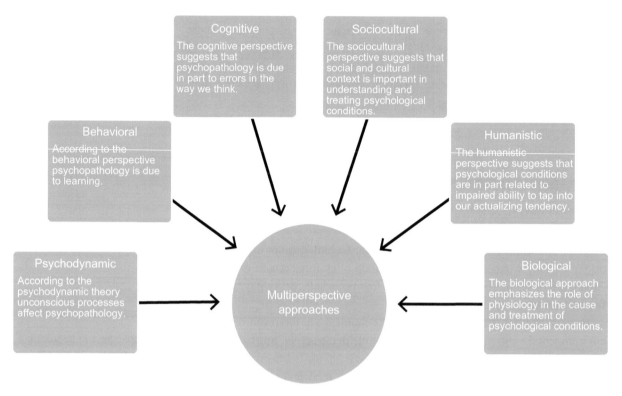

Figure 2.13 The multiperspective approach.

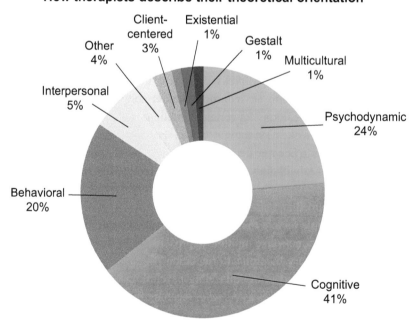

Figure 2.14 How therapists describe their theoretical orientation (numbers do not add to 100 due to rounding).
Source: Data from Prochaska & Norcross (2018).

CONCEPT CHECK 2.7

Choose the response that best explains the case.

1. Whenever he looks toward the sun, Bryson must sneeze. It turns out he inherited this response from his parents. This response is an example of the
   A. Reciprocal-gene environment model
   B. Diathesis-stress model
   C. Eclectic approach

2. Camille has a biological predisposition to become messy whenever she is stressed. But as the semester draws to an end and her room becomes more cluttered, she gets even more stressed because now she has difficulty finding the things she needs. This situation is an example of the:
   A. Reciprocal-gene environment model
   B. Diathesis-stress model
   C. Eclectic approach

3. Sophie's therapist wants to treat her psychological disorder with a mix of CBT and techniques of psychodynamic psychotherapy. This therapist's approach can be described as
   A. Humanistic
   B. Diathesis
   C. Sociocultural
   D. Eclectic

SUMMARY

The Biological Perspective

- The biological perspective suggests that our body and our physiology are the essential components of both our personality and our psychopathology.
- The nervous system is a network of organs and supportive systems that send and receive signals to and from various part of the body.
- The central nervous system integrates and controls the body, and the peripheral nervous system connects the rest of the body to the central nervous system.
- The forebrain is the largest part of the brain and includes the thalamus, hypothalamus, limbic system, and the cerebrum.
- The cerebrum contains about 90 percent of the brain's volume and consists of four lobes: occipital, temporal, frontal, and parietal.
- The neuron is the basic cell of the nervous system; neurons communicate via synaptic transmission.
- The nervous system uses the endocrine system to communicate over larger distances and time.
- Research methods for examining heritability include twin studies.
- Biomedical therapies are a family of therapies that use physiological interventions for the treatment of psychological conditions.

The Psychodynamic Perspective

- The psychodynamic approach suggests that unconscious processes are important for the etiology and treatment of psychological disorders.
- According to Freud, our personality is divided into three structures: an id, ego, and superego.
- The id operates from the pleasure principle, a drive to reduce tension; the ego from the reality principle, deferring pleasure until a reasonable way to obtain it is found; and the superego from the perfection principle, the drive to be the best possible.
- Defense mechanisms are ways a person will attempt to satisfy id instincts indirectly.
- Psychodynamic therapies are a family of treatments that explore unconscious processes and attempt to change them.

The Humanistic Perspective

- The humanistic perspective suggests that psychological conditions are in part related to the disruption of our ability to tap into our actualizing tendency.
- Client-centered approaches utilize the humanistic approach.
- Humanistic therapy relies on genuineness, acceptance, and empathy.

The Behavioral Perspective

- According to the behavioral perspective, psychopathology is due to learning.
- The behavioral perspective includes classical, operant, and observational learning.
- Treatments using the behavioral perspective include systematic desensitization, exposure therapy, and virtual reality therapy.

The Cognitive Perspective

- The cognitive perspective suggests that psychopathology is due in part to errors in the way we think.
- Cognitive therapy is designed to identify and challenge thoughts that might be related to psychological conditions, while third wave cognitive approaches such as acceptance and commitment therapy and dialectical behavioral therapy utilize mindfulness approaches to manage and often integrate thoughts.

The Sociocultural Perspective

- The sociocultural perspective suggests that social and cultural context is important in understanding and treating psychological conditions.
- Systems approaches emphasize the importance of relationships such as family, couples, and friends in the development and treatment of psychological conditions.
- Group therapy uses the power of social situations as a therapeutic tool.

Pulling It Together: A Multiperspective Approach

- Multiperspective approaches to psychopathology recognize the value of each individual theory but also take account of the complexity of psychopathology.
- The diathesis-stress model suggests that biological predispositions may be triggered by environmental events.
- The reciprocal-gene environment model suggests that a feedback loop between stressors and predispositions leads to psychopathology.

DISCUSSION QUESTIONS

1. The biological perspective suggests that psychopathology is due at least in part to our biology. Considering how often people get physical illnesses, why isn't the incidence of psychological conditions *higher* than reported?
2. Psychodynamic therapy is often considered an insight-oriented therapy. What kind of insight does this therapy provide?
3. Compare and contrast traditional psychoanalytic therapy and short-term dynamic therapy.
4. The humanistic approach assumes that people are trying to be the best possible version of themselves. How does this explain why people might want to steal food when they already have it, or why you are accidentally mean to someone but not accidentally nice. Do you think people are inherently good (as the humanists suggest) or inherently bad (as in the psychodynamic approach)?
5. Culture and social factors may influence psychopathology. Consider two or three of these factors and discuss how they can influence a person's behavior.

ANSWERS TO CONCEPT CHECKS

Concept Check 2.1

1. C
2. A
3. B
4. D
5. A
6. E

Concept Check 2.2

1. Repression
2. Superego
3. Sublimation

Concept Check 2.3

1. C
2. A
3. B

Concept Check 2.4

1. Operant conditioning
2. Classical conditioning
3. Observational learning

Concept Check 2.5

1. ACT
2. DBT
3. CBT

Concept Check 2.6

1. F
2. F
3. T
4. T

Concept Check 2.7

1. B
2. A
3. D

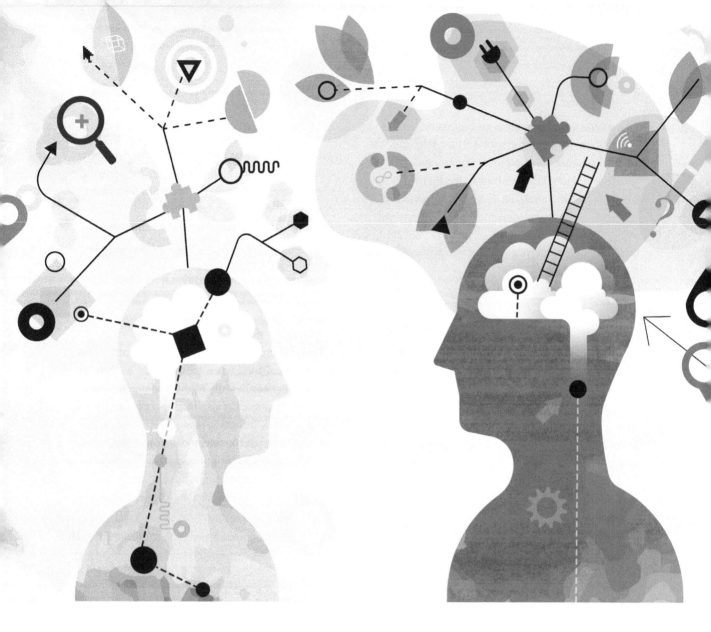

CHAPTER CONTENTS

3

Research, Assessment, Diagnosis, and Treatment

CASE STUDY: Revisiting King George

Let's think back to the case of King George from Chapter 1 and consider what additional information we might need to understand the changes in mood and behavior he was experiencing (Figure 3.1).

To understand their clients, clinicians need to assess symptoms and then come to a conclusion in order to provide the best course of treatment. The first step is an assessment. But what are the components of an assessment, and how are a diagnosis and treatment plan conducted?

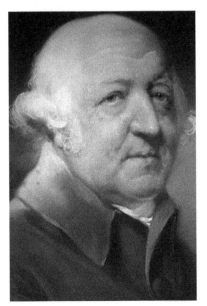

Figure 3.1 Francis Willis was a physician and clergyman who was in charge of the treatment of King George III.

Source: Dr Francis Willis (detail) by John Russell, 1789, National Gallery, London. Licensed under the Creative Commons Attribution-Share Alike 4.0 International license.

Learning Objectives

- Identify the important characteristics of clinical assessment.
- Describe the various tests psychologists use.
- Explain the way psychologists organize information in an intake report.
- Explain the purpose and limitations of diagnosis.
- Summarize the way diagnostic manuals have changed over time.
- Describe the research evaluating the effectiveness of psychotherapy.

3.1 CLINICAL ASSESSMENT

An assessment is an appraisal or evaluation. It requires gathering important data needed to choose the best conclusion and course of action to take. We make assessments all the time when we're solving problems. Let's say your phone is losing power early in the day and you see the dreaded red battery icon. What's the first thing you do? You probably think about the possible reasons why power is low. Maybe you forgot to charge the phone last night. Maybe the screen is too bright. Maybe one of the apps is using up too much energy. When we make an assessment, we are evaluating and making a judgment about what might be happening, and then we take a specific course of action based upon the data.

> **Clinical assessment**: the process of systematically gathering information for diagnosis and treatment planning.

In **clinical assessment**, the process includes systematically gathering information to make a diagnosis and then choosing the best course of treatment. The assessment can also serve as a baseline. Evaluations can be helpful to look for improvements in the symptoms. Making a clinical assessment is a little like solving a mystery or putting together the pieces of a puzzle. Why might the person feel the way they feel or behave the way they do? How might these feelings and actions explain or contribute to the person's symptoms and problems?

The first step is to gather information from as many sources as possible to try to identify what the symptoms are. From there the clinician might rule out some possible diagnoses and start to focus on others that seem more likely. The choice of tools for a clinical assessment depends on the clinician's theoretical orientation. You'll remember that the etiology of a disorder directs the treatment. It also guides our selection of the kinds of assessment tools as well. For example, if you believe the etiology is biological, you're going to need a biological assessment tool; psychodynamic theorists will delve into intrapsychic conflicts; behaviorists will measure and track behaviors.

Characteristics of Accurate Assessments

Regardless of the type of tool, all accurate assessments have a few things in common. These are reliability, validity, and standardization (Ayearst & Bagby 2010).

> **Reliability**: the consistency of a measurement.

Reliability. **Reliability** tells us how consistent our measure is. Does the test obtain the same results over and over again, exhibiting what's called *test-retest reliability*? Another gauge of reliability is that if, for example, five people (raters) administer the same assessment to the same person, they should all get the same result, a quality called *interrater reliability*.

> **Validity**: the degree to which an assessment measures what it claims to measure.

Validity. An assessment has **validity** if it measures what it was designed to measure. A test is said to have high *face validity* if the questions appear to ask about the topic on the surface. *Predictive validity* is an assessment's ability to predict a certain behavior in advance. *Descriptive validity* captures the same results as another established tool.

Standardization. A test is **standardized** if a common set of steps is used to administer and score it. This means that everyone who conducts the test will follow the same instructions. Having a standard protocol reduces the possibility of outside factors influencing the results.

Now let's look at some common forms of assessment, in the form of various psychological tests and inventories.

Standardized: a common set of steps is used to administer and score a measurement.

Psychological Test and Inventories

Psychological tests and inventories are clinical tests intended to collect data on specific aspects of functioning. These are different from the fun personality tests you might see online that will tell you what Harry Potter house you should be sorted into. Some psychological tests focus on a single condition or group of symptoms, such as the Beck Depression Inventory (Beck et al. 1996), while others look at general dysfunction such as the Symptom Check List 90 (SCL90).

THE CLINICAL INTERVIEW

What's the best way to get better acquainted with someone you don't know very well? Sitting down to talk is a pretty straightforward way to gather a lot of useful information. You can even notice nonverbal communication, such as the way the person wrinkles an eyebrow when you ask about their relationship with a sibling. Clinical interviews are often the first contact between patient and therapist, and collecting both verbal and nonverbal information about a client is exactly what they do.

Clinicians use **clinical interviews** to collect a detailed history of a person's life, current and past symptoms, and the **presenting problem**, meaning the reason the person has come in for help. They also gather information about the person's biological, psychological, and social history. Often they assemble this evidence through direct questions and behavioral observations, such as the way the person answers questions. A great many behaviors, symptoms, expectations about treatment, motivations for getting better, and even motivations for maintaining symptoms can be gathered through a clinical interview. Finally, the clinician will also focus on topics and information the client feels are important and wants to make sure the therapist knows about.

Clinical interviews: a procedure used to collect a detailed history of a person's life, including current and past symptoms.

Presenting problem: the reason a person has come in for treatment.

The clinical interview can be quite different depending upon the theoretical orientation of the therapist. Behavioral therapists, for example, will ask questions about triggers to certain actions, cognitive therapists will ask about thoughts, sociocultural therapists will inquire about cultural environments, and family therapists may ask about relationship patterns or create a genogram or family tree (Figure 3.2). Psychopharmacologists will often inquire about medication history and tolerance and preferences for various medications. They may also ask about family history of success or challenges with particular medications.

Structured interviews ask the same specific standardized questions of everyone (like a flow chart or the script of a play). Having the questions laid out can be helpful to ensure all the information is gathered. Structured interviews may ask the client to note how many of a certain list of symptoms they have experienced over

Figure 3.2 Some psychologists use genograms (family trees) to look for patterns in family relationships.
Source: Uwe Krejci/Digital Vision/Getty Images.

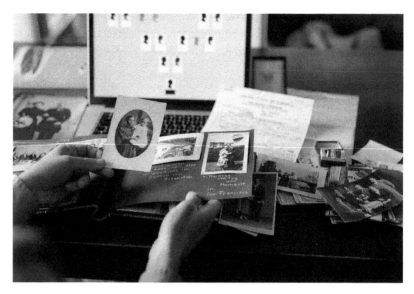

the last two weeks. The Structured Clinical Interview for the DSM-5 (SCID-5) is one of the most commonly used structured interviews in both clinical and research settings (First et al. 2016). However, structured interviews can sometimes seem stilted and too formal. *Unstructured interviews*, on the other hand, are more free-flowing and ask open-ended questions (such as "Please tell me how you've been feeling over the last two weeks"). The questions in an unstructured interview may be adapted or changed to accommodate the client. While this method allows clients to touch on topics that might not typically be asked about, the interviewer needs to be skilled to circle back to relevant topics and be sure to obtain an accurate diagnosis. Combining a bit of both techniques, *semistructured interviews* are much less formal than structured interviews and include a set of themes. The order of the themes is flexible and allows the clinician to establish rapport and let the discussion guide the way the clinical questions are presented.

While clinical interviews can gather a great deal of information, they do have their limits. Sometimes they can have challenges with accuracy (Sommers-Flanagan & Sommers-Flanagan 2013). Clients may misrepresent their symptoms or exaggerate them in order to draw attention to the ones they want the clinician to notice, or they may avoid discussing symptoms that are either embarrassing to them or present them negatively (Curtis et al. 2021). Clients might even overrepresent symptoms because they want the interviewer to understand how much pain they are experiencing, or because they want a particular treatment (like a medication). It's also possible for the experience of symptoms to influence the way the symptoms are expressed.

Clinicians' first impressions may influence the path of follow-up questions, and it is possible to pay too much attention to them. A clinician convinced that a client is depressed may ask a lot of questions about depression and neglect questions that could reveal signs of post-traumatic stress (Wu & Shi 2005). The interviewer's possible age, race, and gender bias may also influence the type and quality of the data collected (Unger et al. 2006). For example, an interviewer who assumes a child's actions in the classroom are due to misbehavior may overlook symptoms of attention deficit hyperactivity disorder or food insecurity, which may lead to behavior that resembles disruptive behavior.

THE MENTAL STATUS EXAMINATION

A **mental status examination (MSE)** is an assessment of cognitive functioning that looks for the presence and sometimes the absence of symptoms. It provides a snapshot of how the client is doing at the moment and includes both objective observations by the clinician and subjective descriptions given by the patient.

Mental status examination (MSE): an assessment of cognitive functioning that looks for the presence and sometimes the absence of symptoms.

Mental status examinations gather information about such patient aspects as appearance, thought processes, mood, intellectual functioning, and orientation (does the person know who and where they are in time and place?). Most of the time mental status exams are structured so clinicians can gather the information quickly and accurately. For example, a client who appears untidy and poorly groomed today but is typically well dressed suggests that something might have interfered with their ability to care for their appearance (Sommers-Flanagan & Sommers-Flanagan 2013). The examination of thought processes assesses whether a client's thoughts are clear, easy to follow, and logical or disorganized. The content of the thoughts also matters: are they delusional or obsessional, for example? Intellectual functioning is the ability to use higher functions such as thinking, logic, and reasoning. Here the clinician might assess consciousness (is the patient alert?), orientation (does the person know where they are?), concentration (can the person focus?), and memory (can the patient store and retrieve information?).

SYMPTOM QUESTIONNAIRES

Symptom questionnaires are tests that measure the presence or absence of certain symptoms. They are easy to administer and interpret, and they may do a good job of establishing a baseline or measuring progress in treatment, but they don't necessarily identify a diagnosis for a particular disorder (Kendall et al. 1987). What's more, because it's so easy to tell what the questions are trying to measure (face validity), a client who doesn't want the clinician to know they are experiencing a condition can readily lie or mask the symptoms. It's also simple to exaggerate or fake them if the client wants to be given a particular treatment or drug. Either way, the questionnaire will not be valid if the client is not honest. It's thus important to garner information from as many different sources as possible, such as different informants or clinical observation.

Symptom questionnaires: tests that measure the presence or absence of certain symptoms.

PROJECTIVE TESTS

As we learned in Chapter 2, psychoanalytic psychologists are interested in assessing intrapsychic conflicts, or the tensions between the desires of the id, the ego, and the superego. They do this by administering **projective tests**, a kind of personality test that uses the interpretation of ambiguous stimuli to uncover unconscious conflicts. These tests operate under the *projective hypothesis*, which suggests that when you

Projective tests: a kind of personality test that uses the interpretation of ambiguous stimuli to uncover unconscious conflicts.

Figure 3.3 Although
controversial, projective tests
are sometimes used by
psychodynamic therapists to
uncover unconscious
information.
*Source: Vitalii Nykolyshyn/
Alamy Stock Photo.*

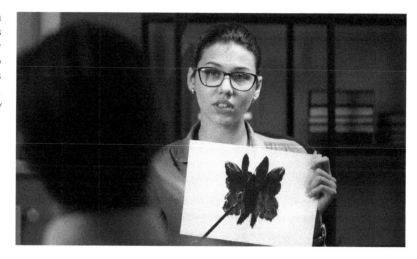

see cryptic material, you describe it in a way that reveals the interplay of your id, ego, and superego desires. "Projective" here refers to the defense mechanism of projection, in which we unconsciously attribute our own threatening impulses to another person or object. In projective tests, a person will unconsciously attribute their own intrapsychic conflicts onto the test material. Examples of projective tests include the Rorschach inkblot test and the thematic apperception test (TAT).

In the *Rorschach inkblot test*, unconscious conflicts are revealed by the client's interpretation of and reaction to ambiguous patterns of ink. The test, developed by Herman Rorschach in 1921, consists of 10 inkblots presented one at a time as the client reports what they see and where. Scoring is complex and uses various criteria, depending on the scoring method used.

The *thematic apperception test* is a projective personality test in which unconscious conflicts are exposed by the interpretation of stories the client tells in response to a series of ambiguous images. Most of the images in the TAT show people interacting with each other. As with other projective instruments, the kinds of stories told reveal intrapsychic and unconscious conflict.

All projective tests are subjectively scored by the examiner. Until the 1950s they were among the most frequently used methods, but more recently they are used more rarely and only to collect secondary information (McGrath & Carroll 2012). While they can reveal a great deal of complex information about a person and can be useful in a therapeutic setting, projective tests can be time-consuming to administer, and interpretation requires extensive training. Some scientists question the tests' validity and reliability as well (Lilienfeld et al. 2000), since the scoring is subjective and can differ depending on the interviewers, and the same test can produce inconsistent results even from the same person (Boinstein 2007). Cultural bias can also influence interpretation. People from some racial and ethnic groups aren't represented in the test, and critics question whether the images should be used at all (Lilienfeld et al. 2000). To improve the reliability and validity of the Rorschach test, John Exner developed a system to score and administer it (Exner

2003). Despite this addition, many clinicians consider the use of projective tests highly controversial because of the lack of empirical support for them.

PERSONALITY INVENTORIES

Personality inventories such as the *Minnesota Multiphasic Personality Inventory (MMPI)* will ask about several personality aspects in a single set of questions. The MMPI is a test that is derived based on research and assesses a range of characteristics. Unlike the results of a TAT or Rorschach test, the results of an MMPI are objective, meaning they are the same no matter who scores it. In fact, most MMPIs are now computer-administered and scored, which yields greater test-retest reliability (Graham 2014) and greater validity than projective tests (Cherry 2015). They are not perfect by any stretch of the imagination, however (Braxton et al. 2007). In fact, some suggest that since many personality inventories are normed on one cultural group, usually whites, they may not necessarily be valid for ethnic minority groups (Dana 2005). The newest iteration of the MMPI is the MMPI 3; it consists of 335 items and takes between 35 and 50 minutes to complete (Whitman et al. 2020).

Some practitioners prefer personality inventories because of their ease of administration, objective scoring system, increased test-retest reliability, and high validity. There are problems with the measures, however. Because they rely on self-reporting, we have to depend on people's own accounts of how they view themselves. Although tests like the MMPI have been translated into hundreds of languages, they can still have cultural limitations. For example, one study showed that the use of the Spanish-language version of the MMPI 2 RF was more likely to produce invalid results with people who spoke Spanish, compared to those who took the English-language version (Benuto et al. 2020).

Personality inventory: a test used to measure an individual's pattern of thinking, feeling, and behaving.

Neuropsychological and Neuroimaging Tests

Neuropsychological tests measure the physiological responses that might be indicators of psychological events (Daly et al. 2014). Measurements can be taken from the brain or from other parts of the body. Neuropsychological tests can confirm or rule out neurological impairment and are helpful in measuring or discovering perceptual, cognitive, or performance differences (Donders 2020; Golden & Freshwater 2001).

One example of a neuropsychological test is the polygraph (Figure 3.4). A *polygraph* is a machine that measures autonomic nervous system responses including blood pressure, pulse, breathing, fidgeting, and galvanic skin response (GSR), which is a measurement of the conductivity of your skin. Why skin conductivity? When you have a sympathetic nervous system spike, the tips of your fingers begin to release tiny beads of sweat. This sweat makes your skin more conductive, and electricity can pass along it more quickly. These sweat glands are deactivated by the parasympathetic nervous system. Because of this relationship, skin conductivity is a good measure of your stress response.

An **electroencephalogram (EEG)** is a device that uses electrodes on the scalp to record the electrical activity or brain waves produced by the neurons. These

Neuropsychological tests: an assessment that measures the physiological responses that might be indicators of psychological events.

Electroencephalogram (EEG): a device that uses electrodes on the scalp to record the electrical activity or brain waves produced by the neurons.

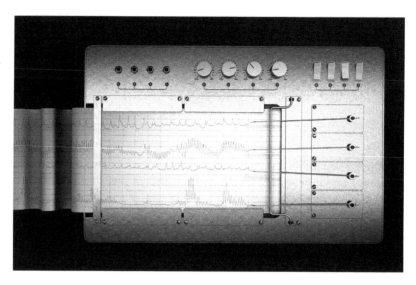

Computerized tomography scans (CT scans): a neuroimaging technique that uses computer-enhanced X-rays in order to examine structures.

Positron emission tomography (PET scan): a neuroscience imaging technique that uses radioactive glucose to indicate areas of activity.

Magnetic resonance imaging (MRI): a non-invasive imaging technique that uses magnets and radio equipment to produce detailed images, particularly of soft tissue.

Functional magnetic resonance imaging (fMRI): an assessment that examines brain activity over time by detecting the differences in blood oxygen between brain areas that are more and less active.

brain waves produce distinct images that can be analyzed. **Computerized tomography scans (CT scans)** are a neuroimaging technique. CT scans are computer-enhanced X-rays useful for examining structures. A computer reconstructs individual CT images into a three-dimensional image that can show brain injuries and tumors. The disadvantage is that CT scans can't show activity, and they expose patients to X-rays which can be harmful over time.

Positron emission tomography (PET scan) is a neuroscience imaging technique that uses radioactive glucose to indicate areas of activity. Patients are injected with glucose that is tagged with small amounts of radiation. The parts of the brain that are more active use more glucose, and the PET scanner can indicate those areas of higher energy with different colors. **Magnetic resonance imaging (MRI)** is a non-invasive imaging technique that uses magnets and radio equipment to produce detailed images, particularly of soft tissue. **Functional magnetic resonance imaging (fMRI)** is like MRI but can also examine brain activity over time by detecting the differences in blood oxygen between brain areas that are more and less active.

Clinical Observation of Behavior

It's common for people to observe the behavior of others. We all do this, and clinicians do too in order to collect information about clients. Sometimes clinicians do this in everyday settings, called *naturalistic observation*, or they may create artificial or *analog environments*, and sometimes they may ask clients to record their own behaviors using *self-monitoring* techniques.

CLINICIAN OBSERVATION

In making *naturalistic observations*, for example, they will examine the behavior of clients in everyday settings such as home or school. A clinician might watch a child in a classroom to see how the child behaves in the school, or at home to see how their behavior changes over time. Parents, teachers, or others could make and record these observations as well and report them to the clinician. This information can be used to help formulate a diagnosis, create a treatment plan, or understand how the person's behavior might be different in different situations. Observation can also show us what situations trigger certain behaviors, and how a behavior is improving (or not) over time in response to treatment.

While most observations focus on children's behavior and are made by people in the child's environment, such as teachers or parents, sometimes it's not practical to do so. In these cases, the observations can be made in an artificial setting such as a playroom, waiting room, or even the clinician's office and be filmed. Sometimes clinicians create *analog* or simulated situations to observe (Haynes et al. 2011). Couples, for example, could be asked to pick a topic that often causes a disagreement, in order to reveal interpersonal dynamics.

Even though it seems you could witness more real behavior by making observations, the method does have some disadvantages, including the fact that the mere presence of the observer can alter the behavior of the person being observed (Antal et al. 2015). Different clinicians may focus on different parts of the observations and draw different conclusions (Meersand 2011). And observing a behavior in one environment doesn't necessarily guarantee you'll see that behavior in other environments (Kagan 2007).

SELF-MONITORING

Clinicians may sometimes ask clients to observe their own behaviors (Figure 3.5). This can be helpful for counting behaviors that occur too infrequently for an observation session, behaviors that occur so frequently they could be difficult to count, and even behaviors that are hidden such as thoughts or impulses (Newcomb & Mustanski 2014). Self-monitoring clients may discover triggers for their own behavior, such as being bored or lonely (Haynes et al. 2011), and build a skill, such as learning ways to comfort themselves when they are feeling anxious, which they can use after therapy is complete. Self-monitoring does have drawbacks

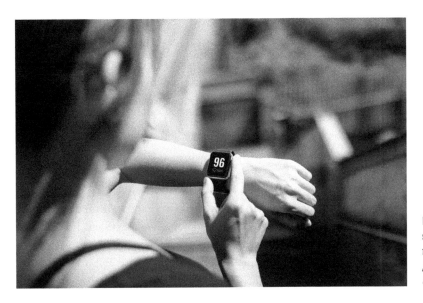

Figure 3.5 Smartphones and smartwatches make self-monitoring tasks much easier.
Source: Oscar Wong/Moment/ Getty Images.

(Huh et al. 2013). People can be inaccurate when they self-monitor and may even change their behaviors as they count them. Smartphone apps can help overcome these drawbacks because they are easily accessible and can generate reports that are simple to interpret or send to their therapist (Gillan & Rutledge 2021).

Physical Examination

Mental health practitioners who are not prescribers may recommend that their clients have a physical examination, to rule out any medical condition that could mimic or even mask a psychological one. For example, low vitamin D can produce symptoms that look a lot like depression. Low thyroid output (also known as hypothyroidism) also can mimic depression. It's sometimes necessary to rule out ingested substances that can mimic psychological conditions, such as excess caffeine from coffee or energy drinks that can look like anxiety, or cocaine, withdrawal from which can produce panic attacks.

Challenges and Limitations of Assessment

Despite their need for an accurate and complete assessment, clinicians sometimes face challenges in obtaining the required information. A person referred to a psychologist by the court system may not want assessment or treatment and may be reluctant to provide any information. Those who feel a negative stigma related to diagnosis may under-report or even fail to report their symptoms. On the other hand, sometimes clients distressed by their symptoms want to be heard and will over-report or exaggerate them.

Cultural differences can present challenges for assessment too, especially differences in language, use of idiom and metaphor, and even the names of symptoms. "I'd shoot myself if I felt that way" is a figure of speech for some people. But it might be interpreted differently by different clinicians based on their cultural background or that of their clients. Some cultures are in fact over-diagnosed because of cultural biases. Black Americans, for example, are often over-diagnosed with symptoms of schizophrenia (Maietta et al. 2020). Some researchers believe this is due, at least in part, to a misinterpretation of symptoms flowing from negative cultural bias or perhaps unconscious bias. For example, Black students are more likely to be perceived as being defiant when not engaged in schoolwork during the classroom day (Fadus et al. 2019). Recognizing and avoiding assessment problems like these requires training and sensitivity.

The Intake Report

Intake report: document that summarizes the patient's relevant history, symptoms, and next steps for the client such as diagnosis, goal setting, and a treatment plan.

Assessments are often summarized into a report called an **intake report**. This report gathers the patient's relevant history, symptoms, and next steps for the client such as diagnosis, goal setting, and a treatment plan. There are many formats for intake reports. Such as a simplified one with five sections (see Table 3.1).

Table 3.1 Elements of a simplified intake report

Section 1	Presenting problem	This outlines the reason the person has come in for treatment or assessment.
Section 2	Signs and symptoms	This summarizes the client's current symptoms.
Section 3	History of the present illness	This section is an account of the symptoms over time.
Section 4	Biopsychosocial assessment	This is typically the longest part of the intake report and outlines the client's biological, psychological, and social history.
Section 5	Diagnosis	This is a summary of the report and explanation of the diagnosis.

A well-written intake report requires that the clinician has identified and evaluated the client's chief complaints and goals, obtained the information that might be related to the client's psychological history, and evaluated the client's current situation and functioning. The clinician should understand when the symptoms first occurred and what antecedent or trigger may make things worse. Since symptoms don't occur out of context, it's important to describe the client's psychosocial history as well.

CONCEPT CHECK 3.1

Indicate the appropriate assessment tool for each of the cases below.
1. A psychoanalytic therapist is curious as to what intrapsychic conflicts might have interfered with Raul's relationships in the past. _____

2. Sam wants to find out how often he bites his nails and under what circumstances. _____
3. While doing a research study, Dr. Miller needs to create an image that indicates the level of active brain activity while his subjects play the piano.
_____
4. Dr. Ford wants to find out whether his 10-year-old client Danielle behaves differently with authority figures at school and at her soccer games. _____.

3.2 DIAGNOSING A PSYCHOLOGICAL DISORDER

Now that the clinician has gathered information from various sources such as interviews, tests, self- and other observations, they have an idea of what might contribute to the client's symptoms, why the client might have come in for help, and what could be contributing to the symptoms. Seen through the lens of the

Diagnosis: a label applied to a disorder whose symptoms tend to occur together.

clinician's particular orientation, this data can enable a **diagnosis**, or a label applied to a disorder whose symptoms tend to occur together.

Predicting from symptoms is complicated. Some people tend to snack a lot when stressed, for example, while others lose their appetite. So lists of symptoms or syndromes don't represent a complete list that everyone with a given diagnosis will have. Rather, they are symptoms that often occur together in people who have the diagnosis. Another challenge is that some symptoms can characterize a number of disorders. Difficulty sleeping, for example, can be a sign of depression, anxiety, or any number of different conditions. Also certain conditions are comorbid. When a condition is **comorbid** it means there is more than one diagnosis. Typically you would only diagnose a person with more than one disorder if they meet the criteria for each condition without double counting the symptoms.

Comorbid: the presence of more than one diagnosis.

Organizing psychological symptoms into a usable set of conditions is no easy task. Imagine you had snapshots of hundreds or even thousands of clients with similar symptoms, an idea of what was likely to happen with those symptoms over time, which ones tend to occur together, and how they might progress. While any person's behavior is an intersection of culture, personality, biology, and environment, you could derive rules from these cases that enabled you to classify the kinds of behaviors you might see in a given individual. This is the precise function of diagnostic manuals in psychology.

Diagnostic manuals help clinicians organize the chaos of the individual symptoms they might see in a client. If a client has symptoms of depression, they may have five or six different symptoms, but they don't have five or six different kinds of disorders.

Diagnostic manuals give us consistent names for and descriptions of disorders and can aid in communication to other professionals. If one therapist sends a report to another about a client with obsessive-compulsive disorder, the second therapist will immediately have an idea about what symptoms to expect, the length of time the client might have had those symptoms, and even which symptoms might be more likely to lead to thoughts of suicide. Diagnosis makes a convenient shorthand to communicate a great deal of information.

One of the reasons a diagnostic system can seem imperfect at times is that it serves many potential constituencies, each of which wants something different from it. For example, researchers use the diagnostic manuals as a tool for clinical investigation and to identify the course and measure the effectiveness of treatments. They want detailed, accurate diagnostic criteria for their research, and they often have the luxury of time. Thus, many researchers prefer a detailed diagnostic manual.

On the other hand, many mental health practitioners use the diagnostic manual to understand conditions, apply treatment plans, and request insurance reimbursement for their time. To reach these goals they want a diagnostic manual that is simple, uncomplicated, and user-friendly. Many mental health care practitioners in private practice don't have the same amount of time as clinical researchers do to make a diagnosis, and often medical professionals in primary care settings have even less. It's a challenge to create a diagnostic manual that's both detailed and user-friendly.

Classification Systems

Imagine for a moment what treatment for any health condition might be like without diagnosis. There would be no real way to feel certain that any one treatment approach might be better (or for that matter even worked at all). Clinicians might not know whether someone else had treated a similar case in another part of the country or the world. It would be difficult to communicate in scientific journals. For all these reasons, in order to make any significant advances in clinical treatment, diagnoses needed to be standardized.

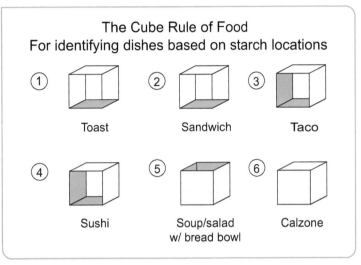

In the United States, diagnosis of psychological disorders was influenced by several independent diagnostic systems and a few outside forces. Understanding the history of these systems might shed some light onto why our current system is sometimes frustrating to the people who use it the most.

Everyone knows what a sandwich is. Something nourishing inside two slices of bread, right? But that's a traditional closed-faced sandwich. But what about burritos, wraps, and hot dogs? Is an ice cream sandwich a sandwich? For people who regulate and tax food purchases, these are important questions. For example, New York State has a special tax category for sandwiches, so it had to categorize what it means to be a sandwich. Some have even proposed the "Cube Rule" as a classification system for sandwiches (see Figure 3.6).

A **classification system** is an attempt to create a set of groups or categories and to sort or assign people or objects to those categories based on their attributes or relationships. There are several ways in which to organize a classification system. We can use a classical categorical, a dimensional, or a prototypical system approach, just to name a few.

CLASSICAL CATEGORICAL APPROACH

In a **classical categorical approach**, categories are distinct. This is the best type of approach when there is a known cause for the disorder and differences between disorders are clear-cut. For example, if your roommate doesn't feel well and thinks they have the flu, they might go to an urgent care center and take a rapid influenza test for the seasonal A and B influenza virus. In 15 minutes, this test will reveal whether your roommate has the flu or not. If they do, they might receive an antiviral treatment such as oseltamivir (also known as Tamiflu) or zanamivir (Relenza) to treat it. Here we see a clear-cut cause and a clear-cut treatment for a specific condition. On the other hand, cold symptoms may be more vague and there currently isn't a specific treatment for the cold.

Figure 3.6 The Cube Rule is a classification system for food. A single starch at the base is "toast," an additional starch on top makes something a "sandwich," and a base plus two parallel walls means it's "taco," for starches all around with two open ends it's "sushi," five sides of starch with an open top and you've got a "bread bowl," and when starches are all round something in the middle it's a "calzone."
Source: Adapted from https://cuberule.com/.

Classification system: an attempt to create a set of groups or categories and to sort or assign people or objects to those categories based on their attributes or relationships.

Classical categorical approach: a diagnostic system in which the categories are distinct.

Emil Kraepelin (1856–1926) employed a classical categorical approach to developing a mental health diagnostic system. The assumption of this approach is that there is an underlying biological etiology for psychopathology, and that every psychological condition is distinct. If this is true, different conditions won't overlap and there should be only one way to define each condition. Each person who sorts into that category will have that condition.

Classical categorical approaches are handy if you do happen to have a clear-cut cause and a clear-cut treatment. That tends to be the case for diagnostic and treatment decisions in most of medicine, like for a roommate with flu symptoms, but in the real world, it isn't as easy to apply a classical categorical approach. To return to our definition of a sandwich, for example, are three pieces of bread a sandwich?

We know that biological ideologies are possible in the study of mental health conditions, and so are psychological and social and cultural factors. Some psychologists employ psychodynamic and humanistic models, and many are eclectic. The classical categorical approaches don't necessarily hold together as nicely under the complexity of the etiology of psychological disorders.

DIMENSIONAL APPROACH

Dimensional approach: a diagnostic classification system which rates the degree to which certain characteristics are exhibited in an individual.

In a **dimensional approach** to classification, instead of looking for the presence or absence of symptoms, we rate the *degree* to which certain characteristics are exhibited in an individual. This approach sometimes sees psychopathology as an extreme version of everyday traits. The important questions for dimensional approaches are which traits to measure, and at what levels to consider them problematic. How much of a sandwich must be bread and how much of it can be non-bread ingredients before it's not a sandwich? In regard to health care, everyone feels sad from time to time and we can think of sadness as a spectrum. At what point on the spectrum does sadness become so severe that we start to consider it depression?

PROTOTYPICAL APPROACH

Prototypical approach: a diagnostic classification system in which the essential characteristics of disorders are identified, and which allows the identification of nonessential variations as well.

A third strategy for classifying and organizing psychological disorders is the **prototypical approach**. In this approach some of the essential characteristics of disorders are identified, and the system allows the identification of nonessential variations as well (sandwiches must have bread but may or may not have mayonnaise). In the prototypical approach, someone is judged to have a certain illness if they are similar enough to someone considered to be a representative example of that condition. Most people have a certain mental image of a sandwich (whether peanut butter and jelly or grilled cheese) in their head. Then they use that mental image to help them decide whether other things are sandwiches. One problem with the prototypical approach is that it suggests some symptoms are just as important as others, when that might be so diagnostically but not clinically. For example, suicidality is just as important as weight loss when diagnosing depression, but any mental health care practitioner will tell you that having a client with active suicidal thoughts is much more serious than having a client with weight loss. As we'll see below, the *DSM* is based on the prototypical approach. Figure 3.7 compares the classical categorical, dimensional, and prototypical approaches.

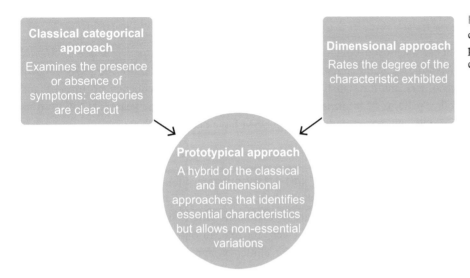

Figure 3.7 The classical categorical, dimensional, and prototypical approaches compared.

Early History of Diagnosis

Early attempts at categorizing psychological disorders would have made learning about diagnostic categories a snap. Fourth-century BCE physician Hippocrates, for example, divided psychological disorders into only a few categories: mania (over-excitement), melancholia (depression), paranoia, and epilepsy.

The 1840 United States Census was an early attempt by the government to classify mental disorders. There was a single category: idiocy/insanity. Forty years later this was expanded to seven categories: mania, melancholia, monomania (extreme preoccupation), paresis (muscle weakness), dementia, dipsomania (craving for alcohol), and epilepsy. In 1917, a committee that later became the American Psychiatric Association and the National Commission on Mental Hygiene created the *Statistical Manual for the Use of Institutes for the Insane*. It listed about 22 disorders.

International Classification of Diseases (ICD)

Meanwhile there was an ongoing effort to create a uniform classification of the causes of death (mortality) in Europe, called the International Classification of Diseases (ICD). The 6th edition of this effort was the first to include information not only about death (mortality) but also about disease (morbidity) (1949). For the first time this manual had a section on mental disorders.

In 1952 the American Psychiatric Association (APA) committee was charged with developing a version of the ICD for use in the United States and helping standardize usage for US psychiatrists. That book was the *Diagnostic and Statistical Manual of Mental Disorders* or the *DSM*. The intention was for it to essentially become a companion guide to the mental health section of the ICD.

Diagnostic and Statistical Manual of Mental Disorders (DSM)

In its diagnostic component, the *Diagnostic and Statistical Manual of Mental Disorders* (*DSM*) contains the information needed to classify the psychological disorders, and the statistical part of the manual lists the frequency, occurrence, and other patterns of information known about them. Over the years that followed its introduction, seven updates to the DSM have been published.

DSM-I

Published in 1952, *DSM-I* was a very different publication from what we have today. It took a very psychoanalytic approach, and most of the disorders were called "reactions." There were no diagnostic criteria in *DSM-I*, only brief descriptive paragraphs, and it wasn't very reliable. In one study of four clinicians who diagnosed 153 patients, different clinicians agreed on the same diagnosis only about half the time (Beck et al. 1962).

DSM-II

When *DSM-II* was published in 1968, the psychoanalytic influence remained in place but the manual was aligned a little more closely with ICD. Disorders were described in paragraphs that allowed for a good deal of interpretation by users, and the result wasn't very reliable. This drawback wasn't very serious for most clinicians, however, since the treatment options were so limited. Patients with psychosis received antipsychotics, those who were severely depressed were prescribed antidepressants, and everyone else got psychotherapy.

THE ROSENHAN STUDY AND THE DEATH OF *DSM-II*

Then something interesting happened. David Rosenhan was a psychologist interested in the medical profession's views of mental health and mental illness, and he oversaw a group of dedicated (perhaps too dedicated) graduate students working on a study of mental health and illness. In 1973 three of the women and five men (including Rosenhan himself) faked psychiatric illnesses at 12 mental hospitals across five states, making a single complaint: "I am hearing a voice that says 'thud.'" While they pretended to have auditory hallucinations in order to enter psychiatric hospitals, they acted normally afterwards and reported to the hospital staff that they felt fine once admitted (Figure 3.8).

Now, however, their everyday behavior was interpreted as abnormal. Though the real patients in each hospital could apparently tell that the pseudo-patients were not ill, the doctors could not. When the experiment was over and Rosenhan published his research, he said, "It is clear that we cannot distinguish the sane from the insane in psychiatric hospitals." The hospitals blamed the error on training, but the episode was very embarrassing for the entire mental health community.

In a follow-up to the study, one hospital challenged Rosenhan to send more pseudo-patients after it had improved the training of its staff. Of 250 new patients,

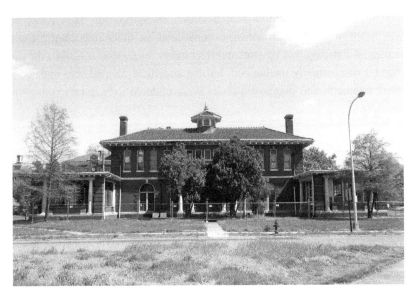

Figure 3.8 Saint Elizabeth's Hospital in Washington DC was one of the sites of the Rosenhan study.
Source: CPC Collection/ Alamy Stock Photo.

the hospital's staff identified 41 potential pseudo-patients whom they suspected Rosenhan had sent their way. Rosenhan had sent none.

Soon after, in 1980 *DSM-III* was released.

But there was much more to the Rosenhan pseudo-patient study. Susannah Cahalan (2019) found inconsistencies in the story and suggested that the conclusions Rosenhan reported may have been exaggerated based on the data he collected. But it was too late. Mental health practitioners' ability to diagnose had been tested and had failed. DSM needed to be revised.

DSM-III AND *DSM-IIIr*

DSM-III was a revolutionary change in psychiatric diagnosis, partly in response to the Rosenhan pseudo-patient study. The goals of *DSM-III* were to improve uniformity of psychiatric diagnosis and bring psychiatry closer to other fields of medicine. Many of the new *DSM-III* criteria were adapted from the Research Diagnostic Criteria or RDC and the Feightner Criteria, moving *DSM-III* to use precise clinical descriptions based on observable phenomena and to move away from the psychoanalytic approach. Over the next several years the *DSM* was refined in *DSM-IIIr* (1987) and categories were removed, added, reorganized, and renamed. For example, a number of controversial diagnoses, such as ego-dystonic homosexuality, were removed, while an effort was made to list more specific symptoms for conditions rather than paragraphs of descriptions of the conditions.

DSM-IV AND *DsM-IVtr*

In *DSM-IV* (1994) the manual was refined, more disorders were added, and diagnostic criteria were tweaked. An important update was the idea that for a condition to be a psychological disorder, its symptoms must cause clinically significant impairment in social, occupational, or other important areas of functioning, a criterion that remains in effect today. In *DsM-IVtr* (2000) the diagnostic manual was virtually unchanged, but the statistical manual was updated with the latest numbers, and diagnostic codes were updated to maintain consistency with the ICD.

DSM-5

While *DSM-III* was a revolutionary change, *DSM-5* (2013) was more of an evolution (Figure 3.9). It was created to correct some of the main problems with the *DSM*, mainly that diagnosis tells little about severity and disability, that the aging *DSM* was starting to hinder the research process, and that researchers wanted more refinement in the diagnoses (such as more biologically oriented descriptions). Those in charge of the *DSM* revision process had a few guiding principles, some of which seemed incompatible. They also wanted the *DSM* to be a "living" document and to be updated more frequently, so they abandoned the roman numbering system and adopted "software style" numbering, so a future update to the *DSM* would be called 5.1.

Similar to the recent edition of ICD, *DSM-5* is organized using a developmental approach. Conditions that have an onset early in life are listed early in DSM (such as neurodevelopment disorders), while conditions that typically have an onset later in life (such as neurocognitive disorders) are listed later.

DSM-5tr

Published in 2022, *DSM-5* text revision (*DSM-5tr*) is the latest version of the *DSM*. *DSM-5tr* includes revised diagnostic criteria and clarifications that were tweaked after the publication of *DSM-5*. *DSM-5tr* includes a new condition, Prolonged Grief Disorder, which we discuss in Chapter 6.

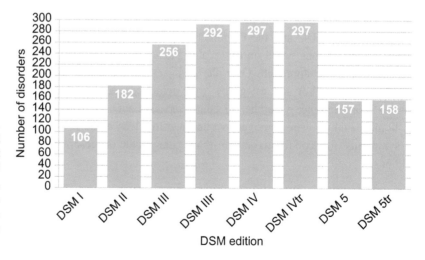

Figure 3.9 Evolution of *DSM*. The *DSM* has grown in size and in the number of disorders it describes. Although *DSM-5* appears to have fewer disorders, many have more specifiers, or types.

Source: Data from Paris (2013).

Although it appears that the number of conditions described in *DSM* has decreased since the publication of *DSM-5* (see Figure 3.9), *DSM-5* includes additional ways to describe features of certain disorders. **Specifiers** are used to further clarify a diagnosis and allow more precision and information about a certain condition. Many of these specifiers were listed as separate conditions in previous versions of the *DSM*. For example, in *DSM-IVtr*, autistic disorder (autism), Asperger's disorder, and childhood disintegrative disorder were listed as separate conditions, while *DSM-5tr* lists a single condition, autism spectrum disorder, and includes a specifier indicating levels of symptom severity (more on this in Chapter 14).

Specifiers: in the DSM an extension to the diagnosis that is used to further clarify a diagnosis and allow more precision and information about a certain condition.

The *DSM-5tr* (APA 2022) contains the following chapters:

- Neurodevelopmental Disorders.
- Schizophrenia Spectrum and Other Psychotic Disorders.
- Bipolar and Related Disorders.
- Depressive Disorders.
- Anxiety Disorders.
- Obsessive-Compulsive and Related Disorders.
- Trauma- and Stressor-Related Disorders.
- Dissociative Disorders.
- Somatic Symptom Disorders.
- Feeding and Eating Disorders.
- Elimination Disorders.
- Sleep-Wake Disorders.
- Sexual Dysfunctions.
- Gender Dysphoria.
- Disruptive, Impulse Control and Conduct Disorders.
- Substance Use and Addictive Disorders.
- Neurocognitive Disorders.
- Personality Disorders.
- Paraphilic Disorders.
- Other Disorders.

Limitations of and Debates about *DSM-5*

Despite the updates, *DSM-5tr* still has limitations. Rather than being guided only by the goal of creating diagnoses based on the best scientific evidence, *DSM-5tr* is a compromise. *DSM* criteria must balance science with ease of use while minimizing stigma, maximizing access to treatment, encouraging research, and maintaining continuity with previous editions of the *DSM* as well as with the ICD (Lilienfeld 2014). Also, some researchers are concerned that *DSM-5tr* may still reflect gender and racial bias; for example, there is a great deal of cross-cultural variability in the expression of anxiety disorders that is not reflected in the *DSM-5tr* diagnostic criteria, such as *ataque de nervios* (which we discuss in Chapter 4)

(Masuda et al. 2020). In the end, it is perhaps better than previous versions, though it is hoped that in each edition the manual will continue to get better over time.

Diagnosis and Labeling – Harmful or Helpful?

However precise, labels are rarely perfect. Anxiety can appear differently in different people. When mental health professionals label disorders – and the people who have them – they risk some consequences. For some clients, a diagnosis can lead to stigma (Parcesepe & Cabassa 2013), and some clients will even identify with that negative stigma (Hinshaw & Stier 2008). Another difficulty is that, often illegally, these diagnoses can influence eligibility for certain jobs, and some can affect a person's ability to get life insurance.

But as you've read throughout this chapter, diagnosis can be beneficial. An official diagnosis can help someone become eligible for accommodations to help them succeed in school and in the workplace. A solid diagnosis is the key to good treatment, it can help clients to understand themselves, and it can help form the foundation for the prognosis toward improvement (Craddock & Mynors-Wallis 2014).

THE POWER OF WORDS

MORE THAN A DIAGNOSIS

Despite the fact that there are many effective treatments for psychological disorders, many people don't seek therapy. One reason is the stigma that some people associate with psychological disorders, and many choose not to seek treatment for their symptoms because they don't want the label of the diagnosis. Regardless of the specific diagnosis or severity of their condition, there is more negative stigma about psychological diagnoses than for other health conditions (Corrigan 2004). Stigma can reduce the likelihood that those with symptoms will seek treatment and can even make the experience of having a psychological condition more severe by creating an artificial "out group" for people with these disorders.

Antistigma programs have been created to help reduce stigma. For example, the "I am more. Facing Stigma" project emphasizes that people are not defined by their diagnosis. This recent traveling exhibit is a collection of about two dozen portraits by photographer Lissy Thomas that explains the life story of people with psychological disorders. Showing a person's life story increases empathy and reduces stigma. Also effective are increasing interaction with people with psychological disorders, focusing on recovery, and finding ways to avoid encouraging and perpetuating stigma. It's important to remember that those who have psychological conditions are more than their diagnosis.

Sources: Campbell (2021); Corrigan (2004).

CONCEPT CHECK 3.2

Indicate the appropriate type of classification system in each case.
1. Best when etiology is clear-cut.
2. Indicates how much or how little a person has of an essential characteristic.
3. Identifies essential and nonessential components of a disorder.

3.3 TREATMENT

After assessment and diagnosis, the next step is choosing a treatment. Treatment decisions and methods are based on a number of factors, as we discuss in Chapter 2. It's the therapist's job to pick the best venue such as inpatient or outpatient therapy, as well as the specific approach that may work best for each client. Choosing a therapy approach isn't a one-size-fits-all approach.

Telehealth

Telemedicine or telehealth is remote clinical care and can be provided over secure phone or videoconferencing applications such as Zoom. Telehealth has some advantages over typical outpatient treatment, including improved access to care and reduction of travel time for clients. Despite these benefits, very few mental health practitioners have traditionally used telehealth, for a variety of reasons including difficulty in detecting nonverbal communication, technical hurdles, and concerns about privacy (secure and encrypted connections are necessary, and clients must be able to participate in their sessions from locations where other people cannot hear them). In 2014 only about 2 percent of mental health clinicians in the United States routinely used telehealth services. In psychiatry, 100 psychiatrists provided 50 percent of all telehealth visits for that entire year (DiCarlo et al. 2021), but trends are changing. The COVID-19 pandemic created shifts in health care delivery, due to the decline of in-person visits and changes in regulations that allowed for expanded insurance reimbursements for a wide range of telehealth visits, including those for mental health care (Patel et al. 2021).

Effectiveness of Treatments

Evidence-based therapies are those that help reduce symptoms of psychological disorders in controlled research studies. Psychotherapy efficacy studies are often conduced in research facilities or research hospitals and use random assignment to compare the effectiveness of the therapeutic intervention. Participants are randomly assigned to several groups that may provide various treatments or no treatment at all, and they and their therapists are unaware of the nature of each group. With these types of research studies, we have found out some general aspects about psychotherapy (see Figure 3.10 in the Pulling It Together feature).

Psychotherapy is an effective treatment for psychological conditions; in general, it is more effective than no treatment. A classic meta-analysis of 375 studies that surveyed more than 25,000 people found that the average person who received treatment was better off than 75 percent of those who didn't (Smith et al. 1980). And more recent meta-analyses of studies looking at depression show similar results (Cuijpers, Karyotaki, et al. 2020; Munder et al. 2019). Despite this, some clients don't improve, and a few (5–10 percent) get worse (Lambert 2010). Although some people prefer therapy over medication, since 1998 the number of people receiving only therapy has dropped by 24 percent, and the number who receive only medication has actually increased by 23 percent (Gaudiano 2013).

Despite the therapist's best efforts, some clients fail to act as advised and even respond negatively to treatment. Sometimes they are oppositional, noncompliant, unmotivated (Bhutta et al. 2015; Dowd 1989), or even resistant to treatment. Interpersonal problems such as lack of social support from family members can also be a source of poor response to therapy (Probst et al. 2020). From a psychoanalytic perspective, resistance is the client's attempt to repress anxiety-provoking memories and insights or block them from conscious awareness. Some therapists see resistance as a process to protect the self from difficult emotions. Confronting negative emotions head-on in therapy can be challenging for some people, and they may put up roadblocks to avoid discussing difficult matters. On the other hand, more contemporary perspectives such as biological and behavioral theories may see resistance simply as noncompliance. Perhaps the client doesn't have the skills necessary to follow the directions or tolerate the side effects of the intervention.

CONCEPT CHECK 3.3

1. Although Peter has been having panic attacks for the last three weeks, he doesn't seem to want to take his medicine for anxiety. His reaction to treatment is known as _____.
2. List one reason a psychotherapist might not be aware of the latest research about treatments for excoriation (skin-picking) disorder.
3. True or false: There are hundreds of known treatments based on sound psychological principles, and the research suggests that one group of treatments is clearly better than the rest.

PULLING IT TOGETHER

Many Effective Therapies Have a Few Factors in Common

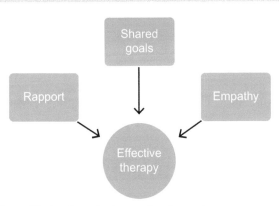

Figure 3.10 Many effective therapies have a few factors in common

By some counts there are as many as 500 known types of psychotherapy. Given that large number, do effective treatments have any elements in common? One study classic (Wampold & Imel 2015) examined more than 200 investigations that compared psychotherapy patients to a no-treatment group and discovered two things. First, most of the therapies provided by a trained therapist and based on psychological principles were better than no treatment. What's more, the 200 therapies had three features in common: The therapists provided empathy for the clients, rapport grew between the therapist and the client, and the therapist and client had shared goals related to the client's concern.

Pim Cuijpers, Mirjam Reijnders, and Marcus Huibers (2019) agree that psychotherapy can be an effective treatment for psychological disorders, but the way it works isn't very well understood. The researchers reviewed hundreds of randomized psychotherapy trials. Their conclusion? Therapy is effective, but the reason could be a technique that's unique to a specific type of therapy, a common factor in all therapies, or a combination of the two.

All other things equal, no one technique tended to be better than another. However, sometimes not all things are equal, and some treatments do tend to help certain disorders better than others, as we will discover in the chapters that follow.

3.4 CHAPTER REVIEW

SUMMARY

Clinical Assessment

- Clinical assessment gathers important data to determine the best diagnosis and identify the best treatment.
- The best assessment tools exhibit reliability, validity, and standardization.
- The variety of psychological assessment tests and inventories includes psychological tests and inventories, neurophysiological tests, clinical observations, and physical examination of behavior.

Diagnosing a Psychological Disorder

- Classification systems in psychology include the classical categorical approach, the dimensional approach, and the prototypical approach.
- Efforts to create a psychological diagnostic system have produced the International Classification of Diseases (ICD) and several editions of the *Diagnostic and Statistical Manual of Mental Disorders* (*DSM*), of which the most current is the *DSM-5*.
- Diagnosis and labeling have both advantages (such as providing a basis for treatment planning) and disadvantages (such as conferring a stigma).

Treatment

- Psychotherapy can be an effective treatment for psychological conditions.

- When considering the best course of treatment, therapists are often limited by their theoretical orientation.
- Patient resistance and noncompliance can hinder the treatment process.
- Rapport, shared goals, and empathy underlie all effective psychotherapies.

DISCUSSION QUESTIONS

1. What kind of assessments would you like to make of King George to identify the psychological disorder he might have, if any?
2. Discuss some of the advantages and disadvantages of the various psychological assessment tools.
3. The Rosenhan pseudo-patient study was a turning point in the history of the *DSM*. However, some wonder whether the study was flawed. What do you suppose the *DSM* would be like today if the Rosenhan study hadn't occurred?
4. Psychological diagnosis is very different from diagnosis of a physical condition. What are some of the challenges in creating a diagnostic system?
5. Discuss some of the reasons why a therapist might not utilize the most effective treatment for a certain psychological disorder.

ANSWERS TO CONCEPT CHECKS

Concept Check 3.1
1. Thematic apperception test
2. Self-observation
3. fMRI
4. Naturalistic observation

Concept Check 3.2
1. Categorical
2. Dimensional
3. Prototypical

Concept Check 3.3
1. Resistance
2. Time constraints
3. False

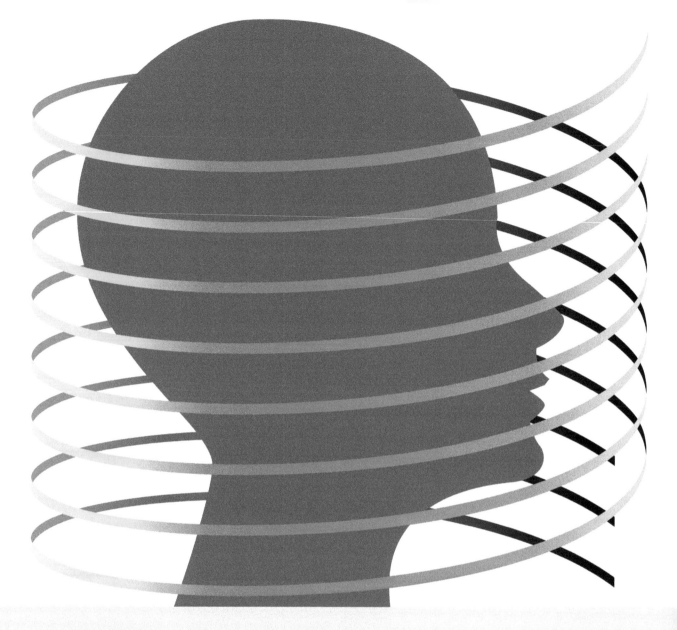

CHAPTER CONTENTS

4

Anxiety, Obsessive-Compulsive, and Related Disorders

CASE STUDY: Agoraphobia – Sara Benincasa

Everything suggested that Sara's life was going to be uneventful. She grew up in a middle-class family in suburban New Jersey (Figure 4.1). Her parents were happily married; she was a good student; she even took a class trip to Italy. But then she started to experience intense episodes of panic. Over time these episodes only got worse and started to increase in intensity and frequency. By the time Sara left for college, her anxiety had become overwhelming.

On the list of triggers that might cause panic: going out alone, driving, being a passenger in a car, flying, taking the bus, having sex, getting pregnant, and thinking about God. Sara didn't have just a passing fear of such things. She described a severe terror, such that she avoided them for fear of having a panic attack.

Too frightened to do anything, Sara retreated to her home and eventually to her bed. If you toured her home, you would have seen piles of garbage and a thin, very unhappy 20-year-old woman hiding cereal bowls filled with urine under her bed. She was too afraid to leave her room even to use the bathroom. We'll talk more about Sara later in this chapter.

Learning Objectives

- Distinguish between adaptive and maladaptive anxiety.
- Describe the essential features of and models and treatments for phobias.
- Describe the essential features of and models and treatments for panic attacks and panic disorder.
- Describe the essential features of and models and treatments for generalized anxiety disorder.
- Describe the essential features of and models and treatments for obsessive-compulsive and related disorders.

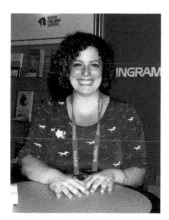

Figure 4.1 Sara Benincasa.
Source: Laura Cavanaugh/Getty Images.

Worry: uneasiness about the past or the future.

Fear: an emotion that is associated with a threat, danger, or pain.

Anxiety: a mood state characterized by concern over an uncertain outcome.

4.1   OVERVIEW OF ANXIETY DISORDERS

Whenever anything comes into the house – groceries, packages, mail, even the occasional jar of fig jam from a neighbor – it goes on the "dirty" table. That means it needs to be cleaned before it can be put away, either washed thoroughly in soapy water, sprayed with disinfectant, or swabbed with disposable wipes. The only other option is that it can sit on the "dirty" table for a few days before being handled.

In the face of the COVID-19 pandemic, television medical correspondents gave tips like these to protect the public from a contagious virus that had swept the globe. If you think back to that time you might recall being filled with a great deal of *stress*, a response to events we see as a challenge. Stress can consist of both worry and fear, and it can be both positive (eustress) and negative (distress). **Worry** is uneasiness about the past or even the future, while **fear** is focused squarely on the present. It's that sense that something is a threat, dangerous, likely to cause pain. Together, worry and fear form the basis of **anxiety**, which is a mood state characterized by concern over an uncertain outcome.

Everyone feels anxious every now and again, like the feeling you might have if you are running late for an appointment, meeting someone special for the very first time, or even doing your best to avoid catching an invisible virus during a pandemic. Most people are no stranger to anxiety. For many of us, anxiety can even be adaptive (Daker et al. 2019; Wu et al. 2019). A bit of anxiety can help motivate us to do our best and to be prepared.

Society and culture can also influence anxiety. We feel anxious when we think we are being left out of something exciting that's going on, often because social media (Elhai et al. 2020) reminds us of how much fun others want us to believe they are having. Anxiety can also be a component of discrimination. Members of racial, ethnic, or gender marginalized groups who face discrimination develop coping strategies such as detachment, because constant exposure to discrimination can increase the amount of anxiety they feel every day (Puckett et al. 2020).

Although anxiety is around us all the time, it can still cause a great deal of distress and impairment. Three chapters in the *DSM* list anxiety as a prominent feature: Anxiety Disorders, Obsessive-Compulsive and Related Disorders, and Trauma and Stressor-Related Disorders (we'll talk about the last category in Chapter 5). Anxiety plays a significant role in a group of conditions called obsessive-compulsive and related disorders, in which people feel overwhelmed by the urge to perform an action in order to reduce their anxiety.

Disorders that include the experience of anxiety are among the more common mental disorders in the United States. Around 19 percent of the US population has been diagnosed with an anxiety disorder, and up to a third will develop one at some point in their lives (NIMH 2019). More than 42 percent of people with anxiety disorders will seek treatment (Alonso et al. 2018) for their conditions.

One characteristic of every condition in which we see anxiety is the **fight, flee, or freeze response** (see Figure 4.2, and see also Figure 4.24 in this chapter's Pulling It Together feature). This is a typical reaction, shared by all animals, to danger or stressful situations. When your brain identifies stress, it prepares your body for vigorous activity and gets it ready to handle stress. Some people call this process the *fight or flight response* because two of the most obvious reactions to immediate dangers are to fight them or to run from them. When these responses are activated, your brain signals your body to release chemicals that help your body face the stress. But sometimes there's no one to fight and no place to run. In many cases people just freeze. So we now call it the fight, flee, or freeze response.

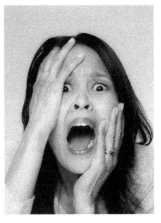

Figure 4.2 The fight, flee, or freeze response is a response to danger or stressful situations. *Source: Rob Lewine/Getty Images.*

Fight, flee, or freeze response: a reaction to danger or stressful situations that prepares your body for vigorous activity and to handle stress.

Let's walk through how it works (see Pulling It Together feature at the end of the chapter). Imagine you are in a scary place and you hear a noise. All of a sudden, your body fires up and your hands become cold and clammy. Your heart races, your blood pressure shoots up. You can thank your sympathetic nervous system for that (take a look at Chapter 2 if you need a review of the central nervous system). Here are just some of the physiological events going on. You breathe more quickly to get oxygen moving around your body. Your heartbeat increases to circulate the oxygen. And at the same time, blood is diverted away from your digestive organs and your bladder relaxes. (This might explain why we feel the need to go to the bathroom and our stomach feels queasy during stressful situations.) Blood is diverted to the major muscle groups so you can fight or flee more easily. In the process it is pulled away from our extremities, which is why our hands can feel cold and clammy. So you are ready to face the challenge, run away from it, or stay as still as possible.

Many of the symptoms of the fight, flee, or freeze response are also the symptoms you saw in Sara and will observe in many of the disorders you will read about in this chapter and the next. People with psychological conditions experience this response more severely, more often, and in response to stimuli that wouldn't typically elicit such a response.

CONCEPT CHECK 4.1

Identify the response in each description.
1. Mood state characterized by a concern of an uncertain outcome. _____
2. A reaction of the sympathetic nervous system activated by danger or stressful situations. _____
3. An unrealistic uneasiness about the past or the even the future. _____
4. Reaction to a threat or something that is dangerous or likely to cause pain. _____

4.2 PHOBIAS

Pretty much everyone is afraid of something. Maybe it is ants (I *hate* ants), or speaking in public, or even having a panic attack. For most people these fears are minor annoyances and don't get in the way of accomplishing the things we want to do. We go about our day as much as possible, and if we encounter the object of our fear, we take a deep breath and endure. A fear becomes a **phobia** only when it is unreasonably great or interferes with your life in some way (this relates to the idea of distress and impairment introduced in Chapter 1).

Phobia: a psychological symptom in which fear is unreasonably great or interferes with a person's life.

Psychologists distinguish three broad categories of phobias that we will discuss in this section: specific phobia, social anxiety disorder, and agoraphobia (fear of being in a situation where escape would be impossible or embarrassing).

Specific Phobias

Nearly everyone has an object that they fear, for me it's ants, Sara Paulson is frightened by closely packed holes (a condition called trypophobia), for Kristen Stewart it's horses, and for Liam Payne it's spoons. However, specific phobias are different than everyday fears because of the intensity and distress they cause.

SYMPTOMS AND DESCRIPTION

Specific phobias: an anxiety disorder characterized by fears of certain objects or certain situations.

Specific phobias are fears of certain objects or certain situations (Diagnostic Overview 4.1). Seeing or even anticipating the objects or situations almost always produces a phobic response. When confronted with the feared object, people will either avoid or endure being around it. For example, if you have a specific phobia of flying, you might avoid taking flights for work or to see distant family or friends and insist on driving or taking a bus or train. Even driving to the airport might create some of the common symptoms of a panic response in someone who fears flying. While many of the objects and events to which people have phobic reactions contain some elements of danger (you can fall from high places, planes can have accidents, and you can become trapped in elevators), the reaction to a specific phobia is out of proportion to the actual danger it poses (Figure 4.3).

Diagnostic Overview 4.1: Specific Phobia

Fear of certain objects or situations that leads to avoidance or endurance with fear or anxiety that is out of proportion to the actual danger.

Impact:	Symptoms must exceed cultural and contextual norms. Symptoms are related to clinically significant distress or create impairment in important areas of life such as with friends and family or at work or school.
Timeframe:	At least six months.

Source: Information from APA (2022).

It's common for specific phobias to affect people's lives so much that they change the way they live to avoid encountering the object of their fear. They may take the train instead of driving long distances, avoid parks because there may be a dog there, or refuse to ever eat food outdoors to avoid the possibility that it might attract flying insects.

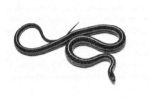

Specific phobias occur in different forms that are listed as specifiers, such as *situational* (fear of enclosed places, flying, driving); *natural environment* (fear of heights, storms, water); *animal* (fear of insects, dogs, birds, snakes); *blood-injec-tion-injury* (fear of blood, seeing injured tissue or wounds, receiving or watching someone have an injection).

Figure 4.3 Specific phobias of snakes are common, but many snakes, such as this common garter, can be quite harmless. *Source: Simon Murrell/Getty Images.*

Most people with a specific phobia actually have more than one (LeBeau et al. 2010), and some types of specific phobias have special qualities. People with blood-injection-injury phobias, for example, exhibit a certain physio-logical response to seeing blood or wounds. Rather than rising blood pressure (which would make it difficult to faint), blood-injection-injury phobias trigger *vasovagal syncope* (vay-zoh-VAY-gul SING-kuh-pee), which causes a drop in blood pressure and a stronger likelihood of fainting (LeBeau et al. 2010).

STATISTICS AND TRAJECTORY

Surveys suggest that as many as 13 percent of the United States population will have symptoms of specific phobias at some point in their lives (NIMH 2019). Rates vary for the subtypes of specific phobias (see Figure 4.4). According to the World Mental Health Surveys, rates are lower in many other countries (see Figure 4.5). Symptoms of specific phobia tend to emerge early, sometimes as young as 5 years of age (Solmi et al. 2021). Women are diagnosed with specific phobia more often than men at a rate of 2:1 (NIMH 2019). Around 32 percent of people with specific phobia will seek treatment for it (McCabe 2018).

Social Anxiety Disorder

It's not that unusual to feel uncomfortable with new people. It can be unset-tling to introduce yourself or make small talk. It can be even more unnerving if you have to perform, like giving a speech, playing the piano, or making a

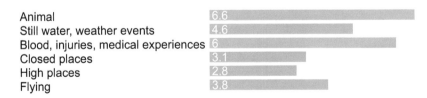

Animal	6.6
Still water, weather events	4.6
Blood, injuries, medical experiences	6
Closed places	3.1
High places	2.8
Flying	3.8

Figure 4.4 Prevalence of specific phobia subtypes in the United States (2017).
Source: Data from Wardenaar et al. (2017).

Social anxiety disorder: also known as *social phobia*, is an anxiety disorder characterized by performance anxiety in social situations.

perfect free-throw in front of people, especially those who might be critical of you. Messing up might be embarrassing or humiliating. People with **social anxiety disorder**, also known as *social phobia*, have an anxiety disorder characterized by performance anxiety in social situations (APA 2022). In contrast with specific phobia, where a particular object or situation is feared, the fear in social anxiety disorder is in essence a fear of embarrassment or humiliation (Figure 4.6). Remember, the anxiety that people experience in social anxiety disorder is more extreme and more distressing than the anxiety most people feel in similar situations.

For some people with social anxiety disorder, the things that make them embarrassed and anxious are fairly narrowly defined and discrete. They have a phobia of eating in public, for example, or of public speaking. For others, the social anxiety disorder is more generalized, meaning they have a fear of nearly any situation that could possibly cause them embarrassment. In every case, the phobia interferes with the person's life. Since more people fall in the generalized range, the disorder took on a new name in *DSM-5*, when it was changed from social phobia to social anxiety disorder to emphasize its general nature.

As for all disorders, it's appropriate to diagnose a person with a specific or social anxiety disorder only if it causes significant distress or impairment.

Figure 4.5 Lifetime prevalence of specific phobia in the World Mental Health Surveys (2002–2017).
Source: Data from Scott, de Jonge, et al. (2018).

SYMPTOMS AND DESCRIPTION

Almost everyone knows someone who might be described as shy and inhibited, who might not be the first person to speak in class or might choose to socialize on

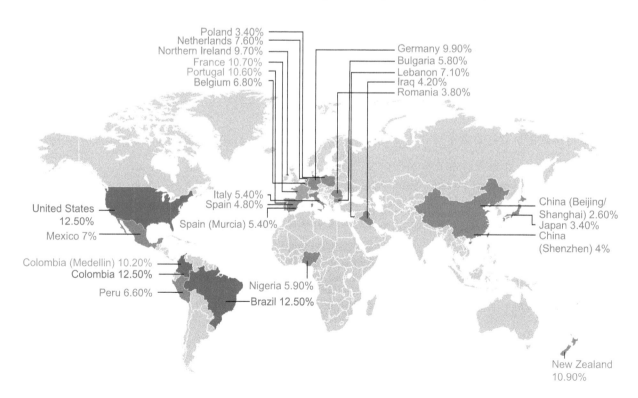

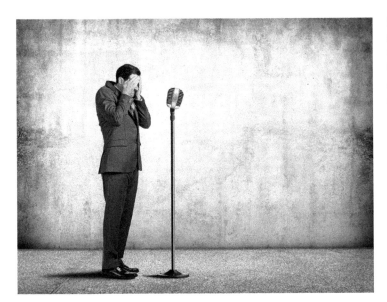

Figure 4.6 Some people with social anxiety disorders experience fairly specific fears, such as fear of public speaking. *Source: DNY59/iStock/Getty Images Plus.*

the side of a party rather than in the middle of the dance floor. In contrast, those with social anxiety disorder have symptoms that cause impairment and distress (Diagnostic Overview 4.2). They will exhibit classic signs of anxiety; they may tremble and perspire, feel confused and dizzy, or have heart palpitations; and some will even have panic attacks or panic-like symptoms. Because of these symptoms, they may avoid dining in public for fear they'll make noise while they eat, drop their food, or otherwise embarrass or humiliate themselves. It's common for people with social anxiety disorder to also feel unattractive, inadequate, or incompetent.

STATISTICS AND TRAJECTORY

Surveys suggest that as many as 12 percent of people in the United States will meet the criteria for social anxiety disorder at some time in their lives (APA 2022). Symptoms of this disorder typically start to emerge in late adolescence, and the age of onset peaks at around 14 years (Solmi et al. 2021). This is not too surprising, since it's the preteen years and adolescence when people start to become more concerned not only with their own appearance but with the way others view them. Most people with social anxiety disorder (nearly 90 percent) report something humiliating that served as a precipitating event to their condition, such as bullying or extreme teasing they experienced as a child (Mei et al. 2021). The humiliation doesn't have to happen in person and can even extend online to the social humiliation of online bullying (Figures 4.7 and 4.8) (Martínez-Monteagudo et al. 2020).

Diagnostic Overview 4.2: Social Anxiety Disorder

Persistent fear or anxiety about being in social situations involving scrutiny by others:

- Fear of acting in a way that will be negatively evaluated.
- Fear or anxiety resulting from being in a social situation.
- Avoidance or endurance of the triggering social situation.
- Reaction that is out of proportion to the context.

Impact: Symptoms must exceed cultural and contextual norms. Symptoms are related to clinically significant distress or create impairment in important areas of life such as with friends and family or at work or school.

Timeframe: At least six months.

Source: Information from APA (2022).

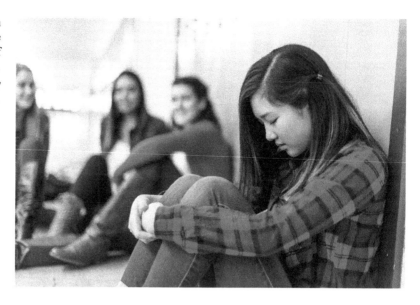

Figure 4.7 Many people with social anxiety disorder have reported earlier episodes of bullying as children.
Source: FatCamera/E+/Getty Images.

Agoraphobia

Figure 4.8 Lifetime prevalence of social anxiety disorder in the World Mental Health Surveys (2002–2017).
Source: Data from Scott, de Jonge, et al. (2018).

Imagine you encountered a terrible but powerful magical incantation. Once read, it guaranteed that you would experience a panic attack sometime in the next 24 hours and there was no way to reverse it. How would you spend the next 24 hours? What would you do? Some people might go about their day normally doing the things they typically do (with worry about having the panic attack). Others might decide to venture out, but

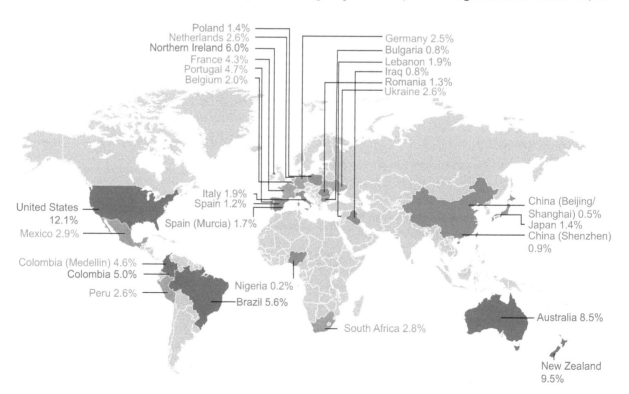

Poland 1.4%
Netherlands 2.6%
Northern Ireland 6.0%
France 4.3%
Portugal 4.7%
Belgium 2.0%
Germany 2.5%
Bulgaria 0.8%
Lebanon 1.9%
Iraq 0.8%
Romania 1.3%
Ukraine 2.6%
Italy 1.9%
Spain 1.2%
Spain (Murcia) 1.7%
United States 12.1%
Mexico 2.9%
China (Beijing/Shanghai) 0.5%
Japan 1.4%
China (Shenzhen) 0.9%
Colombia (Medellin) 4.6%
Colombia 5.0%
Peru 2.6%
Nigeria 0.2%
Brazil 5.6%
South Africa 2.8%
Australia 8.5%
New Zealand 9.5%

only with a safe person to take care of them in case they had the panic attack while out. Most would probably avoid public places where it might be dangerous to have a panic attack. Still others might stay at home, worried about how embarrassing it might be to have a panic attack in public. All these reactions are aspects of agoraphobia.

SYMPTOMS AND DESCRIPTION

While there is no magical incantation (thank goodness), those with **agoraphobia** fear having a panic attack, which causes them to avoid places and situations where having such an attack would be particularly embarrassing or dangerous (Diagnostic Overview 4.3). In a way, people with agoraphobia might live as if there were a magical incantation and there is an impending panic attack on the way that they are trying to avoid or to ease. You may have heard that agoraphobia means "fear of the marketplace" (an *agora* was an open public space in ancient Greece), but it's really more than that. Essentially agoraphobia is a fear of fear.

Because of their fear of experiencing a panic attack, people with symptoms of agoraphobia will avoid situations that might raise their anxiety. These include crowded places such as stores, places far from home, and tunnels. If they travel to these locations, they bring a trusted friend or relative to help keep them safe and calm, but they can often be extremely anxious even so.

It's not unusual for people with agoraphobia to stay in their homes, avoiding all social interaction. Recall Sara from the chapter-opening story, who stayed in her room and didn't leave even to use the bathroom. Fear of having a panic attack doesn't mean the person has actually ever had one. Some people with agoraphobia haven't. If they have, they receive two diagnoses: one for agoraphobia and one for panic disorder.

> **Agoraphobia:** an anxiety disorder characterized by fear of having a panic attack, which causes a person to avoid places and situations where having such an attack would be particularly embarrassing or dangerous.

STATISTICS AND TRAJECTORY

Symptoms of agoraphobia are more likely to be reported in women than in men, by a ratio of almost 2:1 (APA 2022; Bandelow & Michaelis 2015). About 1.3–2.4 percent of people in the United States will be diagnosed with agoraphobia at some point in their lives (NIMH 2019), and the peak age of onset is around 14 years (Solmi et al. 2021). Nearly half those who meet the criteria for agoraphobia (46 percent) will seek treatment (NIMH 2019), and about the same number will also have a history of panic attacks that led to their agoraphobia (Wittchen et al. 2010). Others might have other mental health conditions such as depression (Wittchen et al. 2010).

Models and Treatments of Phobias

Life is much better for Sara. After cognitive-behavioral therapy and trying a few medications things started to improve and she remembers the moment where things

Diagnostic Overview 4.3: Agoraphobia

Fear of being in at least two of the following situations, in which escape would be difficult or embarrassing if panic symptoms occurred:

- Public transportation.
- An open space.
- An enclosed place.
- A crowded place.
- A place way from home.

Impact: Symptoms must exceed cultural and contextual norms. Symptoms are related to clinically significant distress or create impairment in important areas of life such as with friends and family or at work or school.

Timeframe: At least six months.

Source: Information from APA (2022).

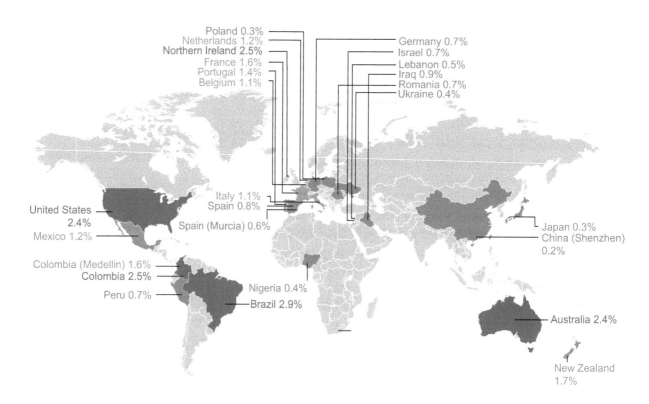

Figure 4.9 Lifetime prevalence of agoraphobia in the World Mental Health Surveys (2002–2017).

Source: Data from Scott, de Jonge, et al. (2018).

started to turn the corner. She returned to school and eventually finished a teaching degree at Columbia University. At 25 she started doing standup comedy, something she never thought she would do.

BIOLOGICAL MODELS AND TREATMENTS

Biological models of phobias are similar to the models suggested for other anxiety disorders, and they adopt similar treatments to relieve symptoms. Most medications for phobias are meant to reduce the fear or worry that clients experience. Prescribers will sometimes use benzodiazepines and medications such as selective serotonin reuptake inhibitors (SSRIs) like paroxetine (Paxil) to relieve persistent anxiety associated with the fear and worry phobias bring (Table 4.1). Benzodiazepines can help quell the fight, flee, or freeze response as it is happening. However, medication isn't helpful for all phobias. It can be modestly effective for

Table 4.1 Some FDA-approved medications for social anxiety disorder

Generic name	Brand name	Class of medication
fluvoxamine	Luvox	Selective serotonin reuptake inhibitor
paroxetine	Paxil	Selective serotonin reuptake inhibitor
sertraline	Zoloft	Selective serotonin reuptake inhibitor
venlafaxine	Effexor	Serotonin norepinephrine reuptake inhibitor

Source: Information from Stahl (2017).

social anxiety disorder, but other conditions such as specific phobias respond better to behavioral interventions (more on that in a bit).

THE POWER OF EVIDENCE

Lavender for anxiety

Lavender has a truly lovely smell. You can find it in detergent, room fresheners, and lotions and soaps. Dried lavender has been used for hundreds of years as a way to calm the nerves. Lately there has been increased interest in the use of essential oils such as lavender to help treat psychological disorders like anxiety (Figure 4.10), but does it work? Let's look at the evidence.

Two meta-analyses have examined the use of various forms of lavender to reduce anxiety (Donelli et al. 2019; Yap et al. 2019). One compared lavender to a placebo and the other to common FDA-approved antianxiety medications. When tested head-to-head against a placebo, lavender looked promising. Many studies in the first meta-analysis used an oral lavender pill called silexan. One group of researchers decided to give a placebo that didn't contain lavender but was coated with a synthetic lavender smell. This worked just as well as real lavender (Donelli et al. 2019).

Against prescription medications, however, lavender didn't do nearly so well. Although it helped reduce stress and allowed many clients to sleep a little better, the researchers didn't see any significant difference in anxiety in various patient samples. They suggested that there is insufficient evidence for the use of lavender as an antianxiety agent (Yap et al. 2019).

The biggest problem with the studies in the meta-analyses was their relative lack of quality. Because of lavender's unique scent, it's hard for people in studies not to know they are receiving it, which makes it difficult to conduct double-blind trials (in which neither the researchers nor the participants know who is in the

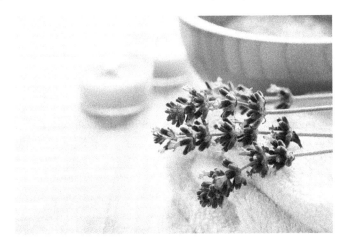

Figure 4.10 Lavender has been used for centuries to calm and relax, but is there evidence that this essential oil is powerful enough for anxiety disorders?
Source: the_burton/Moment/Getty Images.

control group). Double-blind trials are some of the highest-quality studies we have to determine the effectiveness of interventions. So the studies that used a lavender pill to eliminate the telltale scent received the highest quality ratings.

Many people use alternative medicines such as herbs because they are natural and lack side effects, but essential oils such as lavender do have side effects when ingested. The most common are nausea, bad breath, diarrhea, and headaches. And although lavender has a great smell and can be very relaxing, it might not be powerful enough to use against psychological disorders such as panic attacks or the other anxiety disorders in this chapter.

Sources: Donelli et al. (2019); Yap et al. (2019).

PSYCHODYNAMIC MODELS AND TREATMENT

According to insight-oriented approaches such as the psychodynamic and humanistic approaches, anxiety may be based on repressed reactions. That is, the phobia might be not of the ostensibly feared object but of something else, such as the fear of not being in control. Short-term psychodynamic psychotherapy (STPP) was found to be superior to relaxation for treating phobias in some early research (Alström et al. 1984). Some who practice STPP suggest that its advantage over other therapies is the use of more deep examination of a client's life, because unless the actual issue is resolved, it will come up again. A 2014 study followed clients up after two years and found that those who received cognitive-behavioral therapy (CBT) for social anxiety disorder and those given STPP had equal rates not only of reduction of symptoms but also of relapse as well (Leichsenring et al. 2014).

COGNITIVE-BEHAVIORAL MODELS AND TREATMENT

According to the behavioral approach, phobias are learned behaviors. Up to 40 percent of people with phobias can remember a particular event that led to their phobia (Mineka & Zinbarg 2006). Using what we know about classical conditioning, theories of the learning perspective suggest that events can become associated with what later turns into a phobia. The learning model suggests that someone may acquire a response to a previously neutral stimulus that then is paired with a frightening experience. This is known as *phobic acquisition*. The person then maintains the phobia by avoiding the newly acquired conditioned stimulus.

We can also develop anxiety from watching others. A father who has a phobia of storms and forces his children to turn out the lights in their home and unplug all the appliances probably sends the message that storms are dangerous and should be feared. When we react to something fearfully, we can effectively communicate its potential danger to others.

According to the cognitive model, people with social anxiety disorders are preoccupied with applying high standards to their own social behavior and are more likely to want other people to like them. What's more, they tend to focus on and remember the most negative parts of their own interactions with others and to grade those interactions harshly. When observing the reactions of others, they are more likely to notice social cues and interpret them as evidence of their own negative interactions.

To combat their anxiety, they rely on strategies such as avoiding eye contact, rehearsing exactly what they will say, holding back personal information, and even reducing or limiting their interactions with others. All these will absolutely reduce the likelihood of negative events, but they will reduce the quality of social interaction as well and leave an impression on others of aloofness and disinterest (Morrison & Heimberg 2013). After most interactions, people with social anxiety will replay the event in their heads, hunting for clues to everything they feel they did wrong.

Adults with social anxiety describe their parents as having been critical, negative, and controlling (Bogels et al. 2010). However, people with social anxiety disorder might describe everyone as being more critical and negative.

Behavioral therapy focuses on exposing clients to situations that might create anxiety (exposure and response-prevention techniques). Or the therapist will work on skill building, such as role-playing situations that might increase anxiety in order to build resilience, or teaching clients techniques to help calm themselves in social situations. Clients may need to reduce some of their "safety behaviors" such as avoiding eye contact and understand the impact this might have on their interactions with others.

Cognitive techniques focus on identifying the client's negative thoughts about social situations and helping them test out these cognitions, in order to replace them with healthier and more accurate thoughts. CBT is as effective as medications and has lower relapse rates than medications alone (Gregory & Peters 2017). In fact, the research suggests that CBT is perhaps the most helpful of any techniques for social anxiety disorder, while exposure therapies outperform all other treatments that don't include some type of exposure. There have been many attempts at creating virtual reality social anxiety therapy techniques; however, they don't seem to work as well as in-person exposure techniques for social anxiety disorder (Reddy et al. 2020).

SOCIOCULTURAL MODELS AND TREATMENT

Culture has a powerful impact on the things we learn to fear. Social anxiety may be more common in cultures, such as collectivist cultures, in which individual behavior is held to reflect well or poorly on the group (Krieg & Xu 2018). For example, in Japan, *Taijinkyofu sho* or TKS is an intense fear of social situations and is characterized by shame and fear of offending others. It's found more often in young men than in women by a ratio of 3:2 (Ferrão 2019). People with TKS fear blushing, emitting body odors, or irritating other people (Lewis-Fernández et al. 2010). It turns out that symptoms of TKS can be found all over the world.

Negative environmental factors such as poverty and hostile workplaces can increase anxiety as well (Yatham et al. 2018). Children who are already prone to anxiety may be at increased risk of developing social anxiety if they experience constant negative evaluation from, say, caretakers who use shame to shape behavior, or bullying, harassment, or discrimination from others (Zvolensky et al. 2019).

The interpersonal environment of groups may be beneficial to those who have social anxiety disorder. While they may not provide treatment outcomes superior to those of individual therapy, groups can be an effective treatment for phobias including social anxiety disorder (Barkowski et al. 2020).

MULTIPERSPECTIVE MODELS AND TREATMENT

Many therapists don't use a single technique but often combine techniques together. A powerful strategy is to employ CBT in a group setting so group members can help each other, and to provide exposure to the situation that a person might fear but also interpersonal assistance as well. Groups can also be helpful in getting people to change their thoughts.

CONCEPT CHECK 4.2

Match the situation with the correct disorder
A. Specific phobia
B. Social anxiety disorder
C. Agoraphobia
1. Dena has never experienced a panic attack and doesn't plan on having one. She's afraid, however, that if she drives over a bridge, her anxiety will become so high that she'll have a panic attack and will need to stop in the middle of the road to get help. This would be humiliating. So she decides never to drive on bridges and also avoids tunnels and subways for the same reason. She's fine leaving her house as long as she can avoid those things.
2. Rita really loves going outside. However, she is terrified of scorpions, so much so that she won't go camping with her family and friends. Even photographs of scorpions cause her a great deal of anxiety.
3. Tina has a fear of pretty much any social situation. Speaking in public, eating, writing, and performing in front of others all cause her fear. She likes people, but she's afraid of being embarrassed or humiliated and of messing up in public.
4. Alvin tends to freeze up whenever he speaks in public and as a result has been passed over for promotions at work. His reaction has become so much of a problem for him that he has decided to talk to a counselor in order to reduce his fear.

4.3   PANIC ATTACKS AND PANIC DISORDER

Panic Attacks Symptoms and Description

Panic attack: a period of intense fear or discomfort that is linked with specific physical and psychological symptoms.

There are times when anxiety becomes so overwhelming that it boils over. It's what psychologists call a panic attack. A **panic attack** is a period of intense fear or discomfort that is linked with specific physical and psychological symptoms.

Diagnostic Overview 4.4: Panic Attack

A surge of fear with at least four of the following symptoms:

- Heart palpitations or accelerated heart rate.
- Sweating.
- Shaking.
- Shortness of breath.
- Feeling as if you are choking.
- Chest pain.
- Nausea.
- Dizziness or faintness.
- Chills or heat sensations.
- A feeling of pins and needles on the skin.
- A feeling that things are unreal or that you are detached from yourself.
- Fear of losing control.
- Fear of dying.

Impact: Symptoms are related to clinically significant distress or create impairment in important areas of life such as with friends and family or at work or school.

Source: Information from APA (2022).

Remember Sara from the beginning of the chapter? She's had well over 100 panic attacks in her life. She reports that although they don't actually last very long, they're so unpleasant and so intense that she had lost her capacity to realize they won't last forever.

Identifying Panic Attacks

A panic attack is a period of intense fear or discomfort in which four or more of a variety of symptoms are present (Diagnostic Overview 4.4). People with panic attacks often feel a pounding heart, sweating, shaking, feelings of choking, fear of losing control, fear of dying, numbness, and chills or hot flashes. A panic attack can happen quickly, often out of nowhere, and it peaks in intensity within 10 minutes. Panic symptoms can be frightening in themselves, and some people respond to them with intense fear (Figure 4.11). One in three people will experience at least one panic attack at least once in their lives (Olaya et al. 2018), and others (3.1 percent) will experience them over and over to the point where they will change their lives in some dysfunctional way to cope (Bandelow & Michaelis 2015).

Panic attacks are intense bursts of anxiety that often come out of nowhere, though sometimes they can be triggered by the environment, such as the events Sara mentioned. Someone confronted with a panic attack experiences a constellation of anxiety symptoms that are

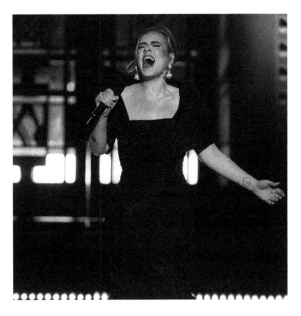

Figure 4.11 Despite performing on stage in front of thousands of people, singer Adele has reported anxiety and described herself as a "walking panic attack."
Source: Cliff Lipson/CBS via Getty Images.

both physiological and psychological. The first time it occurs, the person may have no idea what is happening, and some people feel they are having a heart attack. It's that intense.

Symptoms and Description: Panic Disorder

Panic disorder: an anxiety disorder characterized by the presence of frequent, recurrent panic attacks, along with the fear of panic attacks.

About 28 percent of people who experience panic attacks have them only occasionally (Kessler et al. 2006). Others have them so regularly that they end up changing their lives to try to prevent the attacks. That's the nature of a **panic disorder**. A panic attack itself is not a disorder, but if it happens frequently and the person is in constant fear of having more, a diagnosis of disorder can be made. Panic attacks can be added as a specifier for a number of disorders in the DSM, including depression or generalized anxiety disorder (Diagnostic Overview 4.5).

Statistics and Trajectory: Panic Disorder

Surveys suggest that as many as 7 percent of people in the United States will meet criteria for panic disorder at some point in their lives (NIMH 2019). Rates for panic disorder are lower in many other countries (see Figure 4.12). Like many disorders, panic disorder tends to develop in late adolescence, often around age 15 (Solmi et al. 2021). It is more common in women, as well as in racially marginalized groups (Patel & Hinton 2020), although the symptoms may vary among different groups, as we will discuss later. Panic disorder is not as common as some of the other anxiety disorders. About 59 percent of those with panic disorder will seek treatment for it (NIMH 2019).

Models and Treatments of Panic Disorder

Practitioners use a variety of biological and psychological models to explain and to treat symptoms of panic disorder.

BIOLOGICAL MODELS AND TREATMENT

The biological model suggests that poor regulation of the fight, flee, or freeze response occurs in people with panic disorder. This means that panic attacks are more easily triggered in people with panic disorder (Wittchen et al. 2010). Neuroimaging studies show distinct differences in people with panic disorder, especially in the areas of the limbic system involved in the stress response including the amygdala, hypothalamus, and hippocampus (Lai 2019).

Another part of the central nervous system that might be important for panic attacks is the *locus coeruleus*, located in the brainstem (Figure 4.13). Poor regulation of the locus coeruleus may cause panic attacks, which in turn stimulate the limbic

Diagnostic Overview 4.5: Panic Disorder

At least one panic attack, followed by concern about having additional panic attacks or dysfunctional changes in behavior related to panic attacks.

Impact:	Symptoms are related to clinically significant distress or create impairment in important areas of life such as with friends and family or at work or school.
Timeframe:	At least one month.

Source: Information from APA (2022).

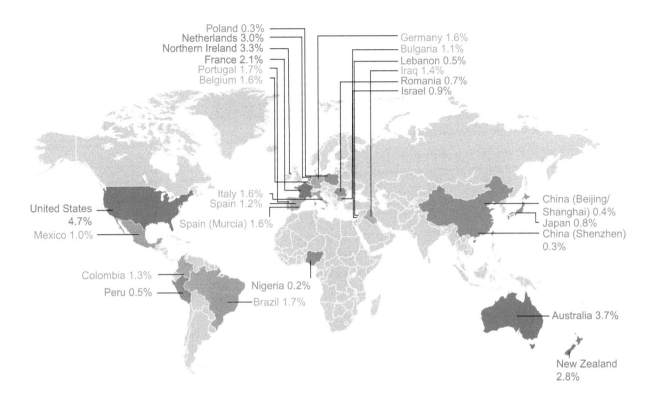

system, lowering the threshold for future attacks. Some early treatments for panic disorder symptoms focused on medications that increased the availability of the neurotransmitter norepinephrine in the locus coeruleus (Table 4.2). More recent evidence points to a brain circuit that connects a number of structures including the amygdala, hippocampus, hypothalamus central gray matter, and

Figure 4.12 Lifetime prevalence of panic disorder in the World Mental Health Surveys (2002–2017).
Source: Data from Scott, de Jonge, et al. (2018).

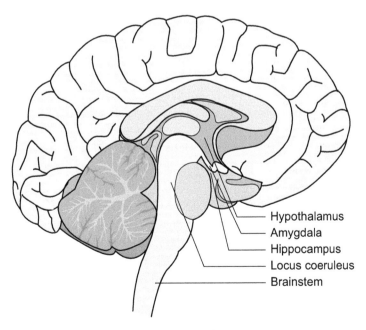

Figure 4.13 Areas of the brain involved in panic disorder include the amygdala, hypothalamus, hippocampus, and locus coeruleus.
Source: Data from Scott, de Jonge, et al. (2018).

Table 4.2 Some FDA-approved medications for panic disorder

Generic name	Brand name	Class of medication
alprazolam	Xanax	Benzodiazepine
fluoxetine	Prozac	Selective serotonin reuptake inhibitor
clonazepam	Klonpin	Benzodiazepine
paroxetine	Paxil	Selective serotonin reuptake inhibitor
sertraline	Zoloft	Selective serotonin reuptake inhibitor
venlafaxine	Effexor	Serotonin and norepinephrine reuptake inhibitor

Source: Information from Stahl (2017).

the locus coeruleus (Elias et al. 2020) is a kind of panic circuit. It's this panic circuit that appears to be overactive in people with panic disorders. Medications such as alprazolam (Xanax) and other benzodiazepines can help, but they aren't used as often because of their side effects such as dependence and grogginess.

PSYCHODYNAMIC MODELS AND TREATMENT

According to a psychodynamic theory of panic attacks, symptoms of panic develop from unconscious fantasies and conflicts, especially those that feature angry and aggressive feelings about important attachment figures such as parents. Some people feel overwhelmed by anger at these important attachment figures, since these attachment figures are often part of what creates our sense of morality. This anger is pushed into the unconscious and experienced as panic, so instead of the anger, people with panic disorder experience fear, which is much less threatening toward the attachment figure than the initial anger. The goal of therapy is to recognize the angry feelings and try to resolve them.

The main type of therapy is called *Panic Focused Psychodynamic Psychotherapy (PFPP)*. Unlike traditional psychodynamic psychotherapy, PFPP is a manualized therapy (a therapy with specific guidelines outlined in an instruction manual) that consists of 24 sessions twice a week for 12 weeks. A study comparing CBT and PFPP for clients with panic disorder showed that PFPP was useful in reducing the severity of panic attacks (Barber et al. 2020).

COGNITIVE-BEHAVIORAL MODELS AND TREATMENT

In the cognitive-behavioral perspective, people who have symptoms of panic attacks and panic disorder are incorrectly interpreting the physical events in their body, like their heart rate or their breathing patterns. They interpret even slight changes in those sensations as dangerous, and fearing the worst, they begin to hyperventilate and believe they are in danger. Then panic sets in. If you stimulate physiological arousal in people with panic disorder by having them do jumping jacks, hyperventilate, take medications to increase their heartbeat, or even think of panic-inducing situations, they tend to feel more upset than people without panic disorder. What's more, they believe their physiological sensations are more dangerous and uncontrollable than do those without symptoms of panic disorder (Perrotta 2019). Treatments focus on helping them analyze their thoughts and interpret them in a more adaptive way.

Anxiety sensitivity is a tendency to interpret bodily sensations as evidence of harmful symptoms. Reducing clients' sensitivity to their bodily sensations can be helpful. How do we do that? Cognitive-behavioral therapy uses a number of techniques. Helping clients understand that they are misinterpreting body sensations is a good start, as is helping them to more accurately interpret their body's reactions, especially during stressful times. Teaching them relaxation or distraction techniques can help squelch the early signs of a panic attack before the anxiety becomes too great.

Anxiety sensitivity: a tendency to interpret bodily sensations as evidence of harmful symptoms.

A typical CBT treatment consists of 12 sessions. One such treatment is called *Panic Controlled Treatment Protocol (PCT)* (Craske et al. 2003). In it, clients learn about panic attacks and their typical causes from the cognitive perspective, as well as how to track their symptoms, recognize triggers, and take helpful actions like relaxation and meditation. Therapy may even include attempts to trigger panic attacks, to show clients techniques to calm themselves (such as slowing their breathing) and to let them practice putting themselves into situations that are bound to set off an attack.

Two of three people who use CBT for panic have become panic-free by using the techniques (compared to 13 percent in a control group). Research examining the effectiveness of CBT techniques find them to be as effective as medications such as benzodiazepines for panic disorder, but without some of the disadvantages (Barlow et al. 2000), and other studies have discovered that most clients treated with CBT (85–90 percent) found symptom relief after 12 weeks (Clark & Beck 2010). Some studies reported that many clients hadn't had a panic attack or symptoms of a panic attack two years after the treatment.

SOCIOCULTURAL MODELS AND TREATMENT

Sociocultural models recognize that society and culture can also play a role in the way the symptoms of panic attacks are expressed. *Ataque de nervios* (attack of the nerves) (Lewis-Fernández et al. 2020) is a condition often described in the Caribbean and Latin America. Symptoms are similar to those of a panic attack and include trembling, a tightness in the chest, fainting, shouting, crying, not knowing who or where you are, and a general sense of being out of control. It often occurs as a response to a stressful event and can sometimes lead to self-harm. *Familismo* is an important culture value in Latin America and the Caribbean and includes dedication, commitment, and loyalty to family. Symptoms of *ataque de nervios* often arise in response to stressful events related to the family and a violation of that value.

CONCEPT CHECK 4.3

1. Lily recently had a panic attack for the first time. Although it was upsetting to her, she hasn't changed her behavior in response. Should Lily receive a diagnosis of panic disorder? _____
2. The biological theory of panic disorder suggests that poor regulation of the locus coeruleus may [increase/decrease] the number of panic attacks a person may experience.
3. List two other evidence-based treatments besides medications for panic disorders.

4.4   GENERALIZED ANXIETY DISORDER

Imagine you are walking to your front door and hunting for your keys in your backpack. You dig around for a few seconds, but you don't see or feel them. Before you know it, you feel a bit of panic. You check in every single pocket you have (and a few you don't). You start thinking about all the places you could have lost your keys, how you'll explain that you lost them, and how you'll get through your day.

If you've had this or a similar experience, it may have felt as if no matter where your mind wandered, it found a problem to land on. Perhaps your stomach hurt, or you were exhausted after it happened. Now imagine you felt that way all the time for months upon months, even when everything was going well. That's what it might feel like to experience generalized anxiety disorder, or GAD.

Symptoms and Description: Generalized Anxiety Disorder

Generalized anxiety disorder (GAD): an anxiety disorder marked by unexplained, excessive worry that's not linked to anything in particular

Generalized anxiety disorder (GAD) is an anxiety disorder marked by unexplained, excessive worry that's not linked to anything in particular. People with GAD find it especially difficult to control their worry (APA 2022). Despite their best efforts, their worry and dread seem to have a life of their own. Sometimes the anxiety is described as "free floating," meaning that it will float and stick to any thought the person might have and infect it with worry. Some even say that GAD is like being in a race without a finish line. In addition, GAD is associated with both psychological and physical symptoms such as restlessness, fatigue, concentration difficulties, irritability, muscle tension, and sleep disturbances (Diagnostic Overview 4.6). This isn't just a rough patch. For a diagnosis of GAD, symptoms must be experienced for at least six months, although many people have them for much longer.

People with GAD are persistently tense (Andrews et al. 2010), sometimes so much that their muscles become sore. They are especially sensitive to stressors in their environment, feel edgy and restless, and have trouble maintaining their concentration. What makes them tense? Nearly every-thing. However, some of the most common worries that occupy their minds are bad things that could happen to their family, their health, their job, chores, the need to be on time, and their performance in school and/or at work. A vast majority of their worries (91.4 percent) turn out to be needless (LaFreniere & Newman 2020). For those with GAD, however, everything is a catas-trophe. They play whack-a-mole with a stream of emer-gencies, which leads to problems sleeping and daytime fatigue that in turn causes forgetfulness and makes matters worse. Their anxiety creates more anxiety and causes problems in their work and social lives (Figure 4.14).

Diagnostic Overview 4.6: Generalized Anxiety Disorder

Excessive anxiety and an inability to control excessive worry, along with three or more of the following symptoms:

- Restlessness.
- Tendency to become easily tired.
- Difficulty concentrating.
- Irritability.
- Excessive muscle tension.
- Problems falling asleep or staying asleep.

Impact: Symptoms are related to clinically significant distress or create impairment in important areas of life such as with friends and family or at work or school.

Timeframe: At least six months.

Source: Information from APA (2022).

Statistics and Trajectory: Generalized Anxiety Disorder

Six to nine percent of the US population meets the criteria for GAD (APA 2022; NIMH 2019). The mean age of onset for GAD is 24, a bit higher than for some other anxiety disorders (Solmi et al. 2021). These rates of GAD are similar around the world, and just under half the people with GAD will seek treatment for it (NIMH 2019). The disorder appears to be more common in women than in men (Jalnapurkar et al. 2018) (Figure 4.15).

Models and Treatments of Generalized Anxiety Disorder

Psychopathologists have created a number of theories about why people develop generalized anxiety disorder including biological and psychological models. And many clients benefit from combination of interventions.

BIOLOGICAL MODELS AND TREATMENT

The fight, flee, or freeze response is a biological response we all have. Many of the symptoms of GAD are symptoms of this response, but people with GAD are so prone to anxiety that they're having the fight, flee, or freeze response even when there isn't an actual threat. In fact, neuroimaging studies of GAD support this hypothesis (Goossen et al. 2019). GAD tends to run in families. Family and twin studies provide evidence for the heritability of these disorders at around 30 percent (Dalvie et al. 2020). This suggests that there may be both specific brain circuits as well as neurotransmitter systems related to anxiety (more on this soon).

People with GAD show more activity in their amygdala, an area in the brain that processes emotions (Suor et al. 2020). And they also seem to have a chronically active sympathetic nervous system, which means their hearts may beat more quickly and they may breathe more heavily

Figure 4.14 For people with generalized anxiety disorder, anxiety can create a feedback loop to more anxiety.

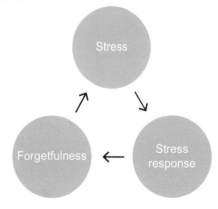

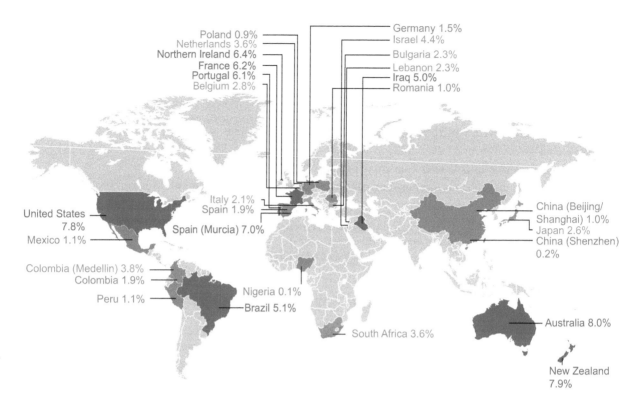

Figure 4.15 Lifetime prevalence of generalized anxiety disorder in the World Mental Health Surveys (2002–2017).

Source: Data from Scott, de Jonge, et al. (2018).

(Brosschot et al. 2007). Some neurotransmitters also might be involved. People with GAD show differences in the GABA neurotransmitter system (Charney 2004). Some theories suggest a deficit in GABA or GABA receptor sites, especially in the areas associated with the limbic system. Since GABA is an inhibitory neurotransmitter, a deficit of GABA would result in overactivation of the limbic system structures responsible for keeping anxiety at bay.

The limbic system also serves as a traffic cop for activity between the cortex and the brainstem area associated with anxiety. The brainstem senses changes in the body and sends these signals to higher brain processes. People who show increased amounts of anxiety may have limbic systems that are overly sensitive to new information (Britton et al. 2013).

Many types of medications have been used to treat GAD, including benzodiazepines and SSRIs (Table 4.3). Benzodiazepines can be helpful in the short term (Gorman 2003), but they do have disadvantages; people can build up a tolerance to and become dependent on them over time. Benzodiazepines can also create problems with thinking and motor functioning (Van Laar et al. 2001), which could cause problems while driving and leave older adults susceptible to slips and falls. Because of these limitations, many prescribers use benzodiazepines cautiously, for only a few days or weeks, and sometimes only as "rescue drugs," to help clients in situations of sudden anxiety.

The most common treatments lately are those that work on the neurotransmitter serotonin, such as SSRIs like paroxetine (Paxil). These improve treatment at

Table 4.3 Some FDA-approved medications for generalized anxiety disorder

Generic name	Brand name	Class of medication
alprazolam	Xanax	Benzodiazepine
duloxetine	Cymbalta	Serotonin norepinephrine reuptake inhibitor
escitalopram	Lexapro	Serotonin reuptake inhibitor
paroxetine	Paxil	Serotonin reuptake inhibitor
venlafaxine	Effexor	Serotonin norepinephrine reuptake inhibitor

Source: Information from Stahl (2017).

similar rates to benzodiazepines in most people (up to 60 percent) who take them (Jakubovski et al. 2019). Although SSRIs are often thought of as antidepressants, the neurotransmitters they act on (serotonin and norepinephrine) often work on the fear and worry circuits in the brain.

PSYCHODYNAMIC MODELS AND TREATMENT

In the psychodynamic perspective, unconscious defense mechanisms may be unable to counteract the anxiety we all experience as we grow and develop (Freud 1933). This view suggests that some children may feel overwhelmed by their own id impulses, and their superegos make them anxious over this.

Contemporary psychodynamic theorists (Sharf 2015) continue Freud's emphasis on the early relationships between children and their caregivers. Some psychodynamically oriented research has supported the idea that overprotective parenting can lead to higher levels of anxiety in some children (Leichsenring et al. 2020).

Psychodynamically oriented therapists use interpretations and working through (as we discuss in Chapter 2) to help clients with GAD. Studies have found these treatments to be of modest success (Leichsenring et al. 2020). Short-term psychodynamic therapy has had more success in reducing the symptoms associated with GAD than traditional psychodynamic therapy (Leichsenring et al. 2020).

COGNITIVE AND BEHAVIORAL MODELS AND TREATMENT

You'll remember that the learning perspective suggests psychological disorders are learned behaviors. From this perspective, all anxiety disorders can be learned and are also maintained through learning.

One theory (Schmidt et al. 1997) suggests that people who are anxious are highly sensitive to the internal sensations associated with anxiety. They are more likely to focus on threatening cues in the environment and to remember threatening events. When presented with ambiguous information, they tend to interpret the events as more threatening than neutral stimuli and more so than other people do (Eysenck et al. 1991).

According to this theory, it's no surprise that people with GAD report feeling more intense negative emotions than others (Aldao et al. 2010) and are more highly stressed during negative events than others (Tan et al. 2012). These maladaptive cognitions also add to their anxiety and lead them to constantly scan their environments for threats (Beck & Emery 1985). When they scan, they find threats and remember them more often.

The first step is helping clients recognize the thoughts that occur when they become anxious. The next step is for them to challenge and modify those thoughts, evaluating them for common errors such as maximization (overestimating their involvement in a situation or overestimating how dangerous a perceived threat might be). Perhaps they are predicting a negative outcome of a situation that might not be negative. Therapists encourage clients to look for patterns in their thoughts and try to create new and healthier patterns of thinking.

CBT is a first-line treatment for GAD and many other anxiety disorders, and randomized controlled trials comparing various types of CBT for GAD have found them to be equally effective (Stefan et al. 2019). CBT is more helpful than benzodiazepines in treating GAD (Borkovec et al. 2003), and the effects may last for years.

SOCIOCULTURAL MODELS AND TREATMENT

Social events both positive and negative, like getting married or having problems with friends, can trigger our psychological and biological responses to anxiety. Even a physical cause like an illness or injury can act as a catalyst for GAD.

Parents who provide a secure home base from which to explore the world tend to have children who more readily feel a sense of control over their environment (Chorpita & Barlow 1998). "Snowplow" parents, in contrast, protect their children from any harm, so the children may develop in an environment where their skills are never tested (Figure 4.16). As a result, they may feel a lack of control over their environment.

Rather than focus on individuals' characteristics, sociocultural models of anxiety such as the Feminist Ecological model emphasize external factors that may be at play (Rodgers et al. 2020). These models examine how external systems may increase risk for certain vulnerable groups. The Feminist Ecological approach, for instance, suggests that for many marginalized groups, anxiety may be increased in some societies that emphasize the individual. Competitive individualism may also act to prevent aspects of cooperation that could decrease levels of anxiety. In addition, the increased prevalence of anxiety disorders in women may be influenced by societal norms that view women as inferior, pay them less for the work they do, and offer few career advancement opportunities. All these factors (and more) may lead to increased worry and stress based on threats to women's financial security.

Sociocultural theories suggest that GAD is more likely to occur in those who live in threatening or dangerous environments. We see higher rates of GAD and other anxiety disorders in people who live in high-crime areas, for example, and in people who live with the stress of poverty (Cerdá et al. 2017). GAD symptoms are

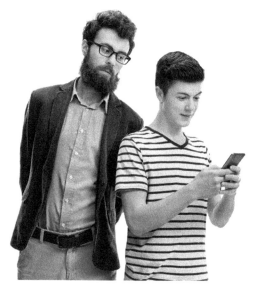

Figure 4.16 Parents who are hovering and controlling may create an environment in which children don't gain a sense of control over their own environments.

Source: Ljupco/iStock/Getty Images Plus.

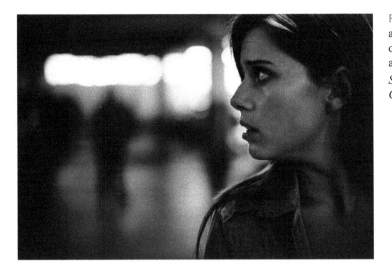

Figure 4.17 The increased alertness or hypervigilance that often accompanies anxiety can also reinforce worry.

Source: PeopleImages/E+/ Getty Images.

exacerbated by not knowing whether your family members will come home safe every day or where your next meal will come from. Therapies that focus only on individual change may not have an impact on these external circumstances, whereas community psychologists and those who focus on prevention may target their interventions to society more broadly by advocating for social justice and working with community organizations to help to solve social problems.

MULTIPERSPECTIVE MODELS AND TREATMENT

The multiperspective theory suggests that a biological and psychological vulnerability may predispose certain people to GAD, such as those who have difficulties with uncertainty and find it hard to tolerate the potential negative consequences of future events. Because of this susceptibility, people set up ways to protect themselves from a perceived uncertain and difficult future. Protective behaviors include frequent checking for or constantly expecting danger, also known as *hypervigilance*, which can make people feel better temporarily but also reinforce their worrying (Figure 4.17). Worry becomes a comforting friend and a torture at the same time.

CONCEPT CHECK 4.4

Fill in the blanks with the correct response.
1. People with generalized anxiety disorder experience an intense burst of anxiety that lasts for at least _____ months.
2. Biological theories of GAD focus on increased brain activity in the _____, the part of the brain that processes emotions.
3. From the cognitive-behavioral perspective, people with generalized anxiety disorder and other anxiety disorders have a tendency to interpret bodily sensations as evidence of harmful symptoms, which is called _____.

4.5   OBSESSIVE-COMPULSIVE AND RELATED DISORDERS

Let's say you are just leaving the house in the morning. You get in your car and are excited to start your day. A moment later you think to yourself, "Do I have my phone?" You always throw it in your bag, but perhaps you only *thought* you put it in there. "Better safe than sorry," you think to yourself as you dig around for it or pat your pockets to make sure it's there. It *is* there. Now you feel much better and you are really ready to start your day.

For a person with obsessive-compulsive disorder (OCD), this need to double-check could be just the beginning. They might feel compelled to engage in a repetitive habit (checking to be sure you have your phone) as a way to relieve the anxiety caused by intrusive thoughts. For example, they might check for the phone a dozen times before they leave, because they think something bad will happen if they don't have it.

In *DSM-5tr* the chapter on Obsessive-Compulsive and Related Disorders identifies several conditions that have, at their root, anxiety created by fear that the person tries desperately to reduce. Unfortunately, many of these attempts result in actions that cause problems themselves. The *DSM* describes five obsessive-compulsive and related conditions: obsessive-compulsive disorder, body dysmorphic disorder, hoarding disorder, hair-pulling disorder (also called trichotillomania), and excoriation disorder (also called skin-picking disorder).

Obsessive-Compulsive Disorder

Obsessive-compulsive disorder (OCD): a psychological disorder associated with obsessions, or obsessions linked to compulsions.

Obsession: an unwanted thought that a person finds disturbing.

The hallmark condition in the Obsessive-Compulsive and Related Disorder chapter of the *DSM* is, of course, obsessive-compulsive disorder (Diagnostic Overview 4.7). In order to be diagnosed with **obsessive-compulsive disorder (OCD)**, a person must have an obsession, or an obsession linked to a compulsion. An **obsession** is an unwanted thought you find disturbing to think about, such as hurting someone you really care about, or thinking you have forgotten something important that will cause harm to another person. These distressing thoughts can enter our minds all the time. Maybe you've left a candle burning in another room, or you've thought about saying something unkind to a dear friend, or you've left your hotel room unlocked. For most people, these thoughts are easy to dismiss. However, for people with OCD the doubts take root, and then the anxiety that something terrible might happen takes over.

Diagnostic Overview 4.7: Obsessive-Compulsive Disorder

Presence of an obsession, a compulsion, or both.	
Impact:	Symptoms must exceed cultural and contextual norms. Symptoms are related to clinically significant distress or create impairment in important areas of life such as with friends and family or at work or school.
Timeframe:	Time consuming (takes up at least one hour a day).

Source: Information from APA (2022).

Compulsions, on the other hand, are behaviors or sometimes mental actions that a person feels they must do as a response to an obsession. An obsession can exist by itself, such as a dislike of dirt, but a compulsion must be linked with an obsession, like handwashing after being exposed to dirt. Other compulsions are meant to neutralize or undo the obsessional thought or mental act, such as counting or praying.

Compulsions: behaviors or mental actions that a person feels they must do as a response to an obsession.

THE POWER OF WORDS

THAT'S SO OCD!

It happens more often than you might think and it happens almost automatically. Let's say you're in the grocery store and you want to do a favor for the cashier . . . turning all the scanning codes face up to make it easier to ring up your order. After all it's something to do, and maybe the cashier will appreciate the extra effort to make their job just a little bit easier. No big deal. Maybe they'll even thank you for the small gesture of kindness.

"OCD much?" the cashier responds.

Some people find it socially acceptable to use psychological disorders such as obsessive-compulsive disorder as a slang expression for being organized and neat. This kind of shorthand is part of our everyday language, and people often mistakenly think having OCD means being super-organized. However, you learned in Chapter 1 that to be a psychological disorder a condition has to cause distress and impairment. People who are super-organized happily use their skills to help them do a better job. In contrast, most people with OCD find their obsessions frustrating and wish they could stop thinking about them. They organize not as a hobby or from a need to be tidy, but from fear that something terrible will happen if they don't.

So what's the consequence of the trivialization? Unfortunately, OCD is often used as comic relief in the media, and this leads to oversimplification of and skepticism about the severity of the symptoms. When OCD is used as a joke, people with this life-altering condition may feel like they can't talk about their experiences without being dismissed, which means they are less able to take advantage of social support, further contributing to the silence, shame, and stigma surrounding mental illness. A great way to build empathy and understanding of the condition is to do what you are doing right now, learning about psychological disorders and reading real cases of people with the conditions.

About 80 percent of people with OCD have both obsessions and compulsions, leaving about 20 percent of people with OCD who have only obsessions. As you can see in the *DSM* criteria listed in Diagnostic Overview 4.7, people with OCD have symptoms that take up a considerable amount of their time (more than an hour each day) or that cause them significant impairment or distress.

In many cases of OCD, the obsessions and compulsions exemplify a theme, such as contamination, violence, orderliness, or sexuality. Although the general

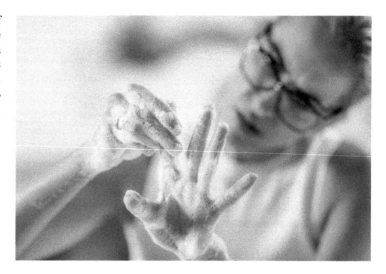

Figure 4.18 Obsessions of contamination often have compulsions that follow a similar theme, such as handwashing.
Source: microgen/iStock/Getty Images Plus.

symptoms of OCD appear consistent across cultures the themes may vary by culture or country. For example, Brazil has a higher rate of obsessions about contamination than other countries, and the compulsions are related to cleaning (Nicolini et al. 2017). Although they don't have to be, compulsions are often linked to the nature of the obsession (Figure 4.18). For example, an obsession with balance and order might be tied to counting or organizing items (Bloch et al. 2008).

OCD often begins at a younger age than some other disorders, and the most common age of onset is around 14 (Solmi et al. 2021). Lifetime prevalence of OCD in the United States ranges from 1.6 percent to 2.3 percent (Calamari et al. 2012; Kessler et al. 2005), and 1–2 percent of people in the United States meet the criteria for the disorder in any given year (Zhou et al. 2019). About 3 percent of the population will develop the condition at some point during their lives. Men and women develop OCD at equal rates.

Case Study: Fletcher Wortmann

Even when he was in the third grade, Fletcher Wortmann would become overwhelmed by anxiety. He was convinced, for example, that the entire planet would soon freeze. To prepare, he starting planning survival strategies for his family. He would spend hours doing so. While some people might just shake off upsetting or distressing thoughts, he couldn't. Soon his obsessive-compulsive disorder took over his life. His mind would settle on something distressing and he couldn't seem to let it go. Despite the fact that his friends, family, and even his therapists tried to reassure him that his thoughts were just that ... thoughts, it didn't seem to ease his deep sense of uncertainty that his worst fears might occur: contamination would lead to disease, that he and his family would be harmed. The condition grew to the point that Fletcher was eventually hospitalized for his OCD. We'll return to Fletcher's story in a bit.

To read more about Fletcher Wortmann, take a look at his book, *Triggered: A memoir of obsessive-compulsive disorder* (2012).

Body Dysmorphic Disorder

Body dysmorphic disorder (BDD) is an obsessive-compulsive and related disorder associated with an imagined defect in appearance and compensatory behaviors (Diagnostic Overview 4.8). The obsession is the imagined defect, and the compulsive behaviors tend to be things such as frequently checking in mirrors and asking friends and family members for reassurance about the person's appearance. People with BDD draw attention to their own perceived flaws and rate photographs of their own faces as less attractive than unfamiliar faces (Möllmann et al. 2020). They spend an average of three to eight hours a day checking their appearance or grooming themselves (Phillips et al. 2010) and will often avoid social activities because of their concern over the way they look. Their concern is not just about their facial appearance; the average number of body areas of concern for people with BDD is seven (Figure 4.19) (Phillips et al. 2005).

The prevalence of clinically significant BDD symptoms was estimated to be between 1 percent and 2 percent in the United States, with a significantly higher prevalence in women than in men. The heritability of body dysmorphic concerns was estimated to be 49 percent at age 15, 39 percent at age 18, and 37 percent at ages 20–28 (Enander et al. 2018). Research in other countries such as Australia shows men and women with similar rates of BDD, although there were differences in which body parts were believed to be flawed (Schneider et al. 2019). For example, one study in Australia reported that women had more concerns than men about their calves and/or thighs, and men had more concerns than women about how muscular their bodies were (Malcolm et al. 2021). For many people, symptoms start in early adolescence (Phillips et al. 2005). They may not seek treatment, although relatives and friends may suggest it and the symptoms do cause stress and impairment (Phillips et al. 2000).

Body dysmorphic disorder (BDD): an obsessive-compulsive and related disorder associated with an imagined defect in appearance and compensatory behaviors.

Hoarding Disorder

Maybe you've seen something about hoarding on television or have been concerned about friends or family members whose collections are taking over their homes. It's only fairly recently (in *DSM-5*) that hoarding disorder has become an official psychological diagnosis (Diagnostic Overview 4.9). **Hoarding disorder** is an obsessive-compulsive and related disorder associated with difficulty discarding unneeded possessions. It's not just that people with hoarding disorder are messy;

Hoarding disorder: an obsessive-compulsive and related disorder associated with difficulty discarding unneeded possessions.

Diagnostic Overview 4.8: Body Dysmorphic Disorder

Preoccupation with an imagined defect in appearance, along with repetitive behaviors or mental acts in response to the perceived defect.

Impact: Symptoms must exceed cultural and contextual norms. Symptoms are related to clinically significant distress or create impairment in important areas of life such as with friends and family or at work or school.

Source: Information from APA (2022).

Figure 4.19 Percentages of people with BDD who have a concern with this part of the body (from a sample of 200).

Source: Data adapted from Phillips et al. (2005).

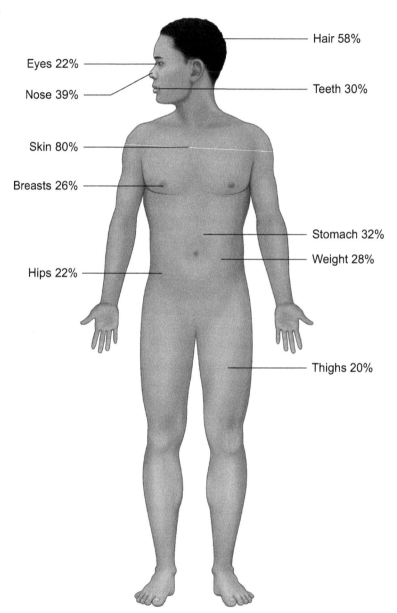

Diagnostic Overview 4.9: Hoarding Disorder

Difficulty discarding possessions and a need to save items even when they have no value:

- A great deal of anxiety when discarding items.
- Living areas cluttered to the point that they cannot be used for their intended purpose.

Impact: Symptoms must exceed cultural and contextual norms. Symptoms are related to clinically significant distress or create impairment in important areas of life such as with friends and family or at work or school.

Source: Information from APA (2022).

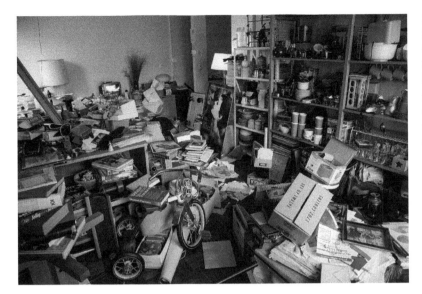

Figure 4.20 People with hoarding disorder don't just clutter up rooms; their disorder renders the rooms useless for their original function.
Source: Kurt Wittman/ Education Images/Universal Images Group via Getty Images

they also show attachments to their possessions (Frost et al. 2012) and will become distressed if asked to discard them, even if the items look worthless to other people. They keep objects to the point that rooms become so cluttered they can't be used for their original purpose. Kitchens might hold boxes of unopened mail, and ovens are stuffed with old magazines. Bedrooms might have stacks of empty grocery bags (Figure 4.20).

Although hoarding disorder and OCD are in the same chapter in the DSM, some research suggests that the two are quite different. For example, people with hoarding disorder don't feel their need to hoard is intrusive or unwanted (Mataix-Cols et al. 2010). They will often fight the interventions of others to clean their homes.

Between 1.5 percent and 6 percent of the population of the United States shows evidence of hoarding disorder (Postlethwaite et al. 2019), and a small group of those will also meet criteria for OCD (Frost et al. 2011). Unlike many psychological disorders that begin when people are younger, hoarding disorder tends to become more prevalent as people get older. Three times as many adults aged 55 to 59 are affected as are adults 34 to 44 years of age (Ayers et al. 2009). Later onset of hoarding disorder is not necessarily due to the fact that people simply possess more items as they get older, since in one study people with hoarding disorder reported both symptoms of urges to save items and difficulty discarding items (Dozier et al. 2016). The later onset of the symptoms may be part of the way hoarding disorder progresses.

Trichotillomania and Excoriation Disorder

The last two disorders in the DSM chapter on Obsessive-Compulsive and Related Disorders are **trichotillomania**, in which an individual repeatedly pulls out their hair, and **excoriation disorder**, in which an individual picks at their own skin and causes skin lesions or wounds (Figure 4.21).

Trichotillomania: an obsessive-compulsive and related disorder in which an individual repeatedly pulls out their hair.

Excoriation disorder: an obsessive-compulsive and related disorder in which an individual picks at their own skin and causes skin lesions or wounds.

Figure 4.21 Excoriation is a condition in which a person picks at their skin to the point where it causes a wound.

Source: Adam Gray/Barcroft Media via Getty Images.

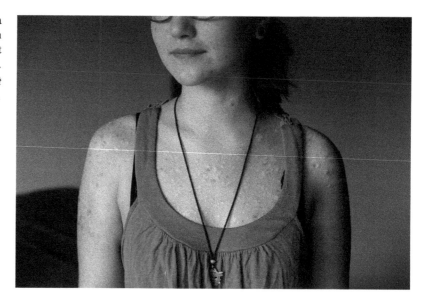

In both these conditions, people report a feeling of tension that builds up and then an almost automatic response that they often don't know they are enacting (Stein et al. 2010). Hair pulling can cause severe social problems for some people, and many with hair-pulling disorder work hard to hide their behavior. Many more feel a great sense of shame about it (Diagnostic Overview 4.10) (Grant et al. 2012; Lochner et al. 2012).

In excoriation disorder, people will feel their face, hands, or arms, searching for an area that doesn't feel right to them, and they will then pick and pick at that area and create a wound (Diagnostic Overview 4.11). They may use their fingers, pin tweezers, or some other object for the purpose. They want to stop, but they can't seem to help themselves, and there may be times when anxiety makes the skin picking worse.

Three in four people with excoriation disorder are women (APA 2022). The prevalence is relatively low, at only about 3.1 percent of individuals (APA 2022). The average age of onset is 13 for hair pulling (Flessner et al. 2010). Prevalence can be up to 5 percent of college students (Scott et al. 2003).

Diagnostic Overview 4.10: Trichotillomania (Hair-Pulling Disorder)

Recurrent hair pulling that results in hair loss, along with unsuccessful attempts to stop the behavior.

Impact: Symptoms must exceed cultural and contextual norms. Symptoms are related to clinically significant distress or create impairment in important areas of life such as with friends and family or at work or school.

Source: Information from APA (2022).

Models and Treatments of Obsessive-Compulsive and Related Disorders

Fletcher sought treatment which included psychotherapy and medication which improved his symptoms dramatically. In an interview, Fletcher reported "I was very hesitant to take medication, and I think because of this cultural myth we have that medication turns you into a zombie or a robot, or it changes who you are. That hasn't been my experience. I found it's been useful in helping me get into a place where the ... therapy was doable." Psychopathologists have created a number of theories about why people develop OCD, including biological and psychological models.

BIOLOGICAL MODELS AND TREATMENT

Many brain structures are involved in obsessive-compulsive and related disorders. The anterior cingulate cortex (Figure 4.22), especially active in OCD, checks for errors, meaning it helps us be aware when we've make a mistake such as hitting the wrong key on our phone or calling someone by the wrong name (Ursu et al. 2003). One theory of OCD suggests that abnormalities in the limbic systems, frontal lobes, and basal ganglia may interfere with the signal your brain sends to let you know you've finished a task. This would cause people with OCD to feel that they need to complete the task again (Fettes et al. 2017; Szechtman & Woody 2004).

Brain chemicals also play a part in obsessive-compulsive and related disorders. Several biological theories point to GABA, an inhibitory neurotransmitter. Some theorists think low GABA can result in a more active nervous system. Medications such as benzodiazepines, which increase the activity of GABA in the synapse, seem to improve anxiety symptoms (Table 4.4) (Stahl 2017). In addition to GABA, the neurotransmitter serotonin has also been implicated in OCD and in generalized anxiety disorder (Stahl 2017). Antidepressant medications such as SSRIs increase the availability of serotonin and decrease symptoms by up to half in as many as 60 percent of those with OCD (Zhou et al. 2019).

Diagnostic Overview 4.11: Excoriation Disorder (Skin-Picking Disorder)

Recurrent skin picking that leads to skin problems along with unsuccessful attempts to stop the behavior.

Impact: Symptoms must exceed cultural and contextual norms. Symptoms are related to clinically significant distress or create impairment in important areas of life such as with friends and family or at work or school.

Source: Information from APA (2022).

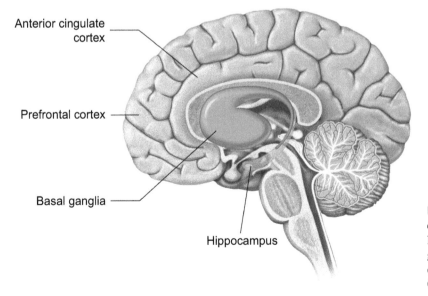

Anterior cingulate cortex

Prefrontal cortex

Basal ganglia

Hippocampus

Figure 4.22 The anterior cingulate cortex is useful in letting us know when we've gotten something wrong. It is especially active in people with OCD.

Table 4.4 Some FDA-approved medications for obsessive-compulsive disorder

Generic name	Brand name	Class of medication
fluoxetine	Prozac	Selective serotonin reuptake inhibitor
fluvoxamine	Louvox	Selective serotonin reuptake inhibitor
paroxetine	Paxil	Selective serotonin reuptake inhibitor

Source: Information from Stahl (2017).

Treatments for excoriation disorder include both SSRIs and a medication called naltrexone. The act of grooming is reinforcing, and neurotransmitters such as dopamine and serotonin help that reinforcement. What SSRIs and naltrexone do is ever so slightly reduce the physiological reinforcement for self-grooming.

The treatment picture isn't as optimistic for every obsessive-compulsive condition. For example, there are few evidence-based treatments for body dysmorphic disorder, although SSRIs such as fluvoxamine (Luvox) can be beneficial (Hadley et al. 2006). People with BDD may be tempted to correct their imagined defects through plastic surgery (Woolfolk & Allen 2011). In one survey, up to 76.4 percent had sought this type of treatment (Phillips et al. 2001). Over 15 percent of respondents in a study of people seeking plastic surgery met the criteria for BDD (Ribeiro 2017), and it's thought that up to a quarter of all patients seeking plastic surgery might do so (Crerand et al. 2004). These procedures do not always relieve the frustration people with BDD have with their bodies, however. In one study of BDD clients who underwent plastic surgery, 81 percent were dissatisfied with the results of their procedures (Phillips et al. 2005).

COGNITIVE AND BEHAVIORAL MODELS AND TREATMENT

Behavioral exposure: a behavioral technique that involves repeated presentation of anxiety-producing stimuli.

The main treatment for obsessive-compulsive and related disorders in the cognitive and behavioral approach is **behavioral exposure**. Behavioral exposures include a repeated presentation of anxiety-producing stimuli when the client is unable to react in their typical maladaptive manner. For example, if being exposed to dirt creates anxiety, then the therapist might ask the client to put dirt on their hands (exposure) but not wash them. What will happen? The client will feel anxious. However, over a period of time, the anxiety will slowly decrease. Repeated exposure sessions will cause the anxiety to *habituate* or decrease over time.

In addition to behavioral exposure, cognitive strategies can be beneficial in helping clients reevaluate their belief systems. CBT is a helpful treatment for most obsessive-compulsive and related disorders and has been found to be helpful in reducing symptoms, even in those who have had difficulty responding to medication (Reddy et al. 2020).

Some clients might not find CBT techniques to their liking. In one study of clients with OCD, some 15 percent refused CBT and 15 percent subsequently dropped out of treatment (Leeuwerik et al. 2019), most often due to poor outcomes. People may also refuse CBT because it can feel overly structured, but for those who do continue, the treatment can be useful. In one study of CBT for body dysmorphic disorder, researchers found a 68 percent reduction of symptoms (Rodgers et al. 2021).

Cognitive strategies such as CBT have been useful for controlling hoarding disorder (Bodryzlova et al. 2019). The main approach helps clients assign different values to objects and then attempt to discard the lower-valued objects first (Grisham et al. 2012). These treatments are only modestly successful.

SOCIOCULTURAL MODELS AND TREATMENT

While biological and psychological theories can explain some of the vulnerabilities people often have for obsessive-compulsive and related disorders, society and culture play a major role as well. This might explain why some individuals are more likely to develop symptoms of some obsessive-compulsive disorders than others. For example, society and culture may create unrealistic standards about the importance of physical appearance that may increase the likelihood of certain conditions such as body dysmorphic disorder (Figure 4.23). Discrimination may also influence the severity of the symptoms of OCD. Studies have revealed a relationship between exposure to everyday racial discrimination and increased severity of these symptoms (i.e. Wilson & Thyer 2020), in part due to the strain discrimination places on the stress response.

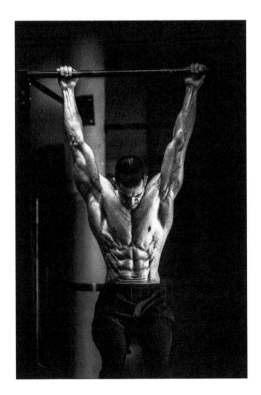
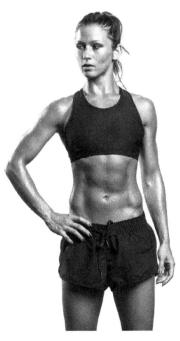

Figure 4.23 Do images of women and men in magazines set unrealistic cultural expectations of body image?
Sources: zeljkosantrac/E+/ Getty Images, and mihailomilovanovic/E+/Getty Images.

CONCEPT CHECK 4.5

Fill in the blanks with the correct obsessive-compulsive and related disorder that fits the short case.

1. Sean loves to go shopping. In fact, he shops so much that his kitchen is too cluttered for him to do any cooking. A therapist might consider that Sean has _____.
2. Roland may have _____ because sometimes he can't help himself as he feels his hands move toward his eyebrows and pull out the hair. Afterward he feels a sense of relief, and then guilt and shame. He has created spots with no hair, not only on his face but on other parts of his head. He has tried to stop many times, but his attempts have not been effective.
3. Madge worries that she will contract a serious illness. This concerns her so much that whenever she touches something, she must wash her hands five times, and if she does not do it in a particular way, she must start over again. Madge's concern about contracting an illness is an example of an _____ and her handwashing is an example of a _____. A psychologist might diagnose her with _____.

PULLING IT TOGETHER

The Symptoms of the Fight, Flee, or Freeze Response

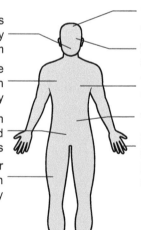

Your mouth becomes dry as blood moves away from digestive system

You breathe more quickly to get oxygen moving around your body

Blood is diverted away from your digestive organs and your bladder relaxes

Blood is diverted to the major muscle groups so you can fight or flee more easily

Your thoughts race as you evaluate the situation

Vision becomes acute so you can pay attention to danger

Your heartbeat increases to circulate the oxygen

Your stomach feels queasy

Blood is pulled away from the extremities, so your hands feel cold and clammy

Figure 4.24 The symptoms of the fight, flee, or freeze response, which is one characteristic of many of the conditions in which we see anxiety.

SUMMARY

This chapter presented the following disorders:

- Specific phobia
- Social anxiety disorder
- Agoraphobia
- Panic disorder
- Generalized anxiety disorder
- Obsessive-compulsive disorder
- Hoarding disorder
- Trichotillomania
- Excoriation
- Body dysmorphic disorder

Overview of Anxiety Disorders

- Anxiety plays a prominent role in three chapters in the *DSM*: the Anxiety Disorders, the Obsessive-Compulsive and Related Disorders, and Trauma and Stressor Related Disorders.
- Many of the symptoms of anxiety are symptoms found in the fight, flee, or freeze response.

Phobias

- A phobia a fear that is unreasonably great or interferes with your life in some way.
- Specific phobias are fears of certain objects or situations.
- Social anxiety disorder is a fear of embarrassment or humiliation.
- Agoraphobia is a fear of having a panic attack or a panic-like feeling in a place where it might be embarrassing.
- Treatments for phobias are similar to other anxiety treatments.

Panic Attacks and Panic Disorder

- A panic attack is a period of intense fear or discomfort.

- People with panic disorder have multiple panic attacks and are either worried about the impact of the attacks or have changed their lives as a response to the attacks.
- The biological model suggests that those with panic attacks are more easily triggered to have them.
- Insight-oriented models of panic focus on helping clients to reinterpret anger.
- Sociocultural models of panic recognize that panic can present itself in different ways in different cultural contexts.
- Cognitive and behavioral models of panic focus on cognitive restructuring to help clients analyze their thoughts and interpret them in a more accurate way.

Generalized Anxiety Disorder

- Generalized anxiety disorder (GAD) is an anxiety disorder marked by unexplained, excessive worry that's not linked to any specific cause.
- Biological models for GAD focus on brain structures such as the amygdala, an area in the brain that processes emotions.
- Cognitive and behavioral models for GAD focus on anxiety sensitivity, which is a tendency to interpret bodily sensations as evidence of harmful symptoms.

Obsessive-Compulsive and Related Disorders

- The disorders in the Obsessive-Compulsive and Related Disorder chapter of *DSM* all lead people to have an unwanted thought or impulse that compels them to do something in order to reduce it.
- In obsessive-compulsive disorder a person has time-consuming obsessions and often companion compulsions.

- An obsession is an unwanted thought that the person finds disturbing.
- Compulsions are behaviors or sometimes mental actions that a person feels they must do as a response to an obsession.
- Body dysmorphic disorder is an obsessive-compulsive and related disorder associated with an imagined defect in appearance and compensatory behaviors.
- Hoarding disorder is an obsessive-compulsive and related disorder associated with having difficulty discarding unneeded possessions.
- Trichotillomania is an obsessive-compulsive and related disorder in which an individual repeatedly pulls out their hair.
- Excoriation disorder is an obsessive-compulsive and related disorder in which an individual picks at their own skin and causes skin lesions or wounds.
- The anterior cingulate cortex is an area of the brain that checks for mistakes and is especially active in people with OCD.
- Differences in the limbic systems, frontal lobes, and basal ganglia may also be related to OCD.
- Cognitive and behavioral models of OCD focus on behavioral exposure strategies.

DISCUSSION QUESTIONS

1. Describe how the various symptoms of the fight, flee, or freeze response manifest in the different anxiety disorders. Do you think these disorders are distinct, or are they just different ways to describe the same stress response?
2. Many people with anxiety disorders ask their prescribers for medications such as Valium or Xanax to reduce their anxiety because they work quickly. But as you've read, these medications also have disadvantages, and there are many other effective treatments. List compelling suggestions a therapist might use to convince a client to try a therapy rather than benzodiazepine to treat one of the anxiety disorders in this chapter.
3. Construct a patient education strategy to use when treating a client with social anxiety disorder. Try to use a multiperspective approach.
4. Many people with hoarding disorder aren't distressed by their possessions, but hoarding does cause a significant amount of impairment. What are some ways that you might assess the impairment of an individual who has hoarding disorder?
5. Describe the difference between obsessive-compulsive disorder and generalized anxiety disorder.

ANSWERS TO CONCEPT CHECKS

Concept Check 4.1

1. Anxiety
2. Fight, flee, or freeze response
3. Worry
4. Fear

Concept Check 4.2

1. Agoraphobia
2. Specific phobia
3. Social anxiety disorder
4. Social anxiety disorder

Concept Check 4.3

1. No
2. Increase
3. Controlled Treatment Protocol (CTP) and Panic Focused Psychodynamic Psychotherapy (PFPP)

Concept Check 4.4

1. 6
2. Amygdala
3. Anxiety sensitivity

Concept Check 4.5

1. Hoarding disorder
2. Trichotillomania hair-pulling disorder
3. Obsession; compulsion; obsessive-compulsive disorder

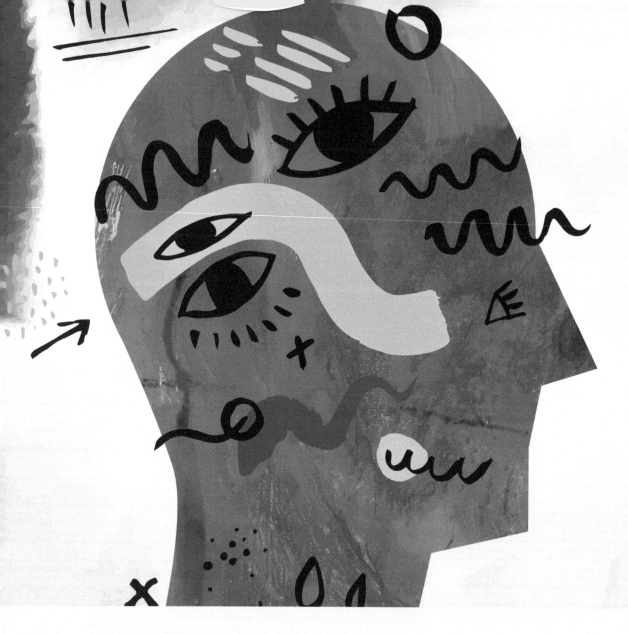

CHAPTER CONTENTS

5

Trauma and Stressor-Related and Dissociative Disorders

CASE STUDY: Post-Traumatic Stress Disorder – TJ Brennan

Not many people have a photograph of the single moment that changed their life. TJ Brennan does.

Sergeant Thomas "TJ" Brennan is a marine who served two tours in the Middle East, and Finbarr O'Reilly, a photojournalist, was right there when an Afghan national police officer fired a rocket that went off target and landed too close to TJ, knocking him unconscious. After that things were fuzzy. TJ couldn't remember the events of the day he was injured, describing his memories as "a jumbled loop of events and conflicting emotions." A medical evacuation was ordered and he was put in the back of an armored vehicle. Along the way someone handed him a satellite phone. Apparently, he called his wife, and according to her, he said, "I got blown up, I've got my arms and legs, I love you, I'll call you, bye," and hung up the phone.

The blast wasn't all that TJ experienced during the tour; he also witnessed other soldiers being wounded and killed. But the explosion left both visible and invisible injuries that lasted for years after his return. TJ experienced persistent symptoms of anxiety, agoraphobia, and insomnia. He was dizzy and disoriented and felt a longing to be alone. Night after night he dreamed about wanting to "kill the enemy" back in Helmand province, and sometimes he was unable to remember the events of that day or separate them from what was going on in the moment.

These symptoms and others pushed TJ away from his family. He was quick to anger, even at small things like eating in a restaurant or waiting in line at the grocery store. He couldn't concentrate, finding it hard to read simple sentences at times. He did whatever he could to avoid being reminded of the traumatic events that he experienced. Nothing seemed to bring him joy. He feared that a diagnosis of a mental condition would give

Learning Objectives

- Describe the symptoms of adjustment disorders.
- Identify the symptoms of post-traumatic stress disorder and acute stress disorder.
- Discuss the various treatments for the trauma and stressor-related disorders.
- Describe the essential nature of dissociative disorders.
- Identify the symptoms of dissociative identity disorder, dissociative amnesia, and depersonalization-derealization disorder.
- Discuss the treatment of dissociative disorders.

his wife an excuse to leave him and wondered whether she deserved better than a "broken man." We'll hear more about TJ later in this chapter.

You can read more about TJ Brennan in his book *Shooting ghosts: A U.S. Marine, a combat photographer, and their journey back from war* (Brennan & O'Reilly 2017).

5.1 TRAUMA AND STRESSOR-RELATED DISORDERS

We've all had a time in our lives when something particularly stressful has occurred. Maybe it's the end of a romantic relationship or the diagnosis of a medical condition. It might even be a positive event like moving to a new city for an exciting job or an education at the college of your dreams. We try our best to cope with these situations. But sometimes the stress creates an emotional and behavioral impact. While most people gradually recover from the psychological effects of the stressors and traumas they experience, some develop psychological conditions. Psychopathologists describe various ways in which trauma and stress can have an impact beyond the initial impact of the event itself.

Two chapters in the *DSM* describe the significant trauma and stress we discuss in this chapter. The first DSM chapter covers the trauma and stressor-related disorders, in which we include adjustment disorders, post-traumatic stress disorder (PTSD), and acute stress disorder. The second chapter in the DSM is the dissociative disorder chapter. Dissociative disorders also tend to have a history of trauma and are often the result of highly aversive events such as child abuse, extreme aloneness, and isolation. These disorders include dissociative identity disorder, dissociative amnesia, and depersonalization-derealization disorder.

Adjustment Disorder

Imagine the excitement of getting the phone call you've been waiting months for, maybe even years. It's the phone call about the job you've always wanted. You celebrate in the last few weeks of college, pack your bags, and leave your friends and family to travel to a town you've never been to before and start a fresh life. It's exciting and new. Once you're there, you realize that as much as you've been raving about this new job, you miss your friends and family and the job is taking up more time that you thought it was going to. Before you know it, months have passed and your friends back home haven't connected as much as they've wanted to and you haven't either. It's no one's fault, but now you feel detached and you haven't done a great job of making friends in your new city. You love going to the movies but you don't relish the idea of going by yourself, so new movies come and go, and just seeing the teaser ads leaves you feeling empty. You end up spending your weekends watching television and working, feeling more and more alone.

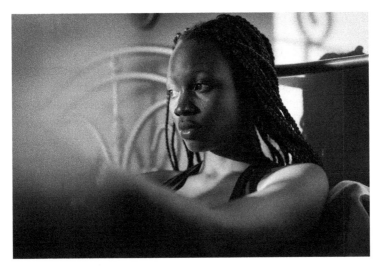

Figure 5.1 Emotional or behavioral problems (such as feeling lonely) that are connected to a specific event are sometimes considered symptoms of an adjustment disorder.
Source: Jasmin Merdan/ Moment/Getty Images.

Life changes and demands adjustments. Sometimes, however, the actions we take in order to adjust cause emotional or behavioral responses that can make our inability to adjust worse (Figure 5.1). In an **adjustment disorder**, a person has experienced a stressor and is having a greater than expected emotional or behavioral response due to the difficulty of coping with it (Diagnostic Overview 5.1).

Adjustment disorder: a trauma and stressor-related disorder in which a person has experienced a stressor and is having a greater than expected emotional or behavioral response due to the difficulty of coping with it.

SYMPTOMS AND DESCRIPTION

Let's think back to the example of moving to a new city for a job. The feelings of detachment and loneliness are related to the specific event of the move. These emotional and behavioral symptoms of an adjustment disorder are thought to come from the stressor (like the move to a new city), so if the stressor goes away, the symptoms of the adjustment disorder eventually dissipate as well. For example, during the COVID-19 pandemic, two out of three people experienced stress over a weakened economy and one out of three showed symptoms of anxiety and nearly 20 percent had physical reactions when they thought about the pandemic. In order to link the symptoms to the stressor, psychopathologists have created some parameters around the diagnosis. For example, the symptoms should appear within three months of the stressor, and if the stressor or the consequences improve, the symptoms should dissipate within another six months. If you move back home or start to make friends in your new city, the stressor of moving, which has led to being disconnected from your friends, has been resolved, and we can reasonably expect complete remission of the emotional and behavioral symptoms. However, some stressors are ongoing, so

Diagnostic Overview 5.1: Adjustment Disorder

- Emotional or behavioral symptoms that occur as a reaction to a known stressor.
- The symptoms do not meet criteria for another psychological disorder and are not related to bereavement.

Impact:	Symptoms must exceed cultural and contextual norms. Symptoms are related to clinically significant distress or create impairment in important areas of life such as with friends and family or at work or school.
Timeframe:	Symptoms must occur within three months of the stressor. After the stress has improved the symptoms should not remain for more than another six months.

Source: Information from APA (2022).

adjustment disorders can last for a long time. In fact, more than one-third of those who receive a diagnosis of adjustment disorder lasting at least three months still have symptoms twelve months later (O'Donnell et al. 2019).

There is some controversy around adjustment disorders as a diagnosis. Some critics view adjustment disorders as a way to pathologize normal reactions to everyday events. It might be expected that someone would feel sad and lonely after a move to a new city, but is it a psychological disorder? Psychologists hoping to be helpful may see it through the lens of pathology. In addition, in settings where clients cannot receive assistance from psychotherapists without a diagnosis, some therapists may feel pressure to diagnose. In some cases, they may choose a diagnosis of an adjustment disorder because it may not carry the stigma of a more severe diagnosis. And many clinicians feel uncomfortable with the official criteria (Maercker & Lorenz 2018), not because adjustment disorder is difficult to diagnose, but because it's so easy (O'Donnell et al. 2019). Adjustment disorders are intended to be diagnosed only when no other diagnosis fits (see Diagnostic Overview 5.1). However, the research does suggest that while the *DSM* isn't very specific about the types of stressors that cause adjustment disorder, practitioners count a wide variety, including interpersonal conflict, unemployment, financial problems, forced migration, illness of self or others, and exposure to actual or threatened death or violence.

The *DSM* uses five different specifiers to describe the nature of the symptoms: with depressed mood, with anxiety, with mixed anxiety and depressed mood, with disturbance of conduct, and with mixed disturbance of emotions and conduct.

STATISTICS AND TRAJECTORY

Adjustment disorders are diagnosed frequently. A study of psychiatrists ranked them seventh among all mental health categories that are used at least once a week in their practices across 44 countries on 6 continents (Maercker & Lorenz 2018). In another survey of clinical psychologists across 25 countries where psychologists diagnosed them at least once a week in their practice (Evans et al. 2013), adjustment disorders were ranked ninth. Prevalence estimates of adjustment disorders vary dramatically based on the population measured. However, a recent study in Canada suggested it could be 1.3 percent (Leclerc et al. 2020).

There is some evidence that adjustment disorders may portend more serious future conditions. Compared to those who experienced a stressor with no major difficulties, those who were diagnosed with adjustment disorder were more than twice as likely to receive a more serious diagnosis (like PTSD or major depressive disorder) a year later (O'Donnell et al. 2019). This view of adjustment disorder is very different from a catch-all diagnosis.

TREATMENT OF ADJUSTMENT DISORDER

While there are many treatments for PTSD and acute stress disorder, few evidence-based treatments are directly geared toward adjustment disorders. By definition, if the stressor or its consequences have been resolved, then the symptoms should also vanish; however, randomized controlled trials (RCT) of adjustment disorders show a variety of interventions that reduce symptoms while the stressor is still present. While no study has shown medication alone to be an effective first-line defense for adjustment disorders, 74 percent of outpatients so diagnosed receive a combination of medications for anxiety (65 percent), depression (10.8 percent), and sleep (8.1 percent) to reduce their symptoms (Greiner et al. 2020).

Post-Traumatic Stress Disorder (PTSD)

After he returned from Afghanistan, things didn't get much better for TJ Brennan (introduced in the chapter opening story). There are times after a painful experience that create an echo of the event in your mind, as if you are trying to work out how you might have prevented the trauma from occurring in the first place. And yet even though it is past, the event is so painful that it continues causing you harm. Imagine continuing to eat spoiled chicken salad so you can figure out what the strange taste was and make sure not to eat it in the future. But the chicken salad just makes you sick all over again. That's what clients with post-traumatic stress disorder describe. For TJ it was like playing the explosion over and over to figure out where he might have gone wrong. **Post-traumatic stress disorder (PTSD)** is a trauma and stressor-related disorder associated with experiencing a traumatic event, re-experiencing the trauma, and exhibiting symptoms of negative changes in mood and chronic arousal (Diagnostic Overview 5.2).

People throw around the word *trauma* a lot. However, the *DSM* is very specific about the kinds of events that meet the definition of trauma (and the kinds that don't). By this definition (see the diagnostic criteria), a person must be exposed to actual or threatened death, serious injury, or sexual violence.

There are a few ways in which this exposure can happen (Figure 5.4 shows the prevalence of exposure to various traumatic events worldwide), and the *DSM* describes four. A person can be directly exposed to a trauma (such as a mugging, or childhood abuse, or waking during surgery) or watch as the trauma occurs to someone else (seeing someone be the victim of a physical attack). Another way is to learn that a traumatic event has happened to a close family member or a friend (such as hearing about a friend who was involved in a serious car accident). A final type is exposure to details of a trauma such as therapists hearing details of traumatic experiences from their clients or police officers who review crime scene photos or videos. There is some controversy around the *DSM* criteria that allows media exposure to count as a traumatic experience only if it's part of a person's job. For example, in one study those who were present during the Boston Marathon bombing experienced fewer symptoms of stress than those who experienced six or more hours of media

Post-traumatic stress disorder (PTSD): a trauma and stressor-related disorder associated with experiencing a traumatic event, re-experiencing the trauma, and exhibiting symptoms of negative changes in mood and chronic arousal.

Diagnostic Overview 5.2: Post-Traumatic Stress Disorder

Trauma: Exposure to either threats of or actual death, injury, or sexual violence through direct experience, witnessing, or learning it happened to someone you know very well. (Exposure to images of trauma on electronic media is excluded unless viewing the images is a requirement of your job.)

At least one recurrent intrusion symptom associated with the trauma event:

- Distressing memories.
- Distressing dreams.
- Flashbacks.
- Psychological distress at exposure to internal or external cues that symbolize or resemble an aspect of the traumatic event (s).
- Physiological reactions to internal or external cues that symbolize or resemble an aspect of the traumatic event(s).

At least one avoidance symptom associated with the traumatic event(s):

- Avoidance of distressing memories, thoughts, or feelings about the event.
- Avoidance of reminders of the event, like people, places, conversations, activities, objects, and situations that could bring on memories, thoughts, or feelings about or closely associated with the traumatic event(s).

At least two symptoms related to negative alterations in thoughts and mood associated with the traumatic event(s):

- Inability to remember an important aspect of the traumatic event(s).
- Persistent and exaggerated negative beliefs or expectations about self, others, or the world.
- Persistent, distorted thoughts about why the event occurred.
- Persistent negative emotional state.
- Markedly diminished interest or participation in significant activities.
- Feelings of detachment from other people.
- Difficulty experiencing positive feelings.

At least two symptoms associated with arousal and reactivity associated with the traumatic event(s):

- Irritability.
- Reckless behavior.
- Hypervigilance.
- Exaggerated startle response.
- Concentration problems.
- Sleep problems.

Impact: Symptoms must exceed cultural and contextual norms. Symptoms are related to clinically significant distress or create impairment in important areas of life such as with friends and family or at work or school.

Timeframe: At least 30 days.

Source: Information from APA (2022).

related to the bombing. In addition, there is evidence that suggests that watching news accounts of violence can contribute to symptoms of trauma, especially in situations such as the terrorist attacks on September 11, 2001 and media coverage of law enforcement officials who have abused or killed Black Americans (Williams et al. 2018). Supporters of the limitation on media exposure as a criterion suggest that traumatic images in the media are so widespread in the United States that nearly everyone would meet the first criterion for

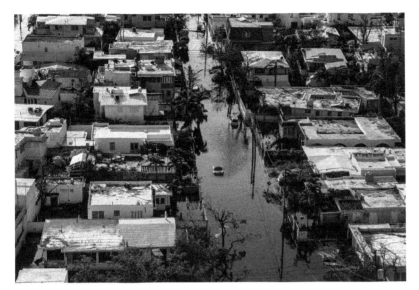

Figure 5.2 Natural disasters such as Hurricane Maria on September 25, 2017 are the kinds of traumatic events that can cause symptoms of PTSD. *Source: Alex Wroblewski/ Bloomberg via Getty Images.*

exposure to trauma, and it would make it difficult for the diagnosis to be useful (see Figures 5.2 and 5.3).

A single traumatic event (such as a hurricane) could produce multiple sources of trauma that could possibly trigger PTSD. Hurricane Maria struck Puerto Rico in the fall of 2017 only two weeks after Hurricane Irma. It was one of the deadliest hurricanes ever to hit the island, and it's estimated that over 3,000 people lost their lives due to the storm. In the aftermath, over a million people lost power, and some 10 weeks after, more than 200,000 people had relocated to Florida. One study showed that rates of PTSD following the storm were 43 percent for those in Puerto Rico (Scaramutti et al. 2019).

Trauma is widespread. A report from the World Health Organization (WHO) found that 70 percent of people worldwide have experienced it (see Figure 5.4 for a breakdown by some selected countries) (Benjet et al. 2016).

The five most common trauma events worldwide, and the percentage of people who have experienced this event (Benjet et al. 2016), are:

- Experiencing accidents/injuries, 36.4 percent.
- Suffering the unexpected death of a loved one, 31.4 percent.
- Witnessing death or a serious injury, 23.7 percent.
- Being mugged, 14.5 percent.
- Being in an automobile accident, 14 percent.

While people respond to trauma in various ways and many have resilient reactions, some do go on to experience grave occupational and personal difficulties from these events. The impact of PTSD is significant. In addition to the many symptoms they experience, those with PTSD are at increased risk of unemployment

Figure 5.3 While watching a horror film might meet some of the criteria of exposure to trauma, such as having a reaction of fear or horror, looking at media images like photographs, television, and film doesn't count as trauma unless your work requires you to view such images.
Sources: SolStock/E+/Getty Images and South_agency/E+/ Getty Images.

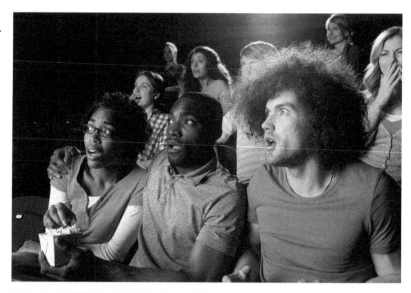

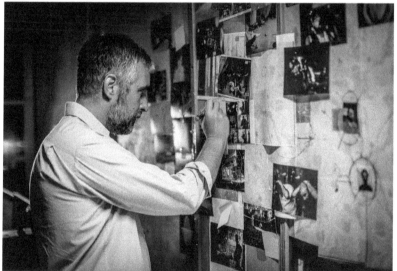

(150 times the rate of those without PTSD) and of relationship instability (more than 60 times). The risk of suicide among those with PTSD is one of the highest among all psychological disorders (Paintain & Cassidy 2018). Fortunately, therapy can help people effectively manage their symptoms.

PTSD is known for producing four types of symptoms related to the trauma (see Diagnostic Overview 5.2):

1. Re-experiencing
2. Avoidance
3. Negative changes in thoughts and mood
4. Hypervigilance and chronic arousal

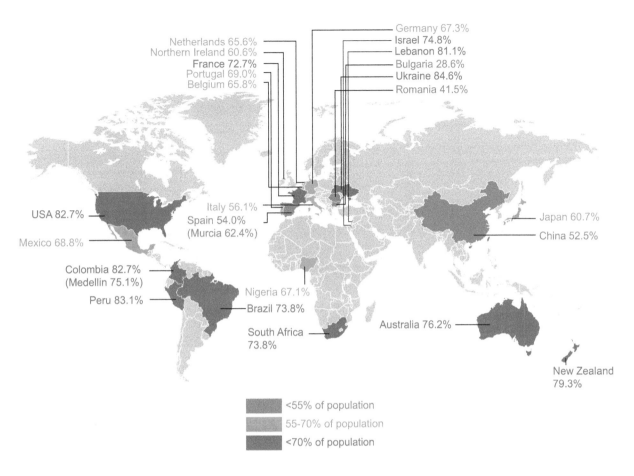

Netherlands 65.6%
Northern Ireland 60.6%
France 72.7%
Portugal 69.0%
Belgium 65.8%

Germany 67.3%
Israel 74.8%
Lebanon 81.1%
Bulgaria 28.6%
Ukraine 84.6%
Romania 41.5%

USA 82.7%

Mexico 68.8%

Italy 56.1%
Spain 54.0%
(Murcia 62.4%)

Japan 60.7%
China 52.5%

Colombia 82.7%
(Medellin 75.1%)

Peru 83.1%

Nigeria 67.1%

Brazil 73.8%

South Africa
73.8%

Australia 76.2%

New Zealand
79.3%

<55% of population
55–70% of population
<70% of population

Figure 5.4 Prevalence of exposure to any traumatic event in a survey of 24 countries.
Source: Benjet et al. (2016).

THE POWER OF WORDS

SHELL SHOCK

PTSD is often associated with the trauma of combat. You may even have heard the term "shell shock" being associated with the trauma of war, but is shell shock the same as what we understand as PTSD?

After World War I, some veterans from the war came back with a mix of symptoms such as paralysis, amnesia, and even difficulty in communication, except they had no injury that might lead to these symptoms (Figure 5.5). One of the early researchers to describe what was then known as shell shock was Charles Myers (Linden & Jones 2014). Myers' early hypothesis was that the symptoms came from blasts leading to concussions as the result of being near wartime explosions, even though many veterans with these symptoms had never

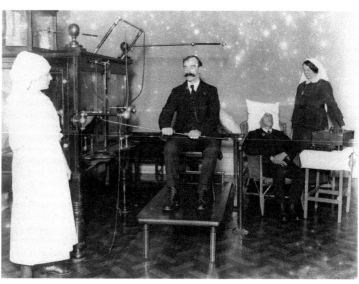

Figure 5.5 Nurses at the Sir William Hospital using experimental medical equipment on soldiers experiencing shell shock.
Source: Central Press/Getty Images.

experienced the blasts. The *British Medical Journal* in 1922 presented a nonphysical explanation of the symptoms and described them as a result of "poor morale."

The idea of shell shock then changed from a physical injury to a sign of weakness. Treatments for it were focused on the assumption that those who experienced the symptoms were weak and needed to be shaken out of their condition. Louis Yealland described some of the common treatments in his 1918 paper (Yealland 1918). They included electric shocks, hot cigarettes to the tongue, hot plates, and instead of support, pleas to the patient with phrases such as, "You must behave as the hero I expect you to be."

Some believed shell shock was at best a sign of cowardice and at worst malingering. Many who displayed symptoms were thought of as military criminals, subject to military discipline, put on trial, seen as deserters, and even executed.

It wasn't until the late 1960s that different thinking around the impact of trauma emerged. Post-Vietnam syndrome, for example, was considered not a sign of weakness but an expected response from war. With this new thinking, a new way to talk about the symptoms emerged. After that, the Veterans Administration lobbied to get post-traumatic stress disorder added to the DSM III.

What we now understand as PTSD has been referred to as combat stress reaction, battle fatigue, soldier's heart, operational exhaustion, and post-concussion syndrome, and of course now we know that it comes not only from combat but from a variety of traumatic experiences. Some people with symptoms of PTSD like TJ Brennan (and some without) still see the symptoms as a weakness, which can have an impact on the way they think about themselves and their willingness to seek treatment.

Sources: Shell shock (1922); Yealland (1918); Yehuda (2002).

The lifetime prevalence of PTSD is 3.9 percent in the general population, according to a 26-nation population survey from the WHO (although the rates vary by country). Even when we consider only the most serious of traumas (such as experiencing accidents/injuries or the unexpected death of a loved one), the prevalence can range from 1.7 percent in countries such as South Korea to 9.2 percent in Canada. The average in the United States is about 8 percent (Koenen et al. 2017).

PTSD occurs later in life than some other disorders, though this statistic can vary by country as well. The median age is 25–43, with younger individuals at greater risk because they are more often exposed to the types of trauma that are themselves likely to carry a greater risk of PTSD. People in their twenties are more likely to be involved in accidents or to join the military, for example (Koenen et al. 2017).

Acute Stress Disorder

In the initial days after a traumatic experience, many people have a flood of symptoms, but the criteria for PTSD don't allow for a diagnosis until a full 30 days of symptoms have passed. For **acute stress disorder (ASD)**, in contrast, the timeframe can be shorter (Diagnostic Overview 5.3). The name means not that the stressor itself is more severe than in PTSD, but rather that the disorder is diagnosed sooner than the 30 days required by PTSD (acute in this instance refers to the shortened timeframe of the diagnosis). Some people with acute stress disorder are at higher risk for developing PTSD (Bryant et al. 2011), but not all.

Acute stress disorder (ASD): A trauma and stressor-related disorder in which people have symptoms of PTSD lasting up to 30 days.

Although many of the symptoms of acute stress disorder are similar to those of PTSD, the diagnosis is a little different. Instead of exhibiting certain symptoms in certain clusters, for a diagnosis of ASD a person has to meet the criteria for a trauma and have nine or more of 14 listed symptoms within the same 30-day period.

Traumatic Events

About 10 percent of people exposed to a traumatic experience will develop PTSD (De Vries & Olff 2009), and the more severe and the longer-lasting the trauma, the more likely is the development of the disorder (Hyland et al. 2017). Some traumas, such as those associated with combat or abuse, are also more likely to produce PTSD than others (Sareen 2014; Sareen et al. 2018).

Elevated rates of both ASD and PTSD have also been discovered by researchers after natural disasters such as floods and tornadoes, and accidents such as serious car accidents and airplane crashes. Between 12 percent and 40 percent of people involved in traffic accidents may develop symptoms of ASD or PTSD within the year following the accident (Sareen et al. 2018). Nearly 30 percent of Vietnam veterans experienced symptoms of either ASD or PTSD (Hermes et al. 2014). In one study, more than half of people who experienced sexual violence went on to develop PTSD, compared to 7.5 percent involved in accidents (Kessler ct al.

Diagnostic Overview 5.3: Acute Stress Disorder

After the presence of a trauma, nine or more symptoms appear from any of the following five categories:

Intrusion Symptoms
- Distressing memories of the traumatic event.
- Distressing dreams of the traumatic event.
- Flashbacks.
- Psychological distress or physiological reactions in response to things that might symbolize the trauma.

Negative Mood
- Inability to experience positive emotions.

Dissociative Symptoms
- Altered sense of the reality of surroundings or self.
- Inability to remember an important aspect of the traumatic event(s).

Avoidance Symptoms
- Avoidance of difficult memories, thoughts, or feelings of the event.
- Avoidance of external reminders that might trigger memories, thoughts, or feelings about the event.

Arousal Symptoms
- Difficulty with sleep.
- Irritability.
- Hypervigilance.
- Problems with concentration.
- Exaggerated startle response.

Impact: Symptoms must exceed cultural and contextual norms. Symptoms are related to clinically significant distress or create impairment in important areas of life such as with friends and family or at work or school.

Timeframe: Duration of symptoms is from 3 to 30 days.

Source: Information from APA (2022).

1994). Events that are less controllable and less predictable are often associated with a more intense trauma response.

Nearly half (46 percent) of people who have been sexually assaulted develop PTSD (Zinzaw et al. 2012), and symptoms can appear shortly after and/or persist four to five years later (Faravelli et al. 2004). Those who have been subjected to abuse have symptoms that linger as well; one-third of victims of physical assault develop symptoms of PTSD, as do nearly half of those who are exposed to terrorism or torture (Sareen et al. 2018).

Sociocultural factors may influence who is the victim of abuse, and trauma exposure can be a reflection of systematic issues. Women, for example are at higher risk for sexual violence. In one study of a college campus, 13 percent of women and 5 percent of men reported a sexual assault, and 20 percent of women and 10 percent of men reported relationship violence (Howard et al. 2019). Sexual and gender minorities are at a particularly high risk for bullying. One study found that 91 percent of LGBTQ adolescents reported at least one experience of bias-based bullying (Lessard et al. 2020), a rate nearly double that for heterosexual adolescents.

Models and Treatments of Post-Traumatic Stress Disorder and Acute Stress Disorder

As with other psychological conditions, researchers have examined biological, psychodynamic, cognitive, behavioral, and sociocultural ways to think about and treat trauma and stressor-related conditions. Despite the distressing nature of the symptoms of PTSD and the variety of treatments available, typically less than two-thirds of those who experience PTSD (58 percent) will seek treatment (Roscoe 2021). Some avoid getting help because they are also avoiding thinking about the trauma. In a study of more than 7,600 veterans who were diagnosed with PTSD, those who sought treatment lived close to a mental health clinic, had knowledge about the signs of PTSD, believed treatment would help them get better, and had greater social support from friends (Spoont et al. 2014). However, many people with PTSD put off seeking treatment. TJ Brennan was no different. Once he returned home, it took him seven months to start therapy for his PTSD, and now he feels stronger after treatment.

BIOLOGICAL MODELS AND TREATMENTS

We know a good deal about how the body handles stressful situations, as we discussed in Chapter 4. But the way the body deals with stress after trauma may be different from the way it handles stress in general, and that may play a role in the development of the symptoms of PTSD. There are several biological findings that help explain post-traumatic stress disorder. Some focus on biochemical aspects, while others focus on neurobiology or genetics.

Biochemical models of PTSD look at the role of chemicals such as hormones and neurotransmitters in the stress response. In Chapter 4 we discussed that when people are stressed, the hypothalamus stimulates both the sympathetic nervous system and the hypothalamic pituitary adrenal (HPA) axis. The HPA axis is a brain/body pathway that is the primary mediator of hormone production for the stress response. Those who develop PTSD or ASD have a heightened reaction in these two stress pathways (Sherin & Nemeroff 2011). This activation can cause increased heart rate and raise epinephrine, norepinephrine, and cortisol levels. High levels of cortisol can in turn damage the hippocampus, which regulates other stress hormones and is important in learning and memory systems. Overexposure to epinephrine, norepinephrine, and cortisol can create the phobic response that causes memories to be overlearned. These overlearned memories in turn may form some of the symptoms of PTSD and ASD (see Figure 5.6).

Neurobiological models of PTSD study brain areas and circuits that might be responsible for the symptoms of PTSD. These include areas that are responsible for fear and panic, such as the amygdala, prefrontal cortex, and the hippocampus. For example, some evidence suggests that an ongoing sense of fear can overwhelm a person's ability to cope.

Some research shows smaller areas of the brain such as the hippocampus in people with PTSD. This reduced size of the hippocampus may be due to chronic

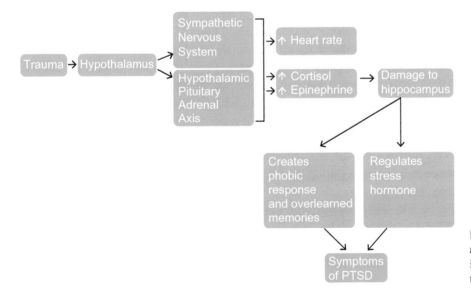

Figure 5.6 Several chemical and biological changes can be influenced by exposure to trauma.

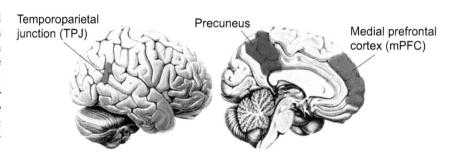

stress to the neurotransmitters and hormones released during stress (Britton &
Rauch 2009). That may explain why those with PTSD can have trouble remembering parts of the traumatic events they experienced, since the hippocampus is
involved in encoding memories.

Neuroimaging techniques have revealed differences in brain activity between
people with and without PTSD in terms of their response to threats. For example,
another part of the brain that's involved in PTSD is the medial prefrontal cortex
(see Figure 5.7), which affects the way the amygdala reacts to emotional stimulation. It is not as active in those with fewer symptoms of PTSD. This means that
those with severe PTSD may be more reactive to emotional stimulation and not as
able to control their reactions (Shin et al. 2011).

Genetic models of PTSD explain the disorder as due at least in part to inherited
predisposition. For example, one study looked at 4,000 twins who had served in
combat; one twin in each pair had PTSD. The researcher found that the other twin
was more likely to also have the disorder if they were monozygotic (identical)
rather than dizygotic twins (Uddin et al. 2012).

Some people may also be at greater risk of developing PTSD than others, based on
accumulated environmental adversity that affects DNA. Although we typically think
we're stuck with the genes we received at conception, there's a bit more to the story.

The Human Genome Project was a $2.7-billion 15-year effort to map out all the
3 billion base pairs that make up human DNA and find out what makes a human.
But what the researchers discovered was that even after they decoded all 3 billion
letters, a task that was completed in 2003, something was missing. It turns out that
DNA sequences are just the beginning when it comes to understanding genetic
traits. Genetics simply determines what genes people have. But a gene has to be
turned on to be helpful; it does nothing if it's silent or turned off. It seems that not
every gene is activated, and some can be switched off or silenced by the body in a
process called **methylation**. In this process, a small marker, just one carbon and
three hydrogen atoms, is attached to a section of DNA and switches it off (see
Figure 5.8). These changes don't involve changes in the specific gene sequences.
What does that mean? It means that the *expression* of the affected gene is changed
without changing the genetic code.

Methylation: a process by which
a gene may be switched on or off
by the body.

What can cause methylation? Many things: food, sleep, exercise, and even
trauma can cause chemical modifications around the genes that turn them on or

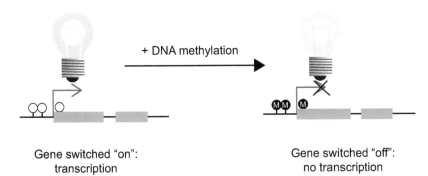

Gene switched "on":   Gene switched "off":
transcription   no transcription

Figure 5.8 Methylation is a process that can either activate or repress gene expression.

off over time. If you think about our DNA as the notes in a song, the notes may always be the same, but the way they are played depends on their expression. The study of these kinds of changes in genes is called *epigenetics.*

Methylation is powerful. For example, when a honeybee is fed royal jelly (a substance secreted by worker bees), methylation causes the bee to grow larger, live longer, develop ovaries, and become a queen bee. Methylation patterns are also affected by behaviors. Let's imagine a mother rat (called a dam) has a mischief (a litter) of pups. There are so many pups that some get lots of attention, like licks and grooming, and others are ignored. Rats change their DNA methylation patterns based on how much attention they are given by their mothers when they are young. In pups whose mothers give them a lot of attention, a gene that helps moderate stress is activated. When a mother rat ignores or neglects the pups, the gene remains silenced. Because of this, pups of attentive mothers grow up to be less stressed, while the pups of neglectful mothers grow up anxious. If you examined the genes themselves, however, they would be identical. What's different? The gene's expression – which is determined by the behavior of the mother.

In one study, researchers compared the genes of combat veterans diagnosed with PTSD to those combat veterans without PTSD. Results showed that those with PTSD had lower levels of methylation on certain key genes involved in the HPA axis (Hossack et al. 2020). The theory is that the trauma may have influenced the way certain key genes are expressed. Of course, resilience plays a pivotal role in who might develop PTSD in the future, and not everyone will develop the disorder because of methylation. But methylation may play a role. Several genes may be implicated in susceptibility to trauma disorders (Sheerin et al. 2017).

From a biological perspective, medication such as SSRIs, which increase the availability of the neurotransmitter serotonin to the serotonin receptor sites, have been used to help relieve the symptoms of PTSD (see Table 5.1). Other medications such as tricyclics, MAOS, and benzodiazepines have been used as well, but the American Psychological Association Clinical Practice

Table 5.1 Some FDA-approved medications for PTSD

Generic name	Brand name	Class of medication
paroxetine	Paxil	Selective serotonin reuptake inhibitor
sertraline	Zoloft	Selective serotonin reuptake inhibitor

Source: Information from Stahl (2017).

Guidelines (Courtois et al. 2017) call for medicines typically thought of as antidepressants such as Prozac (fluoxetine), Paxil (paroxetine), Zoloft (sertraline), and Effexor (venlafaxine) as first-line medications for PTSD.

PSYCHODYNAMIC MODELS AND TREATMENTS

Psychodynamic theories suggest that the symptoms of PTSD are a normal response to an abnormal event. According to one such theory, the intensity of the trauma can create an upheaval of emotions and memory complications in clients. This memory effect produces some of the symptoms of PTSD. It can cause clients to have trouble understanding themselves, while vacillation between flashbacks and hazy recollections of the trauma can also prevent the formation of a narrative that makes sense to the client. From a psychodynamic perspective, without even realizing it, the client may be unconsciously repeating the trauma, or experiences that recall the trauma, in an attempt to reorganize this disorganized memory and seek control over the experience (Figure 5.9).

There is limited evidence for the effectiveness of psychodynamic therapy for PTSD (Paintain & Cassidy 2018). The idea is to confront the trauma and work with the therapist to understand what the event means to the client and to their life. Psychodynamic therapy has been found to be effective, with up to 50 percent of participants diagnosis-free in follow-up (Paintain & Cassidy 2018). However, it tends not to be as effective as exposure-based approaches to trauma (more on this later). Psychodynamic approaches also tend to take longer than other therapies.

One evidence-based psychodynamic treatment for PTSD was developed from the Panic-Focused Psychodynamic Psychotherapy (PFPP) described in Chapter 4 (Busch et al. 2012). The main treatment from this psychodynamic perspective is to help clients create a coherent understanding of the traumatic experience.

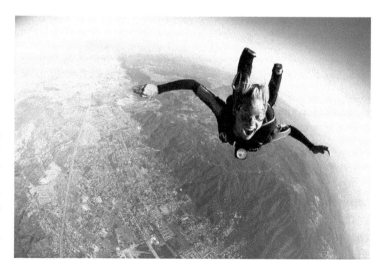

Figure 5.9 The psychodynamic model suggests that clients may seek out ways to repeat trauma without even being aware of it. This may explain the reckless behavior in which some people with PTSD engage.

Source: Joe McBride/The Image Bank/Getty Images.

COGNITIVE-BEHAVIORAL MODELS AND TREATMENTS

From a behavioral perspective, PTSD is, in part, a learned reaction to trauma-related cues. For example, imagine a person involved in a car accident where a certain song was playing in the car. The song started as an unconditioned stimulus and is paired with the emotional and physical pain of the car accident which naturally produced fear (unconditioned response). After the accident the person may react strongly (conditioned response) to the same song (conditioned stimulus) or react with fear to things associated with the song or the neighborhood in the future. The person has learned that the song feels dangerous and is working to protect themselves by eliciting the fight, flee, or freeze response. In addition, operant conditioning can help maintain this behavior over time. If the song produces fear and related sympathetic arousal and behaviors, then the person may avoid such songs or parts of town which removes anxiety from their lives.

A number of treatment guidelines recommend CBT as a first-line therapy for PTSD. Cognitive-behavioral approaches to trauma are some of the most highly researched and frequently used means of understanding PTSD.

Certain personalities and coping strategies may be more likely to lead to ASD and PTSD. For example, children who were more anxious before Hurricane Hugo, which struck the Caribbean and the southeast United States in 1989, were more likely to develop severe stress reactions. People who view negative events as beyond their control (Catanesi et al. 2013) and people who can't seem to find the positive in any negative events also seem to have more difficulty adjusting to traumatic situations (Kunst et al. 2011).

Emotional processing theory suggests that traumatic events can create problems if not processed adequately at the time of the event. According to the theory, fear usually activates an association with the object of the fear, ways to avoid or escape the fear, and what the fear means. For example, if you are attacked by a dog, you may build associative networks to know what the fear is about (the dog), how to avoid or escape the fear (recognizing the dog and staying away from it), and what the fear means (dogs are threatening and should be avoided). Fear becomes problematic when it creates associations that are so intense that they exist even in the absence of danger.

Emotional processing theory: a theory which suggests that traumatic events can lead to problems if they are not processed adequately.

Trauma can lead to chronic avoidance of potentially fearful situations in the environment, or to the creation of meanings about the fear that are maladaptive. For example, rather than thinking that some dogs are dangerous, a person may think, "I should have known that the dog was dangerous, and that means I'm terrible at knowing what's dangerous and what's not." Emotional processing theory suggests that habituation, in the form of prolonged exposure, can counteract trauma. The idea behind prolonged exposure (PE) technique is to help clients activate their fears so they can incorporate new information about the trauma and create a new structure to process it in a more adaptive way.

PE is typically completed in 8–15 sessions of in-person or imaged exposure. Research suggests that exposure techniques in general are more effective for

PTSD. Among PE participants, 41–95 percent no longer had PTSD at the end of their treatment (Jonas et al. 2013). Many therapists worry, however, that exposing their clients to their traumas will increase their distress, and that is one of the biggest reasons it is not used more often (van Minnen et al. 2010). In a survey of 207 licensed psychologists, 83 percent never opted for exposure therapy to treat their clients with PTSD (Becker et al. 2004).

The dropout rate for PE can be high, too, hovering around 28 percent (Swift & Greenberg 2014). In a study of more than 2,000 veterans with PTSD in PE treatment, the dropout rate appeared to be related not to inability to tolerate the treatment, the severity of symptoms, or the specifics of treatment, but rather to avoidance of the treatment itself. Most likely to drop out were those who were younger, especially if they had barriers to treatment such as work obligations and childcare responsibilities (Eftekhari et al. 2020).

Another treatment for PTSD is called Cognitive Processing Therapy or CPT. CPT assumes that people who have experienced traumatic events try to make sense of them and in the process over-accommodate for the trauma, creating maladaptive cognitions about themselves, other people, and the world. These maladaptive cognitions help to maintain the symptoms of PTSD (Scher et al. 2017).

Cognitive processing therapy uses many of the same techniques as CBT. Its goal is to help assess the client's ability to understand current threats and to replace unhealthy coping strategies (symptoms of PTSD) with more adaptive ones (see Figure 5.10). It focuses on identifying and challenging some of the maladaptive thoughts that people with PTSD and ASD often have about themselves and the world. For example, TJ Brennan often talked about how he sometimes blamed himself for what happened to him. CPT therapists can use worksheets such as the one in Figure 5.11 to help clients examine the evidence of their thoughts and show them how these thoughts might be linked to the way they feel and behave.

CPT consists of 12 weekly sessions and is effective, with 30–97 percent of clients no longer meeting the diagnosis of PTSD by the end of their treatment (Jonas et al. 2013). However, it does have a dropout rate of nearly 20 percent (18.28 percent) (Watkins et al. 2018).

Figure 5.10 The CBT framework (A) suggests an interaction between the way we think, feel, and behave. In those with PTSD, maladaptive thoughts such as "I am in danger" when there is no danger can produce feelings of anxiety and cause the person to avoid non-dangerous situations (B). One goal of PTSD is to facilitate change in thoughts, which should also change behaviors and feelings (C).

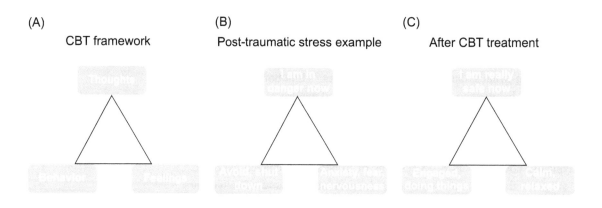

(A) CBT framework
(B) Post-traumatic stress example
(C) After CBT treatment

Your role in the traumatic event: What are the facts?

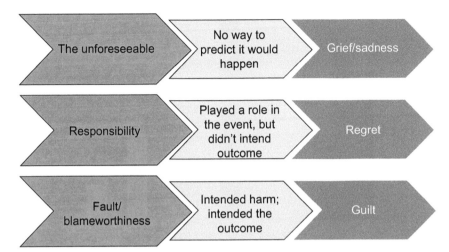

Figure 5.11 A CBT worksheet for helping clients develop more adaptive responses about their role in traumatic events.
Source: Adapted from Williams et al. (2018).

SOCIOCULTURAL MODELS OF PTSD

Culture and systematic inequalities can also play a role in the prevention and development of PTSD. Black Americans have higher rates of PTSD than do white, Hispanic, and Asian Americans (Roberts et al. 2011) (Figure 5.12). Black Americans reported greater rates of trauma from domestic violence and violent assault, and Asian Americans reported greater amounts of trauma related to being a civilian in a war zone. Most racially marginalized populations were less likely to seek treatment for trauma, which may be due to mistrust of physicians (Alim et al. 2006) and reduced access to mental health facilities (Chow et al. 2003) or access to health care (Roberts et al. 2011).

Women are more likely than men to have PTSD; some 20 percent of women who are exposed to a severe trauma develop the disorder (the figure is 8 percent for men). Women may experience more triggers for PTSD, including sexual abuse, and may not have access to the supports they need after the trauma (Resick & Calhoun 2001).

Income and psychological factors can also be related to the way people respond to trauma. People with lower incomes are nearly two times more likely to experience ASD or PTSD (Sareen et al. 2018). And those experiencing depression or anxiety prior to trauma are more likely to develop PTSD (Cardozo et al. 2003).

Clients who have experienced the negative impact of racial discrimination may be more likely to have higher rates of PTSD (Comas-Díaz 2016). Examples include mistreatment in the workplace and harassment by some law enforcement officials. Figure 5.13 shows how racial trauma can lead to symptoms of PTSD (Williams et al. 2018). Some therapists may feel uncomfortable discussing race and may neglect to have conversations with racially marginalized clients who may have experienced racism.

What people do after the trauma can also be related to the incidence of PTSD. Those who choose avoidance strategies such as drinking or isolating from friends

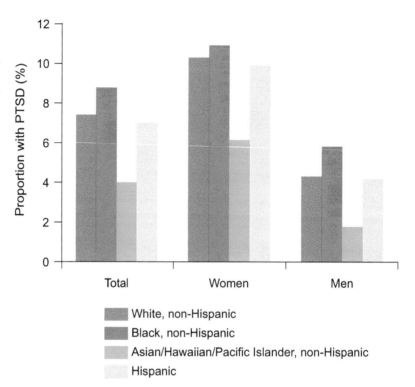

Figure 5.12 US lifetime prevalence of PTSD by race, 2011. There are racial/ethnic differences in the prevalence of PTSD, which may reflect difference in the types of exposure to trauma, access to care, or variations among those seeking treatment.

Source: Adapted from Roberts et al. (2011).

can increase their likelihood of developing PTSD symptoms (Merrill et al. 2001). These include dissociative symptoms such as feeling like they are someplace else, in another person's body, or outside themselves and watching the trauma unfold (Friedman et al. 2011). Those who have the social support of others after a trauma are less likely to develop long-lasting symptoms of PTSD (van der Velden et al. 2012). For example, a meta-analysis examining 15 studies that explored the relationship between social support and psychological wellbeing in people who experienced the violent death of a loved one showed that people with social support had fewer symptoms of PTSD (Scott, Pitman, et al. 2020).

Sociocultural factors and systematic inequity can also influence our development of – or our resilience toward – traumatic experiences. People who have less support and less education are more likely to have a diagnosis of PTSD. Those with weaker support systems are more likely to develop PTSD after being exposed to traumas (Alipour & Ahmadi 2020; Sareen et al. 2018). When those who experience stressors feel valued by their friends and family, they tend to experience the stressor less severely. This is one of the reasons it's important to be a source of social support for the people in your life who are experiencing trauma.

The experience of trauma isn't universal, and many people who experience it can also feel stigmatized. Stigma can be another factor that contributes to the development of PTSD and stress disorders (Bonfils et al. 2018).

There are some limitations on sociocultural research. Research data might be affected by the fact that some people don't respond to surveys, and by the relative

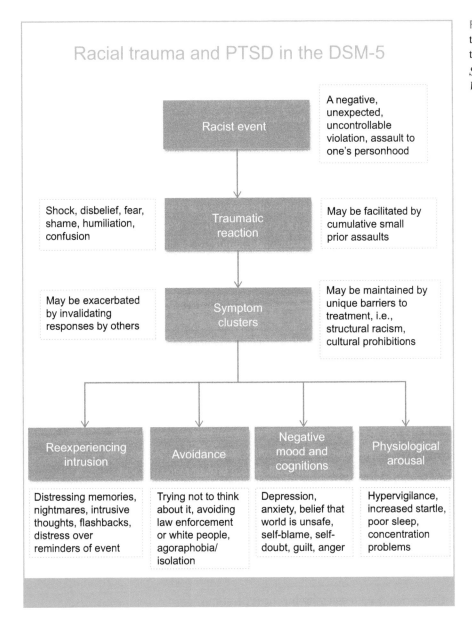

Figure 5.13 Example of racial trauma within the framework of the *DSM*.

Source: Adapted from Williams et al. (2018).

willingness of those who do respond to discuss their traumas with researchers, especially traumas associated with stigma. And some relevant data are understandably hard to collect, such as in the aftermath of mass violence, so this kind of trauma might not be represented sufficiently.

MULTIPERSPECTIVE MODELS AND TREATMENTS

Those with PTSD also have children who are more likely to have PTSD (Cook et al. 2017). For example, women who were pregnant during the September

11 terrorist attack in 2001 and who have developed PTSD (Yehuda et al. 2007) had higher than average levels of cortisol (related to the trauma of the terrorist attack), and their babies did as well.

Other experiences in childhood are also associated with ASD and PTSD (Ross et al. 2017). Poverty and chronic neglect and abuse can lead to overreactive stress pathways and the dysfunctional stress circuits associated with ASD and PTSD (Kraaijenvanger et al. 2020). And those who grow up in a family with significant psychological disorder (Hyland et al. 2017) are also at an increased risk for PTSD.

To sum up, what are the main characteristics associated with PTSD? Clients tend to be younger, female, single, unemployed, and have a lower education level and lower household income (Koenen et al. 2017). Societal inequalities may lead people who are younger, female, and single to be unemployed, achieve lower education levels, and earn lower incomes.

CONCEPT CHECK 5.1

Post-traumatic stress disorder has four different clusters of symptoms. For each example, indicate the type of symptom and the correct cluster (intrusion, avoidance, negative alteration of thought and mood, or arousal and reactivity).

1. Even when walking around, TJ will suddenly remember how his friends were injured in combat. These memories are extremely upsetting to him.
2. TJ has dreams about combat.
3. TJ does whatever he can in order not to think about his time in combat.
4. TJ believes his wife will think he's a broken man.
5. TJ finds it difficult to focus when he reads.

THE POWER OF EVIDENCE

Can moving your eyes help process trauma?

Eye movement desensitization and reprocessing, or EMDR therapy, was developed in 1987 to help clients process traumatic memories. The client is asked to focus on emotionally disturbing material while tracking the therapist's finger taps or movements with their eyes. Shapiro (2001) hypothesizes that EMDR therapy helps to repair the traumatic memory network and create more adaptive associations with the traumatic memory. However, the treatment has critics, with the harshest calling it a pseudoscience. Is EMDR an effective treatment for PTSD and other psychological disorders? Let's look at the evidence.

A recent meta-analysis (Cuijpers, Veen, et al. 2020) included 77 randomized controlled trials (RCTs) of EMDR with 3,309 clients. Most were diagnosed with

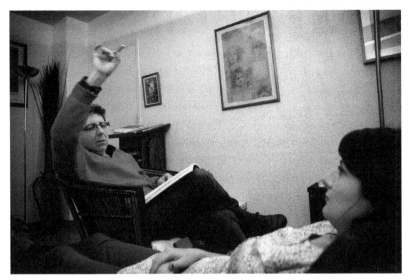

Figure 5.14 Eye movement desensitization and reprocessing (EMDR) might be an effective treatment for PTSD; however, its effectiveness may have nothing to do with the eye movements that are at the heart of the treatment's underlying theory.
Source: BSIP/Universal Images Group via Getty Images.

PTSD and a few from anxiety and depression. The meta-analysis found EMDR to be an effective treatment for PTSD. Why isn't this surprising? One reason is that both the WHO and the APA list EMDR as an evidence-based treatment for PTSD, and more than 60,000 clinicians have been certified in it. Then why the controversy over this treatment? Let's dig deeper.

First, among the 77 studies, only a handful had a low risk of bias. Second, those that did, didn't reveal significant differences between EMDR and other therapies for PTSD. So does this mean EMDR is a unique and useful treatment for PTSD? Sort of.

One of the biggest critiques of EMDR is that it is essentially an exposure technique, in which the finger tapping and eye movements are not essential and asking the clients to remember the trauma is the real therapy (Figure 5.14). This would mean that the eye movements in EMDR have nothing to do with its ability to be helpful for PTSD. What's more, when they looked at the outcomes of EMDR for conditions other than PTSD, such as depression, pain, or obsessive-compulsive disorder, the meta-analysis authors concluded, "There is not enough evidence for the use of EMDR for mental health problems other than PTSD."

If you are disappointed that the 77 randomized controlled trials didn't reveal why EMDR sometimes works for PTSD, that's not what RCTs do. "Trials can show *if* a treatment works, but to show *how* a treatment works is much more complicated" (Cuijpers, Veen, et al. 2020). That's the power – and the limitation – of evidence.

Sources: Cuijpers, Veen, et al. (2020); Shapiro (2001).

5.2 DISSOCIATIVE DISORDERS

Dissociation: a split of your consciousness or attention into separate streams.

Imagine running into someone who knows you well and having no recollection of the dinner you shared with them. Or finding unfamiliar objects in your home, unexpected purchases on your credit card statement, or strange text messages to people with names you don't know. **Dissociation** is a split of your consciousness or attention into separate streams, a feeling of being disconnected or separated from yourself, watching things happen without feeling them. We all dissociate every now and then. Maybe you are doing a presentation and thinking about lunch at the same time, or reading about psychology and wondering how much longer the chapter will be. These are common forms of normal dissociation. Dissociation can also be a way to escape from stressful or traumatic situations.

Dissociative disorders: disorders characterized by a sudden loss of the integration of consciousness, identity, or memory.

Dissociation becomes problematic only when the streams of consciousness become too separate, disjointed, and fragmented, and the integration of the personality is lost. This is what we see in the dissociative disorders. **Dissociative disorders** are characterized by a sudden loss of the integration of consciousness, a change in a person's identity, or even amnesia because the streams of consciousness become so separate and distinct. Sometimes the streams may even take on a life of their own.

Dissociative disorders can occur when a stressful event becomes overwhelming and the individual escapes by diverting awareness from painful memories, thoughts, and emotions. Sometimes in dissociative states individuals escape conflicts by giving up consistency and rejecting a part of themselves. This observation is supported by evidence that many people with dissociative disorders report high rates of trauma. Between 57 percent and 90 percent have reported childhood sexual trauma, 57 percent emotional trauma, and up to 82 percent physical trauma (Sar 2011).

Dissociative symptoms are found in many psychological disorders, including obsessive-compulsive disorder, borderline personality disorder, and functional neurological symptom disorder (conversion disorder) (Sar 2011). And dissociative specifiers are found in conditions such as post-traumatic stress disorder (APA 2022).

Psychopathologists describe three main dissociative disorders: dissociative identity disorder (DID), dissociative amnesia, and depersonalization-derealization disorder.

Dissociative Identity Disorder

Dissociative identity disorder (DID): a dissociative disorder in which two or more distinct identities, sometimes called *alters*, exist inside one person, each with its own unique characteristics.

Dissociation is a splitting of your consciousness and attention, sometimes so extreme that an identity created in the process can take on a life of its own. This is the case in **dissociative identity disorder (DID)**. You might know DID under its older name, multiple personality disorder. However, DID is a more accurate name since it highlights the importance of dissociation in the disorder (Figure 5.15).

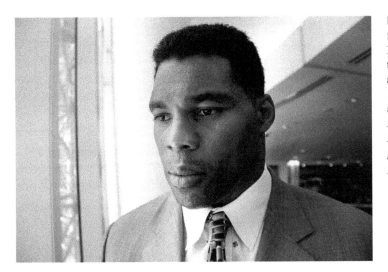

Figure 5.15 Herschel Walker, a former National Football League player who played with the Cowboys, Vikings, Phillies, and Giants and won the 1982 Heisman trophy, is the author of the book *Breaking Free: My Life with Dissociative Identity Disorder* (2008).
Source: Paul Goguen/ Bloomberg via Getty Images.

In DID, two or more distinct identities, sometimes called *alters*, exist inside one person, each with its own unique characteristics. Dramatic differences have been reported in the identities of the alters. The primary or host identity will be in control of the person most of the time. Often memories of the behaviors of the alters are shrouded by amnesia, which may result in gaps in the memories of the other identities. Fortunately, many people with DID do recall some of their alters' information and memory (Allen & Iacono 2001). Alters can have various functions and forms, such as children who might be linked to childhood trauma, or protector and helper personalities. Shifts between alters can often be initiated by stressful circumstances. Some theories suggest that alters are not part of a fractured personality but instead that trauma has prevented the continuity of self that typically would develop over many situations. In this view, a person with DID could have something more like a "never-assembled" personality than a shattered one (Loewenstein 2018).

DID has a long and storied diagnostic history. Some researchers question whether it is a valid diagnosis; after all, before 1980 it was rare to hear of a case and only a few hundred had been reported, but after its inclusion in *DSM-III*, reports of DID started to appear more often. The increase in cases, now reaching into the thousands, was probably due in part to the new diagnostic criteria, which made it easier to categorize clients who might have previously been diagnosed as having a psychotic disorder such as schizophrenia. A series of publications in the 1980s also described cases of clients with DID and piqued the interest of people in the mental health community. Some researchers believe DID may be partially or completely iatrogenic, meaning it is produced (unintentionally) by clinicians (Foote et al. 2006). When clinicians begin to see symptoms that might resemble DID, they may unintentionally encourage them either in therapy or when the client is under hypnosis. They may also give clients more attention when they are expressing symptoms of DID and thus reinforce the DID symptoms. It remains a rare diagnosis, however, and

- Two or more distinct identities or personalities in an individual. This disruption might be described as an experience of possession and could involve a disruption in the sense of self. It could be reported by the person or observed by others.
- Gaps in memory beyond normal forgetting.

Impact: Symptoms must exceed cultural and contextual norms. Symptoms are related to clinically significant distress or create impairment in important areas of life such as with friends and family or at work or school.

Source: Information from APA (2022).

even today people are often definitively diagnosed only after they have received up to three diagnoses before DID (such as for schizophrenia, anxiety disorders, major depressive disorders, or personality disorders) (Dorahy et al. 2014; Rodewald et al. 2011) (see Diagnostic Overview 5.4).

The shift in prevalence of DID may indicate that we are much better at diagnosing it, and that those who need treatment are able to get it. For some, however, the dramatic increase in incidence rates raises suspicion about the existence of the condition, mostly due to the lack of a clear cause for the disorder (Brand et al. 2016).

It's difficult to estimate the prevalence of DID. Some studies find the range to be anywhere between 1 percent and 6 percent of patients. For example, a study of two upstate New York counties found the prevalence of DID to be 1.5 percent of the population (Sar 2011).

Dissociative Amnesia

Dissociative amnesia: a condition in which people forget important personal information much more than you would expect with normal forgetfulness.

Imagine waking up one day with no idea where you are. You are dazed, confused, and unsure of much of anything. A moment later, you also realize you aren't even sure who you are. It's frightening. In **dissociative amnesia**, people forget important personal information much more than you would expect with normal forgetfulness (Diagnostic Overview 5.5). They may not remember their own identity, including their birthday, address, or even their name, even though they haven't had any sort of injury. Some with dissociative amnesia forget all the details of their lives and are found wandering the street confused and bewildered. However, the disorder is fairly self-limiting and doesn't last longer than a week or so, and the person's entire memory soon returns.

Some researchers suggest that dissociative amnesia can be triggered by a severe emotional event such as physical abuse, a natural disaster, combat, or

Diagnostic Overview 5.5: Dissociative Amnesia

Inability to recall important personal information, usually associated with events of a traumatic or stressful nature.

With dissociative fugue:	Travel or wandering that is associated with amnesia.
Impact:	Symptoms must exceed cultural and contextual norms. Symptoms are related to clinically significant distress or create impairment in important areas of life such as with friends and family or at work or school.

Source: Information from APA (2022).

involvement in violence. A type of specifier for the disorder is called **dissociative fugue**. In addition to experiencing amnesia, people with dissociative fugue may drive away from home and start a new life in a new location, often a great distance away (fugue means flight). Like those with dissociative amnesia, people in such fugue states will often recover their memory all at once and have amnesia about the fugue period. As rare as the disorder is (the prevalence of dissociative fugue has been estimated as 0.2 percent), it is even rarer for it to occur more than once in the same person. Details are difficult to come by since those in the fugue state don't realize they are in it.

Dissociative fugue: a specifier for dissociative amnesia where in addition to experiencing amnesia, people may drive away from home and start a new life in a new location.

Depersonalization-Derealization Disorder

People with **depersonalization-derealization disorder (DPDRD)** may feel cut off from their own body, as if they are watching their own body from above (Diagnostic Overview 5.6). Symptoms include feeling robotic, lacking control over speech and movement, and feeling a sense of distortion of time. **Derealization** symptoms include a sense of unreality and detachment from the world, like being in a fog or a dream in which the world around you feels unreal. Dissociation symptoms can also happen when you are sleepy or under the influence of certain drugs, but that doesn't mean you have a dissociative disorder.

Around half of adults have experienced some symptoms of depersonalization or derealization following a stressful situation (APA 2013). The lifetime prevalence of DPDRD is 2.5 percent (Somer et al. 2013) and is linked to a history of emotional abuse more than physical abuse.

Depersonalization-derealization disorder (DPDRD): a dissociative disorder in which people feel cut off from their own body, as if they are watching their own body from above.

Derealization: a sense of unreality and detachment from the world, like being in a fog or a dream in which the world around you feels unreal.

Models and Treatments of Dissociative Disorders

One theory of the cause of dissociative disorders is that the dissociative experience helps to separate and disconnect a person from the awareness of a disturbing experience, and that dissociation acts as a mechanism to help the person cope. Another theory suggests not that the conditions are faked, but rather that the behavior helps people make sense of the many incompatible and contradictory emotions they might experience during and after a trauma. The new identities become real to the client, who behaves accordingly.

It can be difficult to treat DID. The goal is to integrate the alters into a coherent identity and help the client rebuild trusting relationships (Chu 2011). Those who are able to reintegrate their personality can be free of symptoms for quite some time (Ellason & Ross 1997).

Diagnostic Overview 5.6: Depersonalization-Derealization Disorder

- The presence of ongoing depersonalization (experiences of unreality, detachment, or being an outside observer with respect to thoughts, feelings, sensations, body) or derealization (detachment with regards to objects or feeling in a dreamlike state).
- Despite the depersonalization or derealization a sense of reality is in place.
- Feeling unreal, detached, or like an observer to your own body or a sense of being detached from the things around you.

Impact: Symptoms must exceed cultural and contextual norms. Symptoms are related to clinically significant distress or create impairment in important areas of life such as with friends and family or at work or school.

Source: Information from APA (2022).

Many theories of DID point to trauma as one of the precipitating events. The trauma can be sexual or physical abuse and is often an experience the person feels powerless to escape (Ross & Ness 2010).

Unfortunately, there are few studies on models and treatments for dissociative amnesia. As controversial as DID is, dissociative amnesia may be even more so. Some researchers have questioned the existence of the disorder, since trauma is seldom forgotten unless there is brain injury. These researchers suggest that many cases of dissociative amnesia could be due to undetected brain injury, malingering (see Chapter 7), or distressing events clients don't want to discuss (Lynn et al. 2019). Less than 0.25 percent of psychiatrists in the United States and Canada feel there is evidence that dissociative disorders are a valid diagnostic category (Lalonde et al. 2001). However, many studies have provided evidence of amnesia for traumatic events and difficulty recalling details of childhood sexual and physical abuse (Loewenstein 2018).

BIOLOGICAL MODELS AND TREATMENTS

Researchers are still trying to tease out possible biological causes of dissociative disorders (Sutar & Sahu 2019). Some suggest they may be a protective response to danger that leads to the parasympathetic nervous system's response. In some people this leads to a sense of stupor and trance and lack of responsiveness (Loewenstein 2018).

People with dissociative disorders show differences in some brain areas involved in memory and emotion. One study found differences in the brain's metabolic activity among people with depersonalization disorder (Rathee 2020). It's possible that the part of the brain involved in body perception may create the feeling of being disconnected (Rathee 2020). In clients with DID some areas of the brain appear to be larger (the white matter tracts, ganglia, and the precuneus), and some smaller (hippocampus, the amygdala, and the parietal areas associated with perception and personal awareness, and frontal lobe structures invoked in movement and fear learning). These differences are associated with DID symptoms (Blihar et al. 2020).

Very few studies have examined the use of medications for dissociative disorders, since psychotherapy has been the main treatment for most (LaFrance et al. 2014). However, a recent meta-analysis of five studies that reported data on more than 200 participants with dissociative disorders found modest evidence for the effectiveness of paroxetine (Paxil) and naloxone (Narcan) in helping control dissociative symptoms in about 68 percent of those who took these medications (LaFrance et al. 2014).

PSYCHOLOGICAL MODELS AND TREATMENTS

Psychotherapy is the main treatment for dissociative disorders (Subramanyam et al. 2020). Psychodynamic models for dissociation suggest that painful memories get disconnected, split off, and repressed from consciousness so the person can adapt, either by masking the memories as in dissociative amnesia, or by splitting them into another identity as in dissociative identity disorder.

The sociocognitive model, also called the non-trauma related or fantasy model, suggests that sociocognitive symptoms of DID are created by sociocultural influences and not by trauma at all (Reinders et al. 2012). In this view, disorders such as DID are inflated by culture and society. Dissociation is then a learned response, a form of role-playing honed through observational learning and reinforcement (Rathee 2020). Some researchers suggest that alters are created by patients as metaphors to understand their experiences, and that they are playing a role (Piper & Mersky 2004). There's some evidence that people who develop DID are highly suggestible and able to be hypnotized (Kihlstrom et al. 1994), and that their alters may be created to provide a sense of safety (Brand et al. 2016).

Whatever the source of the disorder, the experience of DID *is* influenced by culture. In some cultures, it feels like an experience of possession (Spiegel et al. 2011). The alters take the form of spirits, demons, animals, or mythical figures. These possessions can feel distressing and out of control.

CONCEPT CHECK 5.2

Match the case with type of dissociative disorder.
   A. Dissociative identity disorder
   B. Dissociative amnesia
   C. Depersonalization-derealization disorder
   1. When Arlie walks into the room she feels like she's outside her own body and almost like she's watching what's going on. Her emotions are turned off, she's not in charge of her movements, and everything feels "automatic and mechanical" as if she were a robot.
   2. After a traumatically destructive hurricane, Simon can't seem to remember his wife of 15 years or the names or faces of the people he knows. He was examined by his physician, who found no brain trauma that would explain this phenomenon.
   3. Bryce experiences dramatic changes in his personality and appears to have no memory of some of his past actions. It seems that he is being truthful with his therapist about his memory and there doesn't seem to be evidence of any physical reason for his forgetfulness. At home Bryce often finds evidence of what he describes as "another life he leads."

PULLING IT TOGETHER

Symptoms of PTSD

In addition to exposure to a trauma, individuals with PTSD have symptoms that span four different clusters over a period of at least 30 days (Figure 5.16).
   Symptoms of intrusion (at least one required):

   • Distressing memories.
   • Distressing dreams.
   • Flashbacks.
   • Psychological distress at exposure to internal or external cues that symbolize or resemble an aspect of the traumatic event(s).

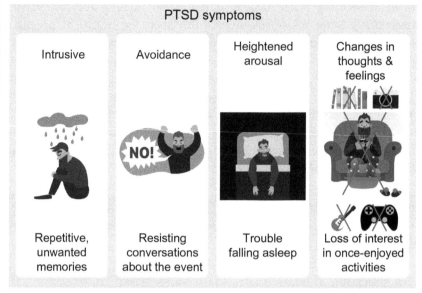

Figure 5.16 Symptoms of PTSD.

- Physiological reactions to internal or external cues that symbolize or resemble an aspect of the traumatic event(s).

Avoidance symptoms (at least one required):

- Avoidance of distressing memories, thoughts, or feelings about the event.
- Avoidance of reminders of the event, like people, places, conversations, activities, objects, and situations that could bring on memories, thoughts, or feelings about or closely associated with the traumatic event(s).

Symptoms related to negative alterations in thoughts and mood (at least two required):

- Inability to remember an important aspect of the traumatic event(s).
- Persistent and exaggerated negative beliefs or expectations about self, others, or the world.
- Persistent, distorted thoughts about why the event occurred.
- Persistent negative emotional state.
- Markedly diminished interest or participation in significant activities.
- Feelings of detachment from other people.
- Difficulty experiencing positive feelings.

Symptoms associated with arousal and reactivity (at least two required):

- Irritability.
- Reckless behavior.
- Hypervigilance.
- Exaggerated startle response.
- Concentration problems.
- Sleep problems.

SUMMARY

This chapter presented the following disorders:

Trauma and stressor-related disorders:
- Adjustment disorders
- Post-traumatic stress disorder (PTSD)
- Acute stress disorder

Dissociative disorders:
- Dissociative identity disorder
- Dissociative amnesia
- Depersonalization-derealization disorder

Trauma and Stressor-Related Disorders

- Adjustment disorders are trauma and stressor-related disorders that are diagnosed when an individual has difficulty dealing with a stressor. They are diagnosed only when the symptoms don't meet the criteria for another diagnosis.
- In post-traumatic stress disorder (PTSD) a person who has experienced a trauma frequently re-experiences it, avoids situations associated with it, exhibits negative changes in thoughts and mood associated with the event, and feels chronic arousal for at least 30 days.
- Symptoms of PTSD experienced for fewer than 30 days may meet the criteria for acute stress disorder.
- Events more likely to lead to PTSD include traumas like the experience of violence and the threat of injury or death. Factors that can influence development of PTSD include the degree of controllability, predictability, and perceived threat of the trauma.
- Biological models of PTSD emphasize the biochemical, neurobiological, and genetic aspects of the condition.
- Biological treatments include many medications that were traditionally used to treat depression such as SSRIs.
- Cognitive-behavioral models of PTSD use treatment techniques similar to those to treat anxiety disorders.

- Sociocultural models of trauma emphasize the impact of trauma on certain populations.

Dissociative Disorders

- Dissociative disorders involve a sudden loss of the integration of consciousness or memory, which may split into separate streams, or a change in identity.
- Psychopathologists describe three main dissociative disorders: dissociative identity disorder (DID), dissociative amnesia, and depersonalization-derealization disorder.
- In dissociative identity disorder, a person has two or more identities.
- In dissociative amnesia, a person experiences loss of memory for important personal information which isn't due to an injury.
- In derealization-depersonalization disorder, a person feels cut off from their own body.

DISCUSSION QUESTIONS

1. The *DSM*'s criteria for PTSD make a specific exception for media exposure to traumatic images through photographs, television, or film (unless your work requires you to view such images). Why do you believe the *DSM* makes this distinction? What do you believe the impact of PTSD diagnosis would be without this exception?
2. Exposure-based treatments for trauma are some of the most effective treatments we have, yet they are underused by clinicians. What are some of the reasons for this, and what do you think could be done to improve their utilization?
3. Adjustment disorders are possibly over-diagnosed conditions and may not fit into the way some clinicians understand psychopathology. How should clinicians utilize the diagnosis of adjustment disorders?
4. What are some reasons for the increase in diagnosis of dissociative identity disorder?

ANSWERS TO CONCEPT CHECKS

Concept Check 5.1

1. Distressing memory; intrusion
2. Distressing dream; intrusion
3. Avoid distressing memory; avoidance
4. Negative beliefs about self or others or the world; negative alteration of thoughts and mood
5. Concentration problems; arousal and reactivity

Concept Check 5.2

1. Depersonalization-derealization disorder
2. Dissociative amnesia
3. Dissociative identity disorder

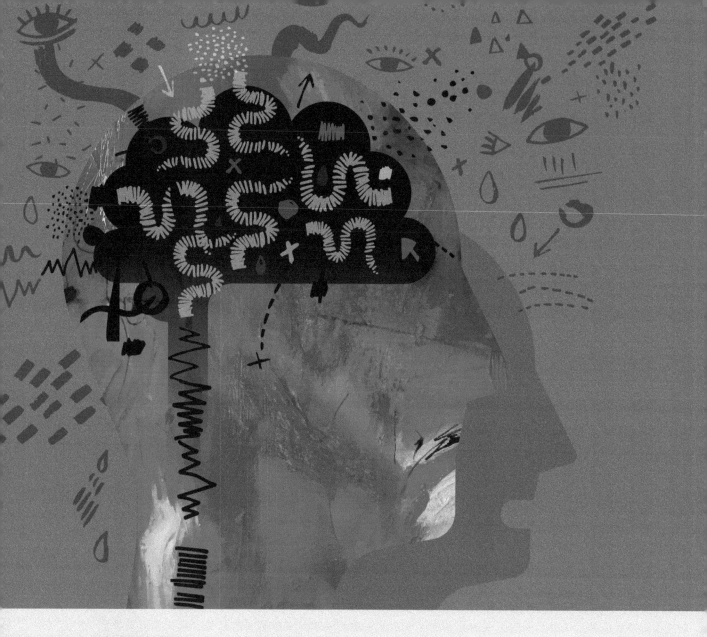

CHAPTER CONTENTS

6

Mood Disorders

CASE STUDY: Bipolar Disorder – Andy Behrman

Andy used to describe himself as "Mister Fun" and "the guy standing with a lampshade on his head, a margarita in each hand and doing the meringue at parties" (Figure 6.1). Sometimes he would want to go "everywhere at once," often impulsively taking walks or drives that might end with him boarding a flight to a random city halfway across the world. Once he took an impromptu trip to see the Berlin Wall because he watched a story about it on CNN one night and felt an intense urgency to see it in person.

During these times Andy spent an excessive amount of money on things. Despite his energy, he reported that he didn't accomplish much that was important and then got himself into trouble with people because he didn't fulfill the promises he had made. His periods of confidence and increased self-esteem would last for weeks at a time, though he had trouble sleeping.

But Andy didn't always feel like this. He had down periods, too, in which he was unable to leave his bed in the morning for weeks at a time. He had no interest in any of his activities and responsibilities, and he felt that his life was out of control, both personally and professionally. He had no energy to do much and felt overwhelmed by a sense of loneliness. Unable to concentrate, he ate only when his friends brought him food.

Weeks later Andy's energy would return. He experienced racing thoughts, got very little sleep, and had problematic drug and alcohol use. He was worried about getting treatment for his problems because he thought it would make him "dull and boring." Eventually he sank into a deep depression again, and he went from being a public relations agent and art dealer to someone unable to take care of himself, staying in bed and watching television. We'll return to Andy's case later in this chapter.

To read more about Andy Behrman take a look at his book, *Electroboy: A memoir of mania* (2002).

Learning Objectives

- Identify the major features of major depressive episodes, dysthymic episodes, manic episodes, and hypomanic episodes.
- Describe the essential features of major depressive disorder and persistent depressive disorder.
- Describe the essential features of bipolar I and bipolar II disorder.
- Describe the essential features of premenstrual dysphoric disorder, disruptive mood dysregulation disorder, and prolonged grief disorder.
- Describe the models and treatments for mood disorders.

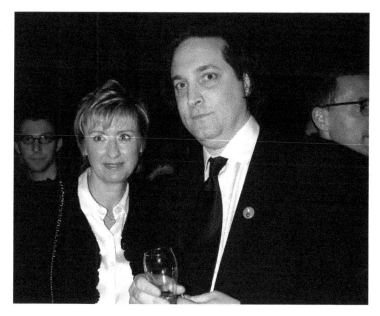

6.1   MOOD DISORDERS OVERVIEW

We've all had our ups and downs. When something amazing happens, it's uplifting, our mood soars, and sometimes we can't wait to tell someone about it. The opposite is true too. When something unexpected, unpleasant, or sad occurs, we might feel blue and down in the dumps. The peaks, valleys, strength, and lengths of our emotional states are usually predictable in relation to the things that happen to us. We tend to feel worse after losing a loved one than after getting a bad grade. That by itself is no surprise. However, such lows and highs move into the category of mood disorder symptoms when they start to interfere with a person's functioning in life. People with mood disorders have more extreme, intense, and long-lasting variations in their emotional states than do people without mood disorders. These fluctuations can create distress and impairment in their personal, social, and work life. They might miss assignments or work or not feel up to social engagements. That was certainly the case for Andy.

Moods are long-lasting, nonspecific emotional states. They aren't the ups and downs we experience during a normal day or even over a few days. Think of a mood like the temperature. In one particular location, the temperature changes throughout the day (like someone emotionally responding to a particular event or trigger), but if we think about multiple locations around the world, they all have average temperatures that hover around a fairly stable range. It's that baseline temperature that resembles someone's mood. When someone's moods are too high or too low over week or months, the person is said to have a mood disorder. **Mood disorders** are psychological conditions marked by tumultuous emotional states that can result in problematic social functioning and thinking behaviors, and in physical symptoms.

Mood disorders are described in two different chapters in the *DSM-5tr*: Depressive Disorders and Bipolar and Related Disorders (APA 2022). **Depressive disorders** are a

Mood disorders: psychological conditions marked by tumultuous emotional states that can result in problematic social functioning and thinking behaviors, and in physical symptoms.

Depressive disorders: a category of mood disorder characterized by sad moods or lack of pleasure.

category of mood disorder characterized by sad moods or lack of pleasure. **Bipolar disorders** are mood disorders in which a person may alternate between a sad, depressive mood and elevated, irritable, or manic episodes (manic episodes are associated with an elevated, expansive, sometimes irritable mood and abnormally increased energy or activity). Because depressive and bipolar disorders share many characteristics, we'll discuss them both in this chapter. We'll learn the criteria that define them, their possible causes, and ways they may be treated (see also Figure 6.17 in the Pulling It Together feature at the end of this chapter).

Bipolar disorders: mood disorders in which a person may alternate between a sad, depressive mood and elevated, irritable, or manic episodes.

Mood Episodes

Psychological diagnosticians use *mood episodes* to help identify mood disorders. Mood episodes have specific symptoms that define them, but they aren't stand-alone disorders. Instead, these episodes serve as the building blocks of mood disorders themselves. Different mood disorders can be diagnosed depending on which kind of episodes someone experiences, how severe the episodes are, and how long they last. There are four distinct mood episodes: major depressive episode, dysthymic episodes, manic episode, and hypomanic episode.

MAJOR DEPRESSIVE EPISODE

A **major depressive episode** is more than just a sad mood. It's a syndrome that carries a number of emotional, motivational, behavioral, cognitive, and physical symptoms (see Diagnostic Overview 6.1).

Major depressive episode: a mood episode that often includes lack of interest and sad moods along with cognitive and behavioral symptoms that lasts at least two weeks.

Diagnostic Overview 6.1: Major Depressive Episode

At least one of the following:

- Depressed mood: Feeling of sadness, emptiness, or hopelessness.
- Lack of interest and feelings of pleasure: reduced capacity to experience pleasure (*anhedonia*). Depression isn't just the presence of negative moods, but also the lack of positive moods.

In addition to at least one core symptom (above), the individual must have five or more symptoms:

- Disrupted sleep patterns: inability to sleep, called *insomnia*, or a pattern of sleeping excessively and not feeling rested, called *hypersomnia*. About 40 percent of people with a major depressive episode sleep more than usual.
- Changes in psychomotor functions: Motion and speech that are faster than when not depressed, called *psychomotor agitation*, or slower, called *psychomotor retardation*.
- Changes in appetite: Tendency to eat too much or too little (which may result in weight changes).
- Inability to concentrate: Reduced ability to think, focus, or make decisions.
- Lack of energy: Feeling of fatigue or listlessness, or like the body is heavy.
- Feelings of guilt and lack of self-esteem: Sense of worthlessness, inadequacy, culpability, undesirability, or inferiority.
- Desire to end one's life (suicidality): Thoughts of death (also called *suicidal ideation*), of the world as better off if the person were dead, consideration of suicide, or of a plan to commit suicide.

Impact:	Symptoms must exceed cultural and contextual norms. Symptoms are related to clinically significant distress or create impairment in important areas of life such as with friends and family or at work or school.
Timeframe:	At least 14 days in a row.

Source: Information from APA (2022).

Diagnostic Overview 6.2: Dysthymic Episode

- Depressed mood: a sad or down mood.
- At least three of the following:
  - Poor or excessive appetite.
  - Disrupted sleep patterns: problems getting to sleep or sleeping too much and not feeling rested.
  - Lack of energy.
  - Low self-esteem.
  - Problems with concentration and decision making.
  - Feelings of hopelessness.

Impact: Symptoms must exceed cultural and contextual norms. Symptoms are related to clinically significant distress or create impairment in important areas of life such as with friends and family or at work or school.

Timeframe: At least four days in a row.

Source: Information from APA (2022).

To meet the criteria for a major depressive episode, a person must have one or both of two core symptoms – lack of interest and depressed mood – and at least three or four other symptoms for a total of at least five symptoms for most of the day, nearly every day for a time period of at least two weeks (APA 2022).

DYSTHYMIC EPISODE

Dysthymic episode: a mild depressive episode that doesn't meet the full criteria for a major depressive episode.

A **dysthymic** (diss-THIGH-mick) **episode** is a mild depressive episode that doesn't meet the full criteria for a major depressive episode (Diagnostic Overview 6.2).

People in a dysthymic episode experience a depressed mood, and just two other symptoms of a major depressive episode. This is a bit different from the five symptoms needed for a major depressive episode.

MANIC EPISODE

Mania: an emotional and behavioral condition associated with an elevated, expansive, sometimes irritable mood and abnormally increased energy or activity.

Manic episode: a type of mood episode where a person's moods are abnormally elevated, and their emotions, thinking, and reactions might be so elevated that they do things that get them into trouble or put them in danger.

Think about the best day you've ever had. Maybe it's a special vacation you spent with your family, or a surprise birthday party. Remember how amazing that felt? Capture that feeling then triple or quadruple it. Think of being in a mood that is "better than good" (Figure 6.2). **Mania** is a condition associated with an elevated, expansive, sometimes irritable mood and abnormally increased energy or activity. A **manic episode** is the polar opposite of a major depressive episode: instead of feeling down and blue, people experiencing a manic episode are abnormally elevated, and their emotions, thinking, and reactions might be so elevated that they do things that get them into trouble or put them in danger (Diagnostic Overview 6.3).

In addition to experiencing an elevated, expansive, and sometimes irritable mood (a core symptom of a manic episode), a person having a manic episode has three or more associated symptoms most days for at least a week. While the *DSM-5tr* suggests that a manic episode has a minimum duration of one week, untreated manic episodes can run an average of three to four months (Miller et al. 2004).

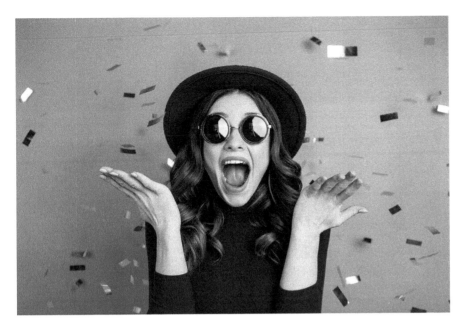

Figure 6.2 People with symptoms of mania often describe feeling "better than good."
Source: Deagreez/iStock/ Getty Images Plus.

HYPOMANIC EPISODE

In Chapter 1 we discussed that in order for something to be a disorder, a syndrome has to cause distress and/or impairment (Figure 6.3). *DSM-5tr* uses the term hypomania to describe a less severe form of mania. In a **hypomanic episode**, a person has symptoms of mania but they do not impair the person's ability to function effectively. A hypomanic episode is not itself a problem, but its presence is characteristic of several mood disorders (Diagnostic Overview 6.4).

Hypomanic episode: a mood episode in which a person has symptoms of mania but they do not impair the person's ability to function effectively.

Diagnostic Overview 6.3: Manic Episode

A mood that is overly elevated or irritable and at least three of the following symptoms:

- Inflated self-esteem: development of elaborate, sometimes outlandish plans for personal or business life.
- Decreased need for sleep: sleep times as short as three hours with a feeling of being completely rested.
- Pressured speech: the need to keep talking and talking.
- Racing thoughts (also called flight of ideas): attempt to rapidly express so many ideas at once that speech becomes incoherent.
- Increase in goal-directed behavior: Focus on a project with such intensity that basic self-care or sleep are neglected.
- Lack of control: over-involvement in activities with a potential for harm such as buying sprees, sexual indiscretions, or participation in get-rich-quick schemes.

Impact: Symptoms must exceed cultural and contextual norms. Symptoms are related to clinically significant distress or create impairment in important areas of life such as with friends and family or at work or school.

Timeframe: Seven days in a row.

Source: Information from APA (2022).

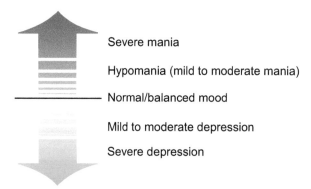

Severe mania

Hypomania (mild to moderate mania)

Normal/balanced mood

Mild to moderate depression

Severe depression

Diagnostic Overview 6.4: Hypomanic Episode

A mood that is overly elevated or irritable and at least three of the following symptoms:

- Inflated self-esteem: development of elaborate sometimes outlandish plans for personal or business life.
- Decreased need for sleep: sleep times as short as three hours with a feeling of being completely rested.
- Pressured speech: the need to keep talking and talking.
- Racing thoughts (also called flight of ideas): attempt to rapidly express so many ideas at once that speech becomes incoherent.
- Increase in goal-directed behavior: Focus on a project with such intensity that basic self-care or sleep are neglected.
- Lack of control: over-involvement in activities with a potential for harm such as buying sprees, sexual indiscretions, or participation in get-rich-quick schemes.

Impact: Symptoms must exceed cultural and contextual norms. The symptoms are not severe enough to cause impairment.

Timeframe: At least four days in a row.

Source: Information from APA (2022).

CONCEPT CHECK 6.1

Indicate the mood episode or symptom associated with each case:

1. Mia has been in an unusually good mood for the last few days. Her mood doesn't seem to interfere with her social life and has helped her get things done at work, but she noticed that she's been sleeping less, feels a pressure to talk, and has been playing video games more often than usual. Mia appears to have the symptoms of a(n) _____ episode.
2. Miriam has been feeling better than good for the past week. She has been productive at work and more socially active than ever before. In fact she's been so active that she hasn't been sleeping and her partying has gotten her into trouble. Miriam appears to have symptoms of a(n) _____ episode.
3. Jayden has been depressed for the last several weeks, staying indoors and avoiding social interaction. He usually likes seeing his friends and family, but

he hasn't lately because he doesn't think he'll enjoy it. The symptom of a depressive episode that is causing him to stay away from his friends and family is most likely _____.

4. Lately, Ethan has had no interest in the things that are usually fun for him. He's been unable to focus and concentrate on his daily tasks. He worries all the time and seems to sleep only three hours a night. During the day he has no appetite and no energy whatsoever. He's been feeling this way for the past four weeks. Ethan's symptoms seem indicative of which mood episode? _____

6.2 DEPRESSIVE DISORDERS

Depressive disorders are a category of mood disorder characterized by sad moods or lack of pleasure. They are also known as *unipolar depressive disorders*, or, more commonly and simply, depressive disorders, because they only occupy one end (or pole) of the mood disorder spectrum. Bipolar disorders occupy both the manic and depressive ends. It's worth noting that although the *DSM* puts the depressive and bipolar disorders in separate chapters, that wasn't always the case. Until *DSM-5* they were in the same chapter (under a series of names of affective disorders then mood disorders) in order to emphasize how connected depressive disorders were to their bipolar counterparts. In *DSM-5* the depressive disorders and bipolar disorders get their own separate chapter. DSM describes several depressive disorders (Figure 6.4). In this section we discuss the two most common: major depressive disorder and persistent depressive disorder.

You'll remember from the previous section that four types of mood episodes are the building blocks of depressive disorders: major depressive episodes, dysthymic episodes

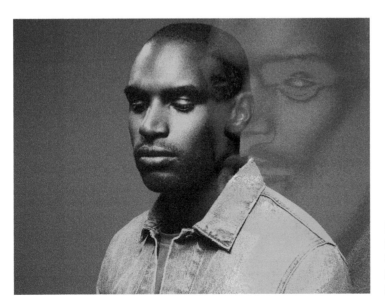

Figure 6.4 Mood disorders are different from the ups and downs of daily living.
Source: Jonathan Knowles/ Stone/Getty Images.

(not described in the *DSM*), manic episodes, and hypomanic episodes. In the discussions that follow, you'll see how these building blocks interact in the depressive disorders.

Major Depressive Disorder

Major depressive disorder: a depressive disorder characterized by two or more weeks of low mood or anhedonia and at least four other symptoms of a major depressive episode.

Major depressive disorder (sometimes referred to as clinical depression or depression) is a depressive disorder characterized by two or more weeks of low mood or anhedonia and at least four other symptoms of a major depressive episode (Diagnostic Overview 6.5). The way depression affects an individual depends on the specific symptoms the person experiences. Symptoms can be so severe that some people lose their ability to be an effective friend, partner, or parent, or their ability to work and take care of themselves. Andy's symptoms, for example, were so debilitating that other people had to shop for him and bring him food.

Some depressed people experience an irritated, anxious, angry depression, while others show a gloomier, sad, and slowed-down version. Regardless of their experience, people cannot simply snap out of depression. Some describe it as being a ghost, or as falling down a dark bottomless shaft and wondering whether anyone will catch them.

Depression has been ranked as the leading cause of illness and disability worldwide, affecting over 300 million people (Friedrich 2017). Those with depression miss work five times more often than people without it (Luca et al. 2014). In 2010 in the United States alone, depression created a financial burden of $210.5 billion in missed work and decreased work productivity (Greenberg et al. 2015). More importantly, depression can reduce the number of healthy years that people experience in their lives (known as disability-adjusted life years or DALY).

Major depressive disorder is the most frequently diagnosed psychiatric disorder in the United States (Smithson & Pignone 2017). Around 19 percent of US adults will experience it at some point in their lives, and prevalence rates are similar in many other countries (see Figures 6.5 and 6.6) (Leclerc et al. 2020). Nearly a third of US college students will experience symptoms of depression at some point in their undergraduate career (Novotney 2014).

Despite its prevalence, major depressive disorder does not occur with equal frequency in all groups. For example, while there are gender disparities in rates of depression, these differences tend to emerge during adolescence. During childhood, boys and girls are equally likely to be depressed, but by adulthood as many as 26.1 percent of women will have had an episode, compared with only 14.7 percent of men (Hasin et al. 2018). And while the rates of depression are similar in different cultures around the world, the constellation of symptoms can vary from country to country. Some countries, for example, report more cognitive symptoms such as guilt and feelings of worthlessness, while

Diagnostic Overview 6.5: Major Depressive Disorder

- A major depressive episode (see Diagnostic Overview 6.1).
- No history of either a manic or hypomanic episode (see Diagnostic Overviews 6.3 and 6.4).

Impact: Symptoms must exceed cultural and contextual norms. Symptoms are related to clinically significant distress or create impairment in important areas of life such as with friends and family or at work or school.

Source: Information from APA (2022).

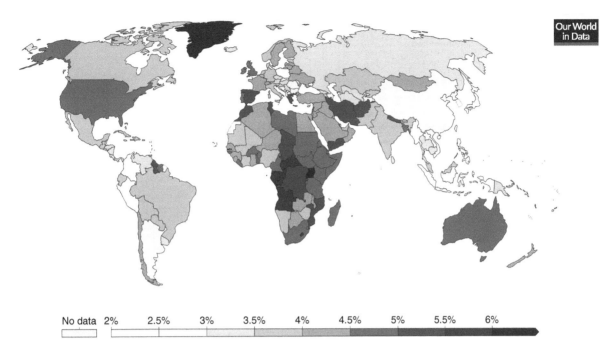

No data 2%   2.5%   3%   3.5%   4%   4.5%   5%   5.5%   6%

Source: IHME, Global Burden of Disease

weakness and somatic symptoms such as sleep problems are hallmarks of depression in others (Haroz et al. 2017; Juhasz et al. 2012).

Figure 6.5 Prevalence of depressive disorders around the world, 2017, by share of the population.
Source: Roth (2018).

Persistent Depressive Disorder

Persistent depressive disorder (PDD) is a depressive disorder characterized by a chronic low mood and other symptoms of depressive mood episodes (Diagnostic Overview 6.6). If someone experiences two straight months without any symptoms, they are no longer eligible for a diagnosis of persistent depressive disorder.

The word persistent indicates how chronic and long-lasting someone's symptoms are, but additional details can also be added to the diagnosis to indicate the severity of symptoms. Those with PDD with milder (dysthymic) symptoms are diagnosed with persistent disorder with dysthymic syndrome. Those with more severe symptoms are diagnosed with persistent depressive disorder with major depressive episode.

The symptoms of persistent depressive disorder can be just as or even more severe than that of major depressive disorder. People with PDD are more likely to lose their jobs (Adler et al. 2004) and are at a higher risk of having poor health in general (Barbui et al. 2006).

Persistent depressive disorder (PDD): a depressive disorder characterized by a chronic low mood and other symptoms of depressive mood episodes.

Diagnostic Overview 6.6: Persistent Depressive Disorder

Either a major depressive episode or a dysthymic episode (see Diagnostic Overview 6.2).

Impact:	Symptoms must exceed cultural and contextual norms. Symptoms are related to clinically significant distress or create impairment in important areas of life such as with friends and family or at work or school.
Timeframe:	At least two years.

Source: Information from APA (2022).

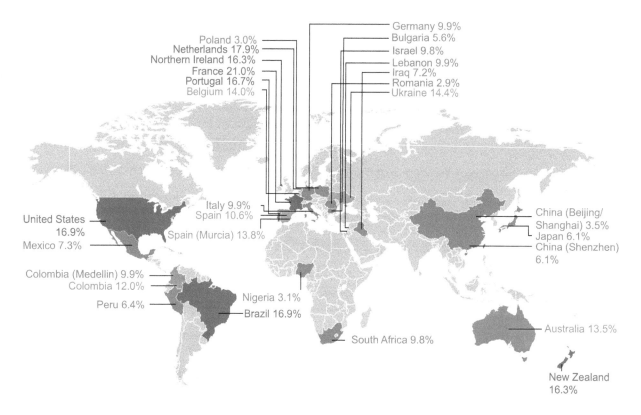

Figure 6.6 Lifetime prevalence of major depressive disorder in the World Mental Health Surveys, selected countries (2002–2017)

Source: Data from Scott, de Jonge, et al. (2018).

Persistent depressive disorder is less common than major depressive disorder and affects about 6.4 percent of the general US population per year (Klein 2010). Around 20 percent of people with major depressive episodes will have the symptoms long enough to meet the criteria for persistent depressive disorder (Klein 2010).

Specifiers for Mood Disorders

Specifiers can be added to many diagnoses in the *DSM* (including depression) to describe someone's condition in greater detail. Below are some of the specifiers *DSM-5tr* uses to describe depressive and bipolar disorders. For example, some individuals who experience symptoms of depression more strongly in the fall and winter may be diagnosed as having "depressive disorder *with seasonal pattern*," and those with depressive symptoms around (*peri*) the time of childbirth would receive a "with peripartum onset" specifier.

Some specifiers for depressive and bipolar and related disorders are:

- With anxious distress.
- With psychotic features.
- With peripartum onset.
- With seasonal pattern.

Major depressive disorder can appear at pretty much any age, but people are most likely to first experience symptoms in their early twenties (Solmi et al. 2021) (see Figure 6.7). Younger adults may have depressed mood, hypersomnia, and increased

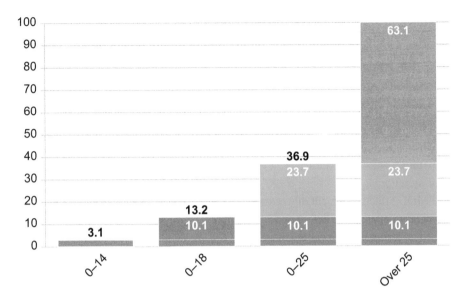

Figure 6.7 Meta-analytic estimates of age of onset of depressive disorders. Although around 19% of people will experience depression at some point in their lives, nearly 37% will have an episode by the time they are 25 years old.

eating (resulting in weight gain). For about 40 percent of people with depression, the symptoms will last about three months. Most of the remaining 60 percent will have symptoms that last at least a year; however, more than half of those who have severe depression will have another episode sometime in their lives (Solomon et al. 2000).

For some, a single episode of depression is all they'll ever experience, and the symptoms won't return. However, the more severe the symptoms are, the more likely they'll occur again.

Premenstrual Dysphoric Disorder, Disruptive Mood Dysregulation Disorder, and Prolonged Grief Disorder

Major depressive disorder and persistent depressive disorder aren't the only unipolar mood disorders described by the *DSM-5tr*. For example, *DSM-5tr* includes premenstrual dysphoric disorder, disruptive mood dysregulation disorder, and prolonged grief disorder.

PREMENSTRUAL DYSPHORIC DISORDER

Those who have **premenstrual dysphoric disorder (PMDD)** show symptoms of depression in most of their menstrual cycles during the weeks around menstruation. Symptoms often include depressed mood, anxiety, irritability and, at times, also disruptions in sleep and appetite. These tend to appear in the week before their menstrual cycle starts, and to improve a few days after their menstrual cycle has begun.

Whereas in premenstrual syndrome (PMS) some people experience changes in appetite, mood swings, headaches, muscle aches, and swollen hands and feet, these symptoms are not too severe and do not generally interfere with daily functioning. PMDD, on the other hand, is a serious condition characterized by severe symptoms

Premenstrual dysphoric disorder (PMDD): a depressive disorder in which a person shows symptoms of depression in most of their menstrual cycles during the weeks around menstruation. Symptoms often include depressed mood, anxiety, irritability and, at times, also disruptions in sleep and appetite.

such as stronger mood disturbances, irritability, anxiety, and even suicidal thoughts, all of which can seriously affect relationships and functioning.

The inclusion of PMDD in the *DSM-5* was controversial because of concerns about over-diagnosing healthy women who experience the usual shifts in hormones related to menstruation, in effect pathologizing normal menstruation. However, PMDD is quite different from the uncomfortable premenstrual symptoms that up to a third of women experience and that are not associated with impairment. Supporters of the diagnosis suggest that the addition of PMDD will help those who do experience severe symptoms to obtain treatment to relieve their symptoms.

PMDD affects 5 percent of women of reproductive age (Mattina & Steiner 2020). It can occur at any time before or after the first menstrual cycle but symptoms tend to improve during pregnancy and after menopause. Another 7.5–13 percent will show mild symptoms that won't meet criteria for PMDD (Eisenlohr-Moul et al. 2020). PMDD can arise at any time during a woman's reproductive years although the average age of onset is 26 years. While there is some evidence that PMS symptoms worsen with age, not enough has been studied regarding PMDD. It is common knowledge that hormone levels fluctuate unpredictably in perimenopause – the transition between regular menstruation cycles and the end of a woman's reproductive years – typically beginning in a female's forties.

PMDD has been diagnosed all around the world but – interestingly enough – the way it's expressed, and the frequency of reporting may be influenced by cultural factors. For example, researchers Cosgrove and Riddle (2003) discovered that women who endorsed traditional US gender roles experienced more menstrual distress. In their study the researchers accessed feminine gender identity using the Bem Sex Role Inventory (BSRI) (Bem 1981), which measures how participants describe their behavior in terms of traditional views of femininity or masculinity. They also assessed the participants' experiences of menstrual distress, including pain, water retention, behavior change, negative mood, and impaired concentration. The researchers discovered that those who endorsed more traditional feminine gender identity items were not only experiencing greater distress, but these individuals also were more likely to expect to have distressing physical and emotional symptoms both during and after menstruation, and to think of menstruation as something negative.

DISRUPTIVE MOOD DYSREGULATION DISORDER

Disruptive mood dysregulation disorder (DMDD): a depressive mood disorder found in children aged 6 to 18 that is characterized by severe temper outbursts and a persistent irritable or angry mood.

Psychological disorders can change over time, manifesting one way when an individual is younger and quite differently later in life. This appears to be the case with depression, and it can pose a dilemma for practitioners. In some children, for example, depressive symptoms can manifest themselves not as sad mood but as newly increased irritability, suggesting other conditions such as bipolar disorder. **Disruptive mood dysregulation disorder (DMDD)** is a depressive mood disorder found in children aged 6 to 18 that is characterized by severe temper outbursts and a persistent irritable or angry mood. Its prevalence is around 2–5 percent and is higher in men than in women (APA 2022).

While some parents might think the "terrible twos" is an example of this disorder, the outbursts of DMDD are not developmentally appropriate and occur more often than you'd expect, even in an angst-filled teen: three or more outbursts per week, with irritable mood sustained between them. Supporters of this diagnosis see DMDD as an early version of depression with the irritability and outbursts of bipolar disorder. Critics of the *DSM* say the diagnostic criteria are too vague and result in poor reliability across various clinicians (Mayes et al. 2015), and that the diagnosis turns typical temper tantrums into disorders (Frances & Nardo 2013). However, other therapists see value in the new diagnosis. They view DMDD as an early warning sign of a major depressive disorder and believe the availability of this diagnosis decreases the over-diagnosis of bipolar disorders.

PROLONGED GRIEF DISORDER

Prolonged grief disorder (PGD) (APA 2022) is a depressive disorder that resembles major depressive disorder and is marked by a pervasive yearning for the deceased. We all know that the death of someone close to us can be emotionally painful, so much so that many people have symptoms that resemble depression for weeks after their loved ones have passed away. However, with time, the pain lessens. In **prolonged grief disorder**, on the other hand, a person experiences persistent grief that both exceeds cultural norms and causes significant distress and impairment (Diagnostic Overview 6.7). Prolonged grief disorder was added to *DSM-5tr* to help distinguish it from depression. According to researchers, there is evidence that the symptoms of prolonged grief disorder are biologically different from those of depression (Boelen & Lenferink 2020), and treating this condition requires grief-specific treatments rather than depression-focused treatments (Shear et al. 2014).

Diagnostic Overview 6.7: Prolonged Grief Disorder

After the death of someone close, a person experiences intense preoccupation or yearning for the deceased person. At least three of the following symptoms:

- Identity disruption (feeling as if a part of them has died).
- Disbelief about the death.
- Avoidance of any reminders that the person has died.
- Emotional pain related to the death.
- Difficulties in moving on.
- Feeling of emotional numbness.
- Loneliness as a result of the death.
- A sense that life is meaningless.

Impact: Symptoms must exceed cultural and contextual norms. Symptoms are related to clinically significant distress or create impairment in important areas of life such as with friends and family or at work or school.

Timeframe: At least 1 month of symptoms that are 12 months after the death of someone close to them.

Source: Information from APA (2022).

Prolonged grief disorder: a depressive disorder in which a person experiences persistent grief that both exceeds cultural norms and causes significant distress and impairment

CONCEPT CHECK 6.2

Indicate the depressive disorder or symptom associated with each case.
1. A 37-year-old woman has felt very down and has had difficulty sleeping for the last three weeks. She also reports having repeated thoughts of death, problems focusing on her work, and too little energy to get her work done. She appears to have _____
2. Sara, a 40-year-old woman, has had a low, depressed mood as long as she can remember. Her energy is low and she always has trouble concentrating. "I guess I'm just a sad person." Sara most likely has _____

3. For the last four weeks Claude hasn't been interested in activities he usually enjoys. Riding his motorcycle hasn't seemed fun to him; nothing has. In addition, he's been very indecisive, has had trouble sleeping, is eating more than he usually does, and has been restless and moving around more than usual. Claude's symptoms suggest _____.

6.3   BIPOLAR DISORDERS

The depressive disorders occupy the unipolar part of the mood disorder spectrum because they don't exhibit a change to the elevated or expansive moods that characterize a manic or hypomanic episode. If the mood episodes cross to the manic pole, then we are in the domain of the bipolar and related disorders. The *DSM-5tr* describes several of these. In this section, we'll discuss the three most common: bipolar I, bipolar II, and cyclothymic.

You'll remember from section 6.1 that there are four mood episodes: depressive, dysthymic, manic, and hypomanic. While unipolar depressive disorders are characterized by symptoms from only two types (depressive and dysthymic), bipolar disorders can be characterized by symptoms from all four.

Bipolar I Disorder

Bipolar I disorder: a bipolar mood disorder in which a person cycles between mania and the other mood episodes.

Bipolar I disorder is a bipolar mood disorder in which a person cycles between mania and the other mood episodes. In bipolar I, the individual has experienced at least one manic episode and may not have experienced a depressive episode (yet) (Diagnostic Overview 6.8). Mania rarely appears alone (Bech 2009); more than 90 percent of those who experience symptoms of mania go on to have depressive episodes, hypomanic episodes, or even additional manic episodes months or years later. In all these cases, the mood episodes that follow the initial manic episode are considered part of the bipolar I disorder.

Most people who experience mania will not seek treatment; in fact, they may resist efforts to rein in their better-than-good moods. If symptoms get out of hand (like wild overspending), however, friends and family may hospitalize the manic person or encourage outpatient treatment. They are often better at identifying the symptoms of mania than the clients themselves, who are frequently unable to notice the impact of their actions during a manic state and who may not remember how they behaved after the episode has passed.

Between their manic and depressive episodes, people with bipolar I disorder may be symptom-free, but about a

Diagnostic Overview 6.8: Bipolar I Disorder

- At least one manic episode and may be followed by subsequent hypomanic or major depressive episodes.

Impact: Symptoms must exceed cultural and contextual norms. Symptoms are related to clinically significant distress or create impairment in important areas of life such as with friends and family or at work or school.

Source: Information from APA (2022).

third have problems finding and keeping work, often resulting in lower income regardless of the education level. Bipolar disorder is also associated with interpersonal problems such as frequent fights, because of the irritability and inflated ego experienced during a manic episode. People with symptoms of mania may also have problems with gambling, sex, hostility, and financial consequences of their tendency to act without considering the consequences. All these can make it difficult to interact productively with friends and family.

Diagnostic Overview 6.9: Bipolar II Disorder

- A past or current depressive episode.
- A past or current hypomanic episode.
- *No* experience of a manic episode.

Impact: Symptoms must exceed cultural and contextual norms. Symptoms are related to clinically significant distress or create impairment in important areas of life such as with friends and family or at work or school.

Source: Information from APA (2022).

Bipolar II Disorder

Bipolar II disorder is a mood disorder in which a person alternates between depressive and hypomanic episodes. Unlike those with bipolar I disorder, people with bipolar II disorder never have full manic episodes (Diagnostic Overview 6.9). You might recall as discussed in section 6.1 that hypomanic episodes aren't as severe as manic episodes, and don't cause significant impairment or distress in one's life.

This cycling between depressive and hypomanic states is not only taxing on the person, but it also affects their social and work lives. About 0.8 percent of the US population has bipolar II disorder; women are more likely to report their hypomanic symptoms. Most people seek treatment during their depressive phase because those symptoms are more likely to disrupt their lives and impair their functioning. The symptoms of hypomania, by definition, do not really create problems for them. In fact, many people in treatment for bipolar II disorder will deny they have a problem once they start cycling into the hypomanic episode and will stop treatment.

Although bipolar II might seem like a milder form of bipolar I, it can affect a person's life nonetheless. Because it is more persistent, and clients spend more time being depressed, they are more likely to experience suicidal symptoms. Indeed, a third of people with bipolar II have reported a suicide attempt, so it's important for clinicians to recognize the symptoms early (Miller & Black 2020).

Bipolar II disorder: a mood disorder in which a person alternates between depressive and hypomanic episodes.

Cyclothymic Disorder

Cyclothymic disorder is a milder but persistent bipolar mood disorder characterized by periods of hypomanic symptoms and mild depressive episodes (Diagnostic Overview 6.10). In cyclothymic disorder, individuals cycle between hypomanic moods and low moods, called dysthymic episodes, that don't meet the criteria for depression. For a diagnosis of cyclothymic disorder, a person's moods need to be disrupted cyclically for at least two years.

Like persistent depressive disorder, cyclothymic disorder is mild and chronic. People may be in one mood or the other for years. The hypomanic symptoms may not be a problem, but the dysthymic episodes can significantly interfere with daily

Cyclothymic disorder: a milder but persistent bipolar mood disorder characterized by periods of hypomanic symptoms and mild depressive episodes.

Diagnostic Overview 6.10: Cyclothymic Disorder

- Two years of hypomanic and depressive symptoms that aren't severe enough to meet diagnostic criteria for mania or major depressive episode.
- *No* symptom-free period longer than two months.
- *No* experience of a major depressive episode, a manic episode, or a hypomanic episode.

Impact: Symptoms must exceed cultural and contextual norms. Symptoms are related to clinically significant distress or create impairment in important areas of life such as with friends and family or at work or school.

Timeframe: At least two years.

Source: Information from APA (2022).

functioning. People diagnosed with cyclothymic disorder are at increased risk for developing bipolar I or bipolar II (Otto & Applebaum 2011).

Statistics and Trajectory of Bipolar Disorders

Lifetime prevalence of any bipolar disorder is estimated to be about 1.9 percent worldwide. Rates for the United States are higher, with the lifetime prevalence being around 4.4 percent (see Figure 6.8). The mean age of onset for bipolar I is 18, but it can occur as late as age 60 or 70. Bipolar II typically begins in late adolescence to early adulthood, with the average age of onset in the mid-twenties (slightly later than bipolar I).

In the United States, prevalence rates for bipolar I are about the same for women and men, but women are more likely to report depressive symptoms. Because the instruments used to measure the symptoms of bipolar I disorder have been developed by English researchers in the United States and Western Europe, it has been difficult to assess whether there are cultural variations in the diagnosis. For example, an item that asks how quickly a person "bounces back" or

Figure 6.8 Lifetime prevalence of bipolar I disorder in the World Mental Health Surveys, selected countries (2002–2017). *Source: Scott, de Jonge, et al. (2018).*

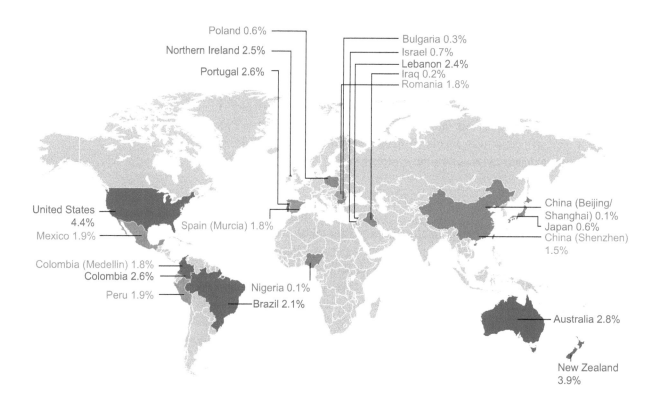

"snaps back" after a difficult experience can easily be translated too literally and confuse the individual taking the questionnaire (Kirmayer & Ryder 2016).

Bipolar II may start as depression and isn't always recognized as a bipolar condition until the hypomanic episode occurs. About 12 percent of people with bipolar II diagnosis are initially diagnosed with major depressive disorder. People experience more depressive episodes in bipolar II than in bipolar I, and these are more enduring and cause more distress and impairment.

CONCEPT CHECK 6.3

Indicate the mood disorder or symptom associated with each case.

1. About two months ago, Sebastian was seriously depressed for a few weeks. He spent most of his time in bed and cried nearly all the time. Over the past two weeks, however, he has emptied his bank account to fund his new idea for selling light bulbs. He's slept only about three hours each night but still feels rested. He's recently checked himself into a hospital because of these symptoms. Sebastian most likely has _____.

2. Mia presents with chronic low mood and decreased energy. In addition, she feels guilty all the time, is having trouble with her co-workers and friends, isn't interested in things that are typically enjoyable to her, and sleeps a lot but never feels rested. She admits she's never felt like this in the past. In fact, several months ago she had a lot of energy and little need to sleep and was more talkative than usual. The increased activity and energy weren't disruptive, and she was getting along fine at work and socially. Mia's symptoms suggest _____.

THE POWER OF WORDS

MANIC DEPRESSION

Maybe you've heard the term manic depressive to describe someone who has bipolar disorder and wondered why it's not used anymore. The terms depression and mania both have their origins in ancient languages. Mania derives from the Greek word *menos* meaning "spirit force or passion," while "depression" derives from the Latin *depriemere* meaning to "sink down."

The phrase "manic depression" was used as early as the first century to describe symptoms of mental illness, most likely thought to be due to an imbalance of bodily humors or fluids. In the 1800s French psychiatrist Jean-Pierre Falret identified what he called "circular insanity," during which an individual had periods of disruptive energy and low moods, and even periods that were symptom-free. Later, in 1902, Emil Kraepelin used the term "manic depressive psychosis" to describe a psychological condition that seemed mostly focused on mood symptoms.

It wasn't until the 1960s that diagnosticians became more nuanced in their distinction between unipolar depression and what came to be known as bipolar disorder. This distinction created more clarity in diagnosis, moved us away from the stigma of the word "mania," and didn't include the other types of conditions in the bipolar spectrum such as bipolar II and cyclothymia. The term manic depression emphasizes the emotional symptoms but doesn't really address some of the physical and cognitive symptoms that are an important part of the condition.

6.4 MODELS AND TREATMENTS OF MOOD DISORDERS

Eventually, Andy (from the chapter-opening case) sought treatment for his bipolar condition, including medication, therapy, and later electroconvulsive therapy (ECT). His doctor was able to find a combination of medications that helped him. Andy reconnected with people and was able to take care of himself again, experiencing years of being free of any mood episodes.

Psychopathologists have identified multiple factors related to the development of mood disorders. In this section we discuss the biological, psychological, social, and cultural factors that can lead to depressive and bipolar disorders.

The symptoms of mood disorders can be treated effectively using biological, psychological, social, and cultural interventions. Often, if one approach isn't effective, another might help to relieve the symptoms, and multiple approaches can be used at the same time. Even if a treatment doesn't eliminate all the symptoms, it can still be useful in making them less problematic or in helping an individual better cope with the disorder.

When left untreated, up to 50 percent of people with depressive disorders will experience another episode and 80 percent of those who have experienced two episodes will experience a third (Burcusa & Iacono 2007; De Zwart et al. 2019); those who receive treatment are less likely to experience future episodes. Despite this, only half of those with bipolar disorder and one-third of those with depressive disorders seek treatment in the United States (Merikangas et al. 2011). Many wait as long as eight years before seeking any help for their symptoms (Wang et al. 2005).

Biological Models and Treatments of Mood Disorders

The biological perspective suggests that symptoms of depressive and bipolar disorders are related to problems in neurological and organ systems. Some of the biological factors implicated in depressive and bipolar disorders include differences in genetics, biochemistry, and differences in organ systems such as brain circuitry, and the neuroendocrine system.

GENETIC MODELS OF MOOD DISORDERS

Mood disorders seem to run in families, which suggests a genetic basis to the condition (Gordovez & McMahon 2020; McIntosh et al. 2019; Sullivan et al. 2000). As we discuss in Chapter 2, family and twin studies can be useful in determining the degree to which genetic factors influence psychological conditions. For example, imagine that you have 100 pairs of identical twins (who share 100 percent of their genes) and 100 pairs of fraternal twins (who share 50 percent of their genes). If there are 50 pairs of identical twins in which both twins have depression, but only 10 pairs of fraternal twins in which both twins are affected, it's likely that depression is genetically influenced. (Note: These numbers are hypothetical. Whenever there are higher concordance rates among identical twins – meaning both twins have the condition – than among fraternal twins, genetic influences are likely at play.)

Studies from multiple sources suggest a connection between genes and risk for depression. For example, the rate of mood disorders among first-degree relatives of people with depression (parents, siblings, and children) is up to three times higher than among the general population (Levinson 2006). A study of 200 pairs of monozygotic twins found that when one twin was depressed, there is a 46 percent chance the other twin was depressed; for dizygotic twins the probability was around 20 percent. Both these rates are much higher than the rate of depression in the general population, which is around 10 percent (Levinson 2006).

Bipolar disorders appear to have a genetic link as well. Someone with a parent or sibling with bipolar disorder is 20 times more likely to have bipolar disorder than someone who doesn't have a relative with the condition (Craddock & Jones 1999). Monozygotic twins are up to 75 times more likely to both experience the symptoms of a bipolar disorder (McGuffin et al. 2003).

BIOCHEMICAL MODELS OF MOOD DISORDERS

In Chapter 2 we learned that neurotransmitters help the nervous system communicate. While no one neurotransmitter accounts for all the symptoms of all mood disorders, researchers have identified a family of neurotransmitters that seem to be involved in the symptoms of depressive and bipolar disorders; specifically: dopamine, norepinephrine, and serotonin, also known as *monoamines.*

Related to this, the **monoamine hypothesis of depression** suggests that symptoms of depression are brought on by malfunction of *monoamines* (Preston et al. 2021).

Monoamine hypothesis of depression: a biological theory of depression that suggests that symptoms of depression are brought on by malfunction of a class of neurotransmitters called monoamines.

Potential causes of chemical imbalance in the brain include:

1. Excessive reuptake of monoamines as being linked to depression. This means that the transport proteins in the synapse reabsorb the monoamines too aggressively and take too many of them out of the synaptic gap. As a result, there are too few monoamines to bind to the receptor site and deliver the message that the next neuron should fire, and the message passes on to the next neuron. Lower activity in one or more of the monoamines will result in less activity in the parts of the brain and yield the symptoms of depression.

2. Neurons do not release enough monoamines, meaning that the "fire" message is not delivered as quickly as it should be.

3. Monoamine oxidase (MAO) – the enzyme responsible for "cleaning up" the synaptic gap – is overactive and breaks down the monoamines too quickly. This also leaves too few monoamines available to bind with neurons to deliver the "fire" message.

4. The receptor site that receives monoamine neurotransmitters is abnormal in some way and needs extra stimulation to send the message to the receiving neuron.

Regardless of the cause, it appears that some form of monoamine malfunction is associated with symptoms of depression.

Among the monoamine neurotransmitters, serotonin has been at the center of attention in treating depressive disorders. It is a neurotransmitter involved in managing emotions, and it's also active in regulating the biological processes that rely on norepinephrine and dopamine.

It's not necessarily the absolute amount of these neurotransmitters in the system that's important, but the balance and interactions among them. For example, the permissive hypotheses suggest that when serotonin is low, the amounts of the other monoamines (dopamine and norepinephrine) are permitted to fluctuate more than they typically would.

Neurochemicals have also been implicated in bipolar disorders. For instance, symptoms of mania can be associated with low serotonin activity (Lan & Mann 2016) and overactivity of norepinephrine (Swann 2009).

THE BRAIN STRUCTURES AND CIRCUITS OF MOOD DISORDERS

On the biological level, our emotional reactions are facilitated (at least in part) by our *brain circuits*, on which depression research has been focusing in recent years.

Brain circuits are networks of interconnected brain regions. They can perform complicated tasks by modifying and transmitting information to other areas of the brain.

Recent studies have shown that dysfunctions in connectivity within and between circuits may contribute to depressive and bipolar disorders. For example, the disruption of monoamines described in the previous section are found in large concentrations in the limbic system, a part of the brain associated with the regulation of sleep, appetite, and emotional processes. Similarly, the prefrontal cortex, anterior cingulate cortex, hippocampus, and amygdala may also be implicated in depression (Treadway et al. 2014).

Prefrontal cortex. You'll remember from Chapter 2 that the prefrontal cortex is a part of the cerebral cortex in the frontal lobe and is associated with tasks such as problem solving and attention. In clients with depressive disorders, neuroimaging studies of the prefrontal cortex have found decreased brain wave activity, blood flow, metabolic activity, and gray matter (the darker tissues of the brain that consists of nerve cells and their dendrites) (Saveanu & Nemeroff 2012). People with the most severe depressive symptoms also had the lowest prefrontal activity.

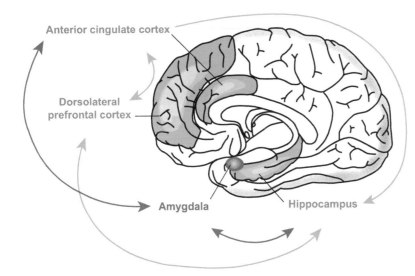

Figure 6.9 The anterior cingulate cortex helps to process the body's reaction to stress and emotional expression. The hippocampus is involved in processing new memories, including fear-related learning, while the amygdala is associated with emotions such as fear and anger and the prefrontal cortex processes motivational responses.

Source: Adapted from Leisman et al. (2012, figure 6).

Anterior cingulate cortex (ACC). This is an area in the frontal part of the corpus callosum and plays a role in the body's response to stress, emotional expression, and social behavior (Lamm & Singer 2010) (see Figure 6.9). Decreased connectivity within the regions of the ACC may be related to symptoms of reduced feelings of pleasure, attention, response planning, and coping (Rolls et al. 2019).

Hippocampus. This is a complex brain structure embedded deep into the temporal lobe. It is part of the limbic system and is involved in processing new memories, including fear-related learning (things we learn while we are stressed or afraid). Stress is correlated with decreased volume in the hippocampus, and decreased hippocampal volume is found in individuals with symptoms of depression (Konarski et al. 2008).

Amygdala. In Chapter 2 we learned that the amygdala is a cluster of neurons in an area of the brain called the temporal lobe. Neurons in the amygdala are linked to emotions such as anger, fear, and also positive emotions. The amygdala integrates the emotional significance of sensory stimuli and guides our behavior. Depressive symptoms are associated with increased volume and elevated activity in the amygdala (Treadway et al. 2014). Likewise, individuals with bipolar disorder sometimes have an overactive and/or enlarged amygdala (Strakowski et al. 2012).

Overall, studies have shown that individuals with bipolar disorder have lower overall brain volume (Maller 2014), including the prefrontal cortex and cerebellum (Wang et al. 2021). These two systems might be associated with the problems in emotion, planning, and judgment that people with bipolar disorder experience. At the same time, individuals with bipolar disorder often have an overactivated striatum, which is associated with hypersensitivity to things that might be rewarding (Caseras et al. 2013).

Just as the brain uses neurotransmitters as chemical messengers, it also uses hormones in the endocrine system. The endocrine system is a collection of glands

Figure 6.10 Overactivity of the hypothalamic pituitary adrenal (HPA) axis has been implicated in depression.

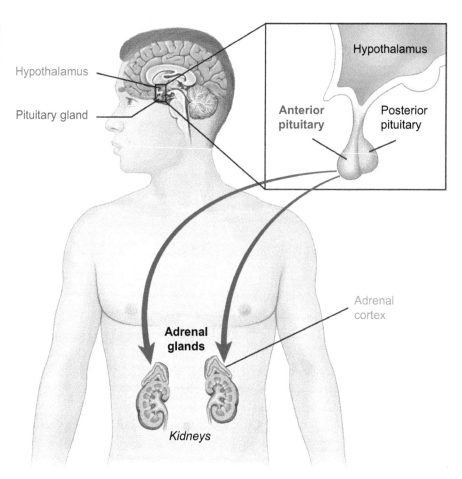

that secrete hormones into the bloodstream to regulate biological processes including sleep, hunger, sex drive, and feelings of pleasure (for more on the endocrine system take a look at section 2.1).

Three key components of this system work together: the hypothalamus, the pituitary, and the adrenal cortex. Together they are called the *hypothalamic pituitary adrenal (HPA) axis*, and they form a brain–endocrine system connection that has been implicated in some psychological disorders (see Figure 6.10). For example, people with depression have higher levels of cortisol than do those without depression. Cortisol is one of the hormones released by the adrenal glands during stressful experiences (Herane-Vives et al. 2016) such as the fight, flee, or freeze response.

Hormones may also play a role in other mood disorders. The release of too much hormone from the HPA (see Figure 6.10) axis can inhibit monoamine receptors in neurons so that an insufficient amount of monoamines is picked up, a process associated with depression. The hypothalamus secretes hormones that help to coordinate body rhythms like sleep and wake patterns, which are sometimes out of sync in people with bipolar disorders.

Biological Treatments of Mood Disorders

Biological therapies use medications or surgery to change the physiological conditions that lead to mood disorders and thus reduce the symptoms of depressive and bipolar disorders. In this section, we focus on biological treatments such as medications, electroconvulsive therapy, magnetic stimulation, and deep brain stimulation.

Table 6.1 Some commonly prescribed monoamine oxidase inhibitors (MAOIs)

Generic name	Brand name
phenelzine	Nardil
tranylcypromine	Parnate
selegiline	Emsam

Source: Information from Stahl (2017).

MEDICATIONS

The most common biological therapies for mood disorders are medications. Prescribers of these treatments assume that mood disorders are due, at least in part, to physiological conditions, including irregularities in neurotransmitters, the chemical messengers in the brain. The medications are prescribed to treat these.

Antidepressants are a category of medications used to reduce the symptoms of depressive mood disorders. There are dozens on the market today, and while there are few differences in effectiveness among them, a particular medication might work better for a particular person than another. Because of this, a prescriber might need to try a few medications (or combinations of medications) to find the one that works well for a client. Antidepressants help more than half of those who take them (Thase & Denko 2008). If one doesn't work, the prescriber will often try another, which can be challenging for clients who are experiencing both the symptoms of their depression as well as the side effects of the various medications.

Medication treatments can also be very effective for bipolar disorders (Galling et al. 2015). More than 60 percent of people with mania, for example, will improve and have fewer relapses as long as they continue their treatment (Malhi et al. 2013). Unfortunately, some people stop taking their medications too soon after beginning to feel better, and the symptoms will often recur.

In this section we cover four types of antidepressant medications used to treat depressive disorders, and two categories of medications used to treat the symptoms of bipolar conditions.

Monoamine Oxidase Inhibitors   Some of the oldest medications used in treating depression are **monoamine oxidase inhibitors** or **MAOIs**, a class of antidepressant drugs whose purpose is to keep the family of monoamine neurotransmitters (serotonin, norepinephrine, and dopamine) in the synaptic gaps in the brain long enough for the monoamines to bind to the receptor sites in order to deliver their message (Table 6.1). MAOIs accomplish this task by preventing (inhibiting) the enzyme monoamine oxidase from doing its job of metabolizing, or destroying, the monoamines (Preston et al. 2021).

MAOIs typically take about four to six weeks to start working and have side effects including dizziness, diarrhea, insomnia, and weight gain (Stahl 2017). One

Monoamine oxidase inhibitors (MAOIs): a class of antidepressant drugs whose purpose is to keep the family of monoamine neurotransmitters (serotonin, norepinephrine, and dopamine) in the synaptic gaps in the brain long enough for the monoamines to bind to the receptor sites in order to deliver their message.

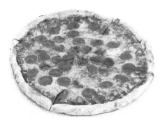

Figure 6.11 Certain foods can be a problematic choice for those on MAOIs.
Source: Tetra Images/Getty Images.

notable side effect is the "cheese effect," or hypertensive crisis. Because MAO helps to regulate blood pressure, destroying it makes it difficult to control blood pressure under certain situations. One of these situations occurs when you ingest tyramine, a naturally occurring substance in many foods and medicines. Ingesting too much tyramine from eating a four-cheese pepperoni pizza (Figure 6.11) or taking cough medicine, for example, can lead to a sudden spike in blood pressure, resulting in a terrible headache or even a stroke. Other foods containing tyramine to avoid with MAOIs include the following:

- All tap beers.
- Matured or aged cheese.
- Fermented or dry sausage like pepperoni, salami, or summer sausage.
- Improperly stored meat, fish, or poultry.
- Fava or broad bean pods.
- Soy sausage or other soybean condiments.

Because many people need to stay on MAOIs for several years, keeping to a tyramine-free diet can be challenging. For this reason MAOIs are not usually the first medicine that prescribers choose, even though they have been shown to decrease symptoms in up to 75 percent of patients with depression (Stein et al. 2005).

Tricyclic antidepressants: a class of antidepressant drugs that have three rings in their molecular structure.

Tricyclic Antidepressants

Tricyclic antidepressants are a class of antidepressant drugs that have three rings in their molecular structure (Table 6.2). You'll remember that serotonin, norepinephrine, and dopamine have been implicated in depression. The tricyclic antidepressants work on two of these monoamines, norepinephrine and serotonin, primarily by preventing the reabsorption or reuptake of them, meaning how they are recycled into the sending neuron. Tricyclics relieve symptoms of depression in 65 percent of those who take them (Arroll et al. 2005).

The tricyclics were once among the most widely prescribed antidepressants (Gitlin 2002), but their use has decreased because of their negative side effects such as weight gain (up to 13 pounds on average), dry mouth, blurry vision, constipation, drowsiness, and sedation. In addition, tricyclics can be fatal in overdose. This is a concern for prescribers who have clients who might be at risk for suicidal thoughts. For all these reasons, tricyclics aren't typically the first line of treatment for depression.

Selective Serotonin Reuptake Inhibitors

The monoamine serotonin is normally removed from the synaptic gaps between neurons by reuptake sites on the presynaptic neuron. Sometimes, however, reuptake can occur too quickly or too much serotonin can be removed from the synapse, and the resulting lack of serotonin is associated with depressive symptoms. While MAOIs increase the amount of monoamines in the synapse by preventing their breakdown,

Table 6.2 Some commonly prescribed tricyclic antidepressants

Generic name	Brand name
clomipramine	Anafranil
amoxapine	Asendin
amitriptyline	Elavil
nortriptyline	Pamelor

Source: Information from Stahl (2017).

Table 6.3 Some commonly prescribed selective serotonin reuptake inhibitors (SSRIs)

Generic name	Brand name
citalopram	Celexa
escitalopram	Lexapro
paroxetine	Prozac
sertraline	Zoloft
vilazodone	Viibryd

Source: Information from Stahl (2017).

selective serotonin reuptake inhibitors (SSRIs) keep monoamines in the synaptic gap by preventing them from being reabsorbed by the presynaptic neuron (Table 6.3). SSRIs are a class of medications that increase the efficiency with which serotonin binds to postsynaptic neurons in the nervous system by blocking its reabsorption into the presynaptic neurons (see Figure 6.12). Doing this causes serotonin to build up in the synaptic gap and increases the likelihood that serotonin will bind with the receptor sites on the postsynaptic neuron. This increase in serotonin availability is associated with a reduction in the symptoms of depression. SSRIs block the serotonin reuptake sites and allow serotonin to remain active in the synapse for a longer time.

SSRIs are generally well tolerated; that is, people do not have as many side effects as they might from other antidepression medications, so they may be more likely to take SSRIs when prescribed. Side effects of SSRIs include high rates of sexual dysfunction, decreased appetite, nausea, diarrhea, insomnia, and headaches; about 38 percent of people taking SSRIs will experience some of these (Cascade et al. 2009). SSRIs are not toxic in overdose and are available as generics, which makes them less expensive than some newer drugs.

Serotonin-norepinephrine reuptake inhibitors (SNRIs) are antidepressants that keep both serotonin and norepinephrine in the synapse longer (Table 6.4). SNRIs have the benefits of SSRIs but treat depression in an additional way by targeting norepinephrine. Unfortunately, they also have

Selective serotonin reuptake inhibitors (SSRIs): a class of medications that increase the efficiency with which serotonin binds to postsynaptic neurons in the nervous system by blocking its reabsorption into the presynaptic neurons.

Serotonin-norepinephrine reuptake inhibitors (SNRIs): a class of medications that aim to keep both serotonin and norepinephrine in the synapse longer.

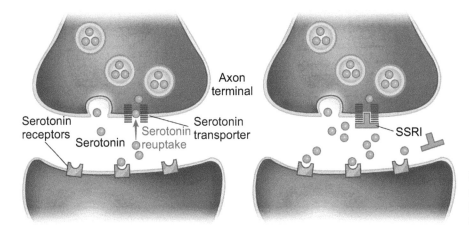

Figure 6.12 SSRIs increase the availability of serotonin to the serotonin receptor sites in the synapse.

Table 6.4 Some commonly prescribed serotonin-norepinephrine reuptake inhibitors (SNRIs)

Generic name	Brand name
desvenlafaxine	Pristiq, Khedezla
cymbalta	Duloxetine
levomilnacipran	Fetzima
venlafaxine	Effexor

Source: Information from Stahl (2017).

additional side effects, including nervousness, insomnia, and increased blood pressure (Stahl 2017).

Some SNRIs offer different kinds of action on serotonin and norepinephrine. Venlafaxine, for example, inhibits the reuptake only of serotonin in low doses, meaning it works just like an SSRI. At moderate doses, venlafaxine inhibits more serotonin and starts to block norepinephrine as well. At high doses, it blocks reuptake of serotonin, norepinephrine, *and* dopamine (Stahl 2017).

THE POWER OF EVIDENCE

Why the best antidepressant isn't always the best antidepressant

Why are there so many antidepressants for treating major depressive disorders? Haven't they been improved over time so prescribers can simply choose the most effective one for their clients? Let's look at the evidence and you'll see why the best antidepressant might not be the best antidepressant.

In 2018 a team of researchers undertook a daunting but impressive task (Cipriani et al. 2018). They conducted a meta-analysis of 21 antidepressant drugs by combing through the literature to find 522 randomized controlled trials that met their criteria and then used them to compare the 21 drugs for two major outcomes. Not only did they measure the medications' effectiveness, but they also examined the tolerability of the medications. In terms of effectiveness they counted medications that reduced the symptoms of depression by at least half. For tolerability they measured the number of people who withdrew from the study for any reason whatsoever; essentially the dropout rate. Here's what they found.

Some antidepressants were more helpful than others (which was to be expected), and all were more effective than placebos. Some of the *most* effective antidepressants were medications such as amitriptyline (also known as Elavil) and mirtazapine (also known as Remeron). You've never heard of them? It's not surprising. Amitriptyline is a tricyclic antidepressant that was discovered back in the early 1950s, and mirtazapine came to market in 1996. If you take a look at the list of the top 50 prescribed psychotropic medications, you might not find them there, and yet these are some of the most effective antidepressants we have.

The researchers found the picture a bit clearer after they looked at their second outcome, tolerability. There were some medications people just didn't seem to like to take, such as . . . you guessed it, these same effective medications. There are often very good reasons, including side effects such as dizziness, memory impairment, and constipation. What's the use of an effective medication if it's not tolerable? Medications with potentially problematic side effects aren't useless, however; sometimes prescribers will use them when other drugs that are easier to tolerate haven't worked that well.

There's another wrinkle. It's difficult to predict what side effects a person might have. One client might have terrible headaches with one antidepressant, but another person on the same medication might have none. Side effects aren't guaranteed to occur in everyone; they are possibilities and so are hard to anticipate.

Choosing a medication for a client is a complicated balance between finding one with minimal side effects that will help a client continue to take it and finding one that will relieve the client's symptoms. The researchers concluded that while antidepressants were better than a placebo, prescribers have to take more into consideration than just effectiveness. Finding the correct diagnosis, understanding client expectations, making sure the medication acts on the client's symptoms, and working with a therapist are important as well.

Source: Cipriani et al. (2018).

Ketamine   There are times when standard medications for depression don't seem to work, and when they do, they can often take weeks for certain clients. Recently a new treatment, esketamine, which focuses on a receptor called N-methyl-D-aspartate (a glutamate receptor also known as the NMDA receptor), has been approved as an in-office nasal spray formulation when used as an add-on to an antidepressant for patients with treatment-resistant depression (Vaccarino et al. 2022).

Lithium   Australian medical scientist Dr. John Cade first used lithium to treat psychological conditions in the 1940s. He discovered its utility almost by accident after delivering the medicine to a group of mice. He thought it calmed them, though it actually made them sick. Luckily, however, lithium treatment did help his patients, and lithium has since been found to be an effective treatment (Gim et al. 2009). In fact, it is one the most effective medications to treat manic episodes in bipolar disorder (Severus et al. 2014) and is particularly helpful at reducing suicide risk in the mood disorders.

It does, however, have some limitations. For instance, up to 55 percent of those who take lithium develop a resistance to it within three years (Hui et al. 2019), and 70 percent of people taking it had a 70 percent chance of relapse (Pinna et al. 2020). Lithium also has a narrow therapeutic window, meaning that if the dose is too low, the medication will not have the desired effect, but a dose that is too high can cause thyroid and kidney damage.

Lithium acts by improving the functioning of the neurotransmitter glutamate, an all-purpose excitatory neurotransmitter that is the "gas" or "accelerator" of the nervous system (Montlahuc et al. 2020). Too much glutamate in the synapse is related to mania and too little to symptoms of depression. By stabilizing the amount of glutamate in the brain, lithium treats both the manic and depressive phases of bipolar disorder (Belmaker 2004). Risk of relapse is 28 percent higher if

Table 6.5 Some commonly prescribed anticonvulsants for bipolar disorder

Generic name	Brand name
valproate	Depakote
lamotrigine	Lamictal
carbamazepine	Tegretol

Source: Information from Stahl (2017).

patients stop taking it (Suppes et al. 1991). Lithium does have some adverse effects: abdominal pain and nausea can be common, and in rare cases lithium treatment can result in low thyroid output and kidney dysfunction.

Anticonvulsants   *Anticonvulsants*, traditionally used to treat seizure disorders like epilepsy, can also be effective treatments for the symptoms of bipolar disorders (see Table 6.5 for some examples of anticonvulsants). Some researchers believe anticonvulsants help to stabilize the neurons in the brain by blocking the sodium channels in the nerve cell's membrane, which cause neurons to fire. But like most medications, anticonvulsants can cause side effects, in this case including blurred vision and fatigue. They can also cause a rare but potentially fatal rash in 3 of 1,000 people. Valproate (Depakote) is one of the most widely used treatments for bipolar disorders (Thase & Denko 2008).

NON-MEDICATION BIOLOGICAL TREATMENTS

When medications don't work for mood disorders, sometimes direct stimulation of the nervous system can help. Such procedures include electroconvulsive therapy (ECT), transcranial magnetic stimulation, vagus nerve stimulation, and deep brain stimulation.

Electroconvulsive therapy (ECT): a biological treatment that uses electricity to induce seizures in anesthetized patients.

Electroconvulsive Therapy and Brain Stimulation   **Electroconvulsive therapy (ECT)** (known in the past as shock therapy) is a biological treatment that uses electricity to induce seizures in anesthetized patients (see Figure 6.13). Back in the 1930s, Ladislas von Meduna noticed that very few people who had epilepsy also had schizophrenia (Dukakis & Tye 2007), and he hypothesized that epilepsy and schizophrenia could not exist in the same body. Perhaps, then, seizures were

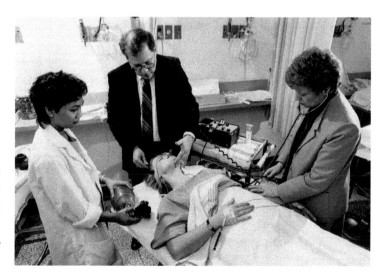

Figure 6.13 Patient undergoing ECT in which seizures are electrically induced in anesthetized patients for therapeutic effect.
Source: David Cooper/ Toronto Star via Getty Images.

curative of schizophrenia. Various substances have been used to induce the seizures including metrazol, insulin, and eventually electricity. Although von Meduna's hypothesis proved false, the connection he saw between seizures and the absence of schizophrenia did lead to an effective treatment for many psychological conditions.

When most people think of ECT, they may think of a barbaric procedure. Improvements in techniques have made ECT a different kind of intervention than it was in the past. Patients are anesthetized and given muscle relaxers to reduce discomfort. A 65–140v electrical charge is given for ½ a second which results in a seizure that lasts for about 25 seconds. Treatments must be repeated up to 12 times over two to four weeks (Fink et al. 2014). About half of patients who fail to respond to medication will respond to ECT, and often medication that didn't work in the past may work once the ECT treatments have been completed. Side effects include memory loss about the treatment, but research suggests that ECT does not produce any brain damage (Eschweiler et al. 2007).

Around 100,000 people receive ECT annually in the United States. While most often used to treat depression, ECT is also effective in treating mania and catatonia (Gitlin 2002; Glass 2001) and treatment-resistant bipolar disorder (Medda et al. 2015).

Unlike antidepressant medication, which can take months to work, ECT may relieve symptoms after only a few days. In fact, about 80 percent of depressed patients who receive ECT improve (Glass 2001) within a few weeks. Unfortunately, however, about half of people treated with ECT will have a recurrence of depression within just six months (Glass 2001). Additional ECT treatments or the addition of antidepressants can stave off these new depressive episodes.

Despite the benefits, ECT is still a rare procedure, prescribed by only 8 percent of all psychiatrists. Some researchers think this low rate is due to the misunderstanding and fears people have about ECT.

Exactly how ECT works is still a mystery. Some theories suggest that it lowers activity in brain areas that might be involved in depression (Nobler et al. 2001) while others suggest that ECT stimulates **neurogenesis** or new nerve growth, which may be the source of symptom relief. The electrical stimulation may increase serotonin, decrease stress hormones and increase growth of neurotransmitters in the hippocampus (Li et al. 2020).

Transcranial magnetic stimulation (TMS) uses electromagnetic coils to deliver a painless electromagnetic pulse that activates or deactivates nerve cells in the brain's prefrontal cortex (a part of the brain often underactive in some people who are depressed) (see Figure 6.14). Depressed moods seem to improve when TMS is

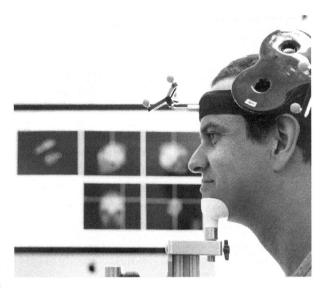

Figure 6.14 Transcranial magnetic stimulation uses electromagnetic coils to deliver a painless electromagnetic pulse.
Source: Monty Rakusen/Getty Images.

Neurogenesis: new nerve growth.

applied daily for two to four weeks (Dunner et al. 2014). While studies suggest that ECT may be more effective than TMS (Micallef-Trigona 2014; Ren et al. 2014), TMS has the advantage of causing few side effects. These include minor headaches, but no memory loss or seizures. About 50 percent of those who have received TMS procedures show an improvement in their symptoms after a few weeks (Modak & Fitzgerald 2021; Schutter 2009).

Vagus Nerve Stimulation   The vagus nerve is the largest nerve in the human body. It runs from the brainstem through the neck down the chest and into the abdomen and transfers signals to several regions of the brain, including the amygdala and hypothalamus (Figure 6.15). **Vagus nerve stimulation (VNS)** is a treatment for depressive disorders in which an implanted pulse generator sends regular mild pulses of electrical energy to the vagus nerve to stimulate the brain. The VNS requires light surgery to implant the device, and the generator results in increased activity in the hypothalamus and amygdala. It reduces depression symptoms in 40 percent of those who haven't responded to previous treatments (Berry et al. 2013). In another study of VNS of patients who didn't experience any improvement from their first medication, those who received a VNS showed improvement on 10 of 14 measures of depression (Conway & Xiong 2018).

Deep Brain Stimulation   Another procedure to treat depression, bipolar disorders, and other illnesses is *deep brain stimulation* (DBS) a surgical treatment in which a medical device is used to send electrical impulses to parts of the nervous system. A small electrode connected to a pulse generator stimulates the junction between the limbic system and the frontal lobe (Brodmann area 25). These electrodes are connected to a pulse generator implanted in the chest or stomach. The resulting stream of low-voltage electricity inhibits abnormal activity and can improve symptoms of depression and bipolar disorder (Holtzheimer et al. 2012).

Vagus nerve stimulation (VNS): a treatment for depressive disorders in which an implanted pulse generator sends regular mild pulses of electrical energy to the vagus nerve to stimulate the brain.

Figure 6.15 Vagus nerve stimulation (VNS) is a treatment for depressive disorders in which an implanted pulse generator sends regular mild pulses of electrical energy to the vagus nerve to stimulate the brain.
Source: Science Photo Library.

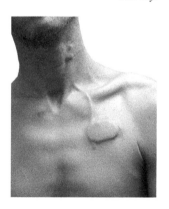

Psychological Models and Treatments of Mood Disorders

Biological treatments aren't the only treatment for mood disorders. A number of psychological treatments for mood disorders focus on the roles of behavior, thoughts, and relationships in determining mood. The effects of psychological interventions for treatment of adult depression have been shown to be comparable to those achieved with pharmacological intervention, and they are probably longer-lasting (Cuijpers & Gentili 2017).

The psychological perspective on the causes of mood disorders recognizes the impact of mental processes on depressive and bipolar disorders. In this section, we discuss evidence-based psychological models that are used to treat depressive and bipolar disorders.

THE ROLE OF ANXIETY, STRESS, AND STRESSFUL LIFE EVENTS

The experience of stressful events is associated with depressive and bipolar conditions. Up to 80 percent of people with depressive disorders report that a specific event (such as a breakup or a job loss) kicked off their depressive symptoms (Kim 2021; Mazure 1998).

Stressful events are also linked with both new bipolar conditions and relapses (Ellicott et al. 2019). And it's not just negative events that have an effect. Positive events such as a new job, a move to a new city, or a great new relationship can be just as stressful and have been associated with new episodes of mania and hypomania (Nusslock et al. 2007).

Stress and stressful events can also lead to increased amounts of cortisol in the bloodstream, and chronic stress may lead to chronically elevated cortisol levels. Such sustained elevated cortisol has been associated with a decrease in volume in brain areas associated with depression. This may explain why those with depressive symptoms have elevated cortisol levels (Saveanu & Nemeroff 2012).

Most people who experience stressful negative events never develop depressive or bipolar conditions. It's the interactions between an individual's genetic and biological processes and environmental influences that determine whether the person will develop symptoms of a mood disorder (Gutman & Nemeroff 2011).

BEHAVIORAL MODELS OF MOOD DISORDERS

In the behavioral perspective, mood disorders are assumed to be the result of the reinforcements and punishments to which a person is exposed (Dygdon & Dienes 2013). Symptoms result from a history of negative life events and systematic responses to depressive behavior. These responses can be complex. It's not simply that people who are depressed are choosing that environment, but rather that they have learned their environment will only bring them misery.

Behavioral theories suggest that stressful life events can initiate symptoms of depression because they reduce the positive things in a person's life (Gotlib et al. 1995). Simply put, people stop doing things that bring them joy. This effect can work the other way too: when people are depressed, increasing positive things around them will typically lift their moods (Bylsma et al. 2011).

Social rewards such as a warm smile and eye contact are thus particularly important in treating depression (Martell et al. 2010), and depressive symptoms develop when a person receives fewer such reinforcements (Coyne et al. 2002). People don't like being around the grim moods of depressed persons and may avoid contact with them. The isolation can create a downward spiral in which social reinforcements wane, and the depressive symptoms increase.

Reinforcements and punishments are also involved in bipolar disorders. There's some evidence that people who are more sensitive to rewards are more likely to develop bipolar disorders (Alloy et al. 2012). Working hard to achieve goals is also associated with manic and hypomanic episodes in people with bipolar disorders (Alloy et al. 2012). You'll remember that people with symptoms of mania and hypomania often are intense in their pursuit of pleasurable activities that could have painful consequences and often exhibit an increase in goal-directed behavior.

Behavioral Therapy   *Behavioral therapies* use learning theory to change moods and actions. These treatments assume that mood disorders are the result of maladaptive behavior patterns, and that if you change the behaviors, you can change the emotions and moods, too. Therapists work with clients on ways to predict and prepare for situations that could trigger depressed moods. They analyze, examine, and modify environmental contributions to depression (such as isolation). For depression, many behavior therapists focus on scheduling and increasing the rewarding events experienced by clients (Martell et al. 2010). In addition, therapists work with clients to improve social skills (like facial expressions and eye contact), which might make behavior less likely to keep others away. After all, many people report that it's depressing to be around someone who is depressed. Training clients on social skills can help to break this cycle.

Behavioral methods can be helpful in reducing symptoms of bipolar disorders as well. To that end, social skills training can help increase sleep, manage stress, improve relationships, increase concentration, and help with adherence to medication regimens (Basco & Rush 2005).

COGNITIVE MODELS OF MOOD DISORDERS

Stress affects everyone differently. Winning a spot on the cross-country team may be exciting to one person, but for another it might mean increased scrutiny and anxiety. According to the cognitive model, the impact of stress is connected to what the stressor means to the individual. The cognitive model of depression thus emphasizes the relationship between thoughts and moods.

People who are depressed, for example, have thoughts that suggest a negative view of three things: themselves, the world, and the future. Aaron Beck calls these the *cognitive triad* (Beck 1967) and posits that it is related to thoughts of inadequacy and hopelessness (Gautam et al. 2020). The more such thoughts people have, the more depressed they tend to be. Either because they occur very quickly in response to events or because people are unaware of having them, these negative thoughts are often automatic. Automatic negative thoughts are associated with the symptoms of depression, and depressed people may ruminate on them to the point of hopelessness. So, not only do the automatic thoughts lead to depressive moods and symptoms; they may also maintain the negative mood (Abramson et al. 2002).

Learned helplessness is a condition associated with being powerless to escape an unpleasant stimulus. The learned helplessness model suggests that when people feel they don't have any control over the things that happen to them, they are more likely to become depressed.

Negative events and thoughts may lead people to believe they are helpless to control the negative things that occur, particularly uncontrollable negative events such as a death in the family, a relationship ending, or a missed promotion (Loftus et al. 2020; Seligman 1975). In Chapter 2 we discuss that this model suggests that people with pessimistic explanatory styles have thinking patterns that are internal, stable, and global. They tend to believe that when unfortunate things occur, it is their fault (internal), it's always going to be that way (stable), and it will affect everything they do (global). This feeling of helplessness results in the lower motivation, passivity, and indecisiveness that often characterize depression.

People with bipolar disorder may demonstrate automatic thoughts as well. Cognitions linked to perfectionism, self-criticism, and over-ambitiousness are associated with the symptoms of mania and hypomania (Alloy & Abramson 2010; Atuk & Richardson 2021).

Cognitive Therapy   **Cognitive therapy** (also known as cognitive behavior therapy or CBT) is a type of treatment that emphasizes the link between thoughts and emotions. Cognitive therapies suggest that thoughts are the etiology, or cause, of mood disorders. The goal of cognitive therapy is to understand these maladaptive thinking patterns and develop healthier ways of thinking: change the way you think and you can change the way you feel. Therapists use specific techniques to recognize patterns of maladaptive thoughts and apply intervention strategies to reshape ways of thinking. One of the many goals of CBT is to help people shift their attributions for some negative events from internal/stable/global to external/temporary/specific.

> **Cognitive therapy (CBT):** a type of treatment that emphasizes the link between thoughts and emotions.

Aaron Beck, who was trained as a psychoanalyst in the Freudian tradition, noticed that his clients' language changed over the course of therapy (Beck et al. 1987). Reflecting on this observation, he wondered whether a therapist could change clients' thoughts more directly using language. As in all forms of cognitive therapy, the basis of Beck's model is that mood disorders result from thoughts. People who are depressed tend to have a pessimistic explanatory style, and when bad things occur, they tend to blame themselves. They are also more likely to discount positive events (Beck et al. 1987). In cognitive therapy (which is short term, lasting around 20 sessions), the goal is to recognize and challenge automatic thoughts linked to depression. The therapist encourages clients not just to think positively but to notice and test their maladaptive or distorted beliefs through questioning techniques and homework.

CBT can also aid in treating bipolar disorders by helping clients better understand their symptoms, become aware of early warning signs of symptom relapse, recognize the cognitive components related to their depressive, manic, and hypomanic symptoms, and smooth out the psychosocial stressors that are related to increased symptoms. CBT is effective and is associated with both fewer symptoms and increased medication compliance (Butler et al. 2006). This is so even when it is delivered in different modes, such as traditional face-to-face psychotherapy or self-directed approaches that require large amounts of homework assignments (López-López et al. 2019).

Sociocultural Models and Treatments of Mood Disorders

We don't exist in a vacuum. Instead, the way we engage with the world, including the moods we experience, is affected by the society and culture around us. Social and cultural models suggest that symptoms of mood disorders stem from social and cultural factors that can influence mood disorders. Culture can also influence diagnosis. Even core symptoms of depression can be shaped by cultural norms. For example, countries such as the United States and Canada have an emphasis on maintaining happiness. When people in those countries become depressed, they tend to have greater symptoms of low and sad moods. At the same time a motivation to pursue happiness is associated with better outcomes in Asia and Russia but more struggles with mood in the United States (Kirmayer & Ryder 2016). We have a number of sociocultural models and treatments for mood disorder.

Interpersonal theories of depression suggest that relational stresses and losses are linked with the symptoms of depression (Coyne 1976) and that symptoms of depression are associated with the presence of fewer social supports, such as family and friends, and greater social isolation (Rueger et al. 2016). These problematic styles may be due to attachment styles, interpersonal stress, or deficits in social skills (Whisman 2017). Social isolation may occur because symptoms of depression lead to significant interpersonal conflict (Hammen 2005), or because depressive symptoms may lead people to seek approval and become sensitive to rejection (Starr & Davila 2008).

Simply being around others will not alleviate or cure a mood disorder, however. The quality of relationships is important, and some research suggests that the symptoms of depression take a toll on interpersonal relationships. Having a depressed partner, for example, is related to the experience of marital dissatisfaction (Whisman 2017). Problematic and unsupportive social networks can also increase the likelihood of depressive, manic, and hypomanic symptoms (Miklowitz & Chung 2016). A third of those who care for people with bipolar disorder report having significant levels of depressive symptoms themselves (Perlick et al. 2016). Those who are divorced or separated are twice as likely to be depressed than those who have never been married (Schultz 2007).

Cultural factors such as racial and gender differences can also contribute to depressive and bipolar disorders. Culture, for example, can influence the way depression is expressed.

In the United States, there don't appear to be significant differences in the rates or expression of symptoms among racial or ethnic groups. There are, however, some big differences in recurrence rates. Hispanic Americans and Black Americans are 50 percent more likely to have a recurrent depressive episode than are white Americans (González et al. 2010), likely because these populations have lower treatment rates rather than because of the specific kinds of mood disturbances experienced. More than half of white Americans (54 percent) receive treatment for their symptoms of depression, while only 40 percent of Black Americans and 34 percent of Hispanic Americans do so (González et al. 2010).

Gender differences in precipitating factors and the expression of depression may also be linked to social and cultural influences. In many countries women are twice as likely to be diagnosed with depression (Hyde & Mezulis 2020). While men are just as likely as women to seek treatment for depression (McSweeney 2004), many related factors (such as poverty, discrimination, and lower control over their environment) are more prevalent in women than men (Hyde & Mezulis 2020). Responses to these factors may also be influenced by social expectations. Men may be more likely to respond with anger and alcohol, while women may respond in ways that are easier for some clinicians to link to depressive symptoms (Nolen-Hoeksema & Hilt 2013).

SOCIOCULTURAL TREATMENTS FOR MOOD DISORDERS

No psychological condition exists in a vacuum. Social systems and cultural approaches suggest that even when an individual has a psychological condition, something in their system is involved in establishing, maintaining, or exacerbating the current psychological state. Systems therapists use the system as an important intervention point in treatment. Families, couples, and friends may participate in the therapy session. Systems approaches also note that people can often play roles in certain social structures, such as being the first born in a family.

Social and cultural therapies may also focus on clients' economic pressures and on marginalized populations' identity, gender, and related cultural issues. Research shows that a culturally sensitive focus can increase psychotherapy success (Griner & Smith 2006).

Patient ethnicity can have an effect on clinical decision making about medications. A study of US adolescents with a diagnosis of bipolar disorder showed no differences between Black Americans and white Americans in number of mood episodes or length of hospital stays. The groups showed no significant differences in the psychotic symptoms they reported. Despite this, Black American adolescents with bipolar disorder were much more likely (nearly twice) to receive treatment with antipsychotic medications than were the other patients. Why? The reason is most likely racial bias among clinical practitioners (Akinhanmi et al. 2018), which leads to increased rates of diagnosis of more severe conditions other than bipolar disorder (such as schizophrenia). Much of the research on bipolar disorders underrepresents marginalized population patients, which leads to problems identifying potential differences in the progression of bipolar disorder in those groups. Solutions include increasing cultural competency in both the clinical and the research communities to try to address the gaps, provide researchers with the appropriate resources and support in order to work with hard-to-reach populations, and to focus on increasing the research on marginalized groups.

Interpersonal Therapy **Interpersonal psychotherapy** is a treatment that examines the changes, reactions, and deficits in an individual's relationships and emphasizes the resolution of relationship stressors as a way to address mood disorders. Changes in relationships over time may be experienced as a loss that causes some clients to become emotionally stuck. For example, depressed people may feel overwhelmed by changes in their roles in a relationship, such as a woman

Interpersonal psychotherapy: a treatment that examines the changes, reactions, and deficits in an individual's relationships and emphasizes the resolution of relationship stressors as a way to address mood disorders.

who has always worked as part of a team but has been promoted and now must work independently and direct teams. An interpersonal therapist may encourage clients to examine their feelings of loss and to develop the tools needed to accept and cope with the loss of the relationship, and to develop new relationships with appropriate expectations.

Therapists work with clients to improve interpersonal skills to make it easier to make and keep relationships and to handle common relationship challenges. Interpersonal psychotherapy can be useful in finding interpersonal blind spots and in helping clients build new skills so they can have smoother relationships.

Interpersonal psychotherapy is an effective treatment that helps 63 percent of depressed clients, a rate similar to CBT and medication treatments. Combining interpersonal therapy with medication is more effective than medication alone (Cuijpers et al. 2011).

Family and Social Rhythm Therapy *Family therapy* is a type of interpersonal psychotherapy that treats an individual's immediate social system, the family, to improve psychological functioning. Family therapy, also known as family systems therapy or couples therapy, is an approach that attempts to change the way individuals in a group (such as a family or couple) relate to each other (Figure 6.16).

Systems approaches emphasize the importance of relationships. Up to 50 percent of those with depressive mood disorders report problems in their family relationships, and the presence of family tension is related to relapse (Park & Unützer 2014). Research suggests that individuals in family therapy show lower relapse rates (Miklowitz & Chung 2016). In addition, family therapy may be as effective as individual cognitive therapy, interpersonal therapy, or drug therapy in helping to reduce depression (Lebow et al. 2012).

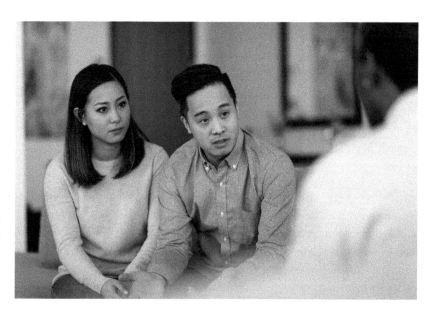

Figure 6.16 Family and couples therapy attempts to change the way individuals in a group relate to one another. *Source: FatCamera/E+/Getty Images.*

Systems approaches such as individual group or family therapy can also be useful in reducing the symptoms of bipolar disorders (Reinares et al. 2016). *Family-focused therapy* works to inform family members and other social support networks about bipolar disorders, to improve family communication, to promote a family's problem-solving skills, to emphasize the importance of taking medication as prescribed, and to improve clients' social skills (Miklowitz & Chung 2016). These interventions can reduce stress and increase the probability of symptom relief. Not only have clinicians had a positive response to family focused therapy, but taking part in at least 12 sessions of family education and skills training reduces the symptoms of bipolar disorder and may reduce the impairment associated with the symptoms clients do experience (Miklowitz & Chung 2016).

Interpersonal and Social Rhythm Therapy (IPSRT)   Another systems approach created to help with bipolar disorders is called **interpersonal and social rhythm therapy (IPSRT)**, a treatment for bipolar disorders that helps clients manage relationships and daily rhythms. Stressful events, including relationship problems and disruptions in daily rhythms, are associated with relapse in bipolar disorders. IPSRT focuses on smoothing interpersonal relationships and daily rhythms (such as by establishing daily schedules for sleep, eating, exercise, and medication; Frank et al. 2005), which can ease the symptoms of bipolar disorders. IPSRT is associated with lower relapse rates and increased medication compliance (Inder et al. 2015). In 2020 Steardo and colleagues found that IPSRT resulted in improvement in symptoms of depression and mania in individuals with bipolar disorder (Steardo et al. 2020).

Interpersonal and social rhythm therapy (IPSRT): treatment for bipolar disorders that helps clients manage relationships and daily rhythms.

CONCEPT CHECK 6.4

Fill in the blanks with the term or condition that correctly completes the statement.
1. Depressive symptoms have been linked to the malfunctioning of a set of neurotransmitters called _____.
2. The permissive hypotheses of bipolar disorder suggest that when _____ is low, the other monoamines are permitted to fluctuate more than they normally do.
3. Stress and stressful events can lead to increased amounts of _____ in the bloodstream.
4. The cognitive triad suggests that people who are depressed have a negative view of three things: _____, _____, and _____.

Fill in the blanks with the type of treatment for mood disorders.
5. _____ is a treatment for bipolar disorders that helps clients manage relationships and daily rhythms.
6. Medicines that block the reabsorption of the neurotransmitter serotonin into the presynaptic neurons, are referred to as _____.
7. _____ is a treatment for depressive and bipolar disorders that helps clients to recognize and challenge automatic thoughts linked to depression.

PULLING IT TOGETHER

Mood Disorders

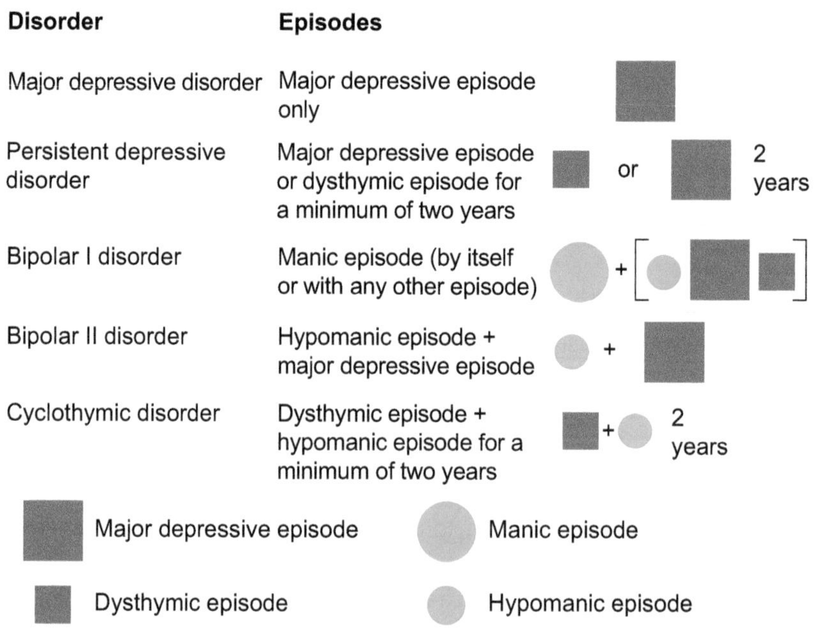

Disorder	Episodes	
Major depressive disorder	Major depressive episode only	
Persistent depressive disorder	Major depressive episode or dysthymic episode for a minimum of two years	or 2 years
Bipolar I disorder	Manic episode (by itself or with any other episode)	+ [ ]
Bipolar II disorder	Hypomanic episode + major depressive episode	+
Cyclothymic disorder	Dysthymic episode + hypomanic episode for a minimum of two years	+ 2 years

■ Major depressive episode   ● Manic episode

■ Dysthymic episode   ● Hypomanic episode

Figure 6.17 The depressive and bipolar chapters of *DSM-5tr* can be challenging. One of the reasons is that it can be hard to tease apart the relationship between mood episodes and mood disorders. Use this chart as a way to remember and to test your understanding.

SUMMARY

This chapter presented the following disorders:

- Major depressive disorder
- Persistent depressive disorder
- Premenstrual dysphoric disorder
- Disruptive mood dysregulation disorder
- Prolonged grief disorder
- Bipolar I disorder
- Bipolar II disorder
- Cyclothymic disorder

Mood Disorders Overview

- Mood disorders are marked by problematic emotional states. Symptoms are not diagnoses but building blocks in the diagnosis of a mood disorder.
- The four distinct mood episodes are major depressive episode, dysthymic episode, manic episode, and hypomanic episode.
- The symptoms of a major depressive episode include sad mood, anhedonia, and other cognitive and emotional symptoms such as changes in appetite and inability to concentrate.
- A dysthymic episode is a mildly depressive mood episode. It is not described as a separate episode in the *DSM-5tr* but is useful in understanding the mood disorders.
- A manic episode is a mood episode associated with an elevated, expansive, or irritable mood and increased activity and energy.
- A hypomanic episode has symptoms similar to a manic episode except the symptoms do not interfere with the person's work or social life.

Depressive Disorders

- When a major depressive episode occurs for a long period, it is diagnosed as a major depressive disorder.
- A persistent depressive disorder is a long-lasting (at least two years) major depressive episode or a long-lasting dysthymic episode.
- In premenstrual dysphoric disorder, a woman shows symptoms of depression in the weeks around menstruation in the majority of her menstrual cycles.
- Disruptive mood dysregulation disorder is a depressive mood disorder found in children and adolescents (between the ages of 6 and 18 years) which is characterized by severe, age-inappropriate temper tantrums and a persistent irritable or angry mood.

Bipolar Disorders

- Bipolar disorders include both depressive/dysthymic episodes and manic/hypomanic episodes.
- Bipolar I is a mood disorder in which a person cycles between mania and either hypomania or depressive episodes. Bipolar II disorder is a mood disorder in which a person cycles between depressive episodes and hypomanic episodes without experiencing mania.
- Cyclothymia is a persistent bipolar disorder in which a person cycles through the symptoms of hypomania and the symptoms of a dysthymic episode over a period of two years.

Models and Treatments of Mood Disorders

- Mood disorders are caused by both biological and environmental factors. They tend to run in families, which suggests a genetic link to the conditions.
- Symptoms of depression and mania are thought to be brought on by differences in the levels of the neurotransmitters serotonin, norepinephrine, and/or dopamine found in the synapse.
- Differences in brain structures and circuits have been found in both depressive and bipolar disorders.

- Biological therapies focus on changing the physiological conditions that lead to depressive and bipolar disorder and can include medications or surgical procedures.
- Stressful life events are also associated with mood disorders.
- Behavioral theories of mood disorders suggest that reinforcements and punishments are involved in establishing and exacerbating mood disorders.
- Behavioral therapies use learning to change moods and actions.
- The cognitive model of mood disorders emphasizes the relationships between thoughts and moods.
- Cognitive therapies emphasize the link between thoughts and emotions.
- Social and cultural factors can exacerbate mood disorders.
- Social and cultural therapies such as family therapy and interpersonal therapy use the social environment as an important intervention point in treatment.

DISCUSSION QUESTIONS

1. Why do you think some people with bipolar disorder may not want to take their psychiatric medications?
2. What are some of the reasons why bipolar disorders are difficult to diagnose? Why do you think that most doctors who see patients with bipolar disorder see them when they are depressed?
3. What are some key ways to distinguish depression from sadness and grief? Why might this be an important distinction?
4. The last section of the chapter presents several effective evidence-based treatments for depressive and bipolar disorders. Why do you believe there are so many effective treatments for depressive and bipolar disorders?
5. With so many effective treatments for depressive and bipolar disorders why don't you think more people seek treatment for these conditions?

ANSWERS TO CONCEPT CHECKS

Concept Check 6.1

1. Hypomanic
2. Manic
3. Anhedonia
4. Depressive

Concept Check 6.2

1. Major depressive disorder
2. Persistent depressive disorder

3. Major depressive disorder

Concept Check 6.3

1. Bipolar I disorder
2. Bipolar II disorder

Concept Check 6.4

1. Monoamines
2. Serotonin

3. Cortisol
4. Themselves, the world, the future
5. Interpersonal and social rhythm therapy (IPSRT)
6. SSRIs
7. Cognitive therapy or CBT

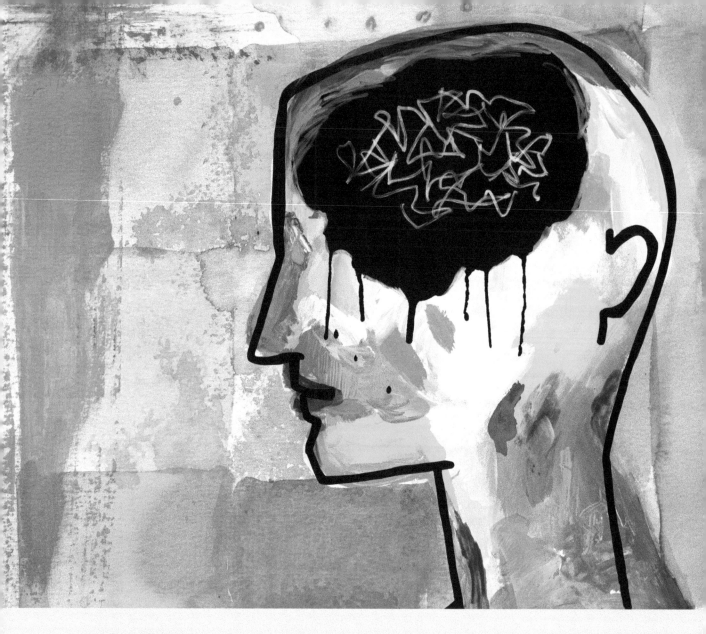

CHAPTER CONTENTS

7

Somatic Symptom, Sleep, and Psychological Factors Affecting Health

Learning Objectives

- Distinguish between malingering, factitious, and somatic symptom disorders.
- Discuss the various models and treatments for somatic symptom disorders.
- Describe the architecture of sleep.
- Discuss the various ways psychologists measure and track sleep.
- Describe the types of sleep-wake disorders.
- Discuss the various models and treatments for sleep disorders.
- Describe some of the techniques psychologists use as primary and adjunctive treatments for medical conditions.
- List some common medical conditions that are treated by psychological means.

CASE STUDY: Illness Anxiety Disorder – Jennifer Traig

Ever since she was four, Jennifer thought there were things wrong with her body. When she was in second grade, her Halloween assignment was to draw something scary. Her choice? A brain aneurysm. It turns out that her grandfather had recently died of a brain aneurysm, so a drawing of a vein exploding was the most frightening thing her seven-year-old mind could summon. By the time of her high school graduation, she was sure she had a slew of conditions – skin cancer, meningitis, and pancreatitis to name a few. The odd headache meant a brain tumor, leg cramps meant Parkinson's, and a stuffy nose must be sinus cancer.

Jennifer was not looking for attention; in fact, she found her trips to the doctor distressing because she really did feel the symptoms she reported. But what she also had was a way to turn the stress of her life into physical symptoms that she believed to be actual medical conditions. Nothing physical was actually going on, but that doesn't mean Jennifer wasn't extremely uncomfortable. She reported severe headaches, swollen arms, mysterious bruising, and rashes. She felt guilty about going to the doctor because she was convinced her frequent visits took time away from people who needed help, people with actual physical problems. Yet when she did visit the doctor, she felt disappointed that no one could ever find anything physically wrong with her. We'll learn a little more about Jennifer later in the chapter.

To discover more about Jennifer (Figure 7.1), take a look at her memoir *Well enough alone: A cultural history of my hypochondria* (2008).

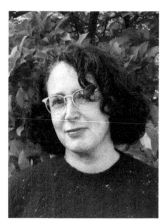

Figure 7.1 Jennifer Traig.
Source: © Jennifer Traig.
Reproduced with permission.

7.1 SOMATIC SYMPTOM AND RELATED DISORDERS

Imagine you just landed a brand-new job as a primary care physician. It's an amazing career but difficult because so many medical conditions come through your office door. Today is no different. Today's patient is much like Jennifer. He has an unexplained stomach problem with sharp pain on the left side pretty much all day, and it becomes much worse whenever he eats. This pain started about three weeks ago after a family argument. Nothing the man does appears to help. You ask a few questions, but none of the answers get you any closer to a diagnosis. The pain is not exercise-related; it doesn't seem to be indigestion or an ulcer. You're baffled, so you run a few more tests ... nothing. It's a mystery. A patient who presents with what appears to be a medical condition but has unexplained symptoms. What could the diagnosis be? Is he trying to get attention, faking symptoms to get pain medication?

Before you book yourself on the next episode of a television medical mystery, you should know that it's not too uncommon for physicians to bump up against unexplained physical symptoms (see Figure 7.17 in Pulling It Together at the end of this chapter). In fact, up to a third of outpatients have symptoms that can't be explained (Bass & Halligan 2014). A few factors might help to explain them, however, and some may even be psychological in nature.

According to psychopathologists, one of the possibilities could lie in the *DSM-5tr* chapter on the Somatic Symptom and Related Disorders. **Somatic symptom disorders** are psychological conditions characterized by excessive focus on physical symptoms or health despite the absence of health concerns. All somatic symptom disorders (*soma* means body) share one essential feature: clients experience symptoms of a physical illness that are not well explained by a medical condition. The presenting problem for most of the disorders is a physical symptom that shadows clients' lives. The *DSM-5tr* describes five somatic symptom disorders: somatic symptom disorder, illness anxiety disorder, functional neurological symptom disorder (conversion disorder), factitious disorder, and psychological factors affecting other medical conditions (which we discuss in section 7.3).

However, before we dive into the somatic symptom disorders, let's consider that some conditions *aren't* in this category. Most unexplained symptoms won't be diagnosed as somatic symptom disorders if they can be accounted for by a medical condition. If a health care provider has missed an important test or diagnosis, or if a patient has neglected to reveal an important symptom, then a medical condition should be considered. In fact, many health care providers who may have been baffled by their patients' initial complaints and who may have thought they were exaggerating symptoms later discovered the patients had legitimate health conditions.

Some providers may respond to certain patients' symptoms in a manner that reflects larger structural inequalities (Figure 7.2). The results of the recent Women

Somatic symptom disorders: psychological conditions characterized by excessive focus on physical symptoms or health despite the absence of health concerns.

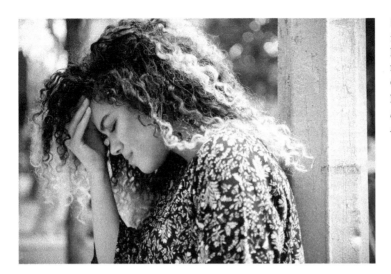

Figure 7.2 Whether intentionally or unintentionally, health care providers may respond to patients' pain differently depending on patients' identity.
Source: JGI/Jamie Grill/Getty Images.

in Pain Survey of more than 2,400 women with chronic pain revealed that over 60 percent of participants reported feeling doctors took their pain less seriously because they were a woman, and 83 percent reported feeling they were discriminated against by health care professionals (Samulowitz et al. 2018). Also, women waited an average of 16 minutes longer than men to receive pain medication at emergency rooms (Chen et al. 2008) and were more likely to be told that pain is linked to their emotions. Other sociocultural factors and structural issues such as patients' socioeconomic status and race can influence the diagnosis of symptoms such as pain (Anastas et al. 2020).

Finally, a diagnosis of somatic symptom disorders shouldn't be driven by a patient's external motivation for being sick. People expressing symptoms have been known to lie, exaggerate, and sometimes even intentionally make themselves sick in order to avoid work, exams, or events, or to get pain medication that can be abused such as hydrocodone (Vicodin).

Malingering

Psychologists refer to faking of illness as malingering (Diagnostic Overview 7.1). **Malingering** is the intentional production or faking of symptoms for *external gain* (also known as secondary gain). It can be mild, such as a person calling in sick to work when not really ill, or more severe, such as when a person decides to add chemicals to a urine sample or even intentionally harm themselves in order to get out of taking an exam.

Malingering is listed in the *DSM* chapter entitled Other Conditions That May Be a Focus of Clinical Attention. This chapter covers conditions or situations that might be the target of treatment but are not by themselves mental disorders. The chapter can also be used to document or draw practitioners' attention to important issues.

Malingering: the intentional production or faking of symptoms for external gain.

Exaggeration or intentional production of health symptoms motivated by external incentives.

Impact: Symptoms must exceed cultural and contextual norms. Symptoms are related to clinically significant distress or create impairment in important areas of life such as with friends and family or at work or school.

Source: Information from APA (2022).

Malingering can be a challenge for many health care professionals. Most are trained to trust clients to report their symptoms truthfully and typically don't expect them to be intentionally deceptive. Malingering can also be a challenge because there are legal and ethical consequences of not providing a patient proper care if they do have a medical condition. The prevalence of malingering can vary depending on the setting. It can be as high as 30 percent for patients claiming personal injury and can reach 50 percent by some estimates in patients with chronic pain who seek financial compensation (Alozai & McPherson 2020).

Factitious Disorder

Not everyone who over-reports or exaggerates symptoms is malingering. Another condition in which a person may exaggerate or internally produce symptoms is nicknamed "hospital hopper syndrome" or Munchausen syndrome, after Karl Friedrich Hieronymus the Baron von Münchausen (1720–1797), who often traveled the taverns of Europe telling false and exaggerated stories (Tatu et al. 2018). Officially, **factitious disorder** is a somatic symptom disorder in which a person will either fake, exaggerate, or intentionally produce symptoms of an illness in order to play the sick role (Diagnostic Overview 7.2). This may seem similar to malingering; however, the motivation in malingering is an external incentive, such as staying home from school or work, while in factitious disorder external incentives are absent and the motivation is internal, to reap the emotional benefits of being ill.

Factitious disorder: a somatic symptom disorder in which a person will either fake, exaggerate, or intentionally produce symptoms of an illness in order to play the sick role.

The motivation of being sick is the primary driver of factitious disorder. Those with this disorder will lie or exaggerate existing symptoms and in some cases will initially make themselves sick. They have been known to inject drugs and take medications such as laxatives, all with the intention of becoming ill (Glick 2021). What is the advantage of being in that sick role? Plenty. Psychologists call these benefits *primary gain*.

It's not uncommon for people with factitious disorder to be very knowledgeable about medical syndromes, and many have been known to spend a great deal of time online researching medical ailments in order to be able to replicate the symptoms they are supposed to have. Some undergo extensive treatments (McDermott et al. 2012). However, when challenged about their illness or when their deception is revealed, they'll often deny and deflect the accusations and may find another health care provider.

Sometimes their behavior has unfortunate consequences. Up to 8 percent have some sort of lasting damage to their health (Braham et al. 2017), and up to

Falsification of symptoms, or induction of injury or disease or injury linked to deception. External incentives are absent.

Impact: Symptoms must exceed cultural and contextual norms. Symptoms are related to clinically significant distress or create impairment in important areas of life such as with friends and family or at work or school.

Source: Information from APA (2022).

30 percent of cases end in unintentional death as a result of the person's attempts to become ill (Akın et al. 2016; Wittkowski et al. 2017).

Those with factitious disorder sometimes target another person, often someone in their care, in whom to produce real or faked symptoms of illness; this is called *factitious disorder imposed on another* (Diagnostic Overview 7.3). Factitious disorder imposed on another may be particularly difficult to diagnose, and law enforcement may see the symptoms as a crime and as a form of abuse (Emerson & Bursch 2020).

Exact estimates of the prevalence of factitious disorder are difficult to determine. The condition appears to be more common among women; however, men typically have more complex cases with more symptoms. Higher rates of factitious disorder can be found among people who received medical treatment as children, those who have negative feelings about the health care industry, and people who have previously worked in the health care field (Yates & Feldman 2016).

Illness Anxiety Disorder

Perhaps you know someone you might call a hypochondriac, someone who always seems to have something wrong or some new illness. This week it's a suspicious food poisoning, next week it might be the flu. When extreme it can become illness anxiety disorder. **Illness anxiety disorder** is characterized by excessive fear of having an illness despite evidence to the contrary. In this disorder individuals are preoccupied with the thought that they have or are getting a disease, and they experience a great deal of anxiety about their health, which may include excessive health-seeking or care-avoidance behaviors (Diagnostic Overview 7.4). They may scan their body for symptoms and interpret everyday body sensations as symptoms of something seriously wrong. As in other somatic symptom disorders, they even insist on invasive medical procedures to find out what they might have. As you might imagine, such tests all come back normal, though they may produce lingering symptoms that the person will interpret as part of the very illness the test disproved.

People with illness anxiety disorder may seek comfort from friends, family, and medical professionals. However, this reassurance never lasts long. Before long they are back at the doctor's office for more examinations looking for what the providers may have missed. Some seek assistance from the Internet to investigate their symptoms, which more often than not increases

Illness anxiety disorder: a somatic symptom disorder characterized by excessive fear of having an illness despite evidence to the contrary.

Diagnostic Overview 7.3: Factitious Disorder Imposed on Another

Falsification of symptoms, or induction of injury or disease or injury linked to deception in another, associated with identified deception.

Note:	The offender, not the victim, receives this diagnosis.
Impact:	Symptoms must exceed cultural and contextual norms. Symptoms are related to clinically significant distress or create impairment in important areas of life such as with friends and family or at work or school.

Source: Information from APA (2022).

Diagnostic Overview 7.4: Illness Anxiety

Preoccupation of either having or getting a serious illness along with anxiety about health. The person may either have avoidance of health-related behaviors or excessive health-related behaviors.

Impact:	Symptoms must exceed cultural and contextual norms. Symptoms are related to clinically significant distress or create impairment in important areas of life such as with friends and family or at work or school.
Timeframe:	At least six months.

Specify if care-seeking type or care-avoidant type.

Source: Information from APA (2022).

their anxiety (Pollklas et al. 2020). During the COVID-19 pandemic, many people with illness anxiety disorder experienced heightened alarm if they experienced a cough or muscle aches, fearing they had been infected (Coelho et al. 2020).

Not everyone with illness anxiety disorder runs to the hospital for tests to determine what's wrong. In fact, some are so worried that they imagine they would be devastated to get confirmation from a health professional, so they avoid doctors altogether. *DSM* specifies both a health-seeking type and a health-avoidant type of illness anxiety disorder.

Between 1 and 5 percent of people in the United States are diagnosed with illness anxiety disorder (Scarella et al. 2019), and while symptoms tend to ebb and flow over time, they can start at any age. Illness anxiety disorder is equally prevalent among men and women (French & Hameed 2021).

Somatic Symptom Disorder

Somatic symptom disorder: a psychological condition where a person experiences significant physical symptoms that cause distress and/or impairment in the absence of a diagnosable condition.

While illness anxiety is focused on a fear of having or getting an illness, **somatic symptom disorder**'s focus is on the symptoms themselves (Diagnostic Overview 7.5). If you ask a person with illness anxiety what they believe is happening, they may tell you very specifically what illness they believe they have, but people with somatic symptom disorder are really concerned about their symptoms.

Their stomach hurts, they may experience shortness of breath, they've got pain in their arm or more general symptoms such as tiredness or weakness. The somatic symptoms cause disruptions in their everyday life, they have constant thoughts and feelings concerning the symptoms, and managing the symptoms takes up a lot of time, money, and energy. These indicators of the disorder have to last for at least six months, and, of course, there needs to be evidence that no actual medical condition is producing the somatic symptoms. One type of somatic symptom disorder is pain-related, and for this reason the *DSM* lists a specifier to indicate that symptom (Witthöft et al. 2018).

Clients with somatic symptom disorder are often baffled as to what actual disorder they have and are in search of relief from their symptoms. In the meantime, they experience depressed moods and anxiety as a result of being unsure of their medical condition (Walentynowicz et al. 2017). Their health concerns are excessive given their symptoms and don't diminish despite the reassurance of health professionals. These clients always think the worst will occur – an abdominal pang is stomach cancer, a raised heart rate is a sign of an impending heart attack, dizziness is a symptom of a stroke. The symptoms can last for years, and some people will consult several doctors, looking for

Diagnostic Overview 7.5: Somatic Symptom Disorder

- Somatic symptoms that cause distress or disruption.
- Thoughts, feelings, or behaviors related to the seriousness of the somatic symptoms, anxiety about health, or time and energy devoted to managing the symptoms.

Impact: Symptoms must exceed cultural and contextual norms. Symptoms are related to clinically significant distress or create impairment in important areas of life such as with friends and family or at work or school.

Timeframe: At least six months

Specify if: with predominant pain. This specifier is used for those whose somatic symptoms are primarily pain-related.

Source: Information from APA (2022).

treatment (Witthöft et al. 2018) and asking for tests or surgeries (Martin & Rief 2011). Some will avoid activities that might make their symptoms worse, which can lead to isolation and exacerbation of the symptoms (Martin & Rief 2011).

In somatic symptom disorder, clients aren't faking the symptoms for attention (as they might in factitious disorder), and they aren't intentionally producing the symptoms for external gain (as they might in malingering). Rather, they actually feel as if they are experiencing symptoms, even though their doctors find no evidence that any medical condition is occurring. Somatic symptom disorder can thus be frustrating for clients because they experience the symptoms but are unsuccessfully treated for what they feel and may not be certain exactly what's wrong with them. They feel sick but don't know why.

It is difficult to measure the prevalence of somatic symptom disorder, because people with symptoms often first appear in primary care settings and may be treated there. In the United States around 12.9 percent of adults experience somatic symptom disorder. Women are diagnosed more than men, and symptoms typically begin in adolescence and young adulthood (Löwe et al. 2021).

Functional Neurological Symptom Disorder (Conversion Disorder)

In **functional neurological symptom disorder** (also known as conversion disorder) psychological worry or concern is transformed (converted) into a physical symptom (Diagnostic Overview 7.6). An early name for this rare condition was hysteria (see The Power of Words feature for more about hysteria). Most of the time in functional neurological symptom disorder, the symptoms suggest a neurological condition such as paralysis, numbness, muscle weakness, or even blindness, yet there is no biological basis.

Functional neurological symptom disorder (conversion disorder): a somatic symptom disorder where a person's psychological worry or concern is transformed into a physical symptom.

Diagnosticians must look for clues to distinguish functional neurological symptom disorders from actual neurological conditions. One clue is the way the symptoms are presented. People with numbness caused by functional neurological symptom disorder, for example, will complain of it only in their hands (called glove anesthesia; see Figure 7.3). But this is impossible given the physiology of the arm. The nerves in the hand provide sensory input along the entire limb; thus people with numbness resulting from neurological damage lose all sensation in their entire arm and hand.

Functional neurological symptom disorder can be difficult to distinguish from a medical condition (Tsui et al. 2017). But another clue to this condition is the blitheness some clients have about their symptoms. You might expect that if you suddenly went blind or had numbness in your arms you would be extremely concerned. However, people with functional neurological symptom disorder seem strangely unworried about their condition (an apathy

Diagnostic Overview 7.6: Functional Neurological Symptom Disorder (Conversion Disorder)

Symptoms of voluntary motor or sensory function that don't fit any medical conditions.

Impact: Symptoms must exceed cultural and contextual norms. Symptoms are related to clinically significant distress or create impairment in important areas of life such as with friends and family or at work or school.

Source: Information from APA (2022).

Figure 7.3 While actual physical damage would cause numbness along the entire arm (A), in functional neurological symptom disorder (conversion disorder) (B) only the hand is numb.

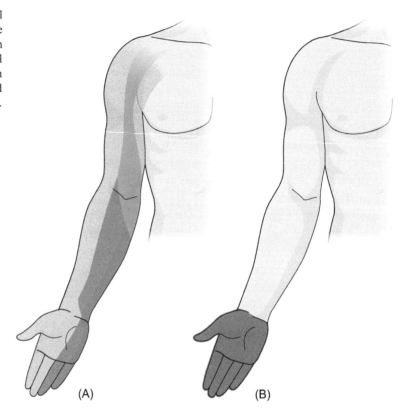

(A)   (B)

sometimes called *la belle indifférence*). Some theories suggest overactivation in the frontal lobes as a reason for the apathy in some people with functional neurological symptom disorder (Aybek et al. 2014; Dattilo 2018).

As is the case for many somatic symptom disorders, in functional neurological symptom disorder the onset or exacerbation of the symptoms is often linked to a stressor or other event in the person's life. When matters get worse, the symptoms do too. Only 1.5 percent of people who seek medical treatment meet the criteria for functional neurological symptom disorder (Carson et al. 2012; Fink 2004).

Functional neurological symptom disorders can come with a number of specifiers:

- Weakness or paralysis.
- Abnormal movement (such as a tremor).
- Difficulty swallowing.
- Speech symptom.
- Seizures.
- Sensory loss.
- Special sensory symptom (such as hearing disturbance).

The prevalence of functional neurological symptom disorder in general hospital settings is about 5 percent (Yakobov et al. 2017). Symptoms typically begin in late childhood and are diagnosed more often in women than in men (Raj et al. 2014).

THE POWER OF WORDS

HYSTERIA

What do hysterical laughter, mass hysteria, the medical procedure called hysterectomy, and one of the oldest psychological disorders ever described have in common? Their names are all related to the Greek word for womb or uterus, *hystera*, and they reveal not only how society views women but also how attitudes about a mysterious and ancient psychological disorder now called functional neurological symptom disorder have changed.

One of the first descriptions of "hysteria," or what we now call functional neurological symptom disorder (or conversion disorder), can be traced back to symptoms of depression or seizures. In Chapter 2, we discussed the idea that the potential cause(s) behind certain conditions can inform the development of treatment strategies. Society once believed (and some still believe) that women's biology, specifically their uterus, made them mentally weak. Thus when nineteenth-century practitioners believed the uterus wandered around the body wreaking havoc, the best solution was thought to be trying to coax it back where it belonged. There was no shortage of techniques for achieving this. A common one was to put nice-smelling items near the mouth and foul-smelling ones near the vagina if the uterus was thought to be too low in the body, and reversing the process if it was too high.

It wasn't until 1895 when Sigmund Freud and Joseph Breuer wrote *Studies on Hysteria* that the definition of the disorder was expanded such that those who had symptoms included men. Freud's theory of hysteria centered on the idea that unconscious fantasies were responsible for the unexplained physical changes in those who had the disorder's symptoms. By 1939 people were also using the word hysteria to describe uncontrollable emotions such as laughter, another way to define women by their biology. Fast-forward to 1980 when the *DSM-III* changed the name of the condition called "hysteria" to "conversion disorder," and then in *DSM5-tr* to "functional neurological symptom disorder" to emphasize that psychological concerns were being converted into physical ones and that the disorder had nothing to do with the uterus after all.

Source: Tasca et al. (2012).

Models and Treatments of Somatic Symptom and Related Disorders

Somatic symptom disorders can have multiple causes. Some researchers speculate that vulnerabilities such as hypersensitivity to physical sensations and a history of illnesses may combine with stressors such as emotional conflicts to produce these disorders (Schulz 2020). Remember the case at the start of the chapter? Your patient, for example, may have always been sensitive to physical sensations.

Treating somatic symptom disorders can be challenging. Because they believe their concerns are medical, people with these disorders rarely seek psychological treatment, and when referred to mental health practitioners they may feel as if their other health care providers don't believe they are experiencing symptoms. It is often difficult to convince clients that they don't need medical treatment (Henningsen 2018). Despite the stress their clients feel and their lack of control over their symptoms, some health care practitioners may in fact be dismissive or annoyed when they realize the symptoms are related to mental health or are created intentionally (as in factitious disorders) (Jafferany et al. 2018).

There are not many effective treatments for somatic symptom disorders. Most treatments focus on the anxiety that leads to the disorders. Many will explore the precipitating events that might have first set the physical symptoms in motion, rather than on the symptoms themselves (Jafferany et al. 2018).

BIOLOGICAL MODELS AND TREATMENT

Biology plays a role in setting up the psychological factors related to somatic symptom disorders. For instance, biological factors may be related to some clients' hypersensitivity to viewing life events as unpredictable, which leads to their persistently being on guard about their health (W. L. Huang et al. 2021).

Biological treatments utilize medications that influence the neurotransmitter serotonin to reduce anxiety and depressed moods in clients (Kurlanski & Maffei 2016). Antidepressant medications can be helpful in the same way as they can be for clients with symptoms of obsessive-compulsive disorder, as we discuss in Chapter 4 (Henningsen 2018).

PSYCHODYNAMIC MODELS AND TREATMENT

Functional neurological symptom disorders are some of the oldest disorders described in the *DSM*, but despite their long history they are still not well explained by or treated with psychodynamic methods (Wright et al. 2016).

From the psychodynamic view, Freud saw what he called "hysteria" as a conversion of emotional conflicts into physical symptoms (Ding & Kanaan 2017). Modern psychodynamic theorists suggest that unconscious conflicts from childhood are the source of these conditions, creating anxiety that is converted into physical symptoms that are easier to deal with (Kaplan 2016).

Psychodynamic psychotherapy focuses on providing insight to the connection between physical symptoms and the emotional world and helping clients investigate what might have created these connections. The goal is for clients to become aware of the underlying fears that lead to the expressed symptoms, in order to reduce the need to express them as physical symptoms (Kaplan 2016).

In illness anxiety, psychodynamic therapists attempt to help clients become aware of their fears, which should help reduce anxiety and the need to convert it into physical symptoms (Kaplan 2016; Stone & Sharpe 2018).

COGNITIVE AND BEHAVIORAL MODELS AND TREATMENT

No one likes to be sick, yet according to the cognitive-behavioral view, illnesses can lead to certain reinforcements. It can relieve us of responsibilities or bring us attention. Over time, then, people with somatic symptom disorders learn this and begin to express symptoms in order to get what they want.

From the cognitive perspective, clients may feel the same physical sensations everyone else does, but they respond with undue alarm because they may feel that having good health means being completely symptom-free. Increased anxiety from this exaggerated response can lead to even more physical symptoms. People with somatic symptom disorder are more likely to believe they are vulnerable to illness and to feel pain and body sensations more intensely. They may also believe serious illnesses are common (Voigt et al. 2010). They also doubt their ability to tolerate any pain (Rief et al. 2010).

The cognitive and behavioral approach focuses on changing thoughts and altering the sometimes-hidden reinforcements to illness. Therapists work to remove these reinforcements and increase those for healthy behaviors. They encourage clients to think in a new way about their physical symptoms and illnesses (Levenson 2018). Cognitive restructuring is one way to do so. Cognitive-behavioral therapists may also utilize exposure treatments in order to help clients habituate to upsetting events rather than expressing them through physical symptoms (O'Hara & Howard 2021; Tsui et al. 2017).

SOCIOCULTURAL MODELS AND TREATMENT

Social, gender, and interpersonal factors are also important in somatic symptom disorders. In some cultures, it's easier to express physical complaints than psychological ones. Somatic symptoms in response to emotion are sometimes quite expected in these societies, including Japan, Latin America, and China (Shattuck et al. 2020). For example, somatic symptom disorder has been diagnosed in over a third (33.8 percent) of patients in general outpatient hospitals in China; however, the rates are lower (19 percent) in Traditional Chinese Medicine departments (Cao et al. 2020).

MULTIPERSPECTIVE MODELS AND TREATMENT

Jennifer (from the chapter-opening story) is much better these days. Treatment for her illness anxiety disorder came about unexpectedly. With a diagnosis of irritable bowel syndrome (IBS), she was prescribed an SSRI that helped both her symptoms. She found that she spent much less time on websites searching for symptoms and treatments. Cognitive-behavioral therapy was effective for Jennifer as well. She finds that she still is afraid, but the fear just "drops away."

> **CONCEPT CHECK 7.1**
>
> Fill in the blanks with the condition that best fits the description.
> 1. Martin is back at his doctor's office again. It's the third time this month. All his appointments are about the pain in his shoulder. _____
> 2. Sarah is video chatting with her doctor for the third time today. She is convinced that she has COVID-19 despite the fact she has tested negative six times this week. Her worry has stopped her from doing any work or anything other than tracking how she's feeling. Her doctor believes her symptoms are most likely seasonal allergies. _____.
> 3. A 44-year-old man talks to his primary care physician because for the last three months he's had frequent headaches. Upon questioning he says no medications appear to be helping with the pain, which starts in his head, extends down both arms, and gets worse as he becomes more stressed. After several tests it appears that there are no physical problems, and the pain doesn't match any kind of headache. _____.

7.2 PSYCHOLOGICAL TREATMENTS FOR PHYSICAL DISORDERS

Psychological factors affecting other medical conditions: a condition diagnosed when physical illnesses are created or exacerbated by the interaction of biological, psychological, and emotional and social conditions.

Behavioral medicine: an interdisciplinary field concerned with health and illness that combines knowledge of social and medical sciences to improve health and combat illness.

Psychoneuroimmunology: a field that examines the relationship between the immune system and the stress response.

Health psychology: a general branch of psychology concerned with the way psychological factors affect wellness, illness, and medical treatments.

Psychological factors affecting other medical conditions are diagnosed when physical illnesses are created or exacerbated by the interaction of biological, psychological, and emotional and social conditions (Diagnostic Overview 7.7). While psychological factors are predominant in factitious, functional neurological symptom, and illness anxiety disorders, in other medical conditions (sometimes called psychophysiological disorders) biological processes are the predominant factor. However, psychological and social factors play a large role in the initiation or exacerbation of the problem and thus can also play a role in treatment and the relief of symptoms.

Three broad areas in psychology focus on this interaction between physical and psychological health. They are **behavioral medicine**, an interdisciplinary field concerned with health and illness that combines knowledge of social and medical sciences to improve health and combat illness, **psychoneuroimmunology**, the study of the relationship between the immune system and the stress response, and **health psychology**, which is a general branch of psychology concerned with the way psychological factors affect wellness, illness, and medical treatments.

Health psychology can help health care practitioners understand that the role personality can play is significant in health and wellness. Maybe you've heard someone say "You'll worry yourself sick." The connection between stress and illness is well established. Links between stress and ulcers (Sharma et al. 2004) as well as headaches (Martin et al. 2007) have been made in the literature. When there is a link between an illness and stress, the person's disorder is thought of as a psychosomatic illness. While it is common to think that a psychosomatic illness is all in your head, stressors can create or worsen illness.

Personality also interacts with stress and illness. Back in the 1960s, cardiologists uncovered a link between reactions to stress and cardiac disease (Friedman & Rosenman 1974). This led to the hypothesis that there are essentially two personality types.

Type A personalities tend to be competitive, hostile, and impatient. They are the type of people who not only will walk up an escalator but be gruff when they are passing you. The Type A personality is so aware of time that even the slightest delays in a schedule will cause a lot of anxiety. Type A's also escalate to anger pretty quickly (Mishra & Srivastava 2018).

On the other hand, Type B personalities are relaxed and patient. Seemingly unflappable, they are more resistant to time pressure, more cooperative, and generally easygoing. Researchers discovered that Type A personalities with greater amounts of impatience and hostility have a greater likelihood for coronary heart disease, a medical condition that results in narrowing of the vessels that supply blood to the heart. Type B's, on the other hand tend to have a lower risk of developing heart conditions. They also tend to have higher immunity response (Tohver & Feher 2020).

While stress causes discomfort and even leads to illness, it can also motivate us to reduce the stress by strategies called coping. While stress is the response to the event you see as a challenge, coping is the way we manage the stress.

Coping doesn't always lead to resolution of the *cause* of the stress. Some forms of coping are escaping or avoiding the stressful situation altogether, or simply hunkering down and bearing with it. Some people under stress engage in behaviors that are unhealthy, known as negative coping. They may blame themselves for the events, blame others, or engage in self-indulgent behaviors like overeating, excessive computer use, or even Internet addiction. Negative coping can just make matters worse.

Others shut down under stress and do not attempt to respond or cope. Learned helplessness occurs when an animal fails to take action to escape a noxious stimulus. The same appears to be true for people (Chapter 2). When in a situation in which you feel you have no control, over time you may learn to tolerate it rather than fight (Peterson et al. 1993).

There are also several constructive ways to cope with stress, which rely on strategizing the way you think and what you do in the environment. Researchers have divided positive coping strategies into two types; one focuses on changing the actual stressor and the other on changing our emotional reaction to the event

Diagnostic Overview 7.7: Psychological Factors Affecting Other Medical Conditions

- A medical symptom or condition is present.
- Psychological or behavioral factors unfavorably impact the medical condition such as influencing the course, interfering with treatment, creating a health risk, precipitating or exacerbating symptoms.

Impact: Symptoms must exceed cultural and contextual norms. Symptoms are related to clinically significant distress or create impairment in important areas of life such as with friends and family or at work or school.

Source: Information from APA (2022).

Figure 7.4 Problem vs emotion coping strategies. Top row: In emotion-focused coping, a person will apply arousal regulation techniques to manage thoughts and feelings. Bottom row: Problem-focused strategies help a person to develop relevant solutions and practical actions.

Sources: Top left: Oscar Wong/ Moment/Getty Images; top center: Ridofranz/iStock/Getty Images Plus; top right: Mayur Kakad/Moment/Getty Images. Bottom left: Constantine Johnny/Moment/Getty Images; bottom center: Daisy-Daisy/ iStock/Getty Images Plus; bottom right: NicoElNino/ iStock/Getty Images Plus.

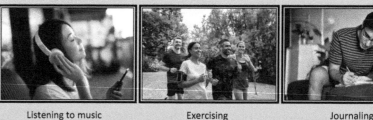

In emotion-focused coping, a person will apply arousal regulation techniques to manage thoughts and feelings

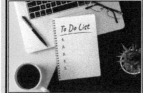 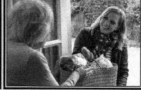 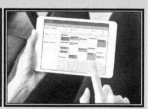

Listening to music   Exercising   Journaling

Problem-focused strategies help a person to develop relevant solutions and practical actions

Creating a to-do list   Asking for help   Improving time management

(Lazarus & Folkman 1984). That is, you can direct your coping skills outward toward the problem causing the stress, or inward to alter your perception of the stressful situation (see Figure 7.4).

Emotion-focused coping directs coping at our response to the event. This coping can be cognitive (varying the way you think about the event) or behavioral (changing the things you do, like distracting yourself). At best, cognitive and behavioral approaches can lead to reappraisal of the stressful situation and help you to see the situation in a new light. At worst, emotion-focused coping can result in drug and alcohol abuse.

You are more likely to employ emotion-focused responses when you think there is not much you can do to change the actual stressor (Lazarus & Folkman 1984). A *problem-focused coping strategy*, on the other hand, directs the coping toward the situation itself. You tend to use problem-focused coping if you think you can influence the situation.

Whether you focus on the stressor or your response to it, employing constructive coping and making healthy efforts to reduce the impact of stress is the best thing you can do to combat stress and make a preemptive strike to keep the effects at bay. Aerobic exercise, physical activity that increases the capacity of the heart and lungs, has been shown to reduce stress, as do getting adequate sleep, meditation, and eating healthy foods. Ironically, these are the very things people often stop doing when they begin to feel stress.

The goals of health psychology (see Figure 7.5) are to prevent illness, promote good health, help with the treatment of illnesses, investigate the correlates of

Figure 7.5 Health is at the nexus of biology, psychology, and social factors. This means that health can be influenced by psychology as well.

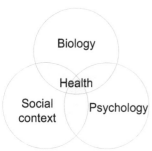

Biology

Health

Social context   Psychology

illness (such as stress) and the motivations to make better health choices (such as nutrition), and improve the health care system and health policy. Common conditions that mental health researchers and practitioners work with include cancer, immune dysfunction, cardiovascular conditions, and chronic pain.

All these health conditions are influenced by psychological and social factors such as smoking, diet, and stress. For example, coronary heart disease is influenced by job stress and high levels of anger and depression (O'Connor et al. 2021), asthma is worsened by stress and anxiety, and chronic headaches are made worse by stress, helplessness, anger, and physiological factors (Dafauce et al. 2021). The leading causes of death in the United States aren't necessarily the ones we focus on. For example, while the media often cover homicide and terrorism and Internet searches focus on cancer, heart disease remains a major cause of mortality in the United States. What's more, there are behavioral modifications that can reduce the likelihood of heart disease (see Figure 7.6).

Models and Treatments of Psychological Factors Affecting Other Medical Conditions

BIOLOGICAL MODELS AND TREATMENTS

Biological factors can be the source of disease, but they can also link to psychological factors and possibly complicate treatments. For example, individuals with autonomic nervous systems that are easily stimulated can be exposed to mildly stressful situations and quickly become overly stressed, complicating their medical conditions (O'Connor et al. 2021).

Another interaction between the body and stress occurs in the immune system. The immune system defends against external invasions such as bacteria and viruses, in part by employing lymphocytes, white blood cells that attack foreign substances. Without your immune system, you would be vulnerable to illness and disease. Hormones such as endorphins and corticosteroids flow into your body during stressful situations, however, and can weaken your immune response in a biological response called *immunosuppression*. In essence, your immune system becomes stressed. Constantly alerting your immune system in this way over time can reduce your ability to react and defend against the foreign substances, which can lead to more illness (Glaser et al. 1987; Seiler et al. 2020).

COGNITIVE AND BEHAVIORAL MODELS AND TREATMENTS

Cognitive-behavioral therapy (CBT) techniques have been used as an adjunctive treatment for many medical conditions, including high blood pressure (Nolan et al. 2018), diabetes, vascular diseases, and the adverse effects of chemotherapy (Ye et al. 2018). Biofeedback has been used to treat headaches, muscular conditions, heartbeat irregularities, high blood pressure, and pain (Kondo et al. 2019).

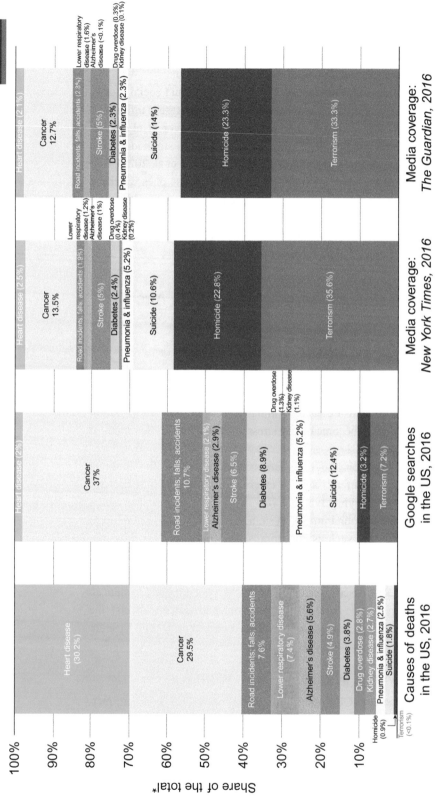

Figure 7.6 The 13 actual leading causes of death compared to Internet searches and media coverage (2016).

Source: Visualization adapted from Ritchie (2019), reproduced under the Creative Commons BY license.

Behavioral medicine, as defined earlier, is an interdisciplinary field concerned with health and illness that combines knowledge of the social and medical sciences to improve health and combat illness. Practitioners who utilize behavioral medicine will often intervene with psychological techniques like biofeedback to reduce their clients' stress. In **biofeedback**, a person is trained to become aware of physiological functions, such as heartbeat or breathing, and attempts to influence those functions. If you are aware of your heart rate, for example, you can use relaxation or meditation techniques to reduce it and activate your parasympathetic nervous system. Biofeedback devices can include portable scalp sensors to monitor brain waves; finger, earlobe, or watch sensors to monitor heart rate; and sensors around the fingertips to monitor sweat glands activity that can be related to anxiety (Badawi & El Saddik 2019).

Biofeedback: a technique in which a person is trained to become aware of physiological functions, such as heartbeat or breathing, and attempts to influence those functions.

SOCIOCULTURAL MODELS AND TREATMENTS

Just as individual behavior can affect our health, structural issues can affect our health in both positive and negative ways. For example, Black women who experienced the stress of daily incidents of racism (such as poor service in stores) were more likely to have lower scores in subjective cognitive functioning (Coogan et al. 2020).

Social factors can also influence our exposure to certain diseases. For example, society can influence what we eat, how or whether we exercise, and whether we are attracted to or repelled by smoking. Social factors can even influence the ways our built environment is constructed, which can in turn alter the way we live, work, and play. Is there easy access to health care, exposure to violence? Something seemingly as simple as sidewalks can be associated with health. In a study using mapping data that analyzed over 430 countries, researchers found a correlation between mortality rates, and access to sidewalks and hiking trails (Levy et al. 2020). However, these amenities can also be associated with more affluent neighborhoods with residents who have better access to health care.

What's more, society can influence the treatments that are prescribed as well as the level of care seeking. Cultural norms can either increase or decrease the use of certain kinds of treatments such as vaccines and mental health treatments, and even whether people access health care at all. For example, a number of Christian denominations such as Jehovah's Witnesses and Christian Scientists are opposed to certain kinds of medical treatment.

Psychological factors can enhance health as well, such as by motivating people to seek treatments for disorders and practice healthy behaviors that may protect them from certain conditions. Social support from family and friends can help people cope with stress and is associated with recovery from illness and protection against psychological concerns. For example, in a study that looked at 169 adolescents in the United States, those with a close friend not only had higher levels of self-esteem; they also had lower levels of depression and anxiety several years later (Narr et al. 2019).

CONCEPT CHECK 7.2

1. Good health is influenced by _____, _____, and _____ factors.
2. Stress can affect the immune system through a process called _____, which makes the immune system work less efficiently.
3. What type of coping directs our energy toward solving the stressful situation _____?
4. Marlin's doctor asked her to wear a brace during the night to help reduce her arm pain. However, the brace was a constant reminder that Marlin wasn't well yet, and because she didn't like to think about that, she decided not to wear it. This is an example of what kind of coping?

7.3   SLEEP-WAKE DISORDERS

You probably heard it from infomercials for space-age mattresses and pillows: we spend a third of our lives asleep. In this section, we investigate sleep, the structure of sleep, and some techniques to help people with sleep-wake disorders.

Sleep-wake disorders may be related to psychological disorders. Poor sleep can be both a precursor and a consequence of mental health conditions. For example, poor sleep can be a result of depressive disorders, bipolar disorder, schizophrenia, and anxiety. Lack of sleep can exacerbate psychological conditions too. Trouble sleeping can be an early sign of depression (Murphy & Peterson 2015).

Before we look at sleep disorders and their treatments, let's take a peek into the architecture of sleep.

Overview of Sleep

Sleep: a state of minimal consciousness associated with reduced motor and sensory activity.

Despite sleep's universality, scientists understand surprisingly little about it. We know that **sleep** is a state of minimal consciousness associated with reduced motor and sensory activity. But why do we sleep? Recent advances in technology have increased what we do understand about this mysterious state.

When most people think about sleep, they imagine that we slowly drift off to sleep, slumber deeply through the night, and then wake up in the morning. They imagine that the body and brain are completely at rest all through the night, and that we wake refreshed and restored because our bodies are being renewed like a set of rechargeable batteries. Measuring the activity of the brain with an electroencephalogram (EEG) during sleep tells a different story entirely, however. In fact, your brain is very active and dynamic during the night, and rather than being dormant, we work our way through several distinct realms of sleep with various levels of activity (see Figure 7.7).

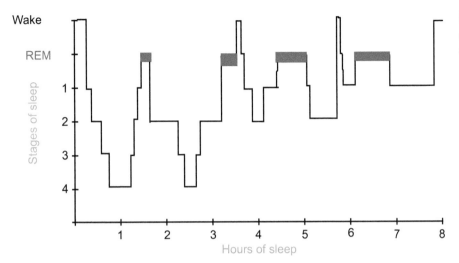

Figure 7.7 Stages of sleep.
Source: Reproduced from Aiton & Silverman (2021).

The truth is, you do "fall" asleep. You can go quite suddenly from being awake and relaxed and emitting *alpha waves* on the EEG (electroencephalogram) to the first sleep stage, Stage 1. Stage 1 is a phase between relaxed wakefulness and sleep. You are calm, your muscles are loose, and your breathing and heart rate have slowed down. You may have strange and wandering thoughts, and your brain also generates an EEG pattern called *theta*. Some people with insomnia may confuse this light sleep with wakefulness.

After a few minutes in Stage 1, you enter Stage 2. In Stage 2, your body is even more relaxed, and it's harder for outside noises to wake you up. The brain emits *sleep spindles*, which are small bursts of brain activity, and K-complexes on the EEG. K-complex patterns are a hallmark of this stage of sleep and have been associated with memory consolidation and the inhibition of activity (Cash et al. 2009; Latreille et al. 2020).

You spend about 45 minutes in Stage 2 before you enter an even deeper sleep – Stage 3 and Stage 4. During these stages, the EEG will show a new kind of pattern called *delta waves*, which begin in Stage 3 and become more prominent in Stage 4. Your breathing, blood pressure, heartbeat, and use of oxygen are at their lowest levels of the night, reflecting the rested state of your body. During this deep sleep, loud noises such as city traffic or even a train won't rouse most people, and it can take some people up to 15 minutes to regain full consciousness from Stage 4 due to the lowered levels of oxygen in the brain during this time.

Stage 4 is your deepest sleep, but you won't be there for long. After around 45 minutes in Stages 3 and 4, you go back to Stage 2. But this time instead of reentering Stage 1, you experience something different. Your eyes dart back and forth under your closed eyelids. If awakened at this point you will probably report having a vivid dream. In addition, your blood pressure, heartbeat, and respiration increase, and penile and clitoral arousal may occur. Although your motor cortex is now hard at work, your brainstem inhibits the signals that come out of it so you remain still. Your brain waves, as measured by EEG, look a lot like they do when you are awake, but you're not. You've entered a mentally active but physically restful state known as **rapid eye movement (REM) sleep**. REM sleep is a period of sleep characterized by darting eye movements and dreams. After a few minutes in this new type of sleep, you make your way back through the stages a second time over a period of about 90 minutes. During a typical night of sleep, you'll have up to six of these cycles.

But the cycles are not all the same. During the start of the night, your Stage 3 and 4 periods are very long, lasting up to an hour, and REM periods are short – only a few minutes. As the night goes on, your Stage 4 periods become shorter and shorter, diminishing altogether by the middle of the night. Your REM periods get longer and longer – up to an hour. This means you get most of your deep sleep at the beginning of your sleep cycle and most of your REM sleep near the end. Because your REM periods occur during lighter sleep, it's pretty normal to wake up after a particularly startling dream. In fact, most people wake up about half a dozen times or so during the night. You end up spending about 5 percent of the night in non-REM or nREM sleep Stage 1, 50 percent in Stage 2, 20 percent in deep Stages 3 and 4, and about 25 percent in REM sleep.

Outside factors can influence your sleep patterns, too. When light enters your eyes during the day, it sends signals to the **suprachiasmatic nucleus**, a part of your hypothalamus involved in sleep and wakefulness (Figure 7.8). This light causes the pineal gland to stop making **melatonin**, a hormone that promotes sleepiness, in the morning, and in the afternoon decreasing light causes it to increase melatonin. So too much nighttime light, such as from a computer screen or tv, can disrupt this sleep regulatory system (Dement & Vaughan 2000; Hastings et al. 2019).

Rapid eye movement (REM) sleep: a period of sleep characterized by darting eye movements and dreams.

Suprachiasmatic nucleus: a part of the hypothalamus which is involved in sleep and wakefulness.

Melatonin: a hormone that promotes sleepiness.

Health Impacts of Poor Sleep

Sleep and health are connected, and the connection may be bidirectional. In other words, the quality of our sleep may influence our overall health and a number of different health conditions may influence our quality of sleep. Although insomnia isn't associated with higher rates of mortality (Lovato & Lack 2019), lack of sleep is associated with higher rates of obesity, cancer, liver disease, and hypertension, among other health conditions and can also weaken the immune system (Irwin & Opp 2017).

Lack of sleep can have psychological impacts as well. It can create problems with memory, learning, verbal processing, and even decision making. Those who reduce their sleep to less than five hours each night for only two nights can experience impairments in creative tasks and math performance,

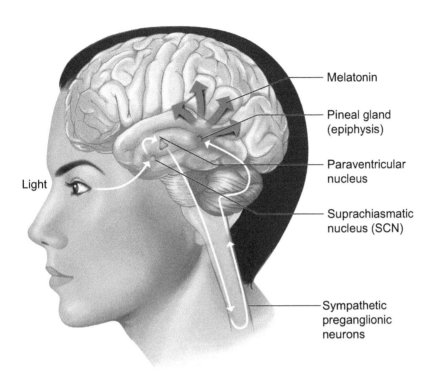

Figure 7.8 Melatonin (red arrows) is a hormone that affects the modulation of sleep patterns in both seasonal and circadian rhythms. It is secreted by the pineal gland (red sphere). The release of melatonin is inhibited during the day by bright light falling on the retina of the eye. However, when decreased levels of light are detected, a signal is sent to the pineal gland via the suprachiasmatic nucleus (green) and the hypothalamus (orange) to begin secreting melatonin.

among other effects. That's why staying up to cram for exams can backfire and impair performance (Keenan & Van Gundy 2021). Anyone who has missed a few good nights of sleep knows that it creates irritability and emotional reactivity. Chronic sleep deprivation is associated with a host of symptoms, including mild hallucinations (Harvey 2008). It can also affect your ability to perceive and react well to emotions in others (Goldstein & Walker 2014; Krizan et al. 2020).

Sleep deprivation can even be deadly. In the United States 16 percent of automobile accidents are related to sleep deprivation (Tefft 2018). More than half of drivers surveyed admitted to drowsy driving in the last 12 months, and nearly one in three people have reported nodding off at the wheel (Connor 2009).

Despite the fact that sleep is important for both mental and physical health, sleep deprivation is common. Over half of people in the United States report being chronically sleepy and may not get the sleep they need (see Table 7.1). Given these statistics, it's clear that sacrificing sleep in order to be more productive may involve a reduction in wellbeing or even safety.

Despite the recommendations of the National Sleep Foundation, The American Insomnia Survey of more than 10,000 participants showed that rates of sleep disorders vary over time, and that people aged over 54 had lower rates of insomnia than did those aged 30 to 44 (see Figure 7.9).

Table 7.1 National Sleep Foundation's sleep duration recommendations

	Newborns (0–3 months)	Infants (4–11 months)	Toddlers (1–2 years)	Pre-schoolers (3–5 years)	School-age children (6–13 years)	Teenagers (14–17 years)	Younger adults (18–25 years)	Adults (26–64 years)	Older adults (65+ years)
Recommended	14–17 hours	12–15 hours	11–14 hours	10–13 hours	9–11 hours	8–10 hours	7–9 hours	7–8 hours	7–8 hours
Maybe appropriate	11–13 hours or 18–19 hours	10–11 or 16–18 hours	9–10 or 15–16 hours	8–9 or 14 hours	7–8 or 12 hours	7 or 11 hours	6 or 10–11 hours	5–9 hours	5–6 or 9 hours
Not recommended	Less than 11 or more than 19 hours	Less than 10 or more than 18 hours	Less than 9 or more than 16 hours	Less than 8 or more than 14 hours	Less than 7 or more than 12 hours	Less than 7 or more than 11 hours	Less than 6 or more than 11 hours	Less than 5 or more than 9 hours	Less than 5 or more than 9 hours

Source: National Sleep Foundation (2019). www.sleepfoundation.org how-much-sleep-do-we-really-need.

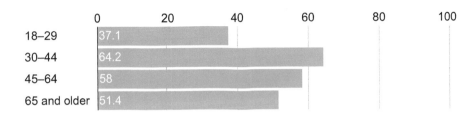

Figure 7.9 Prevalence of any sleep disorder.
Source: Data from Roth et al. (2011).

Assessment of Sleep

A person with sleep difficulties may spend a few nights being monitored in a sleep lab so clinicians can try to identify the problem. The goal is to record brain and body activity during sleep to arrive at a diagnosis and treatment plan (Figure 7.10). A *polysomograph* (PSG) evaluation, a multi-purpose test, might be ordered to measure the following:

- Brain wave activity (via an electroencephalograph or EEG).
- Number and speed of eye movements (via an electrooculogram or EOG).
- Muscle movement (via electromyography or EMG or actigraph).
- Electrical activity of the heart (via electrocardiogram or ECG).
- The number and depth of breathing.
- The amount of oxygen in the blood.
- Sleep latency.
- Sleep duration.
- Sleep efficiency.

The interpretation of these recordings can reveal dysfunctions like sleep apnea and snoring. Low-light video recordings may also be made of the person while asleep in order to observe sleep position, body movements, or respiration.

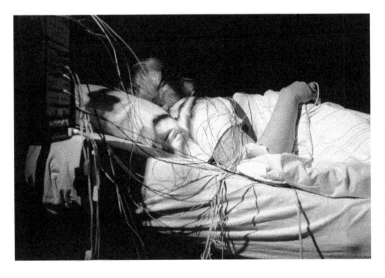

Figure 7.10 Polysomnography is a sleep-lab study of the physiological activity of the body during sleep, including activity in the lungs, heart, and brain.
Source: BSIP/Universal Images Group via Getty Images.

Figure 7.11 Sleep apps on devices such as smartphones and watches can track some useful data during sleep.

Source: Microgen Images/ Science Photo Library/Getty Images.

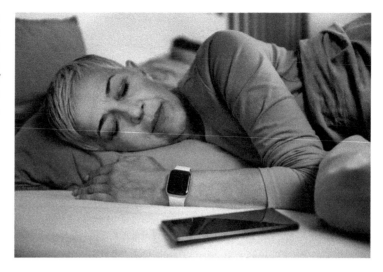

Alternatives to sleep studies include portable sleep-tracking devices such as smartphones or other devices that are worn on the wrist or even a finger. Called *actigraphs*, these devices sense arm movements to measure the quality and length of sleep by detecting when a person has fallen asleep, how often the person woke up, and how restful the sleep was. While these personal devices aren't as reliable as a PSG (Fino & Mazzetti 2019), they can be useful in calculating sleep efficiency as well as patterns of rest and activity (Figure 7.11).

Sleeping isn't always a pleasant experience. According to the National Sleep Foundation, up to 72 percent of us experience some symptoms of a sleep disorder at least a few nights a week, such as difficulty falling or staying asleep. People with chronic symptoms, however, can develop a sleep disorder that interferes with their lives on a daily basis, leaving them impaired and miserable.

Dyssomnias: conditions that can affect the quantity, quality, or timing of sleep, like insomnia, sleep apnea, and narcolepsy.

Parasomnias: abnormal behaviors associated with sleep, such as tremors, nightmares, and sleepwalking.

Sleep specialists have constructed criteria for more than 80 sleep-wake disorders. These disorders are often divided into two broad categories: dyssomnias and parasomnias. **Dyssomnias** are conditions that can affect the quantity, quality, or timing of sleep, like insomnia, sleep apnea, and narcolepsy. **Parasomnias** are abnormal behaviors associated with sleep, such as tremors, nightmares, and sleepwalking. In this next section, we'll examine some common sleep disorders including insomnia, sleep apnea, narcolepsy, and a few parasomnias.

Insomnia

Insomnia: a condition characterized by having difficulty falling asleep or staying asleep, waking up too early, or having non-refreshing sleep.

Insomnia is characterized by having difficulty falling asleep or staying asleep, waking up too early, or having non-refreshing sleep (Diagnostic Overview 7.8). There are various types of insomnia. It can be transient, lasting just a few nights; short term, which might last less than three weeks; or chronic, lasting longer than three weeks.

Much of the time, short-term or *acute insomnia* is due to emotional or physical dysfunction such as an illness or jet lag. Drugs such as caffeine, alcohol, antidepressants, decongestants, and nicotine can also cause problems. Alcohol can enhance the onset of sleep but can lead to sleep disturbances and restless, fitful sleep. Food habits may also affect sleep. Eating high-fat meals, experiencing acid reflux, and dining late at night can all trigger sleep disturbances (Jacobs 2009).

While insomnia can be frustrating during the night, it also has daytime consequences, as you can imagine. Tiredness, lack of energy, difficulty concentrating, and even irritability are common complaints. If insomnia continues, long-term fatigue can set in, along with longer-term mood changes, difficulty concentrating, and greater impairment in daytime functioning.

One in three people report some symptoms of a sleep disorder during any given year (Chung et al. 2015; Hertenstein et al. 2019), and for many, those difficulties are persistent (Lind et al. 2015). As people age, their sleep problems change and include increased nighttime awakening (Brewster et al. 2018). For those who are 55–64 years of age, about 26 percent will complain of sleep problems. Between 65 and 84 the number dips a bit; 21 percent in this age group report having difficulties with sleep. But these disturbances can still cause difficulty. About 15 percent of older adults will experience daytime sleepiness (especially Black men), which can lead to problems with falls and associated injuries (Hayley et al. 2015).

Diagnostic Overview 7.8: Insomnia Disorder

Dissatisfaction with the amount or quality of sleep along with the following symptoms:

- Difficulty falling asleep.
- Difficulty staying asleep (from frequent awakenings or problems going back to sleep).
- Waking up too early.

Impact: Symptoms must exceed cultural and contextual norms. Symptoms are related to clinically significant distress or create impairment in important areas of life such as with friends and family or at work or school.

Timeframe: At least three nights per week for at least three months.

Source: Information from APA (2022).

THE POWER OF EVIDENCE

Is melatonin an effective treatment for insomnia?

When insomnia strikes, often the first thing people reach for is an over-the-counter remedy. Twenty percent of US adults reported trying a natural sleep aid sometime in the last year, and of those, 86 percent chose melatonin, a hormone produced in the pineal gland that helps your body synchronize daily sleep-wake patterns. US consumers spent $408 million on melatonin supplements in 2017 (Loria 2019). However, not everyone gets the results they expect. Let's use the power of evidence to find out why.

Melatonin is effective. A 2013 meta-analysis found that people who took it fell asleep on average seven minutes faster than those who took a placebo. But like all herbal substances in the United States, it isn't regulated. Companies that make it don't have to prove that it has the potency listed on the label, or indeed that their product contains any melatonin whatsoever. A 2017 study found that the potency of melatonin supplements can vary even within the same bottle by as much as 465 percent (Erland & Saxena 2017).

Melatonin does have side effects, including headaches, nausea, dizziness, and sometimes sleepiness the next day. It can also increase the potency of some medications (such as blood-pressure medicines) and lower the potency of others (such as blood thinners). Although the National Institutes of Health suggests that melatonin is safe in the short term, for up to three months' use, a third of people who take it have done so for more than a year (Ferracioli-Oda et al. 2013).

The bottom line is that melatonin won't fix poor sleep habits. To get the best sleep, it's important to develop a good sleep routine, avoid stress and electronics near bedtime, and limit caffeine.

Sources: Erland & Saxena (2017); Ferracioli-Oda et al. (2013); Loria (2019).

Women report insomnia at rates twice those of men and more impact from their lack of sleep (Coelho 2022). But they do not necessarily experience the same types of insomnia. Women report greater amounts of initial insomnia (difficulty getting to sleep) as opposed to terminal insomnia (waking up too early), and these variations in sleep disturbances may be related to differences in hormones in men and women.

Hypersomnolence Disorders

Hypersomnolence disorders: sleep disorders characterized by excessive (hyper) sleepiness (somnolescence) or difficulty maintaining wakefulness.

Hypersomnolence disorders are characterized by excessive (hyper) sleepiness (somnolescence) or difficulty maintaining wakefulness (Diagnostic Overview 7.9). People with hypersomnolence may get adequate or sometimes excessive amounts of sleep. In fact, some may sleep as much as 12 hours and yet feel sleepy throughout the day, take frequent naps, and fall asleep during dull or non-stimulating activities. Not all daytime sleepiness is hypersomnolence; daytime sleepiness is also associated with insomnia or sleep apnea (which we discuss later).

Hypersomnolence often begins in early adulthood (Barateau et al. 2017) and has 1 percent prevalence; the rate is slightly higher among people with depressive disorders (Barateau et al. 2017).

Narcolepsy: a condition characterized by daytime sleepiness and sudden lapses into sleep, called sleep attacks, during the day.

Narcolepsy is a condition characterized by daytime sleepiness and sudden lapses into sleep, called *sleep attacks*, during the day. The sleep attacks usually last 10–20 minutes but can be as long as an hour, and the person will sometimes quickly enter REM sleep and go from wakefulness into a sudden dream (Diagnostic Overview 7.10). The person may even experience *hypnagogic hallucinations*, sensory experiences that occur between being asleep and being awake.

Often those with narcolepsy also have *cataplexy*, an abrupt and temporary muscle weakness following a strong emotional experience (such as being surprised or very upset). This weakness can cause the person to fall and can be dangerous. Luckily, cataplexy tends to decline over time as people learn to avoid situations that would precipitate it (Ahmed & Thorpy 2010).

The symptoms of narcolepsy that people notice first include sleeping a lot and not feeling rested, as well as fatigue, impaired daytime performance, and disturbed nighttime sleep. Recent research has pointed to reductions in *hypocretin*, a hormone linked to regulating wakefulness, as a possible cause of narcolepsy. The absence of hypocretin-producing neurons in those with narcolepsy helps to make the case that it is a possible cause for narcolepsy (Siegel & Boehmer 2006). Stimulants to combat daytime sleepiness, such as modafinil and methylphenidate, may prevent daytime sleep attacks (Stahl 2017).

Narcolepsy is fairly rare, affecting only one in 2,000 people in the United States (Ahmed & Thorpy 2010). It is diagnosed equally in women and men and typically emerges in the teen years, starting as excessive sleepiness. Cataplexy starts later in life (sometimes some 30 years later), and symptoms sometimes diminish with age.

Sleep-Related Breathing Disorders

Sleepiness during the day can be due to low-quality nighttime sleep. In particular, some people have disruptions in breathing at night that can disrupt their sleep. Because of these "micro wakenings," despite being asleep for eight hours they feel tired during the day (Mindell & Owens 2015).

SLEEP APNEA

Associated with snoring, daytime sleepiness, and obesity, **sleep apnea** is a sleep disorder in which breathing stops (*apnea* is from the Greek word meaning "without breath"). Apneas can last from just a few seconds to more than a minute (Kirsch 2020).

During an apnea, the body is starved of oxygen, and the heart has to work harder to keep circulating the reduced amount of oxygen in the blood. This extra burden on the heart puts those with sleep apnea at higher risk for cardiovascular diseases such as high blood pressure.

Why does apnea occur? One reason is that the muscles in the upper airway relax while we are asleep, and it naturally becomes a little harder to breathe (see Figure 7.12). For some people, however, the amount of muscle constriction during sleep is considerable, which leads to breathing that's too slow or too shallow to meet the necessary oxygen levels. As a result, oxygen drops and carbon dioxide levels start to rise. Sometimes breathing stops completely for brief periods of time. You might suppose that if you suddenly stopped

Sleep apnea: a sleep disorder in which breathing stops.

Diagnostic Overview 7.9: Hypersomnolence Disorder

Excessive sleepiness despite adequate sleep (at least seven hours), along with one of the following symptoms:

- Recurrent periods of sleep or lapses into sleep within the same day.
- Unrefreshing sleep.
- Difficulty being fully awake after waking up.

Impact:	Symptoms must exceed cultural and contextual norms. Symptoms are related to clinically significant distress or create impairment in important areas of life such as with friends and family or at work or school.
Timeframe:	Occurs at least three times per week, for at least three months.

Source: Information from APA (2022).

Diagnostic Overview 7.10: Narcolepsy

Recurrent periods of an irrepressible need to sleep, lapsing into sleep, or napping occurring within the same day along with one of the following:

- Episodes of cataplexy occurring at least a few times per month.
- Hypocretin deficiency.
- REM sleep latency of less than 15 minutes.

Impact:	Symptoms must exceed cultural and contextual norms. Symptoms are related to clinically significant distress or create impairment in important areas of life such as with friends and family or at work or school.
Timeframe:	At least three times per week over the last three months.

Source: Information from APA (2022).

Figure 7.12 In adults, sleep apnea is commonly caused by excess weight. During sleep, when the throat and tongue muscles are more relaxed, soft tissue, excess fat deposits, and the weight of abdominal fat pressing on the lungs can interfere with normal sleep.
Source: ttsz/iStock/Getty Images Plus.

Obstructive sleep apnea

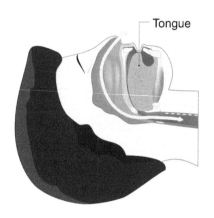
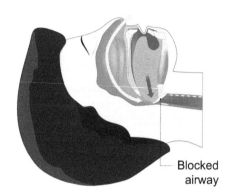

Normal breathing   Sleep apnea

breathing you would know, but many people with sleep apnea are unaware of their breathing difficulties. Bed partners, however, often notice snoring, gasps for air, and at times no breathing whatsoever. Those with sleep apnea may have significant daytime sleepiness. During the day, they may experience headaches or waken covered in sweat.

About 9 percent of women and 24 percent of men have sleep apnea (Ulualp 2010). In a multi-center study highest rates for sleep apnea were found in men in Brazil and the lowest rates were in women in Hong Kong (Lévy et al. 2015) (see Figure 7.13). People tend to have more apneas as they get older and also in certain sleep positions (like sleeping on their back). Some people with severe sleep apnea may have dozens of apneas during the night. Psychopathologists describe three types of sleep apnea, each with its own causes and treatments: obstructive, central, and sleep related hypoventilation.

Diagnostic Overview 7.11: Obstructive Sleep Apnea Hypopnea

At least one of the following:

- Evidence of at least five obstructive apneas and/or hypopneas per hour of sleep along with daytime sleepiness or nighttime breathing problems (like snoring).
- Evidence of at least 15 or more obstructive apneas/apneas and/or hypopneas per hour of sleep.

Impact: Symptoms must exceed cultural and contextual norms. Symptoms are related to clinically significant distress or create impairment in important areas of life such as with friends and family or at work or school.

Source: Information from APA (2022).

OBSTRUCTIVE SLEEP APNEA HYPOPNEA SYNDROME

Obstructive sleep apnea hypopnea syndrome is the most common type of sleep apnea (Senaratna et al. 2017). In obstructive sleep apnea hypopnea syndrome, a person has abnormally slow breathing (hypo means slow or shallow) (Diagnostic Overview 7.11). This may be caused by narrow airways, medical conditions such as obesity, high blood pressure, or diabetes, or damage or an abnormality that restricts airflow such as the inflammation of tonsillitis. Restricted airflow leads to periods of no breathing or too low or too shallow breathing.

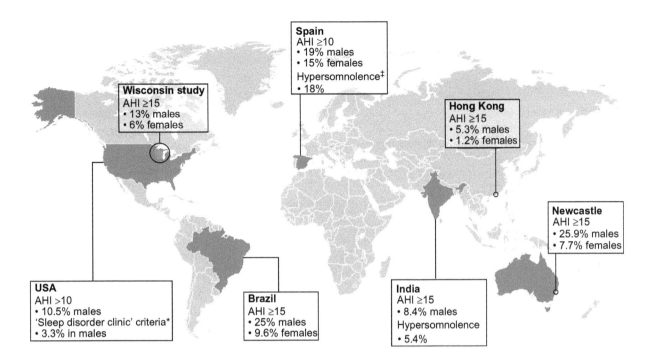

Spain
AHI ≥10
• 19% males
• 15% females
Hypersomnolence‡
• 18%

Wisconsin study
AHI ≥15
• 13% males
• 6% females

Hong Kong
AHI ≥15
• 5.3% males
• 1.2% females

Newcastle
AHI ≥15
• 25.9% males
• 7.7% females

USA
AHI >10
• 10.5% males
'Sleep disorder clinic' criteria*
• 3.3% in males

Brazil
AHI ≥15
• 25% males
• 9.6% females

India
AHI ≥15
• 8.4% males
Hypersomnolence
• 5.4%

Obstructive sleep apnea hypopnea syndrome occurs in 9–38 percent of the population (Senaratna et al. 2017) with more diagnoses in men than in women. Rates also increase as people age.

Figure 7.13 Global prevalence of sleep apnea as measured by the apnea–hypopnea index (AHI).

Source: Lévy et al. (2015).

CENTRAL SLEEP APNEA

While hypopneas refer to shallow breathing, apneas are periods of up to 20 seconds or more with no breathing at all. The brain doesn't send a signal to breathe, perhaps due to head trauma, heart disease, or opioid use. People with this condition may wake up several times during the night but not feel tired the next day, so many are unaware of their condition (Diagnostic Overview 7.12). Central sleep apnea has a prevalence of less than 1 percent (Donovan & Kapur 2016).

SLEEP-RELATED HYPOVENTILATION

In sleep-related hypoventilation (the opposite of hyperventilation), there is slower airflow but not a complete disruption of breathing (Diagnostic Overview 7.13). However, like all apneas, hypoventilation syndrome can create higher levels of carbon dioxide and lower the levels of oxygen in the body. The prevalence rates of sleep-related hypoventilation are unknown but expected to be rare (APA 2022).

Diagnostic Overview 7.12: **Central Sleep Apnea**

Evidence of at least five central apneas per hour of sleep.

Impact: Symptoms must exceed cultural and contextual norms. Symptoms are related to clinically significant distress or create impairment in important areas of life such as with friends and family or at work or school.

Source: Information from APA (2022).

Sleep-Related Hypoventilation

Evidence by polysomnography of five or more central apneas per hour of sleep.

Impact: Symptoms must exceed cultural and contextual norms. Symptoms are related to clinically significant distress or create impairment in important areas of life such as with friends and family or at work or school.

Source: Information from APA (2022).

Circadian Rhythm Sleep-Wake Disorders

Many factors can influence our patterns of sleep and wakefulness. Some are external, like our sleep environment, the relative amounts of daylight and darkness, and the time of day we are sleeping. Some are internal, including the release of substances such as melatonin to help us to be sleepy and others to maintain wakefulness. Many of these occur on a daily cycle called *circadian rhythm*. Circa means "about" and dian refers to "day." So circadian rhythms are biological rhythms that occur on a daily cycle.

One of the parts of the brain that helps us to control sleep and wakefulness is in the hypothalamus. It's called the *suprachiasmatic nucleus*, and it receives light signals via our eyes to help reset our rhythms. When all is going well, these internal and external factors are aligned. When we head to bed in the dark, the clock says it's bedtime and our brain releases the chemicals that make us sleepy. In the daytime it's sunny, the clock says it's time to be awake, and our brain sends signals to the body to keep us alert.

Every now and then, however, internal and external factors aren't aligned. We travel to a new time zone eight hours ahead where the clock says it's time to go to bed, but our brain is still operating on the previous rhythm, pumping out wakefulness chemicals. Typically, in a few days we adjust. But what about people who have persistent misalignments in these influences, or whose rhythms have become disrupted? This problem leads to **circadian rhythm sleep-wake disorder**, a sleep disorder characterized by misalignment between internal and external influences on sleep and wakefulness (Diagnostic Overview 7.14).

A number of sleep-wake disorders are described in the *DSM*.

Circadian rhythm sleep-wake disorder: a sleep disorder characterized by misalignment between internal and external influences on sleep and wakefulness.

DELAYED SLEEP PHASE TYPE

People with *delayed sleep phase type* have persistently late sleep onset and awakening, along with inability to sleep or wake up earlier if they want to. It happens to some people every now and then but should be diagnosed when it causes problems or distress. Of all the circadian rhythm sleep-wake disorders, it's the most common.

Circadian Rhythm Sleep-Wake Disorders

Persistent insomnia or excessive sleepiness caused by change in the circadian rhythms.

Impact: Symptoms must exceed cultural and contextual norms. Symptoms are related to clinically significant distress or create impairment in important areas of life such as with friends and family or at work or school.

Source: Information from APA (2022).

ADVANCED SLEEP PHASE TYPE

People with *advanced sleep phase type* have sleep onset two or more hours earlier than desired, along with early morning insomnia and tiredness during the day (Abbott et al. 2015).

IRREGULAR SLEEP-WAKE TYPE

Irregular sleep-wake type is often associated with neurological conditions; people with this disorder have no consistent sleep patterns.

NON-24-HOUR TYPE

Sleep cycles that are not coordinated with the light/dark cycles of day and night are called *non-24-hour type* disorder. This problem is more likely to occur in people who can't discern day from night because of vision impairments (Flynn-Evans et al. 2017). It's associated with problems in thinking and functioning.

SHIFT WORK TYPE

In *shift work type* disorder, sleep problems are caused by irregular work hours. About 31 percent of people who work at night and 26 percent of those who rotate their work schedules meet the criteria for this condition.

Parasomnia

Parasomnias are sleep disorders characterized by problematic movements and dreams during sleep, or problems with sleep and wake patterns. They are generally of two types: parasomnias that occur during REM periods are also known as *REM parasomnias*, and those that occur during non-REM periods like Stage 3 and 4 deep sleep are called *nREM parasomnias*.

REM PARASOMNIAS

The REM parasomnias are REM sleep behavior disorder and nightmare disorder.

REM sleep behavior disorder is a type of REM parasomnia in which a person will act out their dreams (Diagnostic Overview 7.15). In some ways, it is the opposite of sleep paralysis. In the disorder, while you are asleep, your brain fails to send a signal to your body to inhibit your movement during dreams. Instead of just rapid eye movement, those with REM sleep behavior disorder may kick, punch, or otherwise act in ways that could cause harm to themselves or others while they dream (Figure 7.14). REM sleep behavior disorder affects around 0.5 percent of people in the United States (Avidan & Kaplish 2010).

> **REM sleep behavior disorder**: a type of REM parasomnia in which a person will act out their dreams.

If you do happen to wake and find yourself with a bout of sleep paralysis, try wiggling your toes. The paralysis seems to affect larger muscles more than smaller ones, so a good way to get out of it is to try to make small movements to wake yourself up.

In **nightmare disorder**, a person experiences frequent disturbing dreams (Diagnostic Overview 7.16). Since nightmare disorder occurs during REM sleep,

> **Nightmare disorder**: a sleep-wake disorder in which a person experiences frequent disturbing dreams.

Diagnostic Overview 7.15: Rapid Eye Movement Sleep Behavior Disorder

- During REM sleep, repeated arousal and movement or vocalizations.
- Either: a history of REM sleep without loss of muscle movement, or: a history of a condition that is associated with REM sleep behavior disorders (such as Parkinson's disease).

Impact: Symptoms must exceed cultural and contextual norms. Symptoms are related to clinically significant distress or create impairment in important areas of life such as with friends and family or at work or school.

Source: Information from APA (2022).

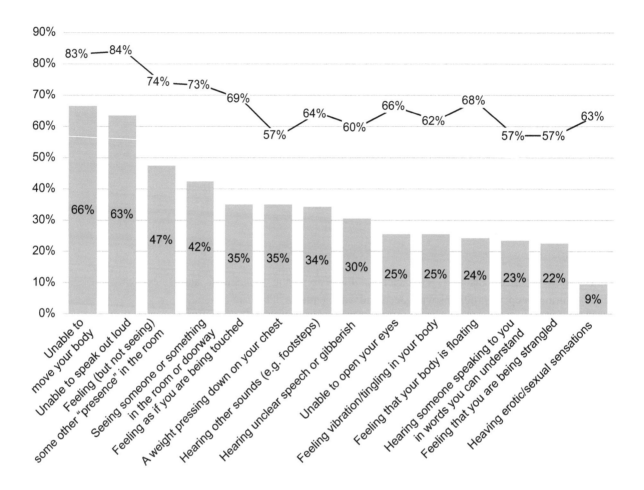

- ▨ Percentage who reported frequently/always having the experience during sleep paralysis
- — Among those who frequently/always have the symptom during sleep paralysis, the percentage who strongly experience the symptom

Figure 7.14 The percentage of sleep paralysis study participants (n = 388) who reported frequently or always experiencing various symptoms at any point in their lives.
Source: Adapted from Benham (2020).

it's more likely to occur in the later part of the night (when there are more REM periods). Some people with nightmare disorders have such frequent bad dreams that going to bed is associated with great anxiety.

NON-REM PARASOMNIAS

Non-REM (nREM) parasomnias occur during nREM sleep and include non-REM movement sleep arousal disorders (sleep walking, sleep eating, and sexomnia) (Diagnostic Overview 7.17).

Sleepwalking is a type of nREM parasomnia in which a person will get out of bed and perform activities while still asleep. It is common among children; up to 17 percent have experienced symptoms at some point. The rate of occurrence decreases to around 3 percent in adults (Avidan & Kaplish 2010). It's safe to wake sleepwalkers, if you can, but it can be difficult to rouse them. The best course of action is to gently guide them back to bed.

Nocturnal sleep-related eating disorder, or *sleep eating*, is a condition similar to sleepwalking in which affected people engage in nightly meals while partially or totally asleep, most commonly by sleepwalking to the refrigerator and having a meal they will probably never remember. Some episodes are more elaborate, with fully asleep people heading to the kitchen and preparing a meal.

Sleep eating is fairly rare, occurring in only about 1.5 percent of the population. Two in three people with sleep eating disorder are women, and three in four of them eat nightly (some up to eight times a night). Most (84 percent) are completely unaware of their behavior. In almost all cases, the behavior doesn't appear to be hunger-related (Howell & Schenck 2009). The food choices of sleep eaters can include cat food, raw chicken, coffee grounds and milk, sandwiches made from fistfuls of salt, and even inedibles such as ammonia or buttered soda cans.

Many precautions can be taken to limit the impact of sleepwalking and sleep eating. Bedrooms should be made safe by blocking windows or locating them on the first floor if possible. It's best for potential sleepwalkers to try to get enough sleep, cut back on alcohol and caffeine, and avoid stressful situations. For more severe conditions, medications that inhibit GABA (an inhibitory neurotransmitter), such as low-dose benzodiazepines (such as diazepam), have been effective (Avidan & Kaplish 2010).

Sexsomnia, or *sleepsex*, is a type of nREM parasomnia associated with engaging in sexual activity while asleep. Sexual behaviors can be classified into three categories. The first involves actions that the researchers describe as "annoying" but not harmful, such as sexual moaning loud enough to be heard in adjoining rooms, attempts to remove clothing, and mumbling of sexually inappropriate phrases. The second category includes behaviors that are also considered annoying but are, at times, harmful to the person suffering from sexsomnia. These can be violent masturbation that causes bruising and soreness the next morning. The last and most severe category is for actions that are harmful to others. These cases involve inappropriate and violent sexual behavior.

Some people think the diagnosis of sexsomnia is used to justify inappropriate sexual advances.

Diagnostic Overview 7.16: Nightmare Disorder

Repeated disturbing dreams typically during REM periods.

Impact: Symptoms must exceed cultural and contextual norms. Symptoms are related to clinically significant distress or create impairment in important areas of life such as with friends and family or at work or school.

Source: Information from APA (2022).

Diagnostic Overview 7.17: Non-REM Sleep Arousal Disorders

Recurrent episodes of behaviors often in the first third of sleep episode along with either sleepwalking or sleep terrors.

Impact: Symptoms must exceed cultural and contextual norms. Symptoms are related to clinically significant distress or create impairment in important areas of life such as with friends and family or at work or school.

Specify if:

Sleepwalking type
With sleep-related eating
With sleep-related sexual behavior (sexsomnia)
Sleep terror type

Source: Information from APA (2022).

However, in nearly every case, doctors were able to document abnormal patterns of REM or nREM sleep, which are impossible to fake (Antelmi et al. 2021). Fortunately, most patients with sexsomnia can be successfully treated with psychotropic medications, which can protect people who might become a victim of assault.

Having a nightmare can be terrifying. You might awaken to your own screaming, remembering vividly disturbing images. But nightmares, which occur late in our sleep cycles and often in REM sleep, are very different from sleep terrors, which happen earlier, during nREM sleep. **Sleep terrors**, also known as night terrors, are a sleep condition in which people experience sudden episodes of panic during Stage 4 sleep.

Sleep terrors: also known as night terrors, are a sleep condition in which people experience sudden episodes of panic during Stage 4 sleep.

To someone else, the person experiencing a sleep terror, though soundly asleep, will seem wide awake. Eyes will be wide open, breathing is intense, and heart rate has shot through the roof. The person might even scream loudly in fear, look panicked, and act as if in excruciating pain. It's okay to wake the person – if you can. But it's very difficult to rouse some sleepers out of these episodes. When they do wake up, most of the time they have no memory of the experience or the emotional upheaval it caused them (and, most likely, the people around them).

Sleep terrors can last between a few seconds and five minutes. The highest rates occur in children aged 4 to 12, with up to 6.5 percent of children in the United States experiencing symptoms. Although many people tend to grow out of sleep terrors as they get older, about 4 percent of adults continue to suffer from them (Avidan & Kaplish 2010).

Case Study: REM Sleep Behavior Disorder – Mike Birbiglia

A few years ago, US actor, writer, and director Mike Birbiglia (Figure 7.15) began to experience what he described as "walking in his sleep." He had recurring dreams of seeing hovering insects and winning sporting events. Soon afterwards he would find that he was awake, striking a karate pose or falling off a bookcase. Despite these incidents he never sought treatment. Then during one work trip Mike fell asleep while watching a news story about war. In the dream that followed, a missile was heading toward his room, so he decided to jump out his second-floor hotel window to escape it.

He woke up running in the street, covered in blood. Three hours and 30 stitches later, he emerged from the emergency room. More about Mike later in the chapter.

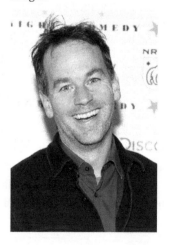

Figure 7.15 Mike Birbiglia. *Source: Gary Gershoff/Getty Images.*

Models and Treatments for Sleep-Wake Disorders

Eventually Mike was diagnosed with a REM sleep behavior disorder, but with medications and behavioral interventions (such as sleeping in a sleeping bag type device to restrict his movement), his sleep improved dramatically. Treatments for sleep-wake disorders focus on the central symptoms or on the biological, environmental, or behavioral conditions that might contribute to the symptoms of the conditions.

BIOLOGICAL MODELS AND TREATMENTS

From the biological standpoint, a sleep-wake disorder has physiological roots and should be treated by altering the biological factors that contribute to it. Some people, for example, may have problems regulating body temperature to the level that would typically initiate sleep (Taylor et al. 2014). Some theories suggest that those with sleep apnea have a central nervous system issue associated with the control of breathing (Chokroverty 2008). Another theory points to physical differences in the throats of those with this condition.

There are many effective treatments for sleep apnea. Avoid sleeping on your back, keep your head elevated, and cut back on alcohol and sleeping pills, which could make the problem worse or even dangerous (Chokroverty 2008). For moderate to severe sleep apnea there are other treatments, including **continuous positive airway pressure (CPAP)** (Figure 7.16), in which a small machine and mask keep the airway open by sending a constant stream of compressed air. About 20–50 percent of those who could benefit from CPAP don't use it because the apparatus can be cumbersome to wear (Patel et al. 2020). More serious cases of sleep apnea may require surgery to increase the size of the airway (Olsen et al. 2010).

Other options for treating breathing-related sleep disorders include medication such as modafinil to increase daytime wakefulness. Modafinil (Provigil) is a stimulant that is also prescribed for people with narcolepsy, hypersomnolence disorders, and circadian rhythm disorders to maintain wakefulness (Kallweit & Bassetti 2017).

For trouble initiating or maintaining sleep, such as in insomnia, many people turn to medications (see Table 7.2). The problem with most sleeping pills, whether over-

Continuous positive airway pressure (CPAP): a treatment for sleep apnea in which a small machine and mask keep the airway open by sending a constant stream of compressed air.

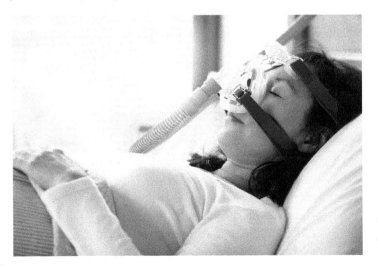

Figure 7.16 CPAP treatments can be helpful for sleep.
Source: cherrybeans/iStock/ Getty Images Plus.

Table 7.2 Some FDA-approved medications for insomnia

Generic name	Brand name	Class of medication
eszopiclone	Lunesta	Non-benzodiazepine hypnotic
lemborexant	Davigo	Dual orexin receptor antagonist (DORA)
ramelton	Rozerem	Melatonin receptor agonist
suvorexant	Belsomra	Dual orexin receptor antagonist (DORA)
zaleplon	Sonata	Non-benzodiazepine hypnotic
zolpidem	Ambien, intermezzo	Non-benzodiazepine hypnotic

Source: Information from Stahl (2017).

the-counter or prescription, is that they decrease Stage 1 and Stage 4 sleep and may lead the user to need higher and higher doses in order to get to sleep. Sleep medications may also produce daytime grogginess, headaches, and an unpleasant taste in the mouth (Stahl 2021).

COGNITIVE AND BEHAVIORAL MODELS AND TREATMENTS

Cognitive-behavioral therapy for insomnia (CBT-I) assumes that insomnia results from personality factors, precipitating events in the environment, and thoughts and behaviors that make insomnia worse. Thus it focuses on teaching clients techniques to modify their sleep behaviors, such as eliminating naps, and cognitions that may disrupt normal sleep and contribute to insomnia (Boness et al. 2020), such as worrying about sleep during the day, and about what the next day will be like if the person doesn't get to sleep. It also includes tweaking the environment to improve sleep quality, such as by removing unnecessary stimuli such as clutter around the room, reminders of work, and phone notifications (Desaulniers et al. 2018).

A recent meta-analysis (Boness et al. 2020) found that CBT-I is an effective treatment for insomnia across many age groups. It has been named a first-line psychotherapy for chronic insomnia by the National Institutes of Health and the American Academy of Sleep Medicine (Boness et al. 2020).

SOCIOCULTURAL MODELS AND TREATMENTS

Sleep-wake disorders can also be influenced by sociocultural factors. Marginalized populations including economically disadvantaged populations have some of the highest rates of sleep disorders. For example, total sleep duration is lower for many racial and ethnic minority populations, particularly for Pacific Island, Black, and Indigenous people. Economic disparity can also influence sleep-wake conditions. The sleep deficiency is higher for those who are unemployed and with only a high school education. Marginalized populations are more likely to have underdiagnosed sleep disorders. Environmental factors can also influence sleep quality. The presence of artificial light, housing conditions, and the availability of green space can affect the quantity and quality of sleep (Shin et al. 2020).

CONCEPT CHECK 7.3

Indicate the sleep-wake disorder described in each case.

1. For the past six months a 50-year-old woman has experienced repetitive movements during sleep. Her wife says they typically occur a few hours before she would normally awaken. ___________
2. Teddy is 16 years old and his parents are concerned about him. For the past three months he has been getting up in the middle of the night and is then found

standing someplace in the house crying and screaming loudly. When his parents wake him up, he seems confused and doesn't report any dream whatsoever. In the morning he can't recall getting out of bed at all. _____

3. A person with nightmares is most likely having them during which stage of sleep? _____

4. A 35-year-old woman contacts her primary care physician because she feels sleepy during the day. She has trouble falling asleep and also wakes up many times during the night. She also becomes frustrated because she can't seem to get to sleep. She has no other medical problems and reports drinking no more than "one cup of coffee" in the morning. _____

5. A 44-year-old man complains of feeling tired all day and unable to get through the day without falling asleep at work. When it's time for bed he isn't tired at all, so he decides to stay up watching TV and looking at his phone. Before his current job, he was a baker and worked evening hours. _____

PULLING IT TOGETHER

Diagnosing Unexplained Health Symptoms or Complaints

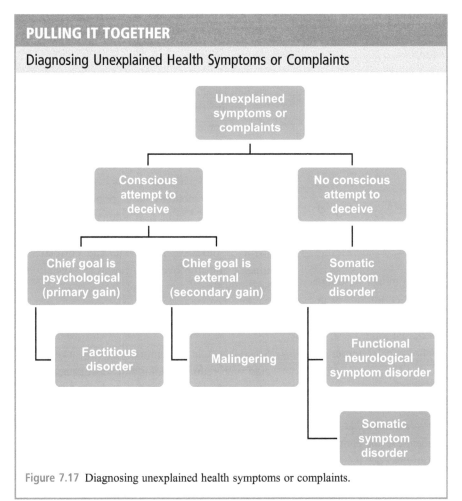

Figure 7.17 Diagnosing unexplained health symptoms or complaints.

7.4 CHAPTER REVIEW

SUMMARY

This chapter presented the following disorders:

- Malingering
- Factitious disorder
- Illness anxiety disorder
- Somatic symptom disorder
- Functional neurological symptom disorder (conversion disorder).
- Insomnia
- Hypersomnolence disorder
- Narcolepsy
- Sleep apnea
- Obstructive sleep apnea hypopnea syndrome
- Central sleep apnea
- Sleep related hypoventilation
- Circadian rhythm sleep wake disorders
- REM sleep behavior disorder
- Nightmare disorder
- Non-REM parasomnias

Somatic Symptom and Related Disorders

- Somatic symptom disorders are psychological conditions characterized by excessive focus on physical symptoms or health despite the absence of health concerns.
- Somatic symptom disorders shouldn't be diagnosed in cases of actual medical conditions or in the case of malingering, intentional production, or faking of an illness for external gain.
- Factitious disorder is a psychological disorder in which a person plays the sick role for emotional gain or attention.
- Illness anxiety disorder is a type of somatic symptom disorder characterized by excessive fear over having an illness despite evidence to the contrary.
- People with somatic symptom disorder focus on the symptoms themselves and feel considerable

anxiety about their health, despite the fact they do not have a physical illness.
- In functional neurological symptom disorder (conversion disorder) psychological worry or concern is transformed (converted) into a physical symptom. People with this condition experience symptoms similar to those of a neurological disorder despite the fact they don't have one.
- Treatment of somatic symptom disorder typically targets the anxiety that might produce the symptoms or the events that may have led to them.

Psychological Treatments for Physical Disorders

- Psychological factors affecting other medical conditions are physical illnesses created or exacerbated by the interaction between biological, psychological, and social conditions.
- Personality can have an impact on health and illness. For example Type A personalities tend to be competitive, hostile, and impatient, while Type B personalities are relaxed and patient.
- Coping styles can also affect health and illness. They can be emotion-focused or problem-focused.
- The goals of health psychology are to prevent illness, promote good health, help with the treatment of illnesses, investigate the correlates of illness, and improve the health care system and health policy.

Sleep-Wake Disorders

- Sleep is a state of minimal consciousness associated with reduced motor and sensory activity.
- Sleep and physical and psychological health are connected, and the connection between sleep and health may be bidirectional.
- While we sleep, our brain goes through distinct and repeated stages of rapid eye movement (REM) sleep and non-REM sleep.

- Psychologists and other health care providers use a number of tools, including tests performed in sleep labs, to assess sleep and diagnose sleep-wake conditions.
- Insomnia is characterized by difficulty falling asleep, difficulty staying asleep, too-early awakening, and non-refreshing sleep.
- Hypersomnolence disorders are characterized by excessive (hyper) sleepiness (somnolescence) or difficulty maintaining wakefulness.
- Narcolepsy is a condition characterized by daytime sleepiness and sudden lapses into sleep, called *sleep attacks*, during the day.
- Sleep apnea is a sleep disorder in which breathing stops. The three types are obstructive sleep apnea hypopnea syndrome, central sleep apnea, and sleep-related hypoventilation.
- A circadian rhythm sleep-wake disorder is a sleep disorder characterized by misalignment between internal and external influences on sleep and wakefulness.
- Parasomnias are sleep disorders noted for problematic movements and dreams while sleeping, or problems with sleeping and wake patterns. There are REM and non-REM types.
- Treatment of sleep disorders can include biological interventions such as medications and CPAP treatments. Some cognitive-behavioral tools can help as well. Sociocultural factors may also influence sleep.

DISCUSSION QUESTIONS

1. Although malingering isn't considered a psychological condition in the *DSM*, it is often described as problematic. Describe some ways in which malingering can be adaptive.
2. Somatic symptom disorders require that there be no medical condition creating the symptoms. But we know from health psychology that there is a connection between physical and mental health. What challenges do you think practitioners have in the diagnosis and treatment of somatic symptom disorders?
3. We know that some of the behavioral treatments for insomnia are very powerful and in the long term may be more effective than medications. Despite this, may people opt for medications such as over-the-counter sleep aids to help them sleep at night. What are some ways to decrease the reliance on medications and increase healthy sleep habits?
5. The role of psychology in health conditions suggests that therapeutic interventions may be a powerful tool for many health conditions, yet there are very few psychologists in primary care settings. What could be some barriers to having psychologists routinely involved in the treatment of health concerns other than those that are seen as mental health conditions?

ANSWERS TO CONCEPT CHECKS

Concept Check 7.1

1. Somatic symptom disorder
2. Illness anxiety disorder
3. Somatic symptom disorder

Concept Check 7.2

1. Biology, psychology, social
2. Immunosuppression

3. Problem-focused coping strategy
4. Emotion-focused coping directs coping at the response to the event.

Concept Check 7.3

1. REM sleep behavior disorder

2. Sleep terrors
3. Rapid eye movement or REM sleep
4. Insomnia disorder
5. Circadian rhythm sleep disorder

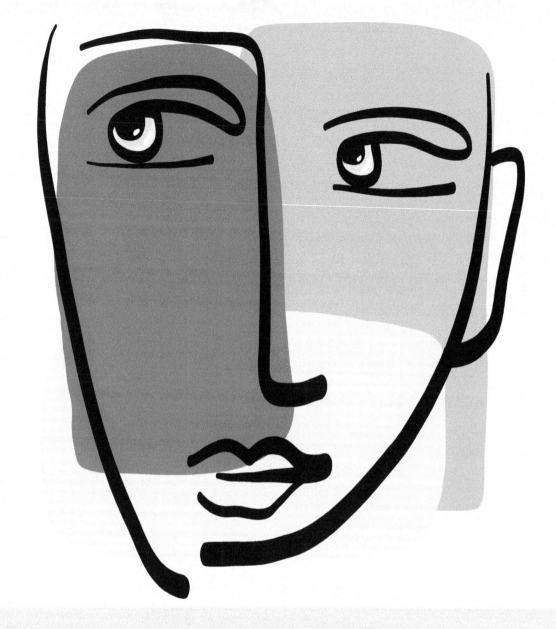

CHAPTER CONTENTS

8

Gender Variation, Sexual Dysfunctions, and Paraphilic Disorders

CASE STUDY: Gender Diversity – Jazz Jennings

"Ever since I could form coherent thoughts, I knew I was a girl trapped inside a boy's body. There was never any confusion in my mind. The confusing part was why no one else could see what was wrong." Jazz Jennings (Figure 8.1) described a nonstop interest in "girly things" that her family thought of as "a phase." Somehow even before she could speak, Jazz figured out how to undo the snaps on her onesie to make it into a dress, and she remembers feeling frustrated, confused, and bothered by her genitals thinking they didn't belong there.

Her family was supportive, and Jazz was allowed to dress in whatever way she wanted to . . . inside the house. But she was forced to wear "boys' clothes" in public and none of the "girl's stuff" she preferred. This left Jazz feeling ashamed and humiliated. She couldn't seem to understand why her parents would make her do that kind of thing. Other relatives tried to prod Jazz toward "boy" things like trucks, but she preferred dolls to G.I. Joes. It was clear that her mother and siblings didn't care, but other relatives were worried about how the world might treat her.

Then around the age of 2, Jazz had a dream that a Good Fairy would appear and use her magical powers to turn Jazz's penis into a vagina. She remembers feeling excited when she woke up and running to her mother to ask when the Good Fairy would come to use her magic powers. That's when her mother realized that what Jazz was going through wasn't a phase. We'll return to Jazz's story later in this chapter.

Learn more about Jazz Jennings by reading her 2017 book, *Being Jazz: My life as a (transgender) teen*.

Learning Objectives

- Describe the differences between gender, sex, and sexual orientation.
- Outline the sexual response cycle.
- Identify the basic features and diagnostic criteria for dysphoria.
- Discuss the various treatments for gender dysphoria.
- Describe the sexual dysfunctions.
- Discuss the treatment approaches for the sexual dysfunctions.
- Describe the paraphilic disorders.
- Discuss the treatment approaches for paraphilia disorders.

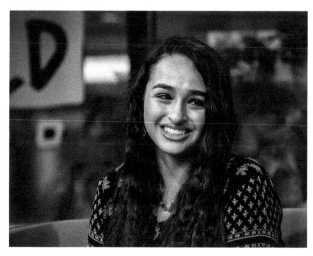

Figure 8.1 Jazz Jennings.
Source: Photo by Anthony DelMundo/WireImage.

8.1   WHAT IS SEXUALITY?

Sexuality is perhaps one of the most private aspects of a person's life. It can be a major focus of our inner thoughts and a source of happiness and pleasure, and it can shape the way we think of ourselves and others. Yet sexuality and sexual behavior are often shrouded in mystery. Despite often being a taboo subject, people are fascinated with the sexual fantasies and behavior of others and even of themselves. It's common to wonder whether your own sexuality is typical and to be concerned when it becomes a source of distress.

This chapter describes three chapters in the *DSM-5tr* that are conventionally presented together in psychopathology textbooks despite being unrelated. The first two of these are **sexual dysfunctions**, in which a person has a concern with one or more areas of the sexual response cycle, and **paraphilic disorders,** in which an individual expresses problematic or inappropriate sexual fantasies, urges, or behaviors.

The *DSM* also has a separate chapter that describes **gender dysphoria**, a condition in which a person experiences distress and/or impairment associated with their gender identity (see below) being different from the *gender assigned* at birth. Note that it's not this incongruence between the assigned and identified gender that is considered a disorder. Rather, any distress or impairment a person might feel as a *consequence* of this incongruence is a disorder that can be diagnosed and treated. There are those who may experience an incongruence and not feel distress or have impairment.

These diagnoses are controversial because, although gender identity, sexual feelings, and sexual expression are common among humans, we are still in the early phases of identifying the cultural and social influences on the way we understand our gender identity and our sexual expression. Thus we tend to rely on our individual feelings or societal stereotypes to decide what's normal and what's not, a strategy that can be problematic (McGoldrick et al. 2007).

Sexual dysfunctions: conditions in which a person has a concern with one or more areas of the sexual response cycle.

Paraphilic disorders: a condition in which an individual expresses problematic or inappropriate sexual fantasies, urges, or behaviors.

Gender dysphoria: a condition in which a person experiences distress and/or impairment associated with their gender identity being different from the gender assigned at birth.

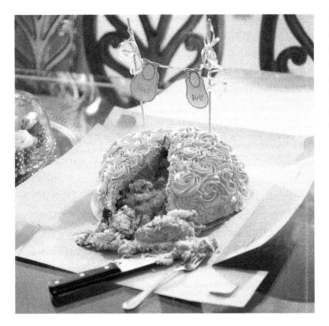

Figure 8.2 Although often considered celebrations to announce the gender of their children, gender reveal parties don't actually reveal much about gender.
Source: Jeneil S/Moment Open/Getty Images.

Every few years a new party phenomenon seems to emerge, and the 2000s have given us the "gender reveal party" (Figure 8.2). The central event of the gender reveal party is a theatrical revelation by expectant parents of whether their infant is going to be a boy or a girl. A variety of pink and blue cakes, confetti blasters, balloons, streamers, and fireworks have been used. But do gender reveal parties actually reveal the *gender* of a future child?

Sex is a set of various biological characteristics, such as hormones, chromosomes, and reproductive organs, that distinguish males and females. Health care professionals can use several of these characteristics to assign sex. These characteristics include:

- Chromosomes.
- Genitalia.
- Internal reproductive organs.
- Sex hormones.
- Gametes (reproductive cells).
- Secondary sex characteristics (such as Adam's apples in males and larger breasts in females). (From Ferber et al. 2016)

Although many people think of sex as either male or female, 1 in 100 people born have bodies that differ from what we think of as male or female (Witchel 2018). And biologists believe that there is a wider spectrum than simple male and female, given that some people experience **intersexuality**, meaning they are born with sexual anatomy that doesn't fit into the categories of male or female. For example, a person might fit the typical male anatomy on the outside but have reproductive organs that are more typical of females on the inside of their bodies (Jorge et al. 2021).

Gender identity is a range of characteristics that characterize the way you think about the biological features that inform who you are. Do you feel as if you are

Sex: a set of various biological characteristics, such as hormones, chromosomes, and reproductive organs, that distinguish males and females.

Intersexuality: a condition in which a person is born with sexual anatomy that doesn't fit into the categories of male or female.

Gender identity: a range of characteristics that characterize the way you think about the biological features that inform who you are.

Gender expression: the way a person behaves and interacts with others, including dress, appearance, and behaviors.

aligned more with the social role of a man, a woman, or neither? Your gender identity is informed by your biology as well as by your environment. You demonstrate that gender identity through your **gender expression**, the way you behave and interact with others, including your dress, appearance, and behaviors. Although it is guided by your gender identity, gender expression can be more fluid; it is heavily influenced by the situation and can change throughout the day.

Sexual orientation: the nature of a person's emotional and physical attractions to others.

Your **sexual orientation** describes the nature of your emotional and physical attractions to others. It can range from *pansexual*, attraction without gender as a factor, to *asexual* or "ace," meaning you may or may not experience romantic feelings but not sexual attractions. Your emotional and physical attraction are independent of your sex and gender identity. They are independent of one another, and all are within the range of normal expression (see Pulling It Together feature at the end of the chapter).

Sexual orientation hasn't always been seen that way. It wasn't until *DSM-II* in 1973 that the American Psychiatric Association removed a diagnosis for homosexuality. Previous editions had suggested it was an "illness," contributing to stigma and unnecessary harm for members of gender and sexual minorities (Drescher 2015).

You probably now realize that "gender reveal" parties use (at most) chromosomes from the mother's blood and perhaps a peek at the baby's genitalia on an ultrasound and employ these biological markers to conflate gender with sex.

CONCEPT CHECK 8.1

Matching: Match the terms with the description.
1. Sex
2. Gender identity
3. Gender expression
4. Sexual orientation

1. Courtney is painting her nails bright colors because they look more feminine to her.
2. Kam has sexual and secondary reproductive organs typical of males.
3. Sam says that he identifies with being a man.
4. Kari doesn't have any sexual attraction to anyone but feels fine about it.

8.2   GENDER VARIATIONS AND GENDER DYSPHORIA

Transgender or gender nonconforming (TGNC): people who have a gender identity that is different from the gender that was assigned to them at birth.

Both when they are children and as adults, most people have a sense of their gender identity and their birth anatomy. Often their sex assigned at birth, whether male or female, is the same as the gender assigned to them at birth, whether boy or girl. However, that's not the case for everyone. There are estimates that 25 million people in the world (0.8 percent of the population) are **transgender or gender nonconforming (TGNC)** (Safer & Tangpricha 2019). People who are TGNC have a gender identity that is different from the gender that was assigned to them at birth. An individual who experiences that inconsistency can either accept it or find a way to change their birth anatomy to be consistent with their experienced identity. Some people who are transgender have extreme distress and impairment associated with the incongruence between their sex and their gender identity. The *DSM-5tr* calls this distress gender dysphoria (see Diagnostic Overview 8.1). The word dysphoria means dissatisfaction or a state of unease.

The diagnosis is controversial. In fact, in 2017 Denmark passed a law saying transgender people shouldn't be diagnosed with a psychological disorder even if their gender identity brings significant distress and impairment (Russo 2017). In ICD-11 you won't find reference to gender dysphoria, and the World Health Organization decided to remove it from the list of mental disorders. Despite this, the *DSM* continues to include gender dysphoria as a psychological condition, which has the disadvantage of contributing to stigma. However, some insurance companies do require this diagnosis in order to proceed with gender-affirming procedures.

Diagnostic Overview 8.1: Gender Dysphoria

- Incongruence between experienced/expressed gender and a person's anticipated or present sex characteristics.
- A strong desire to be rid of the present sex characteristics because they are incongruent with a person's experienced/expressed gender.
- A desire to have sex characteristics of another gender.
- A desire to be of a different gender from the gender assigned at birth.
- A desire to be treated as a gender different from the gender assigned at birth.
- A conviction about having the feelings of a gender different from the gender assigned at birth.

Impact: Symptoms must exceed cultural and contextual norms. Symptoms are related to clinically significant distress or create impairment in important areas of life such as with friends and family or at work or school.

Timeframe: Six months or more.

Source: Information from APA (2022).

Symptoms and Clinical Description

About 90 percent of transgender people have distress and impairment (Billard 2018; Robles et al. 2016), which can include problems at work and with relationship satisfaction. Some feel anxiety and depression or have substance abuse problems or even thoughts of suicide (Mueller et al. 2017; Schulman & Erickson-Schroth 2017).

However, it may not be the incongruence of their assigned sex and assigned gender that leads to this distress and impairment (Robles et al. 2016). Prejudice against transgender individuals may contribute. As many as 80–90 percent of transgender people have experienced harassment or have been attacked in school or at work. Fifty percent have been fired from their jobs or passed over for promotion, and 20 percent have been denied a place to live (Wirtz et al. 2018). In the communities where transgender people are supported by family and friends, they don't seem to experience nearly as many mental health problems (Johns et al. 2018; Seibel et al. 2018).

Statistics and Trajectory

Sometimes, as in Jazz's case (see the chapter-opening story), the feelings of incongruence and dysphoria emerge in childhood (Olson-Kennedy et al. 2018), and for some people they fade by late adolescence. However, some individuals discover they are transgender as adults (Challa et al. 2020). Transgender women outnumber transgender men by 2:1. About 1.5 percent of those assigned as male identify as female and 3.5 percent of those assigned as female identify as male

(Challa et al. 2020), but less than 1 percent of adults are transgender (APA 2022; Zucker 2017). This change in numbers over the years to maturity is one of the reasons many professionals suggest waiting until the age of 14 to 16 to undergo any surgical procedures (Levine 2021), although there are medications considered acceptable before this age (Corathers 2018; Nahata et al. 2017).

Estimates of the number of people who are TGNC are probably under-reports, and the true numbers may be higher than these statistics suggest (APA 2015). And while gender dysphoria is often described in the context of TGNC experiences, it is possible for cisgendered people to experience gender dysphoria as well. For example, while filming *She's the Man*, Amanda Bynes experienced many symptoms of gender dysphoria due to emotional distress while making the movie (Ahlgrim 2018).

THE POWER OF WORDS

MISGENDERING

Have you ever seen email signatures that let you know which pronoun to use to refer to the sender? Or perhaps the question about pronouns arises in an introduction activity at the beginning of class or at a workshop or conference (Figure 8.3). Perhaps you wondered, what's the big deal? The big deal is the power of words.

In this chapter we've learned about how an individual's gender identity may be different from their assigned gender (typically the gender given by medical professionals at birth). *Misgendering* occurs when someone uses a gender pronoun (like him or her) that isn't consistent with a person's gender identity.

People who are transgender already experience a great deal of discrimination in employment, social acceptance, and relationships, and they also report experiencing higher rates of physical and sexual violence. Some people simply respond negatively to those who deviate from what they consider to be expected gender roles. When people who are transgender also experience misgendering, it is associated with feeling more negatively about themselves and their gender identity, and those who are TGNC feel less authentic in their social interactions with others (McLemore 2018).

In one study of 410 TGNC participants whose mean age was 30, a third said they experienced misgendering often and felt consistently stigmatized when it

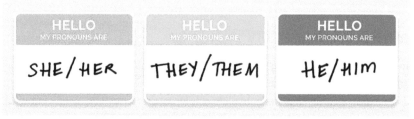

Figure 8.3 Nametags and email signatures often contain gender pronouns.

occurred. About 35 percent felt very stigmatized and looked down on when misgendered (McLemore 2018). The more important their gender identity was to them, the more distress they felt. Taking the time to get a person's gender correct is important because of the distress and impairment that misgendering can cause. As its most basic level, misgendering someone expresses that we are choosing not to treat a person in the way they have asked to be treated. Words are powerful.

Source: McLemore (2018).

Models and Treatments of Gender Dysphoria

In 2018 Jazz Jennings started the first of what were to be three gender-affirming surgeries. She has been open in the media about her journey, and her family continues to be supportive. "I've gone through the whole medical process, and this [the surgery] is really the last thing that will validate my identity as a woman," she said recently (Miller & Nied 2020).

BIOLOGICAL MODELS AND TREATMENTS OF GENDER DYSPHORIA

Biological factors are an important influence on transgender development (Burke et al. 2018). For example, TGNC does run in families (Gómez-Giletal et al. 2010). Twin studies have revealed that in identical (monozygotic MZ) twin pairs, when one twin was transgender, the other was too in 9 of 23 cases (Heylens et al. 2012).

Using MRIs, researchers have found some variations in the brains of transgender individuals. For example, the brains of transgender people are more similar to the brains of others with their gender identity than to their assigned gender (Mueller et al. 2017). In addition, some researchers have found similarities in a few key brain areas that play roles in gender functioning, such as the insula, anterior cingulate cortex, and bed nucleus of stria terminalis (BNST) (Spizzirri et al. 2018).

Biological treatments for gender dysphoria include gender-affirming hormone and medical therapies. Hormone treatment can include feminizing hormone therapy such as anti-androgens and estrogen to decrease facial and body hair, or testosterone to increase erectile tissue, body hair, and muscle mass. It can also include medications such as leuprorelin (Lupron) that may delay the onset of puberty. Medicines such as leuprorelin work to halt the process of puberty. However, once leuprorelin is stopped, puberty begins again. These medications are also commonly prescribed for cis-gendered children who experience early-onset puberty. Psychologists can serve as facilitator to make sure that clients have realistic expectations about the effects and limits of hormone treatments.

Hormone administration (Corathers 2018; Ferrando & Thomas 2018) may not be enough for some, who can then undergo gender affirming surgery consisting of a number of procedures. More than 3,000 such surgeries are performed each year in the United States. Some countries and some states in the United States require surgery for making legal gender-marker changes (such as changing gender on a driver's license or voter registration card). In fact, many TGNC people have problems being allowed to vote because their identification card doesn't match their expected appearance. Gender surgery specialists may recommend no surgery, or they may suggest limited surgery for breast augmentation, tracheal shave (to remove an Adam's apple), voice feminization surgery, feminization or masculinization surgery to change the shape of the face, body contouring procedures, or more invasive procedures such as orchiectomy (removal of testes), penectomy (removal of penis), labiaplasty (construction of labia from scrotal tissue), or removal of the uterus and cervix. In a meta-analysis of 28 studies of 1,822 people who received hormone therapy as gender-affirming procedures, 80 percent also experienced improvement with surgical interventions (Murad et al. 2010).

There is some controversy about the success of these procedures, despite evidence that up to 70 percent of those who undergo them report satisfaction with the outcomes (Ferrando & Thomas 2018). Careful screening is important. And researchers are still working to understand the long-term impact of gender confirmation surgery.

Figure 8.4 Transgender awareness has increased, due in part to the visibility in media, television, and films of TGNC people such as Laverne Cox (left) and actor Elliot Page (right).

Sources: Photo of Laverne Cox by Christophe Polk/Getty Images for Turner. Photo of Elliot Page by Jeff Kravitz/ FilmMagic/Getty Images.

PSYCHOLOGICAL MODELS AND TREATMENTS OF GENDER DYSPHORIA

Transgender awareness has increased, due in part to the visibility in media (Figure 8.4). In addition, the American Psychological Association has established practice guidelines for the treatment of those who are TGNC (American Psychological Association 2015). The guidelines were established to help therapists become culturally competent and provide trans-affirmative experiences, since discrimination and stigma have likely led to increased rates of depression and suicide attempts in this community. Before the guidelines were developed, fewer than 30 percent of psychologists were familiar with many of the issues that TGNC people faced (American Psychological Association 2015). In a recent study of more than 150 TGNC adults,

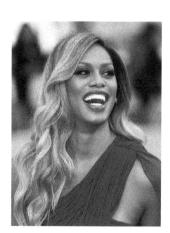
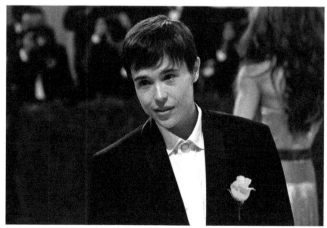

68 percent reported actual mistreatment in medical settings (such as being refused treatment due to being TGNC), and 43 percent had avoided medical treatment in the last year in order to avoid being discriminated against (Hughto et al. 2018). As a consequence, the APA task force developed 16 evidence-based "Guidelines for Psychological Practice with Transgender and Gender Nonconforming People" to assist mental health practitioners (APA 2015). These are as follows:

Foundational Knowledge and Awareness

> **Guideline 1**. Psychologists understand that gender is a nonbinary construct that allows for a range of gender identities and that a person's gender identity may not align with sex assigned at birth.
>
> **Guideline 2**. Psychologists understand that gender identity and sexual orientation are distinct but interrelated constructs.
>
> **Guideline 3**. Psychologists seek to understand how gender identity intersects with the other cultural identities of TGNC people.
>
> **Guideline 4**. Psychologists are aware of how their attitudes about and knowledge of gender identity and gender expression may affect the quality of care they provide to TGNC people and their families.

Stigma, Discrimination, and Barriers to Care

> **Guideline 5**. Psychologists recognize how stigma, prejudice, discrimination, and violence affect the health and well-being of TGNC people.
>
> **Guideline 6**. Psychologists strive to recognize the influence of institutional barriers on the lives of TGNC people and to assist in developing TGNC-affirmative environments.
>
> **Guideline 7**. Psychologists understand the need to promote social change that reduces the negative effects of stigma on the health and well-being of TGNC people.

Life Span Development

> **Guideline 8**. Psychologists working with gender-questioning and TGNC youth understand the different developmental needs of children and adolescents, and that not all youth will persist in a TGNC identity into adulthood.
>
> **Guideline 9**. Psychologists strive to understand both the particular challenges that TGNC elders experience and the resilience they can develop.

Assessment, Therapy, and Intervention

> **Guideline 10**. Psychologists strive to understand how mental health concerns may or may not be related to a TGNC person's gender identity and the psychological effects of minority stress.
>
> **Guideline 11**. Psychologists recognize that TGNC people are more likely to experience positive life outcomes when they receive social support or trans-affirmative care.

Guideline 12. Psychologists strive to understand the effects that changes in gender identity and gender expression have on the romantic and sexual relationships of TGNC people.

Guideline 13. Psychologists seek to understand how parenting and family formation among TGNC people take a variety of forms.

Guideline 14. Psychologists recognize the potential benefits of an interdisciplinary approach when providing care to TGNC people and strive to work collaboratively with other providers.

Research, Education, and Training

Guideline 15. Psychologists respect the welfare and rights of TGNC participants in research and strive to represent results accurately and avoid misuse or misrepresentation of findings.

Guideline 16. Psychologists seek to prepare trainees in psychology to work competently with TGNC people.

CONCEPT CHECK 8.2

Indicate whether each case below is more likely to describe a person with gender dysphoria, a person who is transgender, or someone who should receive no diagnosis.

1. A 17-year-old (male sex assigned at birth) went to an outpatient mental health clinic with complaints of anger and irritability, decreased sleep, and repeated threats over the past seven or eight days to harm himself or run away from home. The patient reports dissatisfaction with their sex assigned at birth and conflicts with family members over this issue.
2. Blake feels as if his gender identity is different from his sex assigned at birth. He has a lot of support from family and friends and as a result does not have significant distress or impairment associated with this incongruency.
3. Kyle, aged 10, is upset with their parents. Although assigned female at birth, Kyle reports wanting to be a boy. In fact, Kyle refused to toilet train until their parents purchased "boy clothes" and was furious when asked to use pink scissors or line up with the girls in physical education class.

8.3 SEXUAL DYSFUNCTIONS

It's not uncommon for people to discuss some of the details of their psychological state, such as their stress level and mood. These are often a topic of everyday conversation. We often share feelings like this with the people who are close to us. However, one segment of our lives remains a mystery even to close friends, family, and many times psychotherapists: our sexuality. Sexual behavior, sexual thoughts, and sexual fantasies are part of most people's experience of being a human. And like our moods and behaviors, they can be disruptive at times and can affect our lives, even causing significant distress and impairment.

Sexual dysfunctions are disorder conditions in which people have difficulty in one or more areas of the sexual response cycle (discussed below). Most people are fairly private about and even embarrassed by sexual dysfunctions, but these disorders are quite common. Some research suggests that up to a third of men and 45 percent of women worldwide will meet criteria for sexual dysfunction at some point in their lives (Cunningham & Rosen 2018). These difficulties can cause distress, frustration, challenges to self-esteem, and interpersonal problems. Sexual dysfunctions can occur among heterosexuals as well as members of sexual and gender minorities.

The Sexual Response Cycle

The **sexual response cycle** is a pattern of biological and psychological events that occurs in response to sexual stimulation (Table 8.1). The classic four-stage model was proposed by William Masters and Virginia Johnson in the mid-1960s (Masters & Johnson 1966). The four phases are desire, excitement, orgasm, and resolution (Shifren 2018).

Sexual response cycle: a pattern of biological and psychological events that occurs in response to sexual stimulation.

- Phase 1 – Desire: The desire phase is characterized by sexual fantasies and the desire to have sex. It can last from a few minutes to several hours.
- Phase 2 – Arousal: In the arousal phase, which extends to the start of orgasm, there is a sense of sexual pleasure along with corresponding body responses.
- Phase 3 – Orgasm: The climax of arousal is the phase during which orgasm and ejaculation occur. The orgasm phase is the shortest of the phases, lasting only a few seconds.

Table 8.1 **The four phases of the classic sexual response cycle**

Phase 1: Desire	Phase 2: Arousal
<ul><li>Blood flow to the genitals increases</li><li>Heart rate and breathing increase</li><li>Lubrication begins in the penis and vagina</li><li>Muscle tension increases</li><li>Nipples harden or become erect</li><li>Skin flushes</li><li>Testicles swell and the scrotum tightens</li></ul>	<ul><li>Breathing, heart rate, and blood pressure increase</li><li>Changes that started in the desire phase increase</li><li>Muscle spasms may begin in the feet, face, and hands</li><li>Tension in the muscles increases</li><li>Testicles are withdrawn up into the scrotum</li></ul>
Phase 3: Orgasm	**Phase 4: Resolution**
<ul><li>"Sex flush," which resembles a rash, may appear on the body</li><li>Involuntary contractions occur in the uterus and muscles of the vagina</li><li>Muscle contractions occur at the base of the penis and result in ejaculation</li><li>Muscle spasms occur in the feet</li></ul>	<ul><li>The body returns to its normal level of functioning in the final stage of the cycle</li></ul>

- Phase 4 – Resolution: In the final stage of the sexual response cycle, the body returns to its normal level of functioning.

Other sexual researchers have divided the sexual response cycle differently. Helen Singer, for example, has proposed a three-phase model of sexual desire, excitement, and orgasm (Magon et al. 2012). Others (Leavitt 2019) have suggested that the Masters & Johnson model is based primarily on men's responses, and that women may progress through the cycle in a nonlinear way. However, for the purpose of discussing sexual dysfunctions, we consider that there are sexual dysfunctions that affect desire and arousal, that interfere with orgasm, and that are related to sexual pain.

People vary in their degree of and even their desire for sexual excitation and responsiveness, and in their ability to inhibit their sexual excitement. Some people move slowly through the stages and others more quickly. It's important to remember that sexual response isn't simply a physical response, but a cognitive and emotional one as well. Sexual response is personal and individual and is influenced by physiological, psychological, and sociocultural influences. Sexual dysfunction in an individual can affect either particular situations or all the person's sexual situations (APA 2022).

Sexual dysfunction is common in women and men alike. In the United States 43 percent of women and 41 percent of men have reported either low sexual desire, low or infrequent arousal, or difficulties with orgasm, and 22 percent of women and up to 25 percent of men have reported significant stress related to a sexual dysfunction (Pozzi et al. 2021; Pyke 2020; Wheeler & Guntupalli 2020). In this section we cover sexual dysfunction, and in the next paraphilic disorders.

Disorders of Sexual Desire and Arousal

Sexual desire disorders: conditions characterized by decreased sexual desire or a total lack of sexual interest or sexual fantasy.

Sexual arousal disorder: a condition where a person has an aversion to sexual contact, which can be experienced in a variety of ways.

The sexual desire and arousal phase is marked by urges or interest in having sex, attraction to others, or sexual fantasies. **Sexual desire disorders** are characterized by decreased sexual desire or a total lack of sexual interest or sexual fantasy. In a **sexual arousal disorder**, a person has an aversion to sexual contact, which can be experienced in a variety of ways. The lack of sexual arousal has an impact on sexual excitement or feelings of pleasure in women and may result in a lack of an erection in men.

The *DSM* lists three disorders in the sexual desire and arousal phase. One occurs in women – female sexual interest/arousal disorder – and two occur in men – male hypoactive sexual desire disorder and erectile disorder.

FEMALE SEXUAL INTEREST/AROUSAL DISORDER

Female sexual interest/arousal disorder: a condition characterized by a lack of interest in sexual activity or a significantly and persistently low level of sexual arousal.

Female sexual interest/arousal disorder is characterized by a lack of interest in sexual activity or a significantly and persistently low level of sexual arousal (Diagnostic Overview 8.2). Women with this condition have a persistent inability to attain sexual excitement and lubrication until completion of sexual activity.

Women with female sexual interest/arousal disorder often report reduced or completely absent interest in all sexual activity and sexual thoughts. Many will be reluctant to engage in or initiate sexual activity and will not have a response to the invitation of sexual activity. They also have reduced or absent arousal, excitement, and sensation during sexual activity.

The diagnostic criteria require these symptoms to be present for a significant number of sexual encounters (75 percent or greater) for at least six months and to be associated with either distress or impairment. Women may be distressed because they feel sexual desire but are not able to feel sexual excitement, which leads to a loss or lack of motivation to participate in sexual activity.

There is some controversy about the name of this disorder, since it incorporates two phases (sexual interest and sexual arousal) into one disorder (Kingsberg & Simon 2020). Some researchers believe this combination obscures what clients are experiencing; they would prefer to have separate disorders (as are listed for men) (Kingsberg & Simon 2020). The combined name may be due to the typical patterns of the conditions. While men with male hypoactive sexual desire disorder have typical physical responses to sex and will have sex, women with female sexual interest/arousal disorder rarely engage in sexual activity.

Lack of sexual interest and arousal can have a profound negative impact on quality of life, causing negative emotional states and personal distress (Kingsberg & Simon 2020).

Female sexual interest/arousal is the most common of the sexual dysfunctions in women, affecting over 7 million women in the United States. About 39 percent of women around the world report reduced sexual arousal and interest, and about half of these feel distressed by their lack of arousal (Kinsberg & Simon 2020). In one international survey, 38.7 percent of respondents reported problems with desire and 26.1 percent experienced low sexual arousal. When we look at purely hypoactive (hypo means under) sexual desire in women, prevalence rates range from 9 to 22 percent, with higher rates among older women and women who are surgically postmenopausal, meaning they've received surgeries to remove their ovaries, the main source of estrogen, as a result of which estrogen levels fall significantly (Kinsberg & Simon 2020). The rates for low sexual arousal are 25.3 percent, with the highest rates occurring 38 percent among women aged 45–64 (Kinsberg & Simon 2020). Rates increase with age; however, distress appears to be more common in middle and early adulthood (Wheeler & Guntupalli 2020).

MALE HYPOACTIVE SEXUAL DESIRE DISORDER

Men with **male hypoactive sexual desire disorder** lack interest in sex but may have typical physical responses to sex and will have sex (Diagnostic Overview 8.3).

Diagnostic Overview 8.2: Female Sexual Interest/Arousal Disorder

Absent or reduced sexual interest and/or sexual arousal in at least three of the following:

- Arousal in response to sexual cues.
- Initiation of sexual activity.
- Sensations during sexual activity.
- Sexual activity.
- Sexual excitement or sexual pleasure during sexual encounters.
- Thoughts or fantasies about sex.

Impact: Symptoms must exceed cultural and contextual norms. Symptoms are related to clinically significant distress or create impairment in important areas of life such as with friends and family or at work or school.

Timeframe: At least six months.

Source: Information from APA (2022).

Male hypoactive sexual desire disorder: a condition associated with a reduced interest in sex but may have typical physical responses to sex.

Diagnostic Overview 8.3: Male Hypoactive Sexual
Desire Disorder

Deficient or absent sexual or erotic thoughts, fantasies, or desire for sexual activity.

Impact:	Symptoms must exceed cultural and contextual norms. Symptoms are related to clinically significant distress or create impairment in important areas of life such as with friends and family or at work or school.
Timeframe:	At least six months.

Source: Information from APA (2022).

They report feeling unaroused by sexual activity, erotic cues, and sexual activity (APA 2022).

Up to 18 percent of men worldwide and about 15 percent in the United States meet criteria for male hypoactive sexual desire disorder (Cunningham & Rosen 2018).

ERECTILE DISORDER

In **erectile disorder**, men are unable to develop or maintain an erection sufficient for sexual activity (Diagnostic Overview 8.4).

Erectile disorder occurs in 15–25 percent of men in the United States (Cunningham & Rosen 2018), mostly men over 50, and can be associated with other medical conditions, particularly heart conditions and diabetes (Bayramova 2018). It can also occur in younger men, however. In fact, about 7 percent of men in their twenties have erectile disorder, compared with more than 70 percent in their seventies and older (Cunningham & Rosen 2018) (Figure 8.5). It can also occur occasionally, and about half of men have experienced some form of erectile dysfunction at some point.

ORGASM DISORDERS

Orgasm is the climax of arousal, during which pleasure leads to ejaculation in men and orgasm in women. Those with orgasm disorders may experience a delayed or absent orgasm following a typical sexual excitement phase. Dysfunctions related to this phase include early ejaculation and delayed ejaculation in men and female orgasmic disorder in women.

Female orgasmic disorder: a condition associated with persistent delay or absence of orgasm following a typical arousal phase.

In women, **female orgasmic disorder** is a condition associated with persistent delay or absence of orgasm following a typical arousal phase (Diagnostic Overview 8.5).

Twenty percent of US women have reported orgasm difficulties and 5 percent have reported distress because of it (Wheeler & Guntupalli 2020). About 50–70 percent of women experience orgasm frequently (Frederick et al. 2018). Women who tend to be more sexually assertive report having more orgasms more frequently (Wheeler & Guntupalli 2020).

Diagnostic Overview 8.4: Erectile Disorder

During most sexual activity (over 75 percent), difficulty in obtaining or maintaining an erection, or a decrease in erectile rigidity.

Impact:	Symptoms must exceed cultural and contextual norms. Symptoms are related to clinically significant distress or create impairment in important areas of life such as with friends and family or at work or school.
Timeframe:	At least six months.

Source: Information from APA (2022).

EJACULATION DISORDERS

Ejaculation and orgasm are distinct but often simultaneous events that occur in the orgasm phase in men. Ejaculations are contractions of the muscles at the base of the penis that cause sperm to be discharged. Men typically have some control over their ejaculation during this phase, and when they don't, they can experience distress. Some men ejaculate consistently early, while

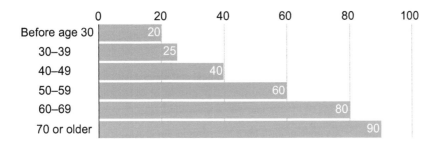

Figure 8.5 Prevalence of erectile disorder by age.
Source: Data from Allen & Walter (2019).

others have a persistent delay in or absence of ejaculation. There are two ejaculation disorders described in the *DSM*: premature (early) ejaculation (Diagnostic Overview 8.6) and delayed ejaculation disorder (Diagnostic Overview 8.7).

When people meet criteria for **premature ejaculation**, they will habitually reach orgasm within two minutes of sexual activity and before they desire to do so. In premature ejaculation a person has a persistent history of premature ejaculation, poor control over ejaculation, and feelings of dissatisfaction and distress. **Delayed ejaculation disorder** is a sexual dysfunction characterized by delayed or absent ejaculation.

Men who ejaculate before or shortly after sexual activity and those who express a lack of control over ejaculation along with significant distress may be diagnosed with premature (early) ejaculation.

Up to 10 percent of men worldwide experience delayed ejaculation (Morgentaler et al. 2017). Up to 25 percent of those with delayed ejaculation report lifetime symptoms, and some have difficulty with delayed or absent orgasm only during partnered sexual activity (Shindel et al. 2020).

Surveys suggest that as many as 30 percent of men worldwide will have symptoms of premature ejaculation in any given year (Pereira-Lourenço et al. 2019). However, few of these men will actually meet the diagnostic criteria for premature ejaculation (experiencing ejaculation within two minutes of sexual activity). When the diagnostic criteria are applied properly, rates for premature ejaculation drop to less than 5 percent (APA 2022). Even among men who experience ejaculation in the typical time period following sexual activity, most of those asked whether they would prefer to delay it will answer yes (Coskuner & Ozkan 2022).

Disorders of Sexual Pain

Physical discomfort and pain during intercourse aren't part of the sexual response cycle, but psychopathologists describe a few conditions in this area. Sexual pain disorders affect women more than men.

Premature ejaculation: a condition where a person has a persistent history of early ejaculation, poor control over ejaculation, and feelings of dissatisfaction and distress.

Delayed ejaculation disorder: a sexual dysfunction characterized by delayed or absent ejaculation.

Diagnostic Overview 8.5: Female Orgasmic Disorder

Infrequent occurrence of or absence of orgasm and/or a reduced intensity of orgasm in more than 75 percent of occasions of sexual activity.

Impact:	Symptoms must exceed cultural and contextual norms. Symptoms are related to clinically significant distress or create impairment in important areas of life such as with friends and family or at work or school.
Timeframe:	At least six months.

Source: Information from APA (2022).

Diagnostic Overview 8.6: **Premature (Early) Ejaculation**

A persistent pattern of ejaculation during sexual activity with another person often within one minute following penetration.

Impact: Symptoms must exceed cultural and contextual norms. Symptoms are related to clinically significant distress or create impairment in important areas of life such as with friends and family or at work or school.

Timeframe: A symptom must have been present for at least six months and must be experienced on 75 percent or more occasions of sexual activity.

Source: Information from APA (2022).

Genito-pelvic pain/penetration disorder: a condition in which the muscles in the outer third of the vagina contract involuntarily and painfully, which prevents sexual intercourse.

Genito-pelvic pain/penetration disorder is a condition in which the muscles in the outer third of the vagina contract involuntarily and painfully, which prevents sexual intercourse (Diagnostic Overview 8.8).

Genito-pelvic pain/penetration disorder encompasses various types of sexual pain, so there are other terms we use to be more specific. The three terms used most frequently to describe sexual pain in women are vulvodynia, dyspareunia, and vaginismus. *Vulvodynia* (chronic vulvar pain) is derived from the combination of the word "vulva" and the name Odyne, the Greek goddess of pain. *Dyspareunia* is general genital pain during intercourse, and *vaginismus* is an involuntary contraction of the musculature of the vagina that interferes with intercourse. Many women with vaginismus enjoy intercourse but fear the pain associated with the spasms.

Those with genito-pelvic pain/penetration disorder experience persistent pain during vaginal sexual intercourse. Persistent difficulty with vaginal intercourse or fear and anxiety regarding pain in anticipation of intercourse can result in tightening of pelvic floor muscles when penetration is attempted. The pain, or anxiety related to anticipation of the pain, results in significant distress and leads to an avoidance of intercourse. In some women even the anticipation of pain will cause painful spasms of the pelvic muscles.

Around 14–16 percent of women and 40 percent of postmenopausal women have experienced dyspareunia to some extent (Shifren 2018), and although they can enjoy sex, pain can limit the experience (Meana et al. 2017). Dyspareunia typically can arise from a physical cause such as injury from childbirth, infectious diseases, cysts, or allergies to latex condoms or contraceptive creams. Psychological conditions such as anxiety (not related to anticipation of sexual pain) may also be a factor, but this is rare (Kelley et al. 2021). Women who experience chronic genital pain may find it difficult to seek help, treatment, or support, and as a result they often experience significant social isolation.

The prevalence rates of dyspareunia and vulvodynia vary by the way we define the disorders and by

Diagnostic Overview 8.7: **Delayed Ejaculation**

A delay in or absence of ejaculation during all or partnered sexual activity.

Impact: Symptoms must exceed cultural and contextual norms. Symptoms are related to clinically significant distress or create impairment in important areas of life such as with friends and family or at work or school.

Timeframe: At least six months.

Source: Information from APA (2022).

geographic region. The global prevalence is estimated to be between 8 percent and 21 percent, but rates vary by country. For example, the prevalence of dyspareunia in the United States is approximately 10 percent to 20 percent, in Brazil 1.2 to 51 percent, and in Puerto Rico between 17 percent and 21 percent (Goldstein et al. 2018; Sorensen et al. 2018).

Studies of vulvodynia have indicated that it is fairly prevalent, with lifetime estimates ranging from 8 percent to 28 percent of reproductive-aged women in the general population. In a study comparing two geographical regions with differing access to health care, there was similar prevalence of about 8 percent (Goldstein et al. 2018). Further, the study's authors show that prevalence rates may differ by race, with nonwhite Hispanic women more likely to report sexual pain (Goldstein et al. 2018). Further research showed that daily pain is worse in Black women than in white women and that they describe their pain differently (Goldstein et al. 2018).

Pain can be reported only by the patient, and the

Diagnostic Overview 8.8: Genito-Pelvic Pain/Penetration Disorder

At least one of the following:

- During intercourse, persistent difficulty with vaginal penetration.
- During vaginal intercourse (or attempts), the experience of persistent or recurrent vulvovaginal or pelvic pain.
- Anxiety about vulvovaginal or pelvic pain in anticipation of or during vaginal penetration.
- As a result of vaginal penetration, tensing of the pelvic floor muscles.

Impact:	Symptoms must exceed cultural and contextual norms. Symptoms are related to clinically significant distress or create impairment in important areas of life such as with friends and family or at work or school.
Timeframe:	At least six months.

Source: Information from APA (2022).

subjective experience of pain can be difficult to describe. Some cultures have different beliefs regarding pain, which also can influence the way people interpret and describe it (Givler & Maani-Fogelman 2020). Some cultures believe that expressing pain is a sign of weakness, while others see it as a sign of progress toward recovery. Evidence suggests that clinicians underestimate patients' pain due to their own prejudices, which can lead them to think it is not as intense as what patients actually experience (Givler & Maani-Fogelman 2020).

Models and Treatments of Sexual Dysfunctions

A major change in the treatment of sexual dysfunctions emerged in 1970 with the publication of a book from William Masters and Virginia Johnson called *Human sexual inadequacy*. The goals of treatment include achieving a higher level of sexual satisfaction (Masters & Johnson 1980; Peterson 2017).

Mood states such as anxiety and anger can all have an impact on sex drive, as can the fear of disease or an unwanted pregnancy (Shifren 2018). Psychological disorders such as depression and OCD can affect sex drive too, and especially conditions where there may be body fluids or unpleasant odors of another person (Cunningham & Rosen 2018).

BIOLOGICAL MODELS AND TREATMENT

Hormones can sometimes be responsible for reducing sexual desire (Cunningham & Rosen 2018). Prolactin and testosterone, for example, can both cause problems if their levels are low. Estrogen can also be problematic,

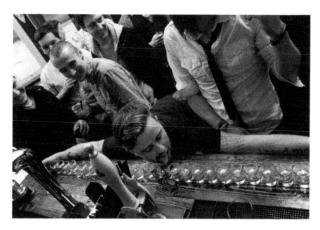

Figure 8.6 While alcohol abuse can cause sexual performance problems, these are separate from the problems caused by psychological disorders.

Source: John Rensten/The Image Bank/Getty Images.

but at high levels. Sex drive can be affected by medications such as birth control pills, hair loss medications, antidepressants, and drugs such as cocaine and heroin (Bala et al. 2018). While alcohol may reduce inhibitions in some people, higher levels may increase them and also impair sexual function (Figure 8.6) (Cunningham & Khera 2018). Similar hormonal culprits can lead to erectile dysfunction that in turn can cause hypoactive sexual desire (Cunningham & Rosen 2018). However, vascular problems can also cause erectile dysfunctions.

Medical procedures like ultrasound can help diagnose medical problems that might be associated with these concerns. Nocturnal penile tumescence (NPT) tests can measure erections at night in order to assess whether psychological or physical factors may be involved (since men typically have erections during rapid eye movement [REM] periods at night). When erections don't occur during this time, it can be a sign of a physical basis for an erectile disorder. NPT assessments consist of a paper band placed around the penis before bed. If the band is broken in the morning, it indicates a nocturnal erection occurred. Newer measures are computer-based and provide measurements of the number of erections during the night (Li et al. 2017).

Medical conditions such as diabetes can affect the nervous system. So can neurological conditions and medications, which can cause problems with orgasm (Hirsch & Birnbaum 2019). Some sexual dysfunctions may be due to an infection such as a urinary tract infection (UTI) or a gynecological disease such as herpes simplex (Kelley et al. 2021). Medical professionals will rule out these conditions before attempting other treatments (Sorensen et al. 2018).

Biology may also play a role in premature ejaculation. Most men who have premature ejaculation (91 percent) have first-degree relatives who do as well. They may also have increased sensitivity to nerve conduction in the penis (Roaiah et al. 2018). Low testosterone can interfere with ejaculation (Abdel-Itamid & Ali 2018), and any substance that can slow the nervous system like alcohol, high blood pressure medicine, and many psychotropic medications can cause delayed ejaculation.

Tricyclic antidepressants such as amitriptyline (Elavil) may be helpful treatments to reduce peripheral nerve sensitization and have been used in the management of neuropathic pain. They can be helpful in improving pain symptoms in clients with sexual pain. However, these medications don't work immediately; it can take up to three weeks to achieve pain control. Other biological interventions include using Botox to reduce spasms (Dahlen 2019).

Viagra (sildenafil), Cialis (tadalafil), and Levitra (vardenafil) are three of the most popular drugs to treat erectile dysfunction (see Table 8.2). Sildenafil was

Table 8.2 Some FDA-approved medications for sexual dysfunction

Generic name	Brand name	Condition	Class of medication
sildenafil	Viagra	Erectile dysfunction	Phosphodiesterase inhibitor
bremelanotide	Vyleesi	Hypoactive sexual desire disorder	Melanocortin receptor agonist
flibanserin	Addyi	Hypoactive sexual desire disorder	Serotonin 1A agonist and serotonin 2A antagonist
tadalafil	Cialis	Erectile dysfunction	Phosphodiesterase inhibitor
vardenafil	Levitra	Erectile dysfunction	Phosphodiesterase inhibitor

Source: Information from Stahl (2017).

originally developed to treat high blood pressure, though men who took it reported more erections. Marketed as Viagra beginning in 1998, it was the first oral medication approved to treat erectile dysfunction in the United States. Along with Cialis, Levitra, and Stendra (avanafil), Viagra is part of a family of drugs called phosphodiesterase type-5 inhibitors (PDE-5 inhibitors). PDE-5 is an enzyme that breaks down a molecule called cGMP, which causes narrowing of blood vessels. Medications to treat premature ejaculation include SSRIs and other medications that influence serotonin (Khera & Cunningham 2018).

Hormone therapy and sildenafil (Viagra) have been less successful in women with sexual desire conditions (Bradford 2017; Shifren 2018; Sorensen et al. 2018).

COGNITIVE-BEHAVIORAL MODELS AND TREATMENT

Cognitive-behavioral explanations for sexual disorders enjoy a fair amount of research support (Metz et al. 2017). Two behavioral approaches are typically used for the spasms in genito-pelvic pain/penetration disorder (Meana et al. 2017; Shifren 2018). Exercises in which a woman tightens and relaxes vaginal muscles can be beneficial, and exposure treatments can help reduce anticipatory anxiety. These two techniques can result in less pain and even pain-free intercourse for some. Psychoeducation can also help couples understand which sexual positions might be best to reduce pain.

Pelvic floor physical therapy is an important treatment given in addition to primary treatments for dyspareunia and vulvodynia. Physical therapy helps the pelvic floor muscles to relax. It can also be helpful in retraining pain receptors. In a systematic literature review, physical therapy including biofeedback, dilators, and electrical stimulation helped to decrease pain during intercourse. From the CBT perspective, avoidance of sexual pain can develop into a learned fear response (Meana et al. 2017).

CBT for dyspareunia and vulvodynia focuses on patterns of thinking and helps identify behaviors associated with negative thoughts and feelings. It has been found to be an effective treatment for reducing the anxiety and fear associated with these conditions (Bergeron et al. 2020).

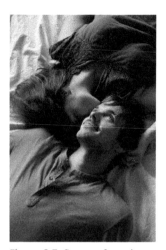

Figure 8.7 Sensate focus is a technique in which couples are encouraged to explore arousal without a focus on orgasm.
Source: Halfdark/Getty Images.

CBT can be useful for treating female orgasmic disorder (Carpenter et al. 2017; Kingsberg et al. 2017). Sexual inhibition can be related to this disorder (Tavares et al. 2018), especially when pain is associated with scars or other injuries. In many cases it's best to adopt a team approach to assess anxiety and physical and other concerns that may lead to pain or lack of arousal (Goodman 2013; Shifren 2018).

Sensate focus introduces both touching and being touched without evaluation while keeping an open mind about the experiences (Figure 8.7). Sensate focus exercises can teach a couple that erections occur naturally in response to stimulation when people don't focus too much on performance, which can help both erectile disorder and delayed ejaculation (Rowland & Cooper 2017).

SOCIOCULTURAL MODELS AND TREATMENT

Sexual attitudes are highly influenced by society and culture, especially religion and norms about women. One common message many women receive is that they should deny their sexuality and sexual attitudes or ideas. It's not surprising, then, that women with arousal and orgasmic conditions often have strict religious backgrounds, were more frequently punished for childhood masturbation, and may relate sexual pleasure to lack of morality (Lentz & Zaikman 2021).

Global differences in the prevalence of ejaculation dysfunction may be due to sociocultural influences, including socioeconomic status, cultural and religious beliefs, and differences in compliance with or access to health care. Some countries are more conservative about discussing sexual matters, which can discourage individuals from seeking help.

Social and cultural factors can have an impact on sexual desire as well. These can include social stressors such as separation, job stress, infertility, and the birth of a baby (Shifren 2018). Cultural standards can affect sexual desire too. In some cultures, as people age they may feel less attractive, which can influence the degree to which they feel desirable.

MULTIPERSPECTIVE MODELS AND TREATMENT

Sexual disorders can be difficult to treat, so many therapists use an eclectic approach (Althof & Needle 2017). Being aware of your emotions, called *affective awareness*, can be useful to reveal the anxiety that might underlie sex. Sex therapy consists of 15–20 sessions that focus on short-term goals and instruction (Peterson 2017) and can emphasize assessment, mutual responsibility, education, identification of emotions, changes in attitude, and reduction of performance anxiety (Bradford 2017; Khera & Cunningham 2018). Other goals include increasing communication skills (Shifren 2018), changing interaction skills (Kingsberg et al. 2017), and addressing any physical and medical conditions (Khera & Cunningham 2018; Shifren 2018).

Cognitive-behavioral techniques can be beneficial to improving clients' reactions to sex and self-statements about sex. Biological treatments such as hormone treatments (Khera & Cunningham 2018; Shifren 2018) have been found to be useful as well.

CONCEPT CHECK 8.3

Identify the sexual dysfunction described below.

1. Brandon has a lack of interest in sex and sexual activity that concerns him as well as his partner. A visit to his physician finds no evidence of a medical concern that might have led to this.
2. Despite being very healthy, Alana experiences very little sexual arousal from any romantic touching. She's experienced this with several partners, and her lack of sexual arousal causes her extreme distress.
3. While Fatimah experiences sexual arousal, she's distressed that she has never been able to experience an orgasm.

8.4 PARAPHILIC DISORDERS

Unusual fantasies are common in adult sexual behavior, and for most people they don't cause problems or lead to a loss of control (Castellini et al. 2018). **Paraphilias** are repeated intense sexual urges or fantasies about situations or objects outside societal sexual norms (Figure 8.8). Some people cannot become sexually aroused without the object, fantasy, or behavior, while others only need it at times. According to *DSM-5tr*, the diagnosis of paraphilic disorder is applied only when the paraphilia either causes the individual distress or impairment or puts the person (or another) at risk of harm. Some paraphilic arousals can be illegal if they are acted on without the consent of the other person (such as frotteuristic disorder, pedophilic disorder, voyeuristic disorder, and exhibitionist disorder), and there are times such sexual arousal may feel unwanted. Some researchers are concerned that medicalizing criminal offences could lead to misusing the diagnosis to absolve the person of legal responsibilities (Yakeley & Wood 2014). Keep in mind that many who may have these urges don't act on them. However, when people do act on their fantasies without consent, it imposes a great deal of harm on the victims of their assault. If you have found yourself a victim, psychological and legal help is available (such as the National Sexual Assault Hotline or your college or university counseling center).

Paraphilias: repeated intense sexual urges or fantasies about situations or objects outside societal sexual norms.

	Overall	Men	Women
Voyeurism	46.3	60	34.7
Exhibitionism	30.6	35	26.9
Frotteurism	26.7	34.2	20.7
Masochism	23.8	19.2	27.8
Sadism	7.1	9.5	5.1
Transvestism	6.3	7.2	5.5
Sex with child	0.6	1.1	0.2

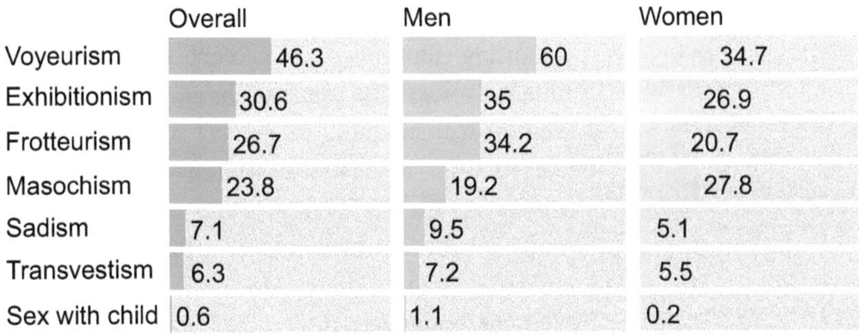

Figure 8.8 Percentage of people in Quebec wishing to experience certain paraphilia behaviors, 2017.
Source: Joyal & Carpentier (2017).

Sex can be filled with stigma and is highly contextualized by society and social and other norms. And psychology has been responsible in part for perpetrating a great deal of harm in the name of diagnosing and treating psychological disorders. For example, homosexual behavior remained in the *DSM* well into the late 1980s, and even today some clinicians recommend conversion therapy to "fix" the sexual orientation of people who might be sexual or gender minorities. For years (and sometimes today), clinicians have utilized these treatments, which harmed their patients.

DSM-5tr describes eight paraphilic disorders: fetishistic disorder, transvestic disorder, exhibitionistic disorder, voyeuristic disorder, frotteuristic disorder, pedophilic disorder, sexual masochism disorder, and sexual sadism disorder. For all paraphilic disorders, the criteria suggest at least six months of intense, recurrent sexually arousing fancies, and significant distress and impairment. Paraphilias are more common in men than in women and begin in adolescence (Bressert 2017; Martin & Levine 2018).

Fetishistic Disorder

If you looked up the word *fetish* in the 1700s, at that time it described religious objects, such as amulets, that were thought to have special powers. Fast-forward to the nineteenth century and that idea of special powers took on a new meaning. By then a fetish could be any idea or object for which a person had an irrational devotion or reverence. In the twentieth century another new meaning emerged – a sexualized desire for a body part (like the earlobe or foot) or even an object (like shoes).

SYMPTOMS AND DESCRIPTION

Fetishistic disorder is a paraphilic disorder in which fantasies, urges, or behaviors related to nonliving objects or nongenital body parts serve for sexual arousal (Diagnostic Overview 8.9). The most common objects are shoes and undergarments (Fisher & Marwaha 2020).

Fetishistic disorder: a paraphilic disorder in which fantasies, urges, or behaviors related to nonliving objects or nongenital body parts serve for sexual arousal.

STATISTICS AND TRAJECTORY

The majority of those with fetishistic disorder are male. In one study, 30 percent of men reported fetishistic fantasies, and about a quarter (24.5 percent) engaged in fetishistic acts (Eusei & Delcea 2020). Of those reporting fantasies, 45 percent said the fetish was intensely sexually arousing. In another study, 26.3 percent of women and 27.8 percent of men reported fantasies about "having sex with a fetish or non-sexual object" (Eusei & Delcea 2020). Fourteen percent of male sexual fantasies involve a fetish including feet or specific clothing items, and 4.7 percent focused on another body part (other than feet) (Eusei & Delcea

---

Diagnostic Overview 8.9: Fetishistic Disorder

Recurrent and intense sexual arousal fantasies, urges, or behaviors from the use of either nonliving objects or nongenital body parts.

Impact: Symptoms must exceed cultural and contextual norms. Symptoms are related to clinically significant distress or create impairment in important areas of life such as with friends and family or at work or school.

Timeframe: At least six months.

Source: Information from APA (2022).

Diagnostic Overview 8.10: Transvestic Disorder

Recurrent and intense sexual arousal from dressing as another gender, as manifested by fantasies, urges, or behaviors.

Impact: Symptoms must exceed cultural and contextual norms. Symptoms are related to clinically significant distress or create impairment in important areas of life such as with friends and family or at work or school.

Timeframe: At least six months.

Source: Information from APA (2022).

2020). Fetishistic disorder is rare; less than 1 percent of the population presents this disorder as their main concern (Eusei & Delcea 2020).

Transvestic Disorder

Those with **transvestic disorder** dress in clothing of another gender and associate it with recurrent and intense sexual fantasies, urges, or behaviors (Diagnostic Overview 8.10). Some will wear the clothes only under their regular clothes, while others dress fully as another gender. Having transvestic disorder is not the same as dressing as another gender as an entertainer or being transgender (Figure 8.9). At the core of transvestic disorder is sexual arousal, and it is diagnosed only when the cross-dressing creates significant distress or impairment.

Transvestic disorder: a condition where a person will dress in clothing of another gender and associate it with recurrent and intense sexual fantasies, urges, or behaviors.

SYMPTOMS AND DESCRIPTION

Most of the time people who dress in the clothes of another gender do not meet the criteria for this paraphilia. For those who do, the condition is associated with intense sexual arousal from wearing clothes typically associated with another gender that also brings with it extreme emotional discomfort. Some will spend a lot of money on clothing and accessories (wigs, undergarments), only to throw them away due to the emotional distress of wearing them. In some cases, transvestic disorder will transform into gender dysphoria.

Transvestic disorder can also include *autogynephilia*, which is sexual arousal in which a person will have fantasies of being another gender (in most cases a woman) while engaging in sexual behavior as themselves in a second gender (a man). For example, a man might fantasize that he is both himself and a woman with whom he will engage in sexual intercourse. For some this is the main or only way to experience sexual arousal.

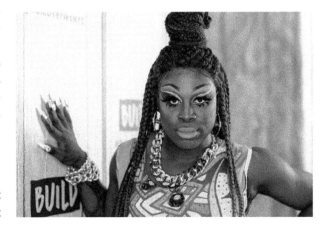

Figure 8.9 Drag performers such as Bob the Drag Queen are engaged in performance art. Most don't dress as another gender for sexual arousal, nor does their dress cause them distress or impairment.
Source: Roy Rochlin/Getty Images.

STATISTICS AND TRAJECTORY

Transvestic disorder is a condition reported almost exclusively in men. Less than 3 percent of men admit having been sexually aroused by wearing clothes of another gender at a given moment in the past (Lescai 2020). Typical in transvestic disorder is a heterosexual male who will start dressing as another gender in childhood or adolescence (Brown 2017; Thibaut et al. 2016). Usually men do so alone or while visiting bars.

Exhibitionistic Disorder

Exhibitionistic disorder: a condition in which a person experiences a sustained, focused pattern of sexual arousal, persistent sexual thoughts, fantasies, urges, or behaviors related to exposing their genitals to an unsuspecting person.

People with **exhibitionistic disorder** have a sustained, focused pattern of sexual arousal, persistent sexual thoughts, fantasies, urges, or behaviors related to exposing their genitals to an unsuspecting person (Diagnostic Overview 8.11). Typically, the exposure will occur in a public place, although those with the disorder don't intend contact with the people who see them. They are aroused by the act itself or by fantasies related to it. Some exhibitionists will engage in sexual acts (such as masturbation) in public places where they don't wish to be seen; however, the risk of being caught is part of the thrill. The diagnosis of exhibitionistic disorder does *not* apply to those who are expecting to be glimpsed, such as people who remove their clothes for the entertainment of others.

SYMPTOMS AND DESCRIPTION

There are gender differences in exhibitionistic disorders. Women with this condition tend to expose themselves in situations in which the victims won't respond by exposing themselves (men tend to respond this way more often than women). Women who have exhibitionistic disorder also tend to expose themselves in a car or to strangers online (Fedoroff 2020), while men will expose themselves in places where contact might occur, as well as from a distance. There is an often an overlap with voyeuristic disorders and problems with social functioning, and lower rates of life satisfaction and higher rates of sexual preoccupation than in men without the condition (Gallo 2020).

STATISTICS AND TRAJECTORY

Exhibitionistic disorder has a 2–4 percent prevalence in the general population, and in men it can be as high as 4.3 percent. Those with this condition typically

Diagnostic Overview 8.11: Exhibitionistic Disorder

- Recurrent and intense sexually arousing fantasies, urges, or behaviors from exposing the genitals.
- The individual has acted on these sexual urges with a nonconsenting person.

Impact:	Symptoms must exceed cultural and contextual norms. Symptoms are related to clinically significant distress or create impairment in important areas of life such as with friends and family or at work or school.
Timeframe:	At least six months.

Source: Information from APA (2022).

begin acting on their urge at around 18 years of age. About 30 percent are married, and another 30 percent are divorced or separated (Brown 2017; Thibaut et al. 2016). The occurrence of exhibitionist behaviors tends to increase with stress.

Published statistics about prevalence may be difficult to rely on, however, because most of those surveyed were in the criminal justice system. Between 30 and 50 percent of women have reported seeing or having contact with an exhibitionist (Marshall et al. 2008), although victims rarely report the acts to authorities (Szumski & Kasparek 2020).

Diagnostic Overview 8.12: Voyeuristic Disorder

Recurrent and intense sexually arousing fantasies, urges, or behaviors from observing an unsuspecting person who is naked, undressing, or engaging in sexual activity.

Impact:	Symptoms must exceed cultural and contextual norms. Symptoms are related to clinically significant distress or create impairment in important areas of life such as with friends and family or at work or school.
Age:	At least 18 years of age.
Timeframe:	At least six months.

Source: Information from APA (2022).

Voyeuristic Disorder

Voyeuristic disorder is a paraphilic disorder in which a person has intense sexually arousing fantasies, urges, or behaviors that involve watching an unsuspecting person naked or engaged in sexual activity.

SYMPTOMS AND DESCRIPTION

In voyeuristic disorder a person has recurrent and intense sexually arousing fantasies, urges, or behaviors about observing people who are either undressing, naked, or engaged in sexual activity (Diagnostic Overview 8.12). The people they watch are usually strangers. Those with voyeuristic disorder don't have an intention to have sexual contact with the person they are watching (although they may have a fantasy of engaging in the sexual activity). In many states, voyeurism (including video voyeurism, in which a person will record others without their knowledge) is a crime (Figure 8.10). The Video Voyeurism Act of 2004 made it a crime to photograph or make a video of a person in a federal building, national park, or military base who is naked or in undergarments, or of their genitals, without their knowledge.

STATISTICS AND TRAJECTORY

The first symptoms of voyeurism occur with sexual curiosity around the age of 15 and often consist of glancing into places where people are undressed (such as at nude beaches), or observing electronically by listening to sexual conversations (Brown 2017). People with the disorder don't typically seek out the people they observe. However, there is a lower age limit for diagnoses of voyeuristic disorder (18) to distinguish it from puberty-related sexual curiosity that might be developmentally appropriate.

Frotteuristic Disorder

In **frotteuristic disorder** a person has sexual urges to touch or rub against an unsuspecting and nonconsenting person and becomes aroused by doing so

Voyeuristic disorder: a paraphilic disorder in which a person has intense sexually arousing fantasies, urges, or behaviors that involve watching an unsuspecting person naked or engaged in sexual activity.

Frotteuristic disorder: a condition in which a person experiences sexual urges to touch or rub against an unsuspecting and nonconsenting person and becomes aroused by doing so.

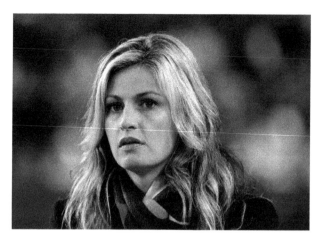

Figure 8.10 Sportscaster and television host Erin Andrews was awarded $55 million in a lawsuit against a man who admitted to making secret nude recordings of her in 2008. The hotel owner and management company were also found at fault for failing to protect Andrews.
Source: Al Messerschmidt/ Getty Images.

(Diagnostic Overview 8.13). The name comes from the French word *frotteur* which means rubbing.

SYMPTOMS AND DESCRIPTION

Frotteuristic behavior can occur in crowded places such as on public transportation (Guterman et al. 2011), in subways and buses, or in other public locations such as elevators or stores. Victims of frotteurism rarely report incidents to police, and prevalence estimates are difficult to acquire since most clients won't admit to the behaviors.

STATISTICS AND TRAJECTORY

Few studies have examined the prevalence of frotteurism, but like many paraphilia disorders, frotteuristic disorders are more likely to be diagnosed in men than in women (Johnson et al. 2014). Four studies have shown rates as high as 35 percent in men. However, perhaps because of variations in assessment methods, other studies ranged from 7.9 to 9.7 percent (Johnson et al. 2014).

Symptoms of frotteuristic disorder tend to emerge in late adolescence and early adulthood (ages 15–25) and often begin when the person watches other people do something similar. Around the mid-twenties, the behavior typically decreases (APA 2000).

Frotteurism can cause significant distress to victims. In a study in South Korea, 20 percent of people reported experiencing it. It was rare for victims to report the incident to police; in fact, of the more than 130 in this study who reported being the victim of frotteuristic behavior, only nine told police and fewer than half reported telling friends and family, although most had

---

Diagnostic Overview 8.13: Frotteuristic Disorder

Intense sexually arousing fantasies, urges, or behaviors that arise from touching or rubbing against a non-consenting person.

Impact:	The person has acted on the urge, or the urge is related to clinically significant distress, or it creates impairment in important areas of life such as with friends and family or at work or school. Symptoms must exceed cultural and contextual norms.
Timeframe:	At least six months.

Source: Information from APA (2022).

distressing feelings about the incident, and for 20 percent these feelings lasted for months (Choi et al. 2020).

Pedophilic Disorder

It can be difficult to relate to someone's sexual attraction to children. The practice of *pedophilia* today is illegal, although sexual attraction to children isn't new. Sexual relationships between men in their late twenties and boys in their mid to late teens were described as acceptable in ancient times, such as in Ancient Greece and during the Roman Empire. Such relationships, called pederasty, were seen as aiding maturity in the boys.

SYMPTOMS AND DESCRIPTION

In **pedophilic disorder** a person experiences sexually arousing fantasies or behaviors involving activity with a prepubescent child and accompanying distress or impairment (Diagnostic Overview 8.14).

STATISTICS AND TRAJECTORY

The prevalence of pedophilic disorder is difficult to estimate since it is rare for people with pedophilic symptoms to seek treatment; however, surveys suggest prevalence rates as high as 3–5 percent in the United States. Rates are higher for men. Symptoms of pedophilic disorder can come and go, and they can be strongest in early adolescence and decrease with age (Khoury et al. 2016; Quinsey 2003; Studer & Aylwin 2006).

Those with pedophilic disorder often develop a pattern of attraction to younger people during adolescence (Thibaut et al. 2016). Many reported experiencing sexual abuse, neglect, or severe punishment as children (Brown 2017), and as adults they may have difficulty planning and anxiety about sexual relationships (Massau et al. 2017). They also show distorted thinking patterns about the appropriateness of their behavior with children (Ciardha et al. 2016; Geradt et al. 2018).

Sexual Masochism Disorder and Sexual Sadism Disorder

The words sadism and masochism are often used in informal ways ("my new boss is a sadist" or "I'm a masochist when it comes to cooking"). The terms have more specific meanings in psychopathology, however (Figure 8.11). They were coined by the nineteenth-century psychiatrist Richard von Krafft-Ebing, after Donatien Alphonse François

Diagnostic Overview 8.14: Pedophilic Disorder

Intense sexually arousing fantasies, urges, or behaviors involving sexual activity with a child (generally under the age of 13).

Impact:	Symptoms are related to clinically significant distress or create impairment in important areas of life such as with friends and family or at work or school. Symptoms must exceed cultural and contextual norms.
Note:	The individual is at least 16 and at least five years older than the child.
Timeframe:	At least six months.

Source: Information from APA (2022).

Pedophilic disorder: a paraphilic disorder where a person experiences sexually arousing fantasies or behaviors involving activity with a prepubescent child and accompanying distress or impairment.

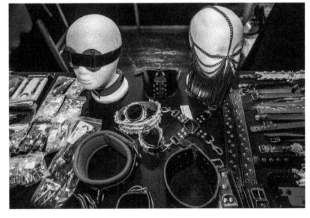

Figure 8.11 Sexual sadism and sexual masochism behavior have been the subject of books and films (such as *Fifty Shades of Grey*) and festivals. Without impairment, it's unlikely this sexual variation could be diagnosed as a disorder.
Source: Celestino Arce/ NurPhoto via Getty Images.

Diagnostic Overview 8.15: Sexual Masochism Disorder

Intense sexually arousing fantasies, urges, or behaviors that involve the act of being made to suffer.

Impact:	Symptoms are related to clinically significant distress or create impairment in important areas of life such as with friends and family or at work or school. Symptoms must exceed cultural and contextual norms.
Timeframe:	At least six months.

Source: Information from APA (2022).

Sexual masochism disorder: a paraphilic disorder where a person experiences recurrent and intense sexually arousing fantasies, urges, or behaviors stemming from the act of being humiliated, beaten, bound, or otherwise made to suffer.

Sexual sadism disorder: a paraphilic disorder where a person is aroused by the suffering of others and may inflict pain on them.

(the Marquis de Sade), who was renowned for his violent erotic writings that often featured abuse and rape, and Leopold von Sacher-Masoch, a journalist who was under Krafft-Ebing's care. Krafft-Ebing suggested Sacher-Masoch was sexually interested in being humiliated, which Sacher-Masoch denied.

Those with **sexual masochism disorder** have recurrent and intense sexually arousing fantasies, urges, or behaviors stemming from the act of being humiliated, beaten, bound, or otherwise made to suffer (Diagnostic Overview 8.15). They may have fantasies about having sex against their will but are distressed and upset about these ideas. Many have sexual partners who fulfill these urges (APA 2022). The disorder is diagnosed only if it becomes problematic and causes distress or impairment. Fantasies often begin in childhood but the person doesn't act on them until early adulthood. Some behaviors can escalate into more dangerous acts, especially during stressful periods (Frías et al. 2017).

Those with **sexual sadism disorder** are aroused by the suffering of others and may inflict pain on them (Diagnostic Overview 8.16).

SYMPTOMS AND DESCRIPTION

Sexual gratification from receiving pain (masochism) and from inflicting pain (sadism) often falls under the category of BDSM (bondage, discipline, dominance, submission, and sadism/masochism). BDSM encompasses a diverse set of sexual interests such as fantasies of control over another person, often a consenting person but not always (Joyal 2017). The suffering of others may be an important part of arousal for people with sexual sadism disorder. Because it has historically been pathologized, people interested in BDSM may hide their sexual proclivities from others. There are several reasons to engage in this behavior, including the use of interpersonal power, the experience of pain, and alterations to the person's state of mind. Some report experiencing pain that creates a trance or altered consciousness (Labrecque et al. 2021).

Diagnostic Overview 8.16: Sexual Sadism Disorder

Intense sexually arousing fantasies, urges, or behaviors that involve the suffering of another.

Impact:	Symptoms are related to clinically significant distress or create impairment in important areas of life such as with friends and family or at work or school. Symptoms must exceed cultural and contextual norms.
Timeframe:	At least six months.

Source: Information from APA (2022).

STATISTICS AND TRAJECTORY

BDSM-related fantasies are fairly common, with up to 70 percent of both men and women expressing this sexual interest. Only about 20 percent reported engaging in BDSM behavior (Brown et al. 2020), which includes sexual behaviors that use pain to elicit sexual gratification.

The exact prevalence of sexual masochism disorder in the population has been difficult to estimate, but the *DSM-5tr* suggests that 2.2 percent of men and 1.3 percent of women may meet the criteria. While paraphilias are not often diagnosed in women, sexual masochism disorder is the most common paraphilia in women (APA 2022).

Models and Treatments of Paraphilic Disorders

Researchers have had difficulty developing models of paraphilic disorders (Martin & Levine 2018), and the research around treatments is thin as well (Thibaut et al. 2016). Neurobiological, sociocultural, and cognitive processes all play a role in the development of paraphilia disorders.

It's uncommon for people to seek treatment. Some may feel humiliation, shame, or discomfort as a result of the disorder, while others concentrate on achieving sexual gratification and are unwilling to stop trying to obtain extreme sexual gratification and ultimate satisfaction. Many may also be too fearful of legal action to come forward for care. Those in care or seeking care are most often either legally mandated or persuaded to do so by relatives, friends, or sexual partners.

Biological treatments focus on removing arousal, while psychological treatments focus on understanding, substituting, or reducing what can sometimes feel like unwanted sexual arousals. Treatment can be court-ordered for certain paraphilias that are also illegal, such as pedophilia, frotteurism, exhibitionism, and voyeurism. Psychological treatments rely on finding ways to modify the paraphilic attractions.

BIOLOGICAL MODELS AND TREATMENTS

Genetic factors are thought to play a role in some paraphilia conditions, and dopamine may feature in many of them. Researchers have suggested that increased levels of serotonin and norepinephrine are found in urine samples of many people with paraphilia disorders (Kamenskov & Gurina 2019). Remember that not all those with increased levels of serotonin and norepinephrine engage in paraphilic behaviors, however.

The focus of most biological treatments is to reduce sex drive and thus reduce the paraphilic behavior. In the past that might have included surgery such as castration to remove the testes and thus eliminate the production of androgens. Modern treatments usually rely on medication. The classifications of medicines used in the treatment of paraphilic disorders include SSRIs, synthetic steroidal analogs, and antiandrogens. Health care providers will choose a treatment based on the risk of the negative impact clients may have on others in their lives and the likelihood they will continue with the treatment. The more negative the impact, the more likely that health care providers may opt for medication treatments.

Medications are effective only when taken regularly, so motivation too can be important.

SSRIs can be useful especially with mild paraphilias, such as exhibitionism. Antiandrogens have also been shown to reduce the frequency and intensity of sexual arousal and behavior. Some treatments, including antiandrogens, lower testosterone and sex drive (Turner et al. 2019), but they may lower *all* sex drive and not just problematic sex drive (Thibaut et al. 2016).

Researchers suggest that those treated with medications do reduce their paraphilic behavior (Holoyda & Kellaher 2016). However, they also experience side effects such as hair loss, breast tissue development in men, leg cramps, fatigue, weight gain, and depression.

COGNITIVE-BEHAVIORAL MODELS AND TREATMENTS

Behavioral perspectives in the treatment of paraphilic disorders suggest that modifying behaviors may help to manage sexual impulses. The learning theory perspective assumes that fetishism, transvestic arousal, and masochism, for example, are learned (Martin & Levine 2018), and some cognitive-behavioral treatments focus on aversion therapy (Thibaut et al. 2016). However, there is limited evidence to support these theories (Keller et al. 2020). Another view from this perspective is that a person with sexual sadism may have unintentionally caused pain to a person or animal in the past and felt a flood of emotions and even sexual arousal (Thibaut et al. 2016).

Cognitive-behavioral therapy can be a helpful treatment no matter the type of paraphilic disorder (Fisher & Marwaha 2020). It can be beneficial for managing sexual fantasies, and for modifying thoughts and replacing them with more socially acceptable behaviors and fantasies. Behavioral modification treatments have also been used to treat paraphilic disorders and are useful in clients who are motivated to change. In addition, some cognitive-behavioral treatments focus on finding new, more socially acceptable ways to interact with those whom clients find attractive.

SOCIOCULTURAL MODELS AND TREATMENTS

Social skills training can also be helpful with certain paraphilias (Tozdan & Briken 2021). It's clear that culture plays a role in the expression of sexuality (McManus et al. 2013), and role-playing techniques that help a person explore their relationships can give those with paraphilic disorders help in approaching and creating positive sexual encounters.

Some sociocultural researchers question the very nature of paraphilic disorders and wonder whether they are disorders at all: "There are people who fervently desire to be rich. These individuals may think about, fantasize about, and have urges to rob banks. They do not receive a diagnosis if, in fact, they rob banks. By contrast, for people with criminal paraphilias who think about, fantasize about, and have urges related to their sexual interests, committing the sexual act inexorably leads to a paraphilic disorder diagnosis" (Moser & Kleinplatz 2020, p. 391). These researchers suggest that those with paraphilic disorders are participating in criminal behavior, and that a psychological diagnosis is not the best explanation for their crime.

MULTIPERSPECTIVE MODELS AND TREATMENTS

Perhaps the most effective interventions for paraphilic disorder are those that combine psychotherapy and medication. For example, when combined with CBT and medication, group work can be particularly effective in treating people who are motivated to change (Kaplan & Krueger 2012). However, treatments are most effective when the client experiences distress about the condition, and less effective when they are court-ordered and the intention is for the client to avoid punishment for a crime.

CONCEPT CHECK 8.4

Indicate the paraphilic disorder (if any) described in the short case.

1. Devan has sexually arousing fantasies about exposing his genitals in public. These fantasies cause him considerable distress and he has exposed himself a few times at a local park.
2. Randal has fantasies of watching women undress without their knowledge. Because he works in a department store, he has set up an area in the changing rooms where he can watch people without their knowledge. He has never been caught.
3. Rahman is sexually aroused by touching or rubbing against a nonconsenting person. He has done this more than a dozen times and has been arrested for the behavior.
4. Josefin's sex assigned at birth is male, but they enjoy dressing as a woman at bars. This behavior doesn't appear to cause Josefin any distress.

PULLING IT TOGETHER

Sex, Gender, and Sexual Orientation

Understanding the social construction of gender is complicated. The Gender Unicorn (Figure 8.12) attempts to break down some of the components, including the elements of gender identity, gender expression, sex assigned at birth, and attraction. These elements are independent and can affect one another, but they do not determine each other. The Gender Unicorn is not an idealized way to view gender, nor is it a diagnostic tool. The model is a way to understand how society constructs gender from the different components that go into it.

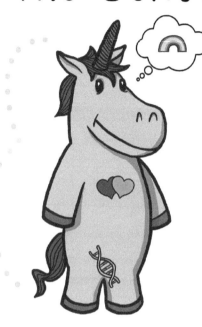

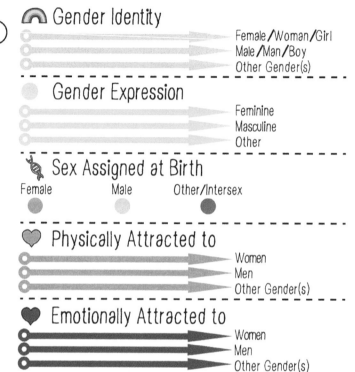

Figure 8.12 The Gender Unicorn.

Source: Design by Landyn Pan and Anna Moore, www.transstudent.org/gender.

SUMMARY

This chapter presented the following disorders:

- Gender dysphoria
- Female sexual interest/arousal disorder
- Male hypoactive sexual desire disorder
- Erectile disorder
- Female orgasmic disorder
- Premature (early) ejaculation
- Delayed ejaculation disorder
- Genito-pelvic pain/penetration disorder
- Fetishistic disorder
- Transvestic disorder
- Exhibitionistic disorder
- Voyeuristic disorder
- Frotteuristic disorder
- Pedophilic disorder
- Sexual masochism disorder
- Sexual sadism disorder

What Is Sexuality?

- Sex is a set of biological characteristics including hormones, chromosomes, and organs.
- Gender identity is a range of characteristics that characterize the way you think about the biological features that inform who you are.
- Gender expression is the way you demonstrate your gender.
- Sexual orientation describes the nature of your emotional and physical attractions to others.
- Although often presented together in discussions of psychopathology, sexual dysfunctions, paraphilic disorders, and gender dysphoria are distinct conditions.

Gender Variations and Gender Dysphoria

- Gender dysphoria is characterized by distress and impairment associated with an inconsistency between a person's birth sex and the gender assigned at birth.
- Gender dysphoria is a controversial diagnosis because the ICD-11 and many countries around the world have removed it from use.
- The distress and impairment associated with gender dysphoria may be related to prejudice that transgender people experience.
- Biological treatments for gender dysphoria include gender-affirming hormone and medical treatments.
- Psychological treatments include trans-affirmative mental health services.

Sexual Dysfunctions

- Sexual dysfunctions are disorders in which people have difficulty in one or more areas of the sexual response cycle.
- The sexual response cycle is a pattern of biological and psychological events in response to sexual stimulation.
- Sexual dysfunctions are common in both men and women.
- Sexual dysfunctions related to the sexual desire and arousal phase include female sexual interest/arousal disorder and male hypoactive sexual desire disorder and erectile disorder.
- Sexual dysfunctions related to the orgasm phase include premature (early) ejaculation, delayed ejaculation, and female orgasmic disorder.
- Genito-pelvic pain/penetration disorder is a condition in which the muscles in the outer third of the vagina contract involuntarily and painfully, preventing sexual intercourse.
- Biological treatments for sexual dysfunction include medications that relieve the symptoms of sexual dysfunction.
- Psychotherapy for sexual dysfunction can include cognitive-behavioral techniques such as

sensate focus that rely on non-evaluative touching.
- Sociocultural models focus on how culture and society view sexuality.
- Many therapists take a multiperspective approach that focuses on psychoeducation, as well as addressing physical and medical concerns for sexual dysfunctions.

Paraphilic Disorders

- Paraphilias are repeated intense sexual urges or fantasies about situations or objects outside societal sexual norms.
- Paraphilic disorders occur when paraphilic urges create distress or impairment.
- Fetishistic disorder is a paraphilic disorder in which fantasies, urges, or behaviors related to nonliving objects or nongenital body parts serve for sexual arousal.
- Those with transvestic disorder dress in clothes of another gender that are associated with recurrent and intense sexual fantasies, urges, or behaviors.
- People with exhibitionistic disorder have a sustained, focused pattern of sexual arousal, persistent sexual thoughts, fantasies, urges, or behaviors that rely on exposing the genitals to an unsuspecting person.
- Voyeuristic disorder is a paraphilic disorder in which a person has intense sexually arousing fantasies, urges, or behaviors that involve watching an unsuspecting person naked, undressing, or engaged in sexual activity.
- In frotteurism a person derives sexual urges from touching or rubbing against an unsuspecting and nonconsenting person.
- In pedophilic disorder a person experiences sexually arousing fantasies or behaviors involving activity with a prepubescent child and accompanying distress or impairment.
- In sexual masochism disorder a person experiences urges to be made to suffer for sexual pleasure. Some may have fantasies about having sex against their will but are distressed and upset about these ideas.
- A person with sexual sadism disorder has recurrent and intense sexually arousing fantasies, urges, or behaviors from the physical or psychological suffering of another person.
- Biological treatments for paraphilic disorders focus on reducing sex drive and thus reducing the paraphilic behavior.
- Psychological treatments rely on unearthing the source of the paraphilic attraction and finding ways to modify the attractions.

DISCUSSION QUESTIONS

1. Individuals who may be asexual might not be interested in any sexual experiences, nor do they experience sexual attraction to others. What questions would you ask to ascertain whether an individual is asexual, or experiencing hypoactive sexual desire?
2. Earlier editions of *DSM* included a diagnosis for homosexuality. These diagnoses were removed, in part because cultural biases against sexual minorities have begun to fade. In what ways, if any, does the diagnosis of gender dysphoria contribute to stigma?
3. Consider the types of conditions currently listed as sexual dysfunctions. What do the conditions say about what's important to our society and about what is considered a healthy sex life? For example, too little sex is listed as a psychological disorder, but not too much.
4. Sexual fantasies can be deeply personal and are influenced by culture. But culture can also influence the distress a person may feel about a sexual fantasy. How much are cultural influences involved in the distress and impairment experienced in disorders?

ANSWERS TO CONCEPT CHECKS

Concept Check 8.1

1. Gender expression
2. Sex
3. Gender identity
4. Sexual orientation

Concept Check 8.2

1. Gender dysphoria
2. Transgender

3. Gender dysphoria

Concept Check 8.3

1. Male hypoactive sexual desire disorder
2. Female sexual interest/arousal disorder
3. Female orgasmic disorder

Concept Check 8.4

1. Exhibitionistic disorder
2. Voyeuristic disorder
3. Frotteuristic disorder
4. No disorder

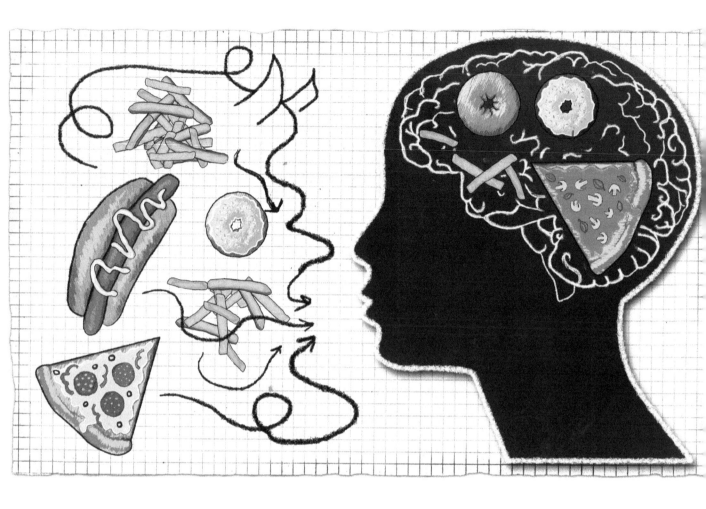

CHAPTER CONTENTS

9

Eating Disorders

CASE STUDY: **Bulimia Nervosa – Stephanie Armstrong**

Stephanie (Figure 9.1) is the youngest of three girls and has had a long-lasting "wonky" relationship with food. She grew up in a family with little money and even less food, and without thinking she would stash food around the house so it was available to her. Sometimes she would gorge herself and eat to the point where it felt like her eating was completely out of control. Because there wasn't much food around her house, she felt a great deal of guilt and shame about this behavior, and she kept the way she ate a secret from everyone.

Stephanie's uncontrolled eating periods were filled with not just emotional pain but physical pain as well. She would eat bowls of ice cream, then doughnuts, then pancakes with jelly, then garlic bread. She barely tasted, much less enjoyed it; her stomach hurt, her jaw hurt, she was exhausted. Then she would use her finger to force herself to throw the food up. Her fingers stung from the stomach acid and her eyes were bloodshot. When all the food she ate didn't come up, she felt a wave of panic. Then she would head back to the kitchen again and repeat this pattern several times a night.

But that wasn't her only pain growing up. When she was 12, Stephanie was sexually assaulted by her uncle. In response, she started to try diet teas and laxatives in order to control her weight. She thought that if she could gain control of her eating, she would be able to control something in her life. She said later that she would eat in order to push down feelings of shame and the way she felt about herself.

Looking back, she didn't get much support for her feelings. "Black women," she thought, "should feel comfortable being large," so she felt like a failure around food. We'll come back to Stephanie's story later in the chapter.

To read more about Stephanie's story take a look at her memoir: *Not all black girls know how to eat: A story of bulimia* (2009).

Learning Objectives

- Describe the symptoms and physical consequences of eating disorders.
- Identify the symptoms of binge-eating disorder, bulimia nervosa, and anorexia nervosa.
- Describe the epidemiology of eating disorders.
- Describe some of the social and cultural factors associated with eating disorders.
- Compare the various treatments for eating disorders.

9.1 OVERVIEW OF EATING DISORDERS

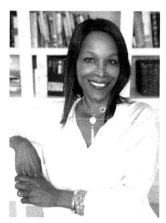

Figure 9.1 Stephanie Covington Armstrong.

Source: Photo by Stephanie Covington Armstrong. Reproduced with permission.

Eating disorder: a psychological condition characterized by severe disturbances in eating behavior.

Many of our day-to-day conversations revolve around food. Eating, cooking, dining, nutrition, fitness, and health are national pastimes. We live in a society preoccupied with food, its preparation, and our enjoyment of it, and we even celebrate chefs, food trucks, and restaurants. What's more, people post photos of food, recipes, and videos of their food experiences using social media. Food is more than a means to live and take in nutrition; it's a cultural and social event.

Let's take a moment now to compare this pastime with our relatively recent ideal of beauty. In the United States, for instance, many people seem to equate beauty and success with thinness (Wagner et al. 2020). While it's true that being overweight can have a number of negative health consequences, many people focus on fitness not because it makes them physically healthy but rather as an aesthetic choice, because they believe being fit means being thin. Thinness is associated with success and positive self-worth, whereas being overweight is viewed by many as signaling personal failure, as well as a lack of self-control and intellect (Puhl & Heuer 2009). This stigma is perpetuated by media images and messages, especially those directed toward women (Nippert et al. 2021).

An **eating disorder** is a psychological condition characterized by severe disturbances in eating behavior which may include limiting the amount of food eaten, eating very large quantities of food, or disruptive attempts to compensate for eating. In this chapter, we focus on *anorexia nervosa*, in which an individual feels they are overweight despite objective evidence to the contrary, *bulimia nervosa*, a disorder characterized by binge eating (eating large amounts of food but maintaining relatively normal weight by engaging in behaviors to compensate for potential weight gain), and *binge-eating disorder*, marked by repeated overeating without the compensatory strategies found in bulimia (see Table 9.2 in the Pulling It Together feature at the end of this chapter).

Eating disorders affect people from all demographics and are caused by multiple factors. They arise from a combination of longstanding behavioral, biological, emotional, psychological, interpersonal, and social factors. While some people may have everyday patterns of eating and compensating for overeating that aren't a problem for them, like many psychological disorders, eating disorders cause some people distress and impairment around activities others engage with to a healthy extent.

Given the current preoccupation with thinness, we might assume that eating disorders are relatively recent phenomena. However, historical evidence shows eating disorders can be traced back to Hellenistic (321 BCE) and medieval times (fifth to fifteenth centuries CE), when deprivation of food was considered a spiritual practice – also referred to as "holy anorexia" – that mostly afflicted women.

Currently, eating disorders affect nearly 16 million people all over the world (Figure 9.2). It's possible that this estimate is low, since the figures are based only on diagnosed anorexia nervosa and bulimia nervosa, and up to 60 percent of

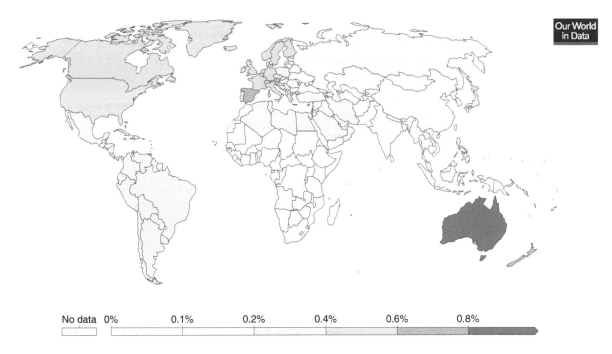

people with symptoms of eating disorders may not fit the standardized criteria (Brooks et al. 2012). This means that even if people do not meet the full criteria to be officially diagnosed with anorexia nervosa or bulimia nervosa, they still may engage in disordered eating that threatens their health and wellbeing.

Eating disorders can affect every organ system in the body (cardiovascular, gastrointestinal, neurological, endocrine), and are serious, potentially life-threatening conditions. In fact, eating disorders have the highest mortality rates of all mental health difficulties. Mortality in anorexia cases is around 6 percent; about half the deaths are attributable to medical complications from the disorder and about a quarter to suicide (Blythin et al. 2020).

Currently **body mass index (BMI)** (Figure 9.3) is the most widely used method for indicating nutritional status in adults. It is defined as a person's weight in kilograms divided by the square of the person's height in meters (kg/m^2). For example, an adult who weighs 70 kg (154 pounds) and whose height is 1.75 m (5 feet 8 inches) will have a BMI of 22.9.

Developed more than 200 years ago, the BMI scale was actually created to describe the "ideal" human size as a means to examine large populations of humans, rather than to assess individual health. What's more, the original data to create the BMI table was collected in Belgium primarily from white European men and afterwards adopted by health and life insurance companies to replace their own height-weight tables. However, over time, it has become more and more tied to individual health measurement. The current BMI tables don't consider ethnicity, and can perpetuate weight bias and stigma.

Figure 9.2 Share of world population with an eating disorder, 2017.
Source: Roth (2018).

Body mass index (BMI): a ratio of height and weight that includes comparison to others.

Figure 9.3 The underweight range, according to the body mass index (BMI), is the yellow area on the chart.

BMI Chart

Weight (*lbs*)	105	115	125	135	145	155	165	175	185	195	205	215
(*kgs*)	47.7	52.3	56.8	61.4	65.9	70.5	75.0	79.5	84.1	88.6	93.2	97.7

Height (*ft'in" – cm*)

☐ Underweight   ☐ Overweight

☐ Healthy   ☐ Obese   ☐ Extremely obese

Height (*ft'in" – cm*)												
5'0" – 152.4	20	22	24	26	28	30	32	34	36	38	40	42
5'2" – 157.4	19	21	22	24	26	28	30	32	33	35	37	39
5'4" – 162.5	18	19	21	23	24	26	28	30	31	33	35	37
5'6" – 167.6	17	18	20	21	23	25	26	28	29	31	33	34
5'8" – 172.7	16	17	19	20	22	23	25	26	28	29	31	32
5'10" – 177.8	15	16	18	19	20	22	23	25	26	28	29	30
6'0" – 182.8	14	15	17	18	19	21	22	23	25	26	27	29
6'2" – 187.9	13	14	16	17	18	19	21	22	23	25	26	27
6'4" – 193.0	12	14	15	16	17	18	20	21	22	23	25	26

While BMI alone isn't enough to make a diagnosis of anorexia, it does serve as a way to gauge the severity of the disorder. For instance, a BMI below 12 can be life-threatening (Figure 9.3).

THE POWER OF WORDS

FAT SHAMING

"Stop saying you're fat, you're beautiful."
"Do you really want to eat that much?"
"Did you lose weight? You look so much better."

It happens more than you might think, in both actions and words. Comments from friends, family members, or people online can range from subtle to aggressive. Insults about weight, also called "fat shaming," can have major impacts on both physical and emotional health.

This shaming can come from health care providers as well. Three in five adults with obesity have experienced weight bias from health care providers (Vogel 2019). Whether they're told to lose weight when they come in for an unrelated medical concern or find that waiting room chairs are too small, subtle cues about their body can lead to anxiety and guilt and take a toll on self-esteem. It appears that fat shaming not only is emotionally harmful but can also create more problems with health and actually increase weight gain. Judgmental responses of disgust, anger, or blame from care providers can discourage people from seeking help (Vogel 2019). Both avoiding exercise and being exposed to weight bias can trigger stress, depression, increased cortisol, lower self-control, and lead to more binge eating (Vogel 2019).

It's important for friends, family, and care providers to be sensitive to unintended judgmental responses. If someone you know is trying to lose weight for health reasons, reach out to ask them how you can be supportive and what statements and behaviors are helpful.

Source: Vogel (2019).

CONCEPT CHECK 9.1

1. Eshan takes in more calories than he burns, mostly because he eats an unhealthy diet consisting of fast food and processed foods. Although he constantly overeats, he doesn't feel his eating is out of control. Does Eshan have an eating disorder? Why or why not?
2. True or false: Eating disorders are a new phenomenon.
3. True or false: Up to 60 percent of people with symptoms of eating disorders may not fit the standardized criteria.

9.2   BINGE-EATING DISORDER

Many people overindulge and have extra helpings during mealtimes when they are already full, or they may "stuff themselves" when eating their favorite foods or celebrating special events such as holidays and birthdays. This is typical overeating. Typical overeating is different from **binge-eating disorder (BED)**, in which a person experiences episodes of uncontrolled eating with distress, but *without* any compensating behaviors (such as purges) to counteract the binges (you'll read more about binging and purging in section 9.3).

Although binge-eating disorder was only recently added to *DSM-5*, researchers identified symptoms of this condition in many people who were overweight in the early 1990s. It's not unusual to find people who meet the criteria for binge-eating disorder in weight-control programs such as Nutrisystem, Weight Watchers, or Jenny Craig.

Binge-eating disorder (BED): an eating disorder in which a person experiences episodes of uncontrolled eating with distress, but without any compensating behaviors (such as purges) to counteract the binges.

Symptoms and Description

People with binge-eating disorder have repeated *binges* during which they consume large amounts of food and feel unable to stop themselves

Diagnostic Overview 9.1: Binge-Eating Disorder

Repeated binge eating along with at least three of the following symptoms related to eating:

- Eating rapidly.
- Eating until uncomfortably full.
- Eating large amounts of food even when not hungry.
- Eating alone because of embarrassment at the amount being eaten.
- Feeling disgusted, depressed, or guilty after eating.

The symptoms are not associated with any compensatory behavior.

Impact: Symptoms must exceed cultural and contextual norms. Symptoms are related to clinically significant distress or create impairment in important areas of life such as with friends and family or at work or school.

Timeframe: At least once a week for at least three months.

Source: Information from APA (2022).

(Diagnostic Overview 9.1). They may eat quickly and to the point of discomfort. Some might seem to be in a daze while eating. They experience a feeling of loss of control while they eat, followed by distress, disgust, guilt, or embarrassment, and they will binge-eat in isolation in order to hide their behavior, just as Stephanie did in the chapter-opening case story. People with binge-eating disorder will have binges at least twice a week for six months or more (see diagnostic criteria), and those with extreme binge-eating disorder will binge up to 14 times per week. The severity of the disorder is based on the number of binges per week (see Table 9.1). About half of those with binge-eating disorder are overweight or obese as a result of their frequent binges (Steinglass & Devlin 2017). However, most people who are overweight don't meet the psychological criteria for binge-eating disorder.

Some people with binge-eating disorder will have binges in response to depression or anxiety (Munsch et al. 2012), while others won't have regular meals but rather will eat throughout the day (Masheb et al. 2011). The consequences of frequent binges in this disorder can create social, emotional, and physical difficulties such as the following (see also Figure 9.9):

- Cardiovascular disease.
- Type 2 diabetes.
- Insomnia.
- Sleep apnea.
- Gastrointestinal difficulties.
- Depression.
- Anxiety.
- Obesity.

People with binge-eating disorder are often overly focused on food, their weight, and their appearance and will have perceptions of their body size that are disordered. They can also struggle with anxiety and depression. Nearly a third of those with binge-eating disorder will have binges that are triggered by negative moods. However, despite the fact that they often misperceive their body size and weight, thinking they are more overweight than they actually are (which leads them to be dissatisfied with both), they aren't as driven to reduce their weight as people with anorexia are.

Table 9.1 Severity of binge-eating disorder

Severity of disorder	Number of eating binges per week
Mild	1–3
Moderate	4–7
Severe	8–13
Extreme	14 or more

Source: Information from APA (2022).

Statistics and Trajectory

Binge-eating disorder is the most prevalent eating disorder in the United States and is more common than anorexia nervosa or bulimia nervosa. The World Mental Health Survey (2018) suggests that as many as 2.6 percent of the United States population will have symptoms of binge-eating disorder at some point in their life. Other estimates suggest similar prevalance (APA 2022). The most common age of onset for binge-eating disorder in the United States is 19.5 years (Solmi et al. 2021). However, this may be an underestimate, because it's easy for those who might meet the criteria to hide the symptoms from family, friends, and health care providers.

Rates for binge-eating disorder are lower in many other countries in the world (Figure 9.4). The lowest rates are in Eastern European countries (0.6 percent), and the highest in the region of the Americas (Colombia, Mexico, Brazil, Peru, and the United States), where the average lifetime prevalence is 2.7 percent. It's likely that sociocultural differences may influence, in part, some of the differences in eating disorder statistics.

Around the world, symptoms of binge-eating disorder tend to emerge later than for some other eating disorders; the median age worldwide is around 24 (Kessler et al. 2018). Women outnumber men; at least 64 percent of people with binge-eating disorder are women (Forman et al. 2016). There are some cultural variations of binge-eating disorder. For example, when compared with white

Figure 9.4 Lifetime prevalence of binge-eating disorder in the World Mental Health Surveys, selected countries (2002–2017). *Source: Data from Kessler et al. (2018).*

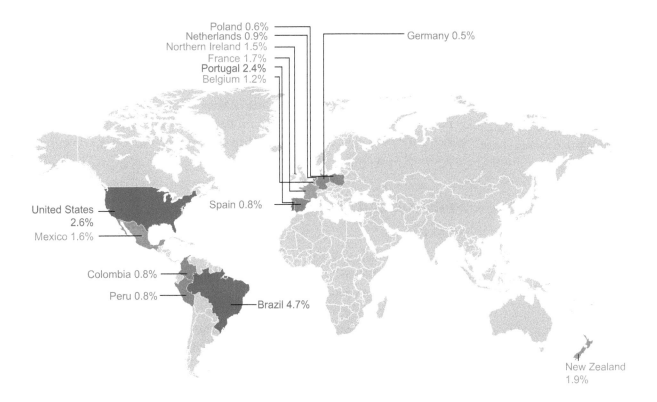

women, Black women have higher rates of binge-eating disorder. Studies suggest the prevalence of binge eating among Black women is around 5 percent, nearly twice the prevalence among non-Hispanic white women (2.5 percent) (Goode et al. 2020).

CONCEPT CHECK 9.2

1. True or false: Binge-eating disorder affects more women than men.
2. Andrea was recently diagnosed with binge-eating disorder. What are some of the common eating behaviors you might expect her to exhibit?
3. What are some of the common events that might trigger a binge-eating episode?
4. Dr. Lawrence is concerned that her patient who was recently diagnosed with binge-eating disorder will be at risk of related health conditions. What are some of the health risks Dr. Lawrence is likely to mention to her patient?
5. True or false: Because binge-eating disorder is new to the *DSM*, that means it is relatively rare.

9.3   BULIMIA NERVOSA

Bulimia nervosa: an eating disorder characterized by recurrent episodes of binge eating and by compensatory behaviors.

Compensatory behaviors: behaviors intended to prevent weight gain or feelings of guilt from eating.

Bulimia nervosa is a disorder characterized by recurrent episodes of binge eating *and* by **compensatory behaviors** intended to prevent weight gain or feelings of guilt from the binges (Diagnostic Overview 9.2). These compensatory behaviors, such as fasting and vomiting, distinguish bulimia nervosa from binge-eating disorder, which is not marked by such actions. People with bulimia nervosa experience their symptoms at normal or elevated weight. However, when the person's weight is significantly low, a diagnosis of *anorexia nervosa* (discussed in section 9.4) is given.

Symptoms and Description

BINGES

In cases of bulimia, individuals have episodes of uncontrollable overeating or binges, such as Stephanie described in the chapter-opening story. During the binge, people will eat considerably more than they typically would and often have a feeling that their eating is out of control (APA 2022). They report feeling like they can't stop eating or control how much or even what they eat. After the binge, they often feel guilt, disgust, shame, and depression (Anderson et al. 2021; Blythin et al. 2020). Binges can last about two hours (APA 2022) and occur at the rate of 1–30 per week (Fairburn et al. 2015). They often occur in secret. The average binge consists of consuming about 2,000–3,400 calories in a single episode, and consumption can go as high as 10,000 (Mourilhe et al. 2021). In contrast, the average moderately active person consumes between 2,000 and 2,500 calories a day.

Stress and negative emotions typically occur before binges. Work and school stressors as well as interpersonal pressures are the most commonly reported worries that precede a binge (Srivastava et al. 2021). During stressful times, the person might feel driven to eat foods they consider "off limits," such as sweets.

COMPENSATORY BEHAVIORS

People with bulimia nervosa engage in compensatory behaviors, acts designed to counteract the binges such as medicines, enemas, diuretics, vomiting, fasting, or extreme exercising. These behaviors are driven by the person's overly negative evaluation of their own appearance, body weight, or body shape.

One of the more common behaviors is to vomit, in the mistaken belief that this will prevent the digestion of the food. In fact, vomiting prevents only about 50 percent of the calories from being absorbed, and repeated vomiting can lead to increased hunger and more binges as well as other negative health effects. For instance, some people with bulimia nervosa will have scarring on their fingers called *Russell's sign* (Figure 9.5). Russell's sign is a callus on the back of the hand or the knuckles caused by contact with the teeth as people induce their own gag reflex. Russell's sign isn't the sole indicator of frequent self-induced vomiting; some people can make themselves vomit without using their hands. Laxatives and diuretics are similarly unhelpful in undoing the effects of binges (Dalle Grave et al. 2021).

Fasting is another technique that people with bulimia nervosa use to compensate for excess food intake. They may go eight or more daytime hours without food in order to reduce their weight.

While compensatory behaviors may not influence the person's weight, they can reduce the feeling of fullness in the stomach and the anxiety that people often have after a binge (Stewart & Williamson 2008). However, as well as interfering with social life and work commitments, these strategies can also begin a cycle that leads to more binges and more compensating purges (Figure 9.6) (Wade 2019).

Overeating and compensating for overeating make it difficult over time for individuals to know when they are hungry and when they are full. After a while these behaviors can affect the body's homeostasis and other biological systems that in turn influence the drive to eat, causing depressed moods, more hunger, and more frequent binge eating. This cycle is called the *bulimic trap* (see Figure 9.6) (Sekuła et al. 2019).

Diagnostic Overview 9.2: Bulimia Nervosa

- Recurrent episodes of binge eating characterized by the consumption of a large amount of food in a discrete period of time and lack of control during the eating.
- Inappropriate attempts to compensate for binge eating.
- Overvaluation of the importance of body shape and/or weight.

Impact:	Symptoms must exceed cultural and contextual norms. Symptoms are related to clinically significant distress or create impairment in important areas of life such as with friends and family or at work or school.
Timeframe:	Binges and compensatory behaviors occur at least once a week for at least three months.

Source: Information from APA (2022).

Figure 9.5 Russell's sign is a callus caused by repeatedly using the fingers to induce vomiting.
Source: Reproduced from https://commons.wikimedia. org/wiki/File:Russell%27s_ Sign.png. In public domain.

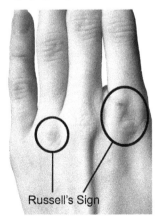

Russell's Sign

Figure 9.6 The cycle
of bulimia.
*Source: Reproduced from
Wade (2019).*

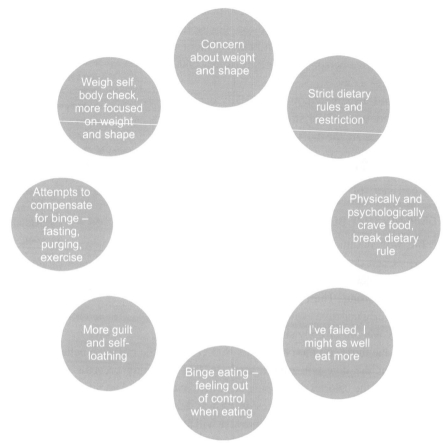

People diagnosed with bulimia nervosa often have difficulty with emotional regulation. They may have problems finding appropriate ways to manage the length and intensity of negative emotions and struggle to inhibit impulsive behavior when they are feeling distressed. They may also be reluctant to accept negative emotional states or to experience emotional distress even if the emotion is important to achieving a goal (such as people who use stress to motivate themselves to complete work) (Wade 2019). Because of this difficulty, those diagnosed with bulimia nervosa have higher levels of impulsivity than people without bulimia or people with anorexia nervosa.

Statistics and Trajectory

Surveys suggest that as many as 1 percent of the United States population will have symptoms of bulimia nervosa at some point in their life (APA 2022; Kessler et al. 2018). Rates are lower in many other countries (Figure 9.7) and may be related to cultural differences in messages about food, body, and self and increased social pressure to meet cultural standards of beauty. Between 75 and 90 percent of

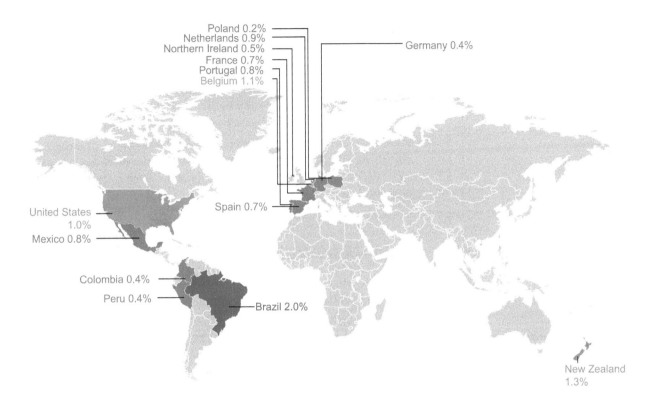

Figure 9.7 Lifetime prevalence of bulimia nervosa in the World Mental Health Surveys, selected countries (2002–2017). *Source: Data from Kessler et al. (2018).*

bulimia cases occur in women (Forman 2016). Symptoms of bulimia nervosa arise in late adolescence and early adulthood, with 19 as the mean age of onset (Wade 2019). Worldwide studies suggest that many people diagnosed with bulimia nervosa have had a previous diagnosis of anorexia nervosa (24–31 percent) (Wade 2019). While a person will only have one disorder at a time, diagnoses can change over time. Movement between diagnoses is referred to as "crossover." About a third of people with anorexia will cross over and have a later diagnosis of bulimia as their weight changes.

Bulimia nervosa often occurs with other psychological disorders. In the United States, the majority of people with this disorder (71 percent) will be diagnosed with another psychological condition, such as an anxiety disorder (50 percent), a mood disorder (40 percent), or a substance abuse condition (10 percent) (Wade 2019).

Although some teenagers experiment with eating binges and occasional purge behaviors such as laxatives, exercise, or vomiting, not all will qualify for a diagnosis of bulimia nervosa. In fact, up to 50 percent of students worldwide report periods of binge and purge behavior (Kato et al. 2011). While only 0.5 percent to 5 percent of women in the United States will meet the criteria for bulimia, the prevalence rate is very high among college students (Jacobson 2018). Fewer than one in three people with the disorder are diagnosed by a professional, however, because of the shame experienced by many who have symptoms (Wade 2019).

CONCEPT CHECK 9.3

Indicate whether the following statements are true or false.
1. Robert has used vomiting and diuretics in an attempt to limit his calorie consumption. This will lead to weight loss.
2. Russell's sign is a necessary diagnostic indicator of bulimia nervosa.
3. Compensatory behaviors are indicators for bulimia nervosa.
4. Wells has recently been diagnosed with bulimia nervosa. If his diagnosis is correct, we can expect his weight to be at or above what is typical for his age, gender, and height.

9.4   ANOREXIA NERVOSA

Anorexia nervosa: an eating disorder characterized by a distortion of body image and an intense fear of weight gain.

While people with binge-eating disorder and bulimia nervosa have disordered eating patterns and will be of average weight or over, those who have eating disorders that push their weight *below* normal weight might meet the criteria for anorexia nervosa. **Anorexia nervosa** is a psychological condition characterized by a distorted body image and an intense fear of weight gain (Diagnostic Overview 9.3). This focus motivates the person to restrict food intake or find other ways to lose weight, including engaging in excessive physical activity or purging. The medical complications that often result can affect all organs in the body due to malnutrition and the unhealthy effects of purging.

Diagnostic Overview 9.3: Anorexia Nervosa

- Restriction of food intake, which leads to a body weight less than minimally normal.
- Behavior that interferes with weight gain, or an intense fear of gaining weight or becoming fat.
- Disruption in the experience of body shape or weight along with an inability to realize the impact of low body weight.

Specify whether:

- Restricting type: weight loss through exercise, fasting, or dieting.
- Binge-eating/purging type: recurrent episodes of binge eating or compensatory behavior.

Severity is based on BMI

- Mild: BMI ≥ 17 kg/m^2
- Moderate: BMI 16–16.99 kg/m^2
- Severe: BMI 15–15.99 kg/m^2
- Extreme: BMI < 15 kg/m^2

Impact: Symptoms must exceed cultural and contextual norms. Symptoms are related to clinically significant distress or create impairment in important areas of life such as with friends and family or at work or school.

Timeframe: Three months.

Source: Information from APA (2022).

The name "anorexia nervosa" means a neurotic loss of appetite. The disorder was first reported by William Gull in the late 1800s (Silverman 1997). People with anorexia nervosa not only fear becoming overweight and try their hardest to achieve low body weight; they also have a distorted view of their weight and body, which influences the way they feel about themselves.

Symptoms and Description

Diagnostic features of anorexia nervosa include restriction of food, intense fear of gaining weight or becoming fat, behaviors that interfere with weight gain, and disruptions in self-perceived weight or shape. Although the *DSM-5tr* suggests that the individual's weight must be significantly below normal, there is no particular cut-off for low weight in anorexia nervosa.

About 50 percent of people with anorexia attempt to control their weight by limiting what they eat, a specifier of the **restricting type** of the disorder, while others adopt compensatory behaviors such as taking laxatives or vomiting after meals, in the **binge-eating/purging type**. (The key difference between bulimia nervosa and anorexia nervosa of the binge-eating/purging type is the person's current weight.) Becoming thin is a key goal, which leads to a preoccupation with food. Some people with anorexia nervosa are constantly thinking and reading about food and spend a lot of time planning meals (Klein & Attia 2017).

Anorexia nervosa, restricting type: a type of anorexia nervosa characterized by limiting food intake in order to control weight.

Anorexia nervosa, binge-eating/purging type: a type of anorexia nervosa characterized by compensatory behaviors to limit weight gain.

Those with anorexia nervosa see themselves as unattractive and will overestimate the size of their body (Klein & Attia 2017). When given a photograph of themselves and asked to adjust the image to their actual body size, more than half overestimated their body size, making the image larger than it should be. These distortions also spill over into attitudes and perceptions. People with the disorder feel driven to be perfect, believe food deprivation will make them a better person, and try to avoid feeling guilty by simply not eating. All these symptoms are associated with signs of psychological distress, including depression, anxiety, decreased self-esteem, and problems with sleep (Klein & Attia 2017). Some people with anorexia nervosa abuse substances, and this correlation might be related to their need for emotional regulation. There is evidence to suggest people with anorexia may use substances to help manage intense and negative emotions they are experiencing (Claudat et al. 2020).

As you can imagine, medical problems can arise from anorexia (Wassenaar et al. 2019) (see Figure 9.9). Some people may develop *amenorrhea* or the cessation of menstrual cycles, lower body temperature, low blood pressure, low bone density, and slower heart rate. Electrolyte imbalances can also cause cardiac problems. Poor eating can lead to nutritional problems that in turn can lead to skin problems, cracked nails, and hair loss.

Statistics and Trajectory

A meta-analysis of 33 studies from around the world found that lifetime prevalence for anorexia disorders is about 1.5 percent for women and 0.2 percent for men. The higher rate for women is most likely due to differences in the cultural messages about weight that are directed toward women (Galmiche et al. 2019). Some researchers suggest this may be due to increased pressure on women to meet current standards of beauty (Mayo & George 2014). Gender can influence an individual's risk of developing an eating disorder. In the United States men account for only 10 percent of the cases of anorexia and bulimia. Others point to the different ways that men and women try to lose weight. Men tend to focus on exercise rather than diet (Thackray et al. 2016), and dieting appears to be a gateway to many eating disorders. That is, many eating disorders start out as "just a diet," but simply going on a diet doesn't mean you are destined to develop an eating disorder.

For many men, eating disorders develop as a result of pressure from work or sports (Freedman et al. 2021). About 37 percent of men in one study of eating disorders played sports or had jobs where their weight was an important aspect. The highest rates of eating disorders in men were found among jockeys, wrestlers, distance runners, body builders, and swimmers (Lavender et al. 2017). But body image was also important among men who wanted a lean, toned shape. For some men with eating disorders, body image often focuses on muscularity (Treasure et al. 2020).

Case Study: Disordered Eating – Tom Daley

Tom (Figure 9.8) won his first diving competition when he was only 10 years old. Fast-forward to 2021 when he was 27 and his Olympic medal count was four (three bronze and one gold). However, heading up to the 2021 Olympics, Tom had something else on his mind. As a diver he knew his body would be clearly on display and he began to feel anxious and exposed. What's more, his coach at the time made comments about his weight.

Tom started to weigh himself daily, cut out carbohydrates, not eat for days, and make himself throw up after eating certain foods like cake. The resulting weight loss and disordered eating left him exhausted.

We'll come back to Tom's story later in this chapter. To read more about Tom Daley take a look at his memoir, *Coming up for air: What I learned from sport, fame and fatherhood* (2021).

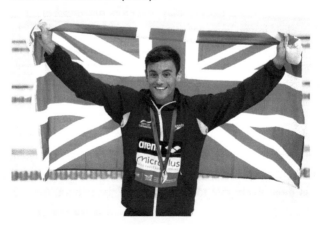

Figure 9.8 Tom Daley.
Source: Clive Rose/ Getty Images.

Higher rates of anorexia nervosa have been reported in Europe and North America, and lower rates in Africa and South America (Wonderlich et al. 2020). Between 75 percent and 90 percent of cases are in women (NIMH 2019), and the age of onset peaks between 14 and 20 years (Solmi et al. 2021). Between 0.06 percent and 4.0 percent of all women in Europe and North America will have symptoms at some point in their lives.

Although there are effective treatments for anorexia, up to 6 percent of people with the disorder become seriously ill and do not recover. They may die from medical complications of malnutrition or by suicide (Fichter et al. 2021; Wassenaar et al. 2019). In the United States the suicide rate among people with anorexia is five times higher than in the general population (Klein & Attia 2017).

Figure 9.9 depicts the physical effects of anorexia nervosa, bulimia nervosa, and binge-eating disorder.

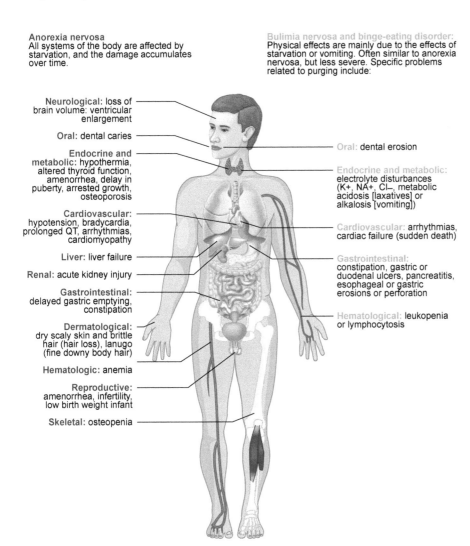

Figure 9.9 Physical effects of anorexia nervosa, bulimia nervosa, and binge-eating disorder. (Left) Anorexia nervosa: all systems of the body are affected by starvation, and the damage accumulates over time. (Right) Bulimia nervosa and binge-eating disorder: physical effects are mainly due to the effects of starvation or vomiting.

Source: Information from Treasure et al. (2020).

CONCEPT CHECK 9.4

Decide whether each case is likely to be anorexia nervosa restricting type or anorexia nervosa binge-eating/purging type.

1. A 22-year-old woman who is significantly underweight appears in her primary care provider's office. Despite her appearance, she reports that she sees herself as very overweight. To cope with this perception, she restricts her food intake to 500 calories a day and exercises three times a day to compensate for the small amount of food she eats.

2. A 28-year-old man who has been struggling in college comes in for evaluation. He is calm, underweight, and dressed in baggy clothes. He reports he exercises five hours a day and tries not to eat "too much" in order to control his weight. He occasionally has periods in which his eating gets out of control and says he would like to lose a little more weight.

3. A 33-year-old woman stopped eating full meals over three months ago. When she eats, she does so in small quantities and only under pressure from others. She is about 20 percent below normal body weight for her height.

9.5 MODELS AND TREATMENTS OF EATING DISORDERS

Despite their struggles with food, both Stephanie and Tom eventually sought help, and Tom says he's "no longer scared of food" (Daley 2021). Tom wanted to speak out about his struggles with eating disorders because not many men do. "I guess there is that stigma around eating disorders that problems with eating only affect women, and it's just not the case," he said. "I have felt the pressure not to talk about things because I didn't want to bother people with it. Or people might not understand. Or they would be like 'oh, don't be silly, you're fine'" (Hosie 2021).

The goals of treatment for eating disorders include correcting dangerous eating patterns and working on psychological influences that may have led to those patterns. However, at the heart of eating disorders is body dissatisfaction. According to Cruz-Sáez and colleagues (Cruz-Sáez et al. 2020), this dissatisfaction is the most consistent factor in the development of eating disorders. In a study of more than 800 adolescents, body dissatisfaction led to lowered self-esteem, negative mood, and disordered eating (Cruz-Sáez et al. 2020). Treatment of eating disorders also addresses nutritional and physical aspects of the person's situation. People with more severe symptoms, or who are not improving in outpatient settings, may be treated at day patient or full hospital inpatient programs.

In one study, a little more than one third of people with binge-eating disorder (37.3 percent) and about 44 percent with bulimia nervosa reported seeking treatment in the last 12 months (Kessler et al. 2018). Treatment can improve the symptoms of eating disorders; without it, these disorders can be persistent and intermittent. For example, for those with bulimia nervosa, with treatment 45 percent of patients in community samples will remain symptom-free for 14 years after their first symptoms (Wade 2019). Forty percent of clients greatly improve by reducing binges and purges and eating more healthily. Another 40 percent improve only moderately, with some binging and purging remaining. Of those treated for bulimia, 75 percent continued their recovery (Engel et al. 2017). However, relapse can occur, especially if there are significant stressors (Liu 2007). Only 23 percent had a chronic course (Voss & Brust 2020); the longer the history of bulimia, the more likely the chance of early relapse. Other factors for early relapse included frequency of binges, the presence of substance abuse, and the degree of trust between clients and their therapists. That is, people who binge more frequently, who abuse substance, or who have limited trust in their therapists are more likely to experience early relapse (Engel et al. 2017; Vall & Wade 2015).

Biological Models and Treatments of Eating Disorders

Eating disorders are complex heritable conditions influenced by both genetic and environmental factors. Today, recent studies suggest that genetic inheritance is a primary driver in eating disorders such as binge-eating disorder, bulimia nervosa, and anorexia nervosa.

Data from over 100 researchers worldwide discovered genetic variations associated with anorexia nervosa. These genetic variations overlap with other psychological conditions such as obsessive-compulsive disorder, depression, anxiety, and schizophrenia (Watson et al. 2019).

Another important aspect to consider is that, like many psychological conditions, eating disorders tend to run in families (see Figure 9.10). Having a sibling or parent with eating disorders increases up to five times the chances that a person will develop an eating disorder in turn. Similarly, twin studies suggest a heritability of 56 percent for anorexia and 41 percent for binge-eating disorder (Bulik et al. 2019), suggesting that these disorders are significantly influenced by additive genetic factors. While the evidence of heritability appears clear, it is harder to identify exactly what is inherited.

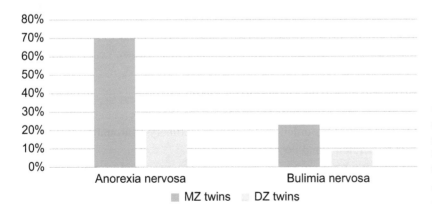

Figure 9.10 Concordance rate of anorexia nervosa and bulimia in monozygotic (MZ) (identical) and dizygotic (DZ) (fraternal) twins.

Source: Data from Bulik et al. (2019).

BRAIN IMAGING AND BRAIN CIRCUITS

Biological models of eating disorders focus on biological processes that influence when and how much we eat (Stice & Shaw 2017). Brain circuits may not only be involved in disruptive eating but also in differences in body perception. Brain imaging has also shown consistently altered activity in the insula – a small region of the cerebral cortex involved in pain, love, emotion, craving, and addiction – and in the prefrontal cortex. While the insula is highly active in many people with eating disorders, the prefrontal cortex appears to be smaller and less active, for instance in response to pictures of food (Uher & Treasure 2003), suggesting the differences in the limbic and cognitive neural circuits in people with eating disorders.

Clinically, people with eating disorders tend to be anxious, and therefore anxiety has been suggested as a key vulnerability factor for the development of eating disorders (Kaye et al. 2004). However, further research is required in order to ascertain the association between eating disorders and areas of the brain such as the insula and the prefrontal cortex (and their interaction with neurotransmitters such as serotonin, dopamine, and glutamate). It's plausible that eating disorders simply co-occur with anxiety and depression but are not related.

THE HYPOTHALAMUS

How do we know when we have had enough to eat? This is the job of the hypothalamus, a small area at the center of the brain that plays a part in many essential body functions such as body temperature, appetite and weight control, and sleep cycles. The hypothalamus processes information about food consumption and lets us know when we've had enough to eat by using neurotransmitters such as serotonin, norepinephrine, and dopamine, and hormones such as cortisol to transmit messages about appetite, hunger, satiation, and limitation of eating. Thus, eating disorders may be influenced, at least in part, by dysregulation of these neurotransmitters, or by disruptions in the hypothalamus that influence the way people notice when they are hungry or that reduce their ability to detect when they are full. The hypothalamus has two areas that regulate eating (Figure 9.11). The lateral hypothalamus (LH) makes us feel hungry, while the ventromedial hypothalamus (VMH) reduces those feelings of hunger. Stimulating the VMH in laboratory animals can lead them to stop eating. Similarly, medications aimed at treating eating disorders tend to target these neurotransmitters.

HORMONES AND NEUROTRANSMITTERS

Hormones and neurotransmitters may also influence eating behavior. When it comes to eating disorders, there are two primary neurotransmitters we need to look at: serotonin and dopamine.

Serotonin helps control everything from memory and learning, to sleep, mood, and appetite. Researchers found that people with anorexia nervosa have significantly lower levels of serotonin than individuals without an eating disorder (Kaye et al. 2018). The same is true for those with bulimia, with the difference that – when

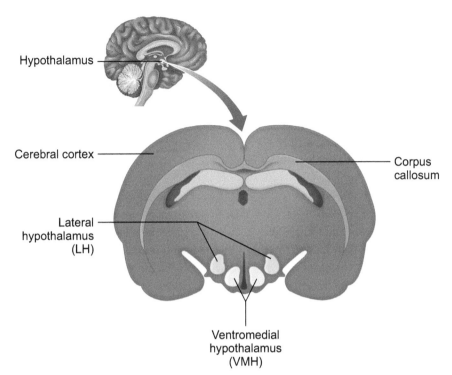

Hypothalamus

Cerebral cortex

Corpus callosum

Lateral hypothalamus (LH)

Ventromedial hypothalamus (VMH)

Figure 9.11 The hypothalamus contains the lateral hypothalamus (LH) and the ventromedial hypothalamus (VMH), which are responsible for triggering our feelings of hunger (LH) and fullness (VMH).

going without food for longer periods of time – their serotonin level drops more acutely than in people without eating disorders. Finally, in individuals with binge-eating disorder, the level of serotonin appears fairly similar to that found in bulimia, although researchers think individuals with binge-eating disorder also have chronically low serotonin levels, which is probably why they binge: to relieve the depressed mood caused (in part) by their low serotonin (Haedt-Matt & Keel 2011).

Dopamine is a neurotransmitter involved in pleasure, memory, and sensory processing (Beaulieu & Gainetdinov 2011). Anorexia nervosa has been associated with high levels of dopamine that can lead to anxiety as well as the ability to abstain from pleasurable activities such as eating (Kontis & Theochari 2012). Bulimia nervosa and binge-eating disorder are also associated with differences in dopamine levels in the brain (Broft et al. 2012). For example, over-responsiveness to dopamine may lead to food feeling more rewarding (Davis et al. 2012) and lead to compulsive overeating (Bello & Hajnal 2010).

TREATMENTS

Appropriate weight and normal eating can be restored through various channels, depending on the physical and mental status of the individual at the time of the treatment.

Like physical rehabilitation following a severe physical injury, nutritional rehabilitation is required as part of eating disorder recovery, and its main initial goal is weight restoration (Peebles ct al. 2017). *Nutritional rehabilitation* is a delicate and complex process that can happen at home, in residential care, or at the hospital if the

Nasogastric feeding tube: a temporary flexible tube that passes through the nose to deliver liquid food to the stomach.

person's health is at risk. In the first case, the individual would participate in normalized mealtimes, slowly increasing solid food intake over the course of several weeks (Zerbe 2010), as well as attending motivational interviews to make changes in their behavior (Macdonald et al. 2012). In the second case, the health provider could use a **nasogastric feeding tube**, a temporary flexible tube that passes through the nose to deliver liquid food to the stomach. This allows the patient to be steadily fed without having to eat huge portions of food, which is initially challenging. Lasting change can be supported by having clients monitor their thoughts and feelings as well as their levels of hunger and food intake during treatment.

Health care professionals can also prescribe antidepressants, not as the sole therapy for eating disorders but in parallel to psychotherapy. These can be helpful to treat bulimia, perhaps even more than for anorexia nervosa (Crow 2017). They can benefit nearly half (40 percent) of those who take them by reducing the urge to binge by more than half (67 percent) and reducing purges such as vomiting by more than half as well (56 percent) (Crow 2017). Medications such as fluoxetine (Prozac), and more recently, stimulant medications such as lisdexamfetamine (Vyvanse) (Hilbert 2020) have been used to treat binge-eating disorder. For anorexia nervosa, olazepaine (Zyprexa), a medication that increases the availability of dopamine and is sometimes classified as a second-generation antipsychotic (Hay 2020), has been shown to be helpful for weight gain. From a treatment perspective, we know that psychotherapy alone is more effective than medications alone. Antidepressants won't have a direct impact on the client's eating disorder but rather will help address it by treating a co-occurring condition such as depression or anxiety (Hay 2020). However, at times, combining medications with effective therapy can produce even better results (Agras et al. 2017).

Biological treatments may also be helpful in addressing low weight and other impacts on the body, such as endocrine levels and sex hormone levels. However, some biological conditions related to eating disorders may be longer-lasting. Bone loss, for instance, may not be reversible, especially when it occurs soon after puberty begins. Thus, some people with eating disorders may never reach typical peak bone mass and may be more prone to bone fractures.

One meta-analysis found that the trajectory of recovery from binge-eating disorder is not always linear. Even though participants experienced significant improvement early in treatment, that progress was not necessarily maintained 6–12 months after treatment ended (Hilbert et al. 2020). These long-term results may be due not to relapse, but rather to the lack of long-term follow-up studies on medications for binge-eating disorder (Hilbert et al. 2020).

Cognitive-Behavioral Models and Treatments of Eating Disorders

CBT for eating disorders is a primary treatment for all eating disorders, with the greatest impact on symptom reduction and other outcomes (Wade 2019). It is a psychotherapeutic approach that involves a variety of techniques. These approaches help an individual to understand the interaction between their thoughts, feelings, and behaviors, and to develop strategies to change unhelpful thoughts and behaviors in order to improve mood and functioning.

CBT for eating disorders (CBT-ED) is typically delivered in 20 weekly sessions for bulimia nervosa and binge-eating disorder, and in 40 sessions for anorexia nervosa. The therapy in all cases consists of many of the same tools but is focused on the thoughts of those with eating disorders (Atwood & Friedman 2020). CBT emphasizes collaboration between therapist and client and requires active participation by the client in order to find appropriate attitudes about weight, eating, and food (Pike et al. 2017). The goal is to move the client away from cognitions around perfection and self-value and to provide education about the distortions that some clients may have around their body size and shape. For example, clients are encouraged to keep diaries of their eating sensations and of their thoughts related to hunger (Wilson 2018). These diaries can help them recognize their cognitive and behavioral patterns related to eating and uncover what might trigger binges. There are now apps to assist in tracking their thinking and eating during the day. Family therapy is often used in addition to other types of therapy (Wilson 2018).

Sociocultural Models and Treatments of Eating Disorders

Standards of beauty in the United States have changed over time, shifting over the last 30 years to greatly value a thin frame (especially for women) (Maymone et al. 2017). Exposure to a thin beauty ideal can lead to body dissatisfaction, negative moods, and dieting behaviors (Vander Wal et al. 2008). It's no surprise that eating disorders are more common in some cultures than others (Keski-Rahkonen 2021).

Your role can have an impact on your likelihood of developing an eating disorder as well. Performers and athletes, for example, are more likely to have anorexia and bulimia. Nine percent of female college athletes have eating disorders, and a third have eating behaviors that would put them at risk for these problems (Kato et al. 2011). Some evidence suggests that social media usage is also correlated with eating disorders, negative body image, dysfunctional eating, and a desire to diet. The COVID-19 pandemic has been especially difficult for those with eating disorders due to fewer treatment options, difficulties with food availability, and limited availability of healthy coping mechanisms. In addition, added stress, changes in routine, and social media messages about weight gain may have contributed to more symptoms of eating disorders during the pandemic (Cooper et al. 2022).

HOW FAMILY INFLUENCES EATING DISORDERS AND THEIR TREATMENT

Family environment can affect eating disorders too (Cerniglia et al. 2017). More than half of those with bulimia or anorexia have families that focused on thinness, appearance, or diets, or parents who dieted and expressed perfectionistic views (Zerbe 2010).

Family-based interventions that focus on drivers of eating are a useful treatment for eating disorders (Treasure et al. 2020), especially for children (Pike et al. 2017). In family therapy, members meet together to identify family patterns that may contribute to the eating disorder. This can help clients separate their own concerns about food and eating from those of family members. Theories about the role of families in the development of anorexia are still being studied. However, the evidence is clear that family support in treatment can be very beneficial (Peckmezian & Paxton 2020).

HOW SOCIETY INFLUENCES EATING DISORDERS AND THEIR TREATMENT

Culture is another factor playing a crucial role in an individual's risk of eating disorders, in part because cultures develop different ideas of beauty. In one recent study (Rosen et al. 2017), 70 percent of Black Americans who responded were dissatisfied with their weight and body shape, as were 90 percent of non-Hispanic white teens. Black American teens were less likely than non-Hispanic white respondents to diet for long periods of time. However, rates of eating disorders have been rising for Black Americans and other marginalized populations (Rosen et al. 2017). About 65 percent of Black Americans who responded to a recent survey said they've been on a diet, nearly 40 percent said food controlled their lives, and 17 percent used laxatives and 4 percent vomited to lose weight, among other unhealthy weight control behaviors and attitudes (Rosen et al. 2017).

Eating is an important social activity, and social support can prove a crucial input for recovery. Group therapy can help as many as 75 percent of those with bulimia (Crowe & Mitchell 2019).

THE POWER OF EVIDENCE

Social media and eating disorders

We usually think of social media as something fun and positive, a great way to keep up with our family, friends, and even celebrities who interest us. However, an emerging literature has been investigating the influence of social media on body image and eating disorders (Figure 9.12). Since it's common to share an idealized

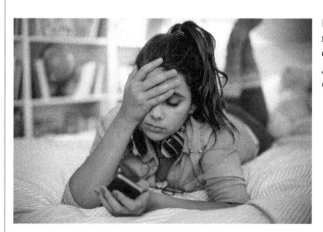

Figure 9.12 Can social media impact eating disorders?
Source: svetikd/E+/ Getty Images.

version of ourselves on social media, it can be hard for others to tell "real" from "edited." Not surprisingly, then, unrealistic standards of appearance and lifestyle can not only affect the way people view and feel about their bodies, but they can also worsen their self-esteem. And for individuals who are particularly vulnerable to the social pressures of thinness and physical appearance, social media messages can aggravate existing eating disorders or trigger the start of a new eating disorder.

In one study, researchers found that those who posted edited social media photos reported a higher number of risk factors for eating disorders. Researchers found that when these participants posted edited photos to social media they experienced increased body weight and shape concerns and increased urges to exercise and restrict their food intake (Wick & Keel 2020).

Another study (Wilksch et al. 2020) recruited nearly 1,000 participants (536 men and 462 women) with an average age of 13 to take a few surveys. The survey questions included measures of the participants' thoughts that might be indicative of eating disorders (such as whether thinking about food, eating, calories, or their shape or weight has made it difficult to concentrate on things they are interested in, or to work or follow a conversation). Also probed were behaviors associated with eating disorders (such as skipping meals or making themselves vomit after meals) and social media use (including the amount of time they spent on social media, the number of social media accounts they maintained, and whether their parents monitored their social media use).

The researchers discovered that the more social media accounts they had, the more disordered eating behaviors and cognitions they reported. This doesn't mean that spending time on social media increases these behaviors or cognitions, but it does suggest that it might be useful for parents, teachers, and therapists to be aware of the impact that social media might have on those who could be vulnerable to eating disorders.

Sources: Wick & Keel (2020); Wilksch et al. (2020).

Multiperspective Models and Treatments of Eating Disorders

The multiperspective approach takes into account the genetic, neurobiological, biochemical, cognitive, and emotional background factors that influence the development of all eating disorders. Therapists must address the client's nutritional, physical, and mental health, and many evidence-based treatments call for a multidisciplinary team consisting of a psychological therapist and a primary care physician. When treatment requires hospitalization, the team may also include a registered dietician, psychiatrist, nurses, and exercise therapists, occupational therapists, family therapists, and social workers (Hay 2020).

Inpatient treatment is multiperspective in its approach and can include **meal support**, a service that helps patients change the way they think about meals and

Meal support: a service that helps patients change the way they think about meals and eating.

eating. With this support patients are encouraged to confront their worries and challenges during meals, in order to gain both the skills and the confidence to successfully follow their meal plans while they are in the hospital and afterwards. Inpatient services sometimes include nasogastric feeding and can also consist of psychological, educational, and pharmacological intervention.

CONCEPT CHECK 9.5

1. The part of the brain associated with feelings of fullness is the _____.
2. True or false: Kurt is taking a medication to help his eating disorder. It's unlikely that he will be prescribed medications that will target mood and anxiety.
3. True or false: Sandra is working with a therapist who uses the psycho-dynamic approach to treating her eating disorder. The therapist will focus on family patterns that may be associated with disordered eating.

PULLING IT TOGETHER

Types of Eating Disorders

Table 9.2 Key diagnostic features of the main eating disorders

	Anorexia nervosa	Bulimia nervosa	Binge-eating disorder
Eating	Severe restriction	Irregular, skipping meals common	Irregular but no extreme restriction
Weight	Underweight	Normal or above normal	Normal or above normal
Body image	Overvaluation with or without "fears of being overweight"	Overvaluation	Overvaluation but not mandatory
Purging, fasting, driven exercise weight control behaviors	One or more is present	Regular as compensatory behaviors	Not regular

Source: Hay (2020).

9.6 CHAPTER REVIEW

SUMMARY

This chapter presented the following disorders:

- Binge-eating disorder
- Bulimia nervosa
- Anorexia nervosa

Overview of Eating Disorders

- An eating disorder is a psychological condition characterized by severe disturbances in eating behavior associated with distress and impairment.
- Eating disorders (as well as obesity) can affect multiple parts of the body and can be disabling and deadly.

Binge-Eating Disorder

- Binge-eating disorder (BED) is an eating disorder in which a person experiences episodes of uncontrolled eating with distress but without any compensating behaviors (such as purges) to counteract the binges.

Bulimia Nervosa

- Bulimia nervosa is a disorder characterized by uncontrolled eating (binges) of large amounts of food and unhealthy behaviors to compensate for the binges, such as enemas, diuretics, vomiting, fasting, or exercising.
- People diagnosed with bulimia nervosa often have difficulty with emotional regulation.

Anorexia Nervosa

- Anorexia nervosa is a disorder characterized by an intense fear of weight gain or a distorted body image.
- In the restricting type of anorexia nervosa, individuals try to control their weight by limiting their intake of calories.

- In the binge eating/purging type of anorexia, individuals try to control their weight by using compensatory behaviors.

Models and Treatments of Eating Disorders

- The goals of treatment for eating disorders include correcting dangerous eating patterns and the psychological factors that may have led to those patterns.
- Biological models of eating disorders focus on biological processes that influence when and how much we eat.
- According to the psychoanalytic perspective, unbalanced parental interactions can lead to ego deficiencies that may create a poor sense of control and independence in children.
- According to the cognitive theory of eating disorders, those with these conditions pay too much attention to body weight and their ability to control it.
- Sociocultural perspectives on eating disorders focus on environmental influences including family dynamics and communication.
- Multiperspective approaches combine nutritional, physical, and mental health solutions to eating disorders.

DISCUSSION QUESTIONS

1. What factors might contribute to the fact that eating disorders are more common in women than in men?
2. Social media can sometimes be a harsh environment. It's easy to criticize others for slight imperfections and we know this can have an impact on a person. What are some ways to help protect those online who have vulnerabilities to eating disorders?

3. Some people may have eating disorders and not realize it. What are some ways to help those who might meet the criteria for eating disorders to recognize the problem and reach out for help?

4. How do cultural and gender-related ideas about body shape affect the risk of developing eating disorders?

ANSWERS TO CONCEPT CHECKS

Concept Check 9.1

1. Eshan doesn't appear to have an eating disorder since his eating is not out of control.
2. False
3. True

Concept Check 9.2

1. True
2. Eating quickly; eat to the point of discomfort; upset or embarrassed by their eating

3. Stress; anxiety; depressed mood
4. High blood pressure; high cholesterol
5. False

Concept Check 9.3

1. False
2. False
3. True
4. True

Concept Check 9.4

1. Anorexia nervosa; restricting type
2. Anorexia nervosa; binge-eating/purging type
3. Anorexia, restricting type

Concept Check 9.5

1. Hypothalamus
2. False
3. True

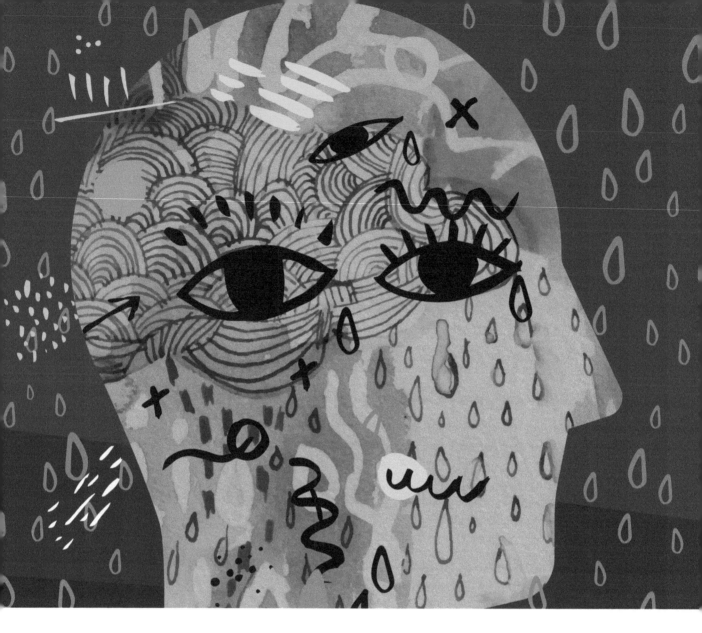

DrAfter123/DigitalVision Vectors/Getty Images Plus.

CHAPTER CONTENTS

10

Disruptive Impulse-Control and Conduct Disorders

CASE STUDY: Conduct Disorder – Michael

Michael had a mostly uneventful childhood until he was 3 years old and his brother Allen was born. After that, Michael's behavior changed dramatically. He would cry at the slightest provocation to the point where his parents couldn't soothe him. It wasn't just the "terrible twos" but instead the beginning of years of disruptive behavioral and emotional difficulties. Michael's tantrums seemed to be unending. "And it would happen for hours and hours each day, no matter what we did," his mother recalled.

For years Michael would scream whenever his parents asked him to get dressed or retrieve a toy from another room. Nearly everything would set off his anger. When getting ready for school he would fly into a fury and kick holes in the door, punch the wall, or slam the toilet seat down again and again until it would break. What's more, he didn't seem to feel any remorse for the destruction he caused. Michael could also change abruptly. He might exhibit angry tantrums and hours of sobbing and screaming, kicking, and hitting things and then calmly explain himself in a calculated way. We'll come back to Michael later in this chapter.

To read more about Michael see Kahn (2012).

Learning Objectives

- Describe the symptoms of intermittent explosive disorder, kleptomania, and pyromania.
- Explain the models and related treatments for impulse-control disorders.
- Describe the symptoms of oppositional defiant disorder and conduct disorder.

10.1 OVERVIEW OF IMPULSE-CONTROL AND CONDUCT DISORDERS

Impulses: strong urges to behave in certain ways.

We all have **impulses**, or strong urges to behave in certain ways. Maybe we are thirsty and in the middle of a conversation and we gravitate to get something to drink. Perhaps a child feels like taking a toy from a friend. Most of our impulses are unplanned and are generated from internal or even external events, such as thirst or the appearance of a new toy at a child's party. Impulses can be so powerful that we react to them without regard to the possibility of negative consequences from our actions. We are usually able to hold back our more dangerous impulses, however; that is, the ones that would cause us to break the law or inflict emotional or physical harm on others.

Sometimes our impulses do cause us to break minor rules. It's not too unusual for people (including children) to lie, speak rudely, or refuse to follow instructions. In fact, it would be out of the ordinary for a person to be obedient at every moment. However, those who constantly engage in disruptive impulses, break rules, or react with hostility to authority figures might meet the criteria for one of the conditions listed in the *DSM-5tr*'s Disruptive Impulse-Control and Conduct Disorder chapter.

Disruptive impulse and conduct disorders: a chapter in the *DSM-5tr* that contains conditions that reflect behaviors that might violate the rights of others or break societal norms.

The **disruptive impulse and conduct disorders** all reflect behaviors that might violate the rights of others or break societal norms. At their core is the person's difficulty resisting urges that can be harmful to the self or to others, including families and communities. The cause is rooted in problems regulating self-control of behaviors and emotions, and in repeated patterns of escalating problematic behaviors. These impulses are driven not by a need for gratification but by the person's hope that acting on the impulse will reduce or prevent distress and anxiety. Another factor might be a feeling of pleasurable tension that leads up to the disruptive act. Some people with these conditions describe a craving to engage in the behavior followed by a sense of relief or guilt afterwards (Frick & Matlasz 2018).

DSM-5tr describes several impulse-control and conduct disorders, including intermittent explosive disorder, kleptomania, and pyromania (described in section 10.2), and some that are exclusively diagnosed in children, including conduct disorder and oppositional defiant disorder (described in section 10.3).

CONCEPT CHECK 10.1

Decide whether each of the following is indicative of an impulse-control/conduct disorder.
1. Jake is 28 years old and for the first time has a strong urge to take a beautiful coin he noticed at a friend's home. He hasn't taken the coin, but does this strong urge mean he has an impulse-control disorder?
2. Diego constantly gives in to his impulses in ways that create distress and impairment not only in his life but in his relationships with his friends and family. He does this despite knowing that the problems may occur. Might Diego have a disruptive impulse/conduct disorder?
3. Kirsten is in a hurry and decides to drive faster than the posted speed limit. Does she have an impulse-control disorder?

10.2   IMPULSE-CONTROL DISORDERS

Most people will every now and then experience a strong and sudden impulse to behave in particular ways. A sudden desire to do something that we know isn't the right thing to do, such as cutting a line in a store or driving over the speed limit, comes over us. At times such an urge can feel overwhelming. We might even need to distract ourselves in order to avoid thinking about or engaging in the behavior. However, the vast majority of these impulses are harmless.

In **impulse-control disorders**, in contrast, people feel overwhelming urges to engage in behaviors that may violate the rights of others or conflict with societal norms. Those with impulse-control disorders may need to make a considerable effort to hold back and manage their desires, yet they are sometimes incredibly difficult to resist. Sometimes the behavior manifests as an emotional reaction (as in intermittent explosive disorder), the taking of things that don't belong to the person (kleptomania), or an urge to set fires (pyromania). These aren't just one-time impulses. Those who have impulse-control disorders engage in these behaviors over and over again, often without thinking through their impact. Impulse-control disorders described in the *DSM-5tr* include intermittent explosive disorder, pyromania, and kleptomania. We look at each of these next.

> **Impulse-control disorders**: a condition in which people feel overwhelming urges to engage in behaviors that may violate the rights of others or conflict with societal norms.

Intermittent Explosive Disorder

Nearly everyone feels angry every now and then. Something disappoints or frustrates us and we lose our temper. While some people are slow to anger, others have a shorter fuse and may get very upset even at a slight provocation. However, people with **intermittent explosive disorder** have sudden episodes of angry verbal outbursts or aggressive, violent behavior that are significantly out of proportion to the situation (Diagnostic Overview 10.1). Essentially, they exhibit repeated uncontrollable temper tantrums. The aggressive outbursts of intermittent explosive disorder aren't calculated to get something (as in a non-disordered behavior called *instrumental aggression*). Instead, people with intermittent explosive disorder have biological and psychological characteristics (more on these later) that trip the switch on their anger and create both emotions and behaviors that are out of control.

> **Intermittent explosive disorder**: a condition in which people have sudden episodes of angry verbal outbursts or aggressive, violent behavior that are significantly out of proportion to the situation.

Diagnostic Overview 10.1: Intermittent Explosive Disorder

Aggressive impulses that lead to behavioral outbursts including verbal and physical aggression.

Impact:	Symptoms must exceed cultural and contextual norms. Symptoms are related to clinically significant distress or create impairment in important areas of life such as with friends and family or at work or school.
Timeframe:	Verbal or physical aggression occurring twice weekly, on average, for a period of three months or three outbursts involving damage to property and/or physical assault within a 12-month period.
Minimum age:	At least 6 years.

Source: Information from APA (2022).

Table 10.1 Intermittent explosive disorder world lifetime prevalence (by subtype), 2020

Description	Prevalence
Intermittent explosive disorder all types	0.8
Destroy property only	0.1
Threaten people only	0.1
Hurt people only (without a threat)	0.2
Destroy property and threaten people	0.1
Destroy property and hurt people	0.4

Source: Data from Scott, De Vries, et al. (2020).

Table 10.2 Intermittent explosive disorder: type and average number of anger attacks in the most violent week of the last year

Type of anger attack	Mean number attacks
Slam a door, kick a chair, or throw clothes in anger	5.5
Break something in anger	3.2
Break several things in anger	2.7
Purposely set fire to or destroy someone else's property	1.8
Purposely injure or torture an animal	2.1
Threaten someone	4.3
Hurt someone badly enough to need medical attention	1.4
Hurt someone badly, but not enough to need medical attention	2.7

Source: Data from Scott, De Vries, et al. (2020).

SYMPTOMS AND DESCRIPTION

Many people with intermittent explosive disorder report feeling irritable or angry almost all the time. They have difficulty resisting their aggressive impulses, and as a result they may assault other people, destroy property, and have frequent verbal aggressive outbursts or tirades. These explosive disruptions can happen suddenly and are usually brief (less than 30 minutes). They also occur frequently, although less severe episodes may occur between more extreme outbursts. After the outburst, the person may feel tired and experience a sense of relief, followed by a wave of embarrassment and resentment over the actions.

Researchers have divided intermittent explosive disorder into different subtypes according to the type of behavior seen during the attack, ranging from only making threats to actually harming others (see Table 10.1).

In one study, people with intermittent explosive disorder symptoms were asked to think back over the last year, and specifically the week in which they had the most violent and aggressive outburst. The respondents were then asked to indicate the type of outburst they experienced. As you can see in Table 10.2, they more often reported less destructive types of anger attacks that involved property (slamming a door, kicking a chair, or throwing clothes), but many also reported breaking something during the outburst, and 42 percent reported injuring a person during that time (Scott, De Vries, et al. 2020).

Those with intermittent explosive disorder have a degree of aggressiveness out of proportion to what they've experienced (Figure 10.1). They will sometimes describe their aggressive periods as "attacks" or "spells," heralded by a building sense of tension followed by the outburst of aggression. They feel intense impulses toward aggression, rage, increased energy, racing thoughts, and adult temper tantrums, resulting in throwing objects, fighting for no reason, giving vent to road rage, or committing domestic abuse. Symptoms can lead to legal problems, as well as problems with relationships and difficulty getting and keeping employment.

STATISTICS AND TRAJECTORY

Surveys suggest that as much as 2.7 percent of the United States population will have symptoms of intermittent explosive disorder at some point in their lives (Scott, Lim et al. 2018). Rates are lower for many other countries (see Figure 10.2). Lifetime prevalence of intermittent explosive disorder in all countries was 0.8 percent, ranging from less than 0.1 percent in Nigeria to a highest in the United States (Scott, De Vries, et al. 2020).

Intermittent explosive disorder is most commonly found in people under 40 and rarely begins after that age. Initial symptoms of the disorder usually occur in the early teens, but they can be seen in children as young as 6. The onset of the full disorder usually occurs in late adolescence, with a median age of onset in all countries of 17 years (Silva et al. 2020). More than 80 percent of people with intermittent explosive disorder have another psychological condition; anxiety disorders are the most common co-occurring conditions, appearing in just over 55 percent of cases (Scott, De Vries, et al. 2020).

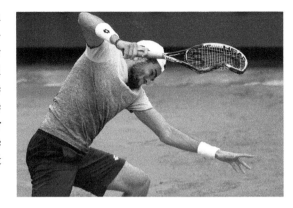

Figure 10.1 Some people will break property when they are frustrated, but those with intermittent explosive disorder have difficulty controlling their anger and some feel angry all the time.

Source: Eric Feferberg/AFP/ Getty Images.

Kleptomania

Case Study: Kleptomania – Joseph

Joseph loves the way stores feel. He's particularly enthralled by the selection of items. Once while shopping he noticed a coffee maker and was fascinated by its compact design. He felt a rush of power and a sense of invincibility as he removed the packaging and tossed it away. He then tucked the glass carafe into his right jacket pocket and the rest of the machine into the left. He felt a mixture of fear, pleasure, and cleverness.

On the way out, Joseph bought toilet paper, smiling at the security guard as he left the store. A feeling of intoxication poured through his body. But the feeling didn't last long. Soon after he felt an enormous amount of shame and guilt.

Joseph didn't have to steal the coffee maker; he already had three at home, and if he had really needed it, he could have easily purchased it. As the owner of a computer consulting business he has plenty of money, in spite of which he steals items he doesn't need nearly every week. This wasn't the first time he'd shoplifted merchandise he didn't need, and over the course of the next few years he was arrested several times for doing so.

Read more about Joseph in Jacobs (1997).

You may have had an impulse to take something that wasn't yours, perhaps something on display in a store that you wanted to put in your pocket. Most people can resist these impulses. However, **kleptomania** is a condition in which people *can't* resist the impulse to take items, usually of nominal value like cosmetics, even when they don't really need them (Figure 10.3). Stealing needed items such as food or medicine is not considered kleptomania, according to the *DSM-5tr* (Diagnostic Overview 10.2).

Kleptomania: a condition in which people can't resist the impulse to take items, usually of nominal value like cosmetics, even when they don't need them.

SYMPTOMS AND DESCRIPTION

Like many people with impulse-control disorders, those with kleptomania may feel an increase of tension or arousal before they act on their urge, in this case

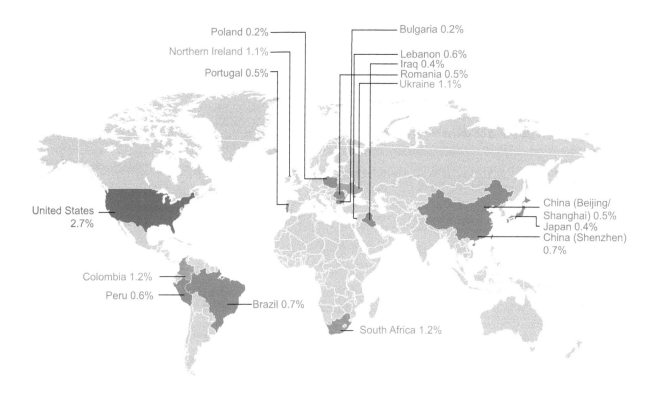

Poland 0.2%
Northern Ireland 1.1%
Portugal 0.5%
Bulgaria 0.2%
Lebanon 0.6%
Iraq 0.4%
Romania 0.5%
Ukraine 1.1%
United States 2.7%
China (Beijing/Shanghai) 0.5%
Japan 0.4%
China (Shenzhen) 0.7%
Colombia 1.2%
Peru 0.6%
Brazil 0.7%
South Africa 1.2%

Figure 10.2 Lifetime prevalence of intermittent explosive disorder in selected countries, from the World Mental Health Surveys (2002–2017).

Source: Data from Scott, Lim, et al. (2018).

to take an item, usually in a public space like a store or at a social event like a party. The tension or arousal is followed by an inability to resist the impulse, which in turn yields to a feeling of relief or pleasure once the item has been stolen.

The items that are taken are usually not needed or used, and sometimes they end up hidden, hoarded, or even discarded. Some people with kleptomania may put the items back a few days later; others may not even remember taking them. Soon after they may feel a sense of guilt, or shame or anxiety about being arrested. This reaction doesn't last too long, however, because people with kleptomania often will repeat the cycle. The majority (up to 87 percent) have been arrested as a result of their behavior (Grant & Chamberlain 2018).

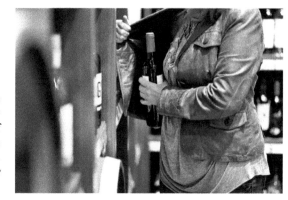

Figure 10.3 When people consistently steal items they don't need, it is a symptom of kleptomania according to the *DSM-5tr.*

Source: industryview/iStock/ Getty Images Plus.

STATISTICS AND TRAJECTORY

Surveys suggest that as many as 6 percent of the United States population will have symptoms of kleptomania in any given year, However, this estimate may be low, given that many with symptoms of kleptomania are embarrassed to report them (Fariba & Gokarakonda 2021). Kleptomania appears to be more prevalent in women, reportedly occurring three times more frequently among women than among men. These rates may not demonstrate actual differences between men and women, however. Instead, they might reflect the fact that courts are more likely to require female shoplifters to undergo psychiatric evaluation than male shoplifters (Fariba & Gokarakonda 2021). Kleptomania typically has an onset in late adolescence or early adulthood, most often between the ages of 16 and 20 (Grant & Chamberlain 2018).

Diagnostic Overview 10.2: Kleptomania

- Theft of objects that are not needed.
- Increasing sense of tension immediately before committing the theft.
- Pleasure, gratification, or relief at the time of committing the theft.
- Absence of anger or vengeance.

Impact: Symptoms must exceed cultural and contextual norms. Symptoms are related to clinically significant distress or create impairment in important areas of life such as with friends and family or at work or school.

Source: Information from APA (2022).

Pyromania

Fires are magical. They can be used for cooking, warmth, and even protection and comfort. People can stare into campfires or lit fireplaces for hours. But fire can be dangerous, and most people follow safety procedures about handling fire so it doesn't get out of control. Some people are so enamored of and fascinated by fire, though, that they deliberately set fires that often get out of control. **Pyromania** is an impulse-control disorder associated with an irresistible drive toward deliberate and purposeful fire-setting that recurs on multiple occasions (Figure 10.4) (Diagnostic Overview 10.3).

Pyromania: an impulse-control disorder associated with an irresistible drive toward deliberate and purposeful fire-setting that recurs on multiple occasions.

SYMPTOMS AND DESCRIPTION

People with pyromania describe a buildup of tension or excitement about starting a fire, which is related to the fascination and attraction they feel to fires and items about fire. This impulse to start fires brings a rush of excitement after starting or seeing the fire, followed by a sense of guilt for setting it.

People with the disorder may start fires frequently, around every six weeks. They may seem obsessed with fires, set off false fire alarms, collect objects associated with fires (such as lighters and matches), and derive pleasure from being around people associated with fires (such as firefighters). Some may set small fires and burn holes in rugs, furniture, or bits of fabric, while others set larger fires than can burn out of control. They don't intend to hurt people or have any secondary goals other than starting the fire, but they may also be indifferent to the financial or physical effects of the fire despite the fact that intentional fires have destructive consequences for both people and property. Between 2010 and 2014, an estimated 261,333 intentional fires were reported in the United States that resulted in an economic cost of $325.5 billion per year in property damage, well over 400 deaths, and thousands of severe injuries (NFPA 2021).

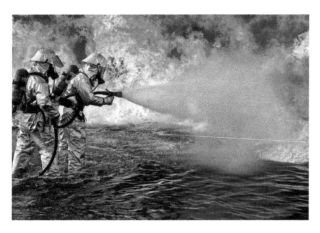

Figure 10.4 People with pyromania can't resist the impulse to start fires despite the devastating impact their actions can create.
Source: Stocktrek Images/ Getty Images.

Not everyone who sets a fire has pyromania. People don't receive a diagnosis if their fire-setting is done for personal gain (as in a scheme to collect insurance money), out of anger, to cover a criminal act, or as a result of impaired judgment (such as when intoxicated). When fire-setting is done willfully or maliciously, in many states it is known as arson.

STATISTICS AND TRAJECTORY

Curiosity about fire typically begins around 6 years of age, leading some children to experiment with matches and fire. Symptoms of pyromania tend to emerge in late adolescence or early adulthood and are more likely to occur in males than in females (Lejoyeux & Germain 2012). Adolescent fire setters outnumber adult fire setters (Johnson & Netherton 2016). Of those incarcerated for arson, only 3 percent meet the criteria for pyromania (Fariba & Gokarakonda 2021).

Models and Treatments of Impulse-Control Disorders

Joseph created a support group for people with kleptomania. More recently, he started avoiding shopping at stores to eliminate temptation. He's even changed the way he dresses, opting for loose-fitting boxers that make it difficult for him to stash stolen items in his underwear.

Unfortunately, evidence-based models and treatments for impulse-control disorders aren't as well developed as for some other psychological disorders. Few randomized controlled clinical trials have been conducted for these conditions. Because of this lack of an evidence base, many clinicians draw upon general treatment options for impulse-control disorders.

Diagnostic Overview 10.3: Pyromania

- Repeated and deliberate fire-setting.
- A build-up of tension before setting fires.
- Feeling drawn to fire.
- A sense of release when setting fires.
- Lack of motive related to monetary gain, cover-up of criminal activity, expression of anger, or impaired judgment.

Impact: Symptoms must exceed cultural and contextual norms. Symptoms are related to clinically significant distress or create impairment in important areas of life such as with friends and family or at work or school.

Source: Information from APA (2022).

BIOLOGICAL MODELS AND TREATMENTS OF IMPULSE-CONTROL DISORDERS

Psychopathologists have considered the influence of brain areas, neurotransmitters, and hormones on impulse-control disorders. It appears that in people with intermittent explosive disorder, there is a relationship between the way they recognize emotions and their amygdala and orbitofrontal cortex function. They seem to have increased activity in the amygdala but lower orbitofrontal cortex activation in response to angry faces. Intermittent explosive disorder was associated with structural differences as well as significant loss of neurons in both the amygdala and the hippocampus (Coccaro et al. 2015). We also see biological differences in people with other impulse-control disorders. For example, some people with kleptomania have lower activity in the inferior temporal region, an area in the brain associated with making decisions, and some people diagnosed with pyromania have shown variations in the frontal lobe (Gannon et al. 2022).

The Food and Drug Administration (FDA) has approved few treatments for impulse-control disorders. They include serotonin and norepinephrine reuptake inhibitors and mood stabilizers such as lithium. These medications are associated with reduction in impulsive actions, although not everyone responds to drug therapy. Naltrexone, an opioid antagonist used in the treatment of alcoholism, is somewhat effective in reducing the urge to steal in people diagnosed with kleptomania. Topiramate, escitalopram, sertraline, fluoxetine, and lithium have been demonstrated to be effective in case studies of pyromania.

Some researchers have suggested that kleptomania behaviors might be risk-taking behaviors clients used to alleviate depression. Several reports suggest that antidepressants improve the symptoms not only of depression but also of klepto-mania (Torales et al. 2020).

COGNITIVE-BEHAVIORAL MODELS AND TREATMENTS OF IMPULSE-CONTROL DISORDERS

According to the principles of operant conditioning, impulse-control disorders may be reinforced by the positive emotions people feel while engaging in them. Kleptomania, for example, is positively reinforced by the taking of items and increased by intermittent reinforcement (since there are times when store security might be watching and sometimes not).

Cognitive-behavioral interventions for impulse-control disorders act to disrupt this pattern of reinforcement (Grant et al. 2011). For example, cognitive-behavioral interventions in intermittent explosive disorder try to help clients learn to identify and avoid triggers for their outbursts and focus on reducing anger and aggression. Cognitive-behavioral treatment for pyromania consists of helping clients identify the signals that initiate their urges and teaching coping strategies to resist the temptation to start fires. Most also focus on a number of methods to reduce the temptation to set fires, including challenging cognitive distortions around the seriousness of starting fires and improving self-regulation of impulses. (For instance, a client might be asked to imagine a situation in which they might have an impulse to set a fire, and to consider the consequences of the fire on other people.) Treatment will also include fire safety education (Johnson & Netherton 2016).

SOCIOCULTURAL MODELS AND TREATMENTS OF IMPULSE-CONTROL DISORDERS

A number of sociocultural aspects are important for impulse-control disorders. It has been hypothesized that intermittent explosive disorder might be more prevalent in countries with higher rates of violence, trauma exposure, and civil conflict (Rees et al. 2013).

Certain environmental aspects can be risk factors for impulse-control disorders such as lower socioeconomic status, frequent changes in caregivers, and exposure to neighborhood violence such as weapons use (Fadus et al. 2019). Youth who are exposed to higher levels of danger and violence may be more likely to view strangers as hostile and as threats, and they may respond in aggressive ways (Fadus et al. 2019). Environmental aspects, sociocultural influences, and structural factors can affect the diagnosis a person might receive. Even when exhibiting similar behaviors, for instance, some racial and ethnic marginalized populations are more likely to be diagnosed with certain disorders such as oppositional defiant disorder and conduct disorders even when the researchers account for adverse childhood experiences. The ways in which society fosters racial and ethnic discrimination (structural racism) may also influence the diagnosis (Ballentine 2019). For example, Black American boys are viewed as less innocent (Goff et al. 2014) and more dangerous and aggressive, and because of this their behaviors may be seen, and a diagnosis given, through that lens. Some researchers are concerned about medicating impulse-control disorders if the cause of the behavior is a problem in society rather than in the person (Hock & Karnik 2017).

MULTIPERSPECTIVE MODELS AND TREATMENTS OF IMPULSE-CONTROL DISORDERS

Due to the limited empirical evidence for the treatment of impulse-control disorders, many treatments will combine multiple psychotherapeutic perspectives, such as family or group therapy and CBT. Some treatment programs will also use medication to target the most troubling symptoms. A person diagnosed with intermittent explosive disorder, for example, might participate in CBT to help reduce anger and aggression and increase anger control, and practice some of these strategies in a group setting.

CONCEPT CHECK 10.2

Indicate whether each case is likely to be intermittent explosive disorder, kleptomania, pyromania, or not an impulse-control disorder.

1. Saffron hasn't been able to get enough food for several days since she lost her job. While in the grocery store she decides to slip a few candy bars in her pocket without paying for them. She feels guilty about taking them.

2. All Belle's friends will tell you she has a "bad temper." She gets angry at the slightest provocation and will throw and break items in her house. She states that her anger is "out of control" and that she is angry "almost all the time."

3. Carla has always wanted to be a firefighter. She reads books about firefighters, knows all about the chemistry of fires, and engages with firefighters on social media. She even has a fire-engine red car. After high school she plans to go to the academy to become a firefighter.

10.3 OPPOSITIONAL DEFIANT DISORDER AND CONDUCT DISORDER

Children as well as adults break the rules at times. Oppositional defiant disorder and conduct disorder, however, are characterized by patterns of disruptive behaviors in children that are not typical for their age and that cause impairment.

Oppositional Defiant Disorder

Oppositional defiant disorder is a childhood disorder marked by repeatedly irritable, angry, defiant, argumentative, and often vindictive behavior (Diagnostic Overview 10.4). While irritable and argumentative behaviors are often demonstrated in childhood, they are more persistent in those with oppositional defiant disorder. As is the case for those with an impulse-control disorder, defiant behavior is linked to a person's inability to regulate negative emotions and behaviors. These children have a marked pattern of hostile, defiant, and disobedient behavior that lasts at least six months and is usually directed at authority figures. The behavior causes considerable impairment in social functioning and in educational settings.

Oppositional defiant disorder: a childhood disorder marked by repeatedly irritable, angry, defiant, argumentative, and often vindictive behavior.

SYMPTOMS AND DESCRIPTION

Children with oppositional defiant disorder argue with adults and ignore rules, and they may annoy others on purpose. They feel much more anger and resentment than their peers without the disorder.

There are both emotional and behavioral symptoms for this condition. Children with oppositional defiant disorder don't destroy property, steal, or act aggressively toward animals or people; rather, they actively defy commands and requests made by authority figures. They are easily angered and struggle to take any responsibility for their actions. In some children these symptoms are manifested at home, in school, and in other activities such as sports, while in others their oppositional defiant disorder symptoms occur in only a single setting. These differences may be based on what limits are set for children in these various settings. Children with the disorder may blame others for their mistakes or misbehaviors and think of their own actions as responses to unfair situations. Because of this, they find their behavior less upsetting and disturbing than do their friends, family, and teachers.

DSM-5tr separates oppositional defiant disorder symptoms into clusters based on whether they have an

Diagnostic Overview 10.4: Oppositional Defiant Disorder

Angry and irritable moods, argumentative or defiant behavior, or vindictiveness that results in at least four of the following symptoms:

Angry/Irritable Mood

- Loses temper.
- Is easily annoyed.
- Is angry and resentful.

Argumentative/Defiant Behavior

- Argues with authority figures.
- Defies or refuses to follow rules.
- Deliberately annoys others.
- Blames others for their mistakes or misbehavior.

Vindictiveness

- Has been spiteful or vindictive.

Impact: Symptoms must exceed cultural and contextual norms. Symptoms are related to clinically significant distress or create impairment in important areas of life such as with friends and family or at work or school.

Timeframe: At least six months.

Source: Information from APA (2022).

emotional component (angry, irritable resentful behaviors), a behavioral component (argumentative defiant behaviors), or a spiteful/vindictive component (see diagnostic criteria). The more emotional symptoms of oppositional defiant disorder such as anger and irritability are associated with the later development of mood and anxiety disorders. Behavioral components, on the other hand, are more likely to lead to a later diagnosis of ADHD, and spiteful or vindictive actions are associated with an increased risk of conduct problems (Rowe et al. 2010).

For a diagnosis of oppositional defiant disorder to be given, the behaviors must be directed toward people who are not siblings. Even so, they will negatively affect relationships not only with teachers, peers, and others in the community but with family members as well.

STATISTICS AND TRAJECTORY

Surveys suggest that as many as 10.1 percent of the United States population will have symptoms of oppositional defiant disorder at some point in their lives (Turner et al. 2018). Rates are lower in most areas of the world, as you can see in Figure 10.5, which may be explained by sociocultural differences. For example, the prevalence of oppositional defiant disorder may be affected by the degree to which its symptoms are considered dysfunctional. In cultures where suppression of anger and aggression are important, parents may have a lower threshold for accepting oppositional behavior (Canino et al. 2010).

Between 6 and 8 years is the most common age of onset for oppositional defiant disorder; earlier onset of oppositional defiant disorder is associated with a later

Figure 10.5 Lifetime prevalence of oppositional defiant disorder in selected countries, from the World Mental Health Surveys (2002–2017).
Source: Data from Turner et al. (2018).

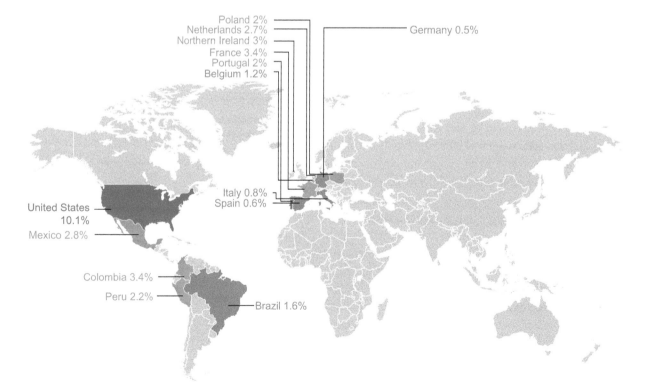

diagnosis of conduct disorder (discussed below). Behaviors in oppositional defiant disorder first manifest at home, and over time they will spread to additional places such as in sports or among friends at school.

The impact of oppositional defiant disorder is clear, and 25 per cent of those with the disorder are identified as being in need of treatment. Only about 30 percent of those diagnosed will still exhibit the symptoms by the time they are 18 (Turner et al. 2018). Children with disruptive mood dysregulation disorder (see Chapter 6, section 6.2) are more likely to develop oppositional defiant disorder (Le et al. 2020). Those with oppositional defiant disorder are more likely in later life to meet criteria for conduct disorder (see the next section), substance use disorder (see Chapter 11) and mood and anxiety disorders (described in Chapters 4, 5, and 6).

Conduct Disorder

It's common for some teens and children to have behavioral problems. Most of the time the problems don't last long. However, children like Michael at the start of this chapter who consistently behave in ways that break rules and violate society's norms might meet the criteria for **conduct disorder** (Diagnostic Overview 10.5). Children and adolescents with conduct disorder exhibit physically violent behavior toward others. Their actions may include physical abuse and destruction of property and often lack regard for the property or rights of others. As in other disorders in this chapter, the symptoms are due in part to the individual's reduced ability to exert successful control over negative emotions and impulses.

Conduct disorder: a condition associated with children and adolescents where they exhibit physically violent behavior toward others.

SYMPTOMS AND DESCRIPTION

DSM-5tr describes 15 behaviors that characterize conduct disorders, organized into four symptom groups:

1. Aggression against people or animals.
2. Destruction of property.
3. Deceitfulness or theft.
4. Serious violation of rules.

Conduct disorder symptoms can appear at different times. When they occur before the age of 10, the disorder is referred to as the childhood-onset type, and when symptoms begin after 10, it is called the adolescent-onset type. The adolescent-onset type is associated with an overall better outcome, even without treatment. (See also Table 10.3 in the Pulling It Together feature at the end of this chapter.)

Some people with conduct disorder feel remorse about their behavior. Others don't; they are repeatedly aggressive and physically cruel to people and animals and destroy property or set fires on purpose. They may lie, steal, run away from home, or threaten or harm others. People with the **callous-unemotional type of conduct disorder** are insensitive to the feelings of others, have shallow emotions, and don't feel guilty or have empathy for the things they might do to others. They also appear to lack concern about not doing well in school (Colins et al. 2021).

Callous-unemotional type of conduct disorder: a specifier for conduct disorder associated with children who are insensitive to the feeling of others, have shallow emotions, and don't feel guilty or have empathy for the things they might do to others.

Diagnostic Overview 10.5: **Conduct Disorder**

A repetitive and persistent pattern of behavior in which the basic rights of others are violated or major laws are broken via at least three of the following:

Aggression to People and Animals

- Bullies, threatens, or intimidates others.
- Initiates fights.
- Has used a weapon that can cause serious physical harm.
- Has been physically cruel to people.
- Has been physically cruel to animals.
- Has stolen while confronting a victim.
- Has forced someone into sexual activity.

Destruction of Property

- Has set fires with the intention of causing serious damage.
- Has deliberately destroyed others' property.

Deceitfulness or Theft

- Has broken into someone else's house, building, or car.
- Often lies to obtain object they want, favors or to avoid duties.
- Has stolen items without confronting the person.

Serious Violations of Rules

- Often stays out at night despite being told not to.
- Has run away from home twice.
- Frequently misses school.

Impact: Symptoms must exceed cultural and contextual norms. Symptoms are related to clinically significant distress or create impairment in important areas of life such as with friends and family or at work or school.

Timeframe: At least three of the criteria were present in the past 12 months with at least one criterion present in the past six months.

Source: Information from APA (2022).

Prosocial emotions: feelings such as responsibility, remorse or guilt for hurting someone, and empathy.

Prosocial emotions are feelings such as responsibility, remorse or guilt for hurting someone, and empathy. Children with conduct disorder who don't have prosocial feelings might be more likely to meet the criteria for antisocial personality disorder in the future. The *DSM* outlines a *limited prosocial emotion* specifier for children with conduct disorder who meet at least two of the following criteria: lack of remorse or guilt, lack of empathy, lack of concern about problematic performance, and lack of or lowered expression of emotions.

STATISTICS AND TRAJECTORY

Conduct disorder is one of the most common diagnoses within child psychopathology. Surveys suggest that as many as 9.5 percent of the United States population will have symptoms of this disorder at some point in their lives (Turner et al. 2018). Based on various studies, boys diagnosed with conduct disorder outnumber girls by a factor estimated at anywhere from 2:1 to 4:1 (Moore et al. 2017). Boys and girls may vary in the kinds of disruptive behaviors they enact. Boys tend to exhibit disruptive behavior, while girls sometimes exhibit less aggressive behavior than boys (Lindner et al. 2016). Rates of conduct disorder tend to be higher in the Americas and in high-income countries and significantly lower in most other countries in the world (see Figure 10.6). Reasons for the differences may be that conduct disorder is more likely to be diagnosed in the Americas, and/or that it is seen there as a mental health condition as opposed to a behavioral or legal problem (Polanczyk et al. 2015).

Symptom onset for conduct disorder can occur between the ages of 7 and 15. It's difficult to predict the course of the condition, but it rarely persists into adulthood. The majority of those with conduct disorder (90 percent) no longer show serious symptoms when they are adults (Turner et al. 2018). However, they may have problems including educational difficulties, financial and work problems, and higher rates of substance disorders. People with early diagnoses of conduct disorders are more likely to have anxiety, mood, eating, and substance disorders as adults (Turner et al. 2018).

Many with conduct disorders are in the juvenile justice system; they may be using, selling, or buying illegal substances and have a lifelong history of breaking rules. Many people with antisocial personality disorder (Chapter 12) have had conduct disorder as children. A recent systematic review of the literature suggests that around 40 percent of children with conduct disorder show the characteristics of the specifier for limited prosocial emotions (Colins et al. 2020).

Figure 10.6 Lifetime prevalence of conduct disorder in selected countries, from the World Mental Health Surveys (2002–2017).

Source: Data from Turner et al. (2018).

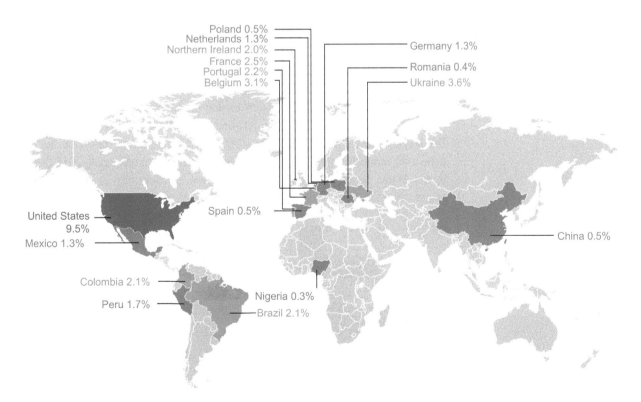

THE POWER OF EVIDENCE

Do video games cause aggression?

Many of the conditions described in this chapter include aggressive and destructive behavior. Evidence from social psychology suggests that observing aggressive behavior can lead to aggression, which has led some to wonder about the effects of video games on children (Figure 10.7). The video game industry is enormous. Consumers in 2019 spent $120 billion on video games, including mobile games, console games (like Xbox and Nintendo), and augmented reality games. One game, Fortnite, accounted for $1.8 billion alone. Fortnite is an action-packed game in which players compete to be the last one standing in player vs player conflict. Players can use assault rifles, tactical submachine guns, grenade launchers, and hand cannons against their opponents.

Violence isn't unusual in video games. With the exception of Animal Crossing (which includes gentle scenarios in which you customize an island and village and talk with kind animal neighbors), the top five games in 2020 were aggressive violent games. And children and teens spend a great deal of time playing these games. In one study, girls aged 12–15 spent around 9 hours per week gaming and boys of this age spent over 16 hours per week.

The American Psychological Association suggests that parents limit the time that children and teens play video games. Most of the concern about violent video games is that repeated exposure to violent media might increase aggressive thoughts, which could make kids more aggressive. But what does the evidence say?

Andrew Przybylski and Netta Weinstein (2019) surveyed a large sample of just over 1,000 British adolescents aged 14 and 15. The teens reported how much they played games and their parents provided evaluations of any aggressive behaviors. What did the researchers find? There was no evidence that video games were related to aggressive behavior. Another study of more than 3,000 youth in Singapore showed that early exposure to aggressive games wasn't associated with emotional difficulties such as anxiety or depression (Ferguson & Wang 2021). The Media Psychology and Technology Division of the APA has concluded that there is no actionable evidence linking aggressive behavior to gaming. In 2011 the United States Supreme Court judged that there is insufficient evidence that games cause harm to uphold laws restricting the sale of violent games to minors.

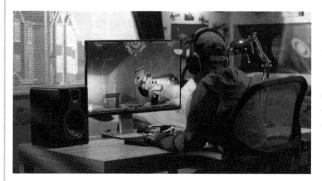

Figure 10.7 Violent video games are popular with kids, but do they create violent kids?

Source: Evgeniy Shkolenko/iStock/Getty Images Plus.

Although many video games are full of violence and aggression, they don't necessarily lead to aggressive behaviors in real life.

Sources: Coyne & Stockdale (2021); Ferguson & Wang (2021); Lejoyeux & Germain (2012); Przybylski & Weinstein (2019); Sinclair (2019); VentureBeat (2020).

Models and Treatments of Oppositional Defiant Disorder and Conduct Disorder

In the summer of 2012 Michael's parents took him to a treatment program to help him with his disruptive behavior. Oppositional defiant disorder and conduct disorder are thought to be related to a number of biological, environmental, and social factors, but, as with impulse-control disorders, there is limited empirical research about these conditions.

BIOLOGICAL MODELS AND TREATMENTS OF OPPOSITIONAL DEFIANT DISORDER AND CONDUCT DISORDER

People with oppositional defiant disorder and conduct disorder do show some biological differences. For example, they have slower heart rates in reaction to frightening events, and their frontotemporal-limbic connections and prefrontal cortex and amygdala, areas of the brain responsible for regulating affect, are different. Some fMRI studies in children diagnosed with conduct disorder have shown lower reactivity of the anterior cingulate cortex and amygdala to normally highly emotional stimuli. This means that when children with conduct disorder were shown anxiety-provoking stimuli, their amygdalas didn't react as much as in children without the disorder. Researchers also found lower amounts of gray matter in several areas of the brain, including the insula, amygdala, and frontal cortex (Rogers & De Brito 2016).

Medications are not the primary treatment for the symptoms of oppositional defiant disorder and conduct disorders. In the United States no medication has been approved as a primary treatment; however, some medications are used off-label to reduce disruptive behaviors and symptoms such as impulsivity, hyperactivity, aggression, and mood disturbances. Medicine to treat comorbid conditions such as ADHD, depression, and anxiety can also be helpful, such as methylphenidate, atomoxetine, and atypical antipsychotics such as ariprizole and risperdone.

COGNITIVE-BEHAVIORAL MODELS AND TREATMENTS OF OPPOSITIONAL DEFIANT DISORDER AND CONDUCT DISORDER

Cognitive-behavioral treatments of conduct disorder and oppositional defiant disorder focus on teaching parents and children anger management skills and problem solving, and improving social interaction.

The development of conduct disorder and oppositional defiant disorder is associated with harsh and inconsistent parenting. While it is impossible to know with certainty that inconsistent parenting leads to oppositional defiant disorder and

Parent management training (PMT): a behavioral treatment that aims to help parents learn successful discipline techniques, increase structure and predictability, and manage their child's behavior more effectively to promote desired behavior.

conduct disorders, there are cognitive-behavioral techniques that can help parents improve the quality and consistency of their parenting skills. **Parent management training (PMT)** is a behavioral treatment that aims to help parents learn successful discipline techniques, increase structure and predictability, and manage their child's behavior more effectively to promote desired behavior.

Parents may learn, for example, how to break large or unwieldy chores into smaller, bite-sized tasks for children, to use positive reinforcement as children accomplish the tasks, and to do their best to ignore minor misbehaviors so that the interventions don't escalate (Axelrod & Santagata 2021). CBT techniques also focus on helping children learn perspective-taking to increase their positive interpersonal interactions and reduce conflict, and to find less destructive ways to handle conflict if it occurs. Parents are often included in order to change family interactions and model ways to handle disruptive behaviors.

SOCIOCULTURAL MODELS AND TREATMENTS OF OPPOSITIONAL DEFIANT DISORDER AND CONDUCT DISORDER

Sociocultural models suggest that certain environments may be risk factors for the development of conduct disorder and oppositional defiant disorder. Some researchers use evidence of the differences rates of these conditions over time, neighborhoods, or cultures to support this hypothesis (Zimring 2020). However, implicit bias may also influence who receives a diagnosis of conduct disorder or oppositional defiant disorder. Even when researchers account for behavioral indicators, Black males are 40 percent more likely and Black females 54 percent more likely to be diagnosed with conduct disorder than whites (Baglivio et al. 2017). Clinicians should also be sensitive to cultural differences in behavior norms and recognize the importance of extended families, who in many cultures can be active in raising children and thus have an impact on parenting styles.

Some researchers are concerned that the diagnosis of oppositional defiant disorder may create more harm than benefits if it affects the way people view themselves and are treated by others. Parents and clinicians who are aware of the diagnosis show pessimistic expectations and are therefore less likely to look for other explanations for their behavior. This leads to lower self-esteem, responses to low expectations, and further disruptive behaviors. In addition, cultural factors, including racial and ethnic bias, can affect the way others interpret and respond to children's behavior (Potter et al. 2014). Also, minoritized youth are subject to more toxic stress (including racism), and their trauma responses may be incorrectly pathologized. Racial stereotyping may lead to the same behavior being seen as more disruptive or as a sign of psychopathology in minoritized populations (Potter et al. 2014). Because of these factors, some researchers suggest a revision of the oppositional defiant disorder diagnosis to reduce the stigma around the diagnosis and to promote racial trauma sensitivity (Beltrán et al. 2021).

MULTIPERSPECTIVE MODELS AND TREATMENTS OF OPPOSITIONAL DEFIANT DISORDER AND CONDUCT DISORDER

Multiperspective models examine the many layers of conduct disorder and oppositional defiant disorder. For example, there is evidence that poor quality of parenting and low levels of parental involvement are related to a diagnosis of conduct disorder (Cox et al. 2018). Children with uninvolved parents may turn to peers for escape or emotional connection, and peers may encourage disruptive behaviors. Further, children with conduct disorder are sometimes described as difficult, irritable, disobedient, and demanding, temperament differences that may have biological origins and that may interact with both environmental and parenting differences. Most treatments of conduct and oppositional defiant disorder include interventions on multiple levels including the family, the school, peers, and the community, and multiperspective models reflect this complex interaction.

CONCEPT CHECK 10.3

Identify the condition most likely associated with each case.
1. Anna is worried about her son Ray, who is very aggressive and always fighting with his brother. Ray's behavior is different at school, where he doesn't seem to have problems.
2. Amilcar's son has been difficult for the last year. He throws temper tantrums, doesn't follow his father's wishes, and fights with his teachers and coaches.
3. Amy's teachers have asked for a parent-teacher conference because of Amy's behavior at school. She's been bullying some of the other children, stealing their money and lunches, and deliberately destroyed another child's project. Amy's mother isn't too surprised. A few months ago, Amy was caught shoplifting and has gotten into fights with some of the members of her sports team.

PULLING IT TOGETHER

Impulse Control and Conduct Disorders

Table 10.3 Age of onset of various impulse control and conduct disorders

Disorder	Age of onset
Intermittent explosive disorder	Six years and older
Kleptomania	Any age
Pyromania	Any age
Oppositional Defiant Disorder	Diagnosis typically assigned to individuals under age 18
Conduct Disorder	Diagnosis typically assigned to individuals under age 18

SUMMARY

This chapter presented the following disorders:

- Intermittent explosive disorder
- Kleptomania
- Pyromania
- Oppositional defiant disorder
- Conduct disorder

Overview of Impulse-Control and Conduct Disorders

- Impulses are strong urges to behave in certain ways.
- The disruptive impulse and conduct disorders all reflect things that a person does that might violate the rights of others or break societal norms.

Impulse-Control Disorders

- Impulse-control disorders are conditions where a person engages in behaviors that may violate the rights of others or conflict with societal norms.
- People with intermittent explosive disorder have sudden episodes of angry and verbal outbursts or aggressive, violent behavior that are significantly out of proportion to the situation.
- Symptoms can lead to legal problems, and problems with relationships and difficulty in getting and keeping employment.
- Kleptomania is a condition where people can't resist the impulse to take items, usually of nominal value, even when they don't need them.
- Items that are taken are usually not even used and hidden, hoarded, or discarded. Some people with kleptomania may even put them back a few days later.
- The majority of those with kleptomania have been arrested as a result of their behavior.

- Pyromania is an impulse-control disorder associated with a person's irresistible drive toward deliberate and purposeful fire-setting that recurs on multiple occasions.
- According to the biological model, brain areas, neurotransmitters, and hormones may influence impulse-control disorders.
- According to the operant conditioning model, impulse-control disorders may be reinforced by the positive emotions people feel while engaging in them.

Oppositional Defiant Disorder and Conduct Disorder

- Oppositional defiant disorder is a childhood disorder marked by repeatedly irritable, angry, defiant and argumentative, and often vindictive behavior.
- Conduct disorders involve patterns of disruptive behaviors that are not typical for that age and cause impairment.
- Conduct disorder is characterized by a persistent pattern of serious violations of rules, norms, and the rights of others.
- There are some biological differences in people with conduct disorder and oppositional defiant disorder including lower resting heart rates, and differences in parts of the brain that are responsible for regulating affect.
- Medications are not primarily used to treat the symptoms of oppositional defiant disorder and conduct disorders.
- Cognitive-behavioral treatments of conduct disorder and oppositional defiant disorder focus on anger management skills, problem solving, and improving social interaction.
- Parent management training (PMT) is a behavioral treatment that aims to assist parents on how to create strategies to increase structure and predictability.

- Most treatment of conduct and oppositional defiant disorder includes interventions on multiple levels including the family, schools, and peer and community.

DISCUSSION QUESTIONS

1. The *DSM* includes specific criteria for impulse-control disorders such as fire starting and theft, likely because of their destructive impact on the lives and property of others. Yet these aren't the only ways that impulses can create problems. What other types of contemporary behaviors might fit into this category, and how would you defend adding a new condition describing them to the *DSM*?

2. Helen's daughter never had any behavior problems when she was younger, but as a teenager, she has become very defiant and is constantly arguing. How can Helen tell whether this is a disorder or just a phase?

3. How would you answer this question from a parent? "Doesn't most misbehavior and defiance in children occur because parents don't discipline them enough?"

ANSWERS TO CONCEPT CHECKS

Concept Check 10.1

1. No
2. Yes
3. No

Concept Check 10.2

1. Not an impulse-control disorder

2. Intermittent explosive disorder
3. Not an impulse-control disorder

Concept Check 10.3

1. Not conduct disorder if only in one area

2. Oppositional defiant disorder
3. Conduct disorder

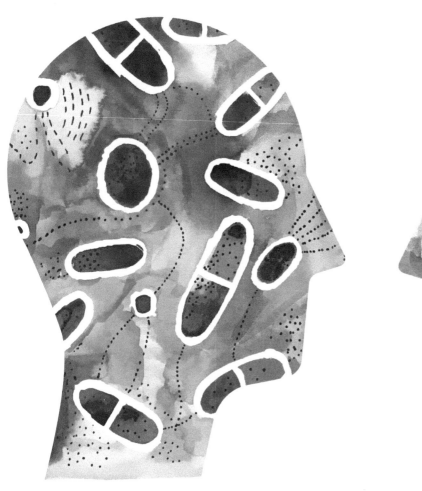
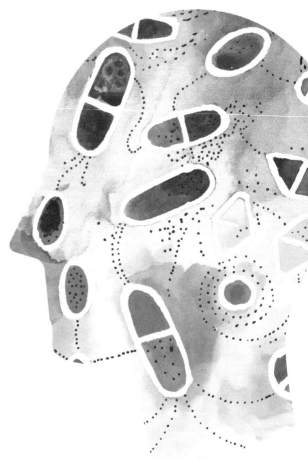

CHAPTER CONTENTS

11

Substance-Related and Addictive Disorders

CASE STUDY: Substance Use Disorder – Demi Lovato

In July 2018, Demi Lovato (Figure 11.1) woke up in an intensive care unit. The night before, they had used what they thought was heroin. This isn't Demi's first time using substances. They started using cocaine at 17, soon taking combinations of Xanax and codeine, followed by other substances such as methamphetamines, molly, marijuana, alcohol, OxyContin, and heroin.

When their assistant found them in the morning, Demi was unresponsive, naked, and blue from oxygen deprivation. Another 10 minutes and they might have died. The overdose led to three strokes, a heart attack, lasting vision impairment, and multiple organ failure. Recovery took months.

Since the age of 6 Demi has been in the entertainment industry in multiple roles, including on a children's television show, in recurring roles on other successful shows, and as a judge in a television competition show. They also recorded six successful albums, two platinum and four gold. Demi admits to being physically dependent on heroin, making multiple attempts at substance rehabilitation, and experiencing relapses into substance use. We'll come back to Demi's story later in the chapter.

Learn more about Demi Lovato in their 2021 documentary, *Demi Lovato: Dancing with the devil* (www.youtube.com/watch?v=EAg69LaLlS0).

Learning Objectives

- Describe the categories of psychoactive drugs.
- Describe the effects of psychoactive drugs on the nervous system.
- Identify diagnostic symptoms associated with intoxication, withdrawal, and substance use disorders.
- List the various models and treatments for substance use disorders.

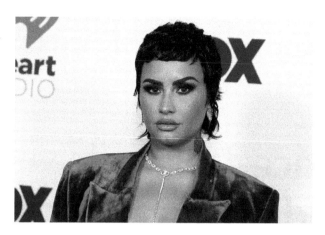

Figure 11.1 Demi Lovato.
Source: Emma McIntyre/Getty Images for iHeartMedia.

11.1 OVERVIEW OF SUBSTANCE USE DISORDERS

According to the Substance Abuse and Mental Health Services Administration (SAMHSA), more than 22 million people aged 12 and over in the United States abuse or are dependent on a nonprescribed psychoactive drug (www.samhsa.gov/). A **psychoactive drug** is a chemical used to alter behavior, mood, thoughts, or consciousness, such as tobacco, alcohol, and cannabis. Psychoactive drugs are used by millions of people in the United States; for example marijuana is used by over 43 million people (see Figure 11.2 for estimates of other psychoactive substances). The COVID-19 pandemic has led to an increase in substance use. Thirteen percent of people in the United States have either started using a psychoactive drug or increased the use of a substance because of the emotions or stress they experienced during the COVID-19 pandemic (Czeisler et al. 2020).

Many psychoactive drugs can have a beneficial aspect. For example, many people use caffeine for alertness, and prescription medication can help reduce pain. But misuse can lead to *tolerance*, a reduction in a person's sensitivity to a drug over time, which can cause the person to need more of the drug to generate the original effect. Misuse can also lead to *addiction*, which is a compulsive need for the substance. Such compulsive use of or craving for a drug in turn can lead to **substance use disorders** and cause distress or impairment in social, work, or school functioning.

These disorders can also tear families apart and cause significant health, financial, and social problems. Though there are many ill effects of psychoactive drugs, stopping their abuse is difficult. Many substances have strong *withdrawal symptoms*, which are distressing side effects and cravings associated with sudden discontinuation. *Drug rebound effects* can also occur, so that stopping the use of a drug makes the user feel even worse. All these symptoms combine to explain drug dependence. Dependence can come in many forms, including *physical dependence*, a condition in which a drug must be taken continually to avoid symptoms of withdrawal, and *psychological dependence*, in which a person's use of a substance leads to cravings, distress, and impairment even in the absence of physical dependence.

Psychoactive drug: a chemical used to alter behavior, mood, thoughts, or consciousness, such as tobacco, alcohol, and cannabis.

Substance use disorders: psychological conditions associated with compulsive use or craving of a drug that leads to impairment in social, work, or school functioning.

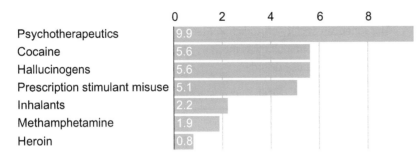

Figure 11.2 Number of people using psychoactive drugs in the United States (2018).
Source: SAMHSA (2018).

The *DSM-5tr* describes substance-related disorders that result from a number of separate classes of drugs: depressants (such as alcohol and sedative hypnotics), stimulants, (such as tobacco, caffeine, and methamphetamines), opioids, cannabis, and hallucinogens. The *DSM* also describes a category of non-substance addictions that includes gambling disorder. In this chapter we cover the general diagnostic criteria for substance use disorders, as well as the criteria and the models and treatments for each of the specific substances described in *DSM-5tr* and for gambling disorder (see Table 11.6 in the Pulling It Together feature at the end of this chapter).

Criteria for Substance Use Disorder

The *DSM-5tr* diagnostic criteria for substance use disorder include impaired control; continued use of the substance despite negative social, occupational, and health consequences; risky use; and evidence of tolerance or withdrawal (see Figure 11.3).

THE POWER OF WORDS

SUBSTANCE USE DISORDER

Before the publication of *DSM-5*, psychopathologists categorized substance use into the two categories of substance abuse and substance addiction. In *DSM-5* they combined these different terms into a single condition called *substance use disorder* that describes problematic substance use along a continuum of severity. But why the shift in language? The reason was the power of words.

Terms like alcoholic, addict, substance addiction, and substance abuse are certainly still in use. There is evidence, however, that using these terms can create stigma, since they highlight personality aspects of an individual rather than putting the focus on the disorder itself. Referring to someone as an addict labels them as a person who is choosing that behavior. Such labels can also have an impact on the way family and friends see the person's behavior, the person's willingness to seek treatment, and even the treatment they receive. For example, in one recent study of more than 500 mental health practitioners, participants reviewed two case studies, identical except that the subject of one case was described as a "substance abuser" and the subject of the other as "having a substance use disorder." The participants were then asked for treatment recommendations. Those who received the case featuring a "substance abuser" were more likely to suggest jail or community service rather than continued treatment.

> The American Society of Addiction Medicine has encouraged using precise and non-stigmatizing terminology as much as possible, such as the *DSM* does by using the term substance use disorder.
>
> *Sources: Botticelli & Koh (2016); Saitz et al. (2021).*

Mechanism of Action of Psychoactive Drugs

Mechanism of action (MOA): a description of the way a drug functions.

The **mechanism of action (MOA)** of a drug describes the way the drug functions. The mechanism of action of most psychoactive drugs is their effect on neurotransmitters, the chemical messengers of the nervous system (see Chapter 2 for more information about neurotransmitters). Psychoactive drugs can influence the functioning of the nervous system in various ways. They can:

- Block the action of neurotransmitters.
- Prevent reuptake, causing excess neurotransmitters to flood the synaptic gap.
- Increase the effect of a neurotransmitter.
- Decrease the effect of a neurotransmitter.
- Bind to receptor sites normally used by neurotransmitters.

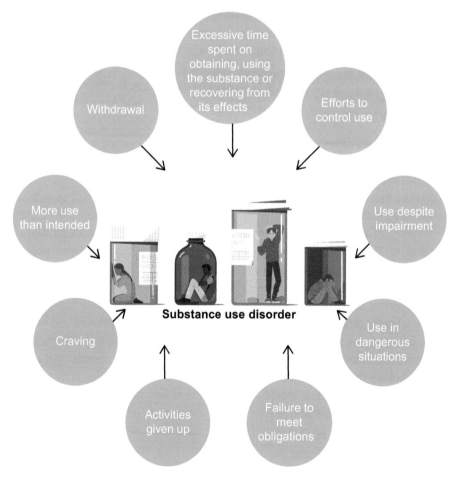

Figure 11.3 Criteria for substance use disorders.

Many psychoactive drugs influence the neurotransmitter dopamine, associated with the nervous system's reward structure, which can make the drugs highly addictive. In general, there are three main classes of psychoactive drugs: depressants, which reduce activity in the nervous system; stimulants, which increase activity in the nervous system; and hallucinogens, which distort conscious experiences. *DSM* organizes the substance use disorders into 10 substances in several different classes, as listed below.

- Central nervous system depressants (alcohol, barbiturates, benzodiazepines, and inhalants).
- Central nervous system stimulants (cocaine, amphetamines, nicotine, and caffeine).
- Opioids (includes heroin and morphine).
- Hallucinogens and phencyclidine (PCP).
- Cannabis.
- Others.

Controlled Substances

Many substances in this chapter are *controlled substances* in the United States; that is, they are drugs regulated by the Controlled Substances Act (1970). This Act sorts substances that have the potential for abuse and dependence into five different lists, or schedules, based on their danger (risk for abuse and addiction) (Table 11.1). Schedule I includes the drugs with the highest risk. However, other factors also influence the way certain drugs are classified, and it's important to be aware of the

Table 11.1 Schedules of controlled substances

Schedule	Definition	Federally accepted medical use?	Examples
Schedule I	High potential for abuse	no	Gamma-hydroxybutyric acid (GHB) Heroin Lysergic acid diethylamide (LSD) Marijuana
Schedule II	High potential for abuse but also accepted medical use, often with severe restrictions	yes	Cocaine Methadone Methamphetamine Morphine Phencyclidine (PCP)
Schedule III	Less potential for abuse	yes	Anabolic steroids Barbiturates Codeine Hydrocodone
Schedule IV	Lower potential for abuse	yes	Darvon Valium Xanax
Schedule V	Low potential for abuse but may result in limited physical or psychological dependence	yes	Cough medicines with codeine

Source: www.dea.gov/drug-information/drug-scheduling

way these policies may affect minoritized communities in unequal ways, increasing stigma and leading to more scrutiny by law enforcement. In the following sections we discuss the substance use disorders as described in the *DSM-5tr*.

CONCEPT CHECK 11.1

Identify the symptom of substance use disorder in each example below.
1. Brad has been drinking two pots of coffee every morning. When he doesn't, he experiences severe headaches, tiredness, and irritability to the point that it interferes with his work.
2. Although Kelvin said he would smoke marijuana only on the weekends, he finds that he smokes it every day.
3. Lisa goes to parties nearly every weekend with her friends. While there she drinks to the point of intoxication, and most weekends she drives while still intoxicated.
4. Stan has been on pain medication (opioids) for several months. He has obtained prescriptions for his pain medication from several different prescribers in order to increase his supply. Because of his opioid use, he has missed work and has neglected his family

11.2 DEPRESSANTS

Depressant: a psychoactive substance that reduces activity in the nervous system.

Depressants work by reducing the level of activity in the nervous system. Those who use these drugs report feelings of reduced inhibition, reduced anxiety, and lethargy. Moderate use of depressants is associated with listlessness, confusion, slowed pulse and breathing, and impairments in coordination, memory, and judgment. Abuse of depressants can lead to addiction, insomnia, brain damage, and stress or damage to the liver as it attempts to clear the substance from the body. Heavy abuse of depressants can interfere with nervous system function, shut down the cardiovascular system, and cause death.

Depressants are among the drugs most likely to be associated with tolerance, withdrawal, and dependence. Some of the most commonly used depressants are alcohol and sedative-hypnotics and anxiolytics (antianxiety drugs).

Alcohol Use Disorder

Alcohol is an ethanol-containing beverage that may be wine, beer, or a liquor such as vodka, gin, or whiskey. The stomach's lining absorbs alcohol into the blood, which carries it into the central nervous system where it acts on the brain. Stimulation is an initial effect of drinking alcohol. People often feel a sense of wellbeing and reduced inhibitions, and some may feel more outgoing. Over time, however, alcohol starts to depress more areas of the brain and can begin to interfere with the judgment and functions of other parts of the body, including motor coordination and sensory functions such as vision and hearing.

The intoxicating effects of alcohol begin to decline as the liver metabolizes the alcohol and blood alcohol levels go down. While the rate of metabolism varies from person to person, alcohol is typically removed at a rate of 25 percent of an ounce per hour. A pint of beer can take about two hours to metabolize, while a glass of wine takes about three hours to metabolize. The more drinks you have, the longer it can take for the alcohol to be removed from your blood. Those with *alcohol withdrawal* experience a number of symptoms, from mild to serious (Diagnostic Overview 11.1). Mild symptoms can appear as soon as six hours after the last drink and can include sweating, vomiting and nausea, headache, inability to sleep, shaking hands, and anxiety. Serious withdrawal symptoms can occur later (within 12–24 hours) and can include hallucinations or seizures. *Delirium tremens* (DT) can begin 48–72 hours after the last drink and include confusion, fever, or racing heart.

The brain and nervous system make use of a few all-purpose neurotransmitters: gamma aminobutyric acid (GABA) for inhibition and glutamate for excitation. Alcohol increases the power of GABA, making it work better. In addition, it can reduce the effectiveness of glutamate, an all-purpose excitatory neurotransmitter. The result is that alcohol will depress activity in certain regions of the brain and generally inhibit the nervous system, slowing everything down. This results in the telltale symptoms of alcohol intoxication, including slurred speech, impulsiveness, and impairments in balance. Heavy use of alcohol can cause a slowing down of the central nervous system, including the nerves that control breathing and the gag reflex. Large enough amounts of alcohol can stop these functions, which is why passing out from excessive alcohol use can be so dangerous.

One factor that can affect a person's ability to become intoxicated is whether the stomach is filled with food or not. The fuller a person's stomach, the longer it takes to absorb alcohol into the bloodstream, slowing any effects of intoxication. This is why it's dangerous to drink on an empty stomach.

Alcohol can have long-term effects on the brain and the body. MRI scans of those with chronic drinking problems show some evidence of damage to structures that regulate balance, attention, and memory.

Diagnostic Overview 11.1: Alcohol Use Disorder

A problematic pattern of alcohol use is manifested by at least two of the following:

- Consumption of more alcohol or drinking over a longer period of time than intended.
- Unsuccessful efforts to cut down or control alcohol use.
- A great deal of time spent in activities necessary to obtain or use the substance or recover from its effects.
- Craving for alcohol.
- Alcohol use that results in missed obligations at work, school, or home.
- Continued alcohol use despite interpersonal problems caused by it.
- Alcohol use in situations in which it is dangerous.
- Tolerance: a need for more alcohol for intoxication or less of an effect when using the same amount of alcohol.
- Withdrawal: Characteristics of withdrawal syndrome for alcohol or alcohol use to relieve or avoid withdrawal symptoms.

Severity is gauged by the number of symptoms:

- Mild: 2–3 symptoms.
- Moderate: 4–5 symptoms.
- Severe: 6 or more.

Impact: Symptoms must exceed cultural and contextual norms. Symptoms are related to clinically significant distress or create impairment in important areas of life such as with friends and family or at work or school.

Timeframe: 12 months.

Source: Information from APA (2022).

SYMPTOMS AND DESCRIPTION

Alcohol use disorder: a substance-related disorder associated with impaired control over the amount and frequency with which they drink and often experience negative emotional states when they aren't drinking.

Those with **alcohol use disorder** have impaired control over the amount and frequency with which they drink and often experience negative emotional states when they aren't drinking. Their use of alcohol affects their ability to work and engage effectively in social interactions. They regularly fail to meet work or social obligations and experience an often-escalating pattern of use despite the negative consequences.

Case Study: Alcohol Use Disorder – "Buzz" Aldrin

Edwin "Buzz" Aldrin, Jr. (Figure 11.4), member of NASA's Apollo 11 mission, was the second human ever to step on the moon. Yet he reports having sometimes felt particularly worthless since then, especially in regard to his career, and turning to alcohol when things weren't going well. He says he was in a cycle in which he would drink to feel "less down," which would, in turn, make him feel even worse, so he would drink even more. He frequently drank in the morning to avoid hangovers from drinking the previous day.

Aldrin first began to have periods of increased stress after the Apollo mission, when he felt pressure to talk about his experience with NASA and was under more scrutiny than ever before. He began drinking as a social activity, for fun or to celebrate an accomplishment, and occasionally to help him relax from a long or stressful day at work. Over time his alcohol use stopped being recreational, and he started using alcohol to temper his moods. When others were drinking coffee, he might have a scotch. He also increased his drinking after his father's death and admits to driving while intoxicated, causing a car accident when his wife was in the car with him.

Source: Aldrin & Abraham (2009).

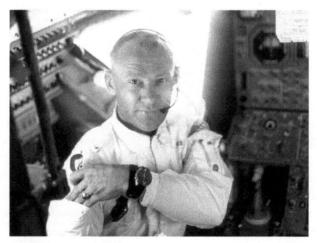

Figure 11.4 Buzz Aldrin.
Source: Neil Armstrong/Space Frontiers/Getty Images.

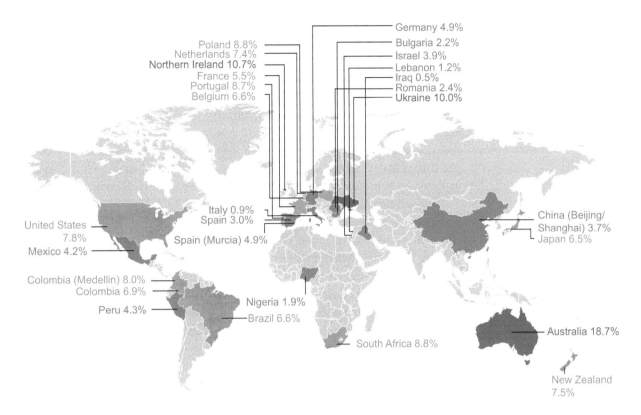

Figure 11.5 Lifetime prevalence of alcohol disorders in selected countries, from the World Mental Health Surveys (2002–2017).

Source: Data from Glantz et al. (2020).

STATISTICS AND TRAJECTORY

Alcohol use is common over the world. The World Health Organization (WHO) estimates nearly 2 billion people worldwide use alcohol (SAMHSA 2017). Surveys suggest that as much as 7.8 percent of the United States population will have symptoms of alcohol use disorder in any given year (Glantz et al. 2020). As Figure 11.5 shows, rates for other countries can range from 0.5 of the population (Iraq) to 18.7 (Australia) (Glantz et al. 2020).

Symptoms of alcohol use disorder tend to emerge between 16 and 20 years worldwide. Men diagnosed with the disorder outnumber women about 5 to 1 (Glantz et al. 2020). However, alcohol use among women, including binge drinking, and alcohol use disorder, is increasing (Glantz et al. 2020). Rates of alcohol use disorder differ among racial and ethnic groups. For example, they are around 6.1 percent for non-Hispanic whites, 6.4 for Hispanic Americans, 4.9 for Black Americans, and 9.7 for American Indians (SAMHSA 2017).

Sedative-Hypnotic-Anxiolytic-Related Disorders

Alcohol isn't the only commonly used depressant substance. The class of depressant substances also includes anxiolytic sedatives such as benzodiazepines (which are calming and can reduce anxiety) and tranquilizers such as hypnotics (which induce sleep), as well as barbiturates.

Sedatives include the barbiturates and sedative hypnotics that are often prescribed for insomnia. *Barbiturates* are a type of depressant drug that reduces stress and induces sleep. Barbiturates such as pentobarbital (Nembutal) and secobarbital (Seconal) have been available for well over 150 years. They were most popular in the early 1900s to help with anxiety and sleep problems and were seen as alternatives to alcohol and opium. By the 1950s, however, their safety record had become tarnished as people began to understand the risks of tolerance and dependence; barbiturates were then some of the most abused substances in the United States. Although they are still prescribed today, they have been largely replaced by benzodiazepines as the most prescribed sedative hypnotic.

Tranquilizers are medications often prescribed to treat muscle spasms and anxiety. The most common substances in this category are the benzodiazepines. *Benzodiazepines* are a group of central nervous system depressants used for treating insomnia, anxiety, and seizures and include medications such as diazepam (Valium), alprazolam (Xanax), and lorazepam (Ativan). Although they are safer than barbiturates, they can still be abused. By 2019 more than 85 million prescriptions for benzodiazepines were being written in the United States each year (Hirschtritt et al. 2021). In 2021 the United States FDA updated its warning for all benzodiazepines to address the serious risk of abuse, addiction, physical dependence, and withdrawal reactions (Knopf 2021).

At lower dosages, both barbiturates and benzodiazepines produce a calming effect. They can relax the muscles, and some people report a general feeling of wellbeing. At higher doses, however, they produce intoxication symptoms similar to those from higher doses of alcohol (see Diagnostic Overview 11.1).

Barbiturate withdrawal can include agitation, anxiety, nausea, tremors, hallucinations, fever, and even death. Symptoms of benzodiazepine withdrawal include low mood, anxiety, muscle spasms, insomnia, nausea, and seizures. Symptoms can begin on the second day after cessation and may last several weeks. Between 10 and 25 percent of persistent benzodiazepine users re-experience withdrawal symptoms that can last for months but often resolve within a year.

Medications such as barbiturates and benzodiazepines act on the GABA system in a different way than alcohol does. Unlike alcohol, benzodiazepines can reduce anxiety without making people feel sleepy or reducing breathing, so they are less likely to cause problems with overdose. However, like barbiturates, benzodiazepines can also lead to decreases in blood pressure, heart rate, and respiratory rate. For this reason, people who use alcohol with either barbiturates or benzodiazepines can experience a potentially dangerous additive effect. Benzodiazepines increase the frequency of GABA receptor openings, and barbiturates increase the duration of opening, both actions that result in increased stimulation of the neuron. Over time the GABA-A response changes, leading to symptoms of withdrawal and tolerance. Symptoms of benzodiazepine intoxication include slurred speech, lack of coordination, impairment in attention or memory, stupor, and coma.

SYMPTOMS AND DESCRIPTION

High doses of benzodiazepines can lead to symptoms of sedative-hypnotic use disorder, in which a person experiences increases in cravings for the substances. People who stop using these substances experience symptoms much like those of alcohol withdrawal (anxiety and insomnia). The diagnosis of **sedative, hypnotic, or anxiolytic use disorder** is similar to the diagnoses of other substance use disorders. People experience both behavioral and physical symptoms, as you can see from the diagnostic criteria in Diagnostic Overview 11.2. Sedatives, hypnotics, and anxiolytics are also associated with symptoms of intoxication and withdrawal (Table 11.2).

Sedative, hypnotic, or anxiolytic use disorder: a substance-related disorder associated with impaired control over the amount and frequency of sedatives, hypnotics, or anxiolytics use and the experience of negative emotional states when not using those substances.

STATISTICS AND TRAJECTORY

According to the National Survey on Drug Use and Health, in 2017 about 15 percent of adults in the United States reported having used prescription benzodiazepines in the last year, and 6.5 percent reported using barbiturates or sedative hypnotics (SAMHSA 2018). Of those who reported using this class

---

Diagnostic Overview 11.2: Sedative, Hypnotic, or Anxiolytic Use Disorder

---

A problematic pattern of sedative, hypnotic, or anxiolytic use as manifested by at least two of the following:

- Use over a longer period of time than intended.
- Unsuccessful efforts to cut down or control use.
- A great deal of time spent in activities necessary to obtain or use the substance or recover from its effects.
- Cravings for the substance.
- Recurrent use which results in missing obligations at work, school, or home.
- Continued use despite interpersonal problems caused by it.
- Reduced or missed social, occupational, or recreational activities because of sedative, hypnotic, or anxiolytic use.
- Recurrent sedative, hypnotic, or anxiolytic use in situations in which it is dangerous.
- Continued sedative, hypnotic, or anxiolytic use despite problems caused by it.
- Tolerance: a need for more sedative, hypnotic, or anxiolytic or less of an effect when using the same amount of sedative, hypnotic, or anxiolytic.
- Withdrawal: Characteristics of withdrawal syndrome for sedative, hypnotic, or anxiolytic use (see Table 11.2) to relieve or avoid withdrawal symptoms.

Severity is gauged by the number of symptoms:

- Mild: Presence of 2–3 symptoms.
- Moderate: Presence of 4–5 symptoms.
- Severe: Presence of 6 or more symptoms.
- **Impact:** Symptoms must exceed cultural and contextual norms. Symptoms are related to clinically significant distress or create impairment in important areas of life such as with friends and family or at work or school.
- **Timeframe:** 12 months.

Source: Information from APA (2022).

Table 11.2 Symptoms of depressant intoxication and withdrawal

Substance	Intoxication	Withdrawal
Alcohol	Slurred speech Lack of coordination Unsteady gait Involuntary eye movements affecting vision (nystagmus) Impairment in attention or memory Stupor or coma	Hyperactivity Sweating Hand tremor Insomnia Nausea or vomiting Transient visual, tactile, or auditory hallucinations or illusions Psychomotor agitation Anxiety Seizures
Benzodiazepines	Sleepiness	Hand tremor
Barbiturates	Slurred speech Lack of coordination Unsteady gait Involuntary eye movements affecting vision (nystagmus) Stupor Coma	Insomnia Nausea Vomiting Hallucinations Anxiety Seizures
Sedative, Hypnotic, or Anxiolytic	Behavioral or psychological changes (such as inappropriate sexual or aggressive behavior, impaired judgment) Slurred speech. Lack of coordination Unsteady gait Involuntary eye movements affecting vision (nystagmus) Impaired cognition Stupor Coma	Sweating Increased heartbeat Hand tremor Insomnia Nausea or vomiting Transient visual, tactile, or auditory hallucinations or illusions Psychomotor agitation Anxiety Grand mal seizures

of prescription drugs, 14.8 percent did so in ways that weren't directed by doctors (SAMHSA 2018). Misuse of benzodiazepines accounted for 17.2 percent of total use.

Clinicians play an important role in providing patients access to these substances. Among those who misused sedatives, 42.6 percent reported obtaining them from a health care provider and 50.9 percent from a friend (sometimes without asking, but also often by purchasing from a friend or family member). Tranquilizers were obtained from a health care provider more than 80 percent of the time (SAMHSA 2018). Even when these medicines are needed, there can be unequal access to them. For example, there is evidence of racial bias in both the assessment and treatment recommendations for pain, based on longstanding false beliefs about differences in experience of pain in Black people. Such beliefs can lead health care workers to write fewer prescriptions for certain medications (Hoffman et al. 2016).

CONCEPT CHECK 11.2

For questions 1–3, indicate the symptom of alcohol use disorder described.
1. Buzz Aldrin admits driving while intoxicated and causing a car accident when his wife was in the car with him.
2. Finbar knows his alcohol use causes problems in his life. He has tried several times to cut back on the amount he drinks but finds that it is difficult to do so.
3. When Jane is at work and unable to drink, she craves alcohol and thinks about getting a drink for most of the morning.
4. True or false: barbiturates have been illegal drugs since their discovery.
5. True or false: benzodiazepines are prescribed to treat anxiety, seizures, and insomnia.

11.3   STIMULANTS

Stimulants are a group of psychoactive substances that increase activity in the central nervous system. This category includes caffeine, nicotine, amphetamines (such as methamphetamine), and cocaine. Small doses of stimulants can produce feelings of increased energy and euphoria, as well as lack of appetite and decreased need for sleep. Moderate doses can lead to *stimulant-induced psychosis*, marked by hallucinations and delusions (to read more about psychotic disorders, take a look at Chapter 13). Larger doses can bring about convulsions, cardiovascular failure, and even death. Stimulants are also associated with symptoms of intoxication and withdrawal (Diagnostic Overview 11.3).

By interacting with the central nervous system, stimulants can alter the electrical activity of the heart, increase blood pressure and heart rate, and cause a dangerous constriction of blood vessels, leading to heart attacks and seizures. They are some of the most used and abused substances in the United States. More than half of drug-related hospital visits are related to stimulant use (SAMHSA 2013).

Stimulants: psychoactive substances that increase activity in the nervous system.

Caffeine Intoxication

Caffeine is one of the most widely used stimulants in the world. It's present in a variety of products including chocolate, coffee, tea, nonprescription medications, and energy drinks. Caffeine stimulates the cerebral

Diagnostic Overview 11.3: Caffeine Intoxication

Consumption of caffeine along with five or more of the following symptoms:

- Increase in urination.
- Increase in excitement.
- Feelings of warmth and rapid reddening of neck, upper chest, or face.
- Gastrointestinal problems.
- Problems getting or staying asleep.
- Muscle twitching.
- Nervousness.
- Periods of inexhaustibility.
- Psychomotor agitation.
- Rambling flow of thought and speech.
- Restlessness.
- Rapid heartbeat.

Impact: Symptoms must exceed cultural and contextual norms. Symptoms are related to clinically significant distress or create impairment in important areas of life such as with friends and family or at work or school.

Source: Information from APA (2022).

cortex and boosts energy and alertness. Even small doses can stay in your system for up to four hours. Mild doses taken too late in the day can impair sleep, and higher doses can lead to anxiety, headaches, and digestive problems. If you feel like you need to reduce your caffeine intake, do it slowly; rapid decreases in caffeine consumption can lead to lethargy, headaches, and difficulty concentrating.

Tobacco Use Disorder

About one in four US adults smoke or vape tobacco. The psychoactive substance in tobacco is a naturally occurring amount of *nicotine*, which reduces activity in many areas of the brain including the amygdala, hippocampus, and frontal lobes (Sharma & Brody 2009). A dose of nicotine can stimulate the central nervous system in less than seven seconds and boost release of the neurotransmitter dopamine, increasing energy, pain tolerance, and alertness and reducing anxiety, appetite, and anger (Heishman et al. 2010) (Diagnostic Overview 11.4). The use of tobacco is also related to the onset of many preventable diseases, such as lung cancer and chronic obstructive pulmonary disease (COPD), and each year 4.5 million tobacco users die from a variety of tobacco-related illness. It is very difficult to stop using tobacco products. Quitting can cause days or weeks of anxiety, irritability, and cravings, while the mood-boosting effects of nicotine last only about 30 minutes.

Diagnostic Overview 11.4: Tobacco Use Disorder

A problematic pattern of tobacco use including at least two of the following:

- Tobacco used over a longer period of time than intended.
- Unsuccessful efforts to cut down or control tobacco use.
- A great deal of time spent in activities necessary to obtain or use tobacco.
- Cravings for tobacco.
- Tobacco use resulting in failure to meet obligations at work, school, or home.
- Continued tobacco use despite problems.
- Missed social, occupational, or recreational activities because of tobacco use.
- Tobacco use in situations in which it is dangerous.
- Continued tobacco use despite problems associated with it.
- Tolerance: a need for more tobacco for intoxication or less of an effect when using the same amount of tobacco.
- Withdrawal: Characteristics of withdrawal syndrome for tobacco or tobacco use to relieve or avoid withdrawal symptoms.

Severity is gauged by the number of symptoms:

- Mild: Presence of 2–3 symptoms.
- Moderate: Presence of 4–5 symptoms.

Impact: Symptoms must exceed cultural and contextual norms. Symptoms are related to clinically significant distress or create impairment in important areas of life such as with friends and family or at work or school.

Timeframe: 12 months.

Source: Information from APA (2022).

Cocaine and Methamphetamine

Cocaine is a powerful natural stimulant. It is derived from the flowering coco plant of South America, where the early Andean people had found that chewing the leaves reduced fatigue and hunger. In the United States in the late 1800s, cocaine was widely available in cigars, cigarettes, and even beverages, including the original formulation of Coca-Cola (Figure 11.6). When processed it becomes a white, fluffy powder that today is inhaled (snorted), injected, or smoked (Biondich & Joslin 2016).

Cocaine, a Schedule II drug, confers increased energy, feelings of euphoria, and decreased appetite, alertness, and anxiety. Long-term use and abuse can result in dependence, depression, tremors, hallucinations, and convulsions. At higher doses people are more impulsive and more sexual and feel increased agitation, panic, and paranoia.

Cocaine can increase the availability of dopamine and norepinephrine in the body by blocking the transport proteins that normally clear these neurotransmitters from the synaptic cleft. This allows dopamine, a neurotransmitter linked to pleasure, to bind with the dopamine receptor sites over and over, which in turn creates a sense of pleasure.

Methamphetamine is a stimulant drug associated with increased nervous system activity and elevated libido and self-esteem. Like cocaine, methamphetamine also interacts with the neurotransmitter dopamine. Methamphetamine resembles dopamine, and for that reason it is easily reabsorbed into the presynaptic neuron by the same reuptake transport proteins that normally recycle dopamine neurotransmitters. Once inside the presynaptic neuron, methamphetamine gets packaged into synaptic vesicles and displaces the dopamine. Dopamine then builds up at the end of the presynaptic neuron, causing the transport proteins to reverse and pump it back into the synaptic gap. Once the dopamine gets trapped in the synaptic gap, it binds to receptor sites on the postsynaptic neuron over and over again and overstimulates the system.

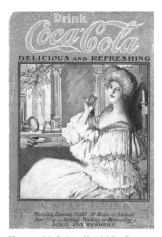

Figure 11.6 Until 1903, Coca-Cola contained small amounts of cocaine. This advertisement is from 1880.
Source: Bettmann/Getty Images.

Symptoms and Description: Stimulant Use Disorder

Stimulant use disorders are characterized by symptoms similar to those of other substance use disorders (see Diagnostic Overview 11.5 and Table 11.3).

Diagnostic Overview 11.5: Stimulant Use Disorder

A problematic pattern of stimulant use manifested by at least two of the following:

- Stimulant used over a longer period of time than intended.
- Unsuccessful efforts to cut down or control use.
- A great deal of time spent in activities necessary to obtain or use stimulants or recover from their effects.
- Cravings for stimulants.
- Stimulant use that results in missed obligations at work, school, or home.
- Continued stimulant use despite interpersonal problems caused by it.
- Stimulant use in situations in which it is dangerous.
- Tolerance: a need for more of the stimulant for intoxication or less of an effect when using the same amount of stimulant.
- Withdrawal: Characteristics of withdrawal syndrome for stimulants (see Table 11.3) or stimulant use to relieve or avoid withdrawal symptoms.

Severity is gauged by the number of symptoms:

- Mild: Presence of 2–3 symptoms.
- Moderate: Presence of 4–5 symptoms.
- Severe: Presence of 6 or more symptoms.

Impact: Symptoms must exceed cultural and contextual norms. Symptoms are related to clinically significant distress or create impairment in important areas of life such as with friends and family or at work or school.

Timeframe: 12 months.

Source: Information from APA (2022).

Table 11.3 Symptoms of stimulant intoxication and withdrawal

Drug	Intoxication	Withdrawal
Amphetamine-type substance, cocaine, or other stimulant	Euphoria Flat moods Changes in sociability Hypervigilance Interpersonal sensitivity Anxiety, tension, or anger Impaired judgment Dilated pupils Elevated or lowered blood pressure Perspiration or chills Nausea or vomiting Evidence of weight loss Psychomotor agitation or retardation. Muscular weakness, respiratory depression, chest pain, or cardiac arrhythmias Confusion, seizures, or coma	Dysphoric mood Fatigue Vivid, unpleasant dreams Insomnia or hypersomnia Increased appetite Psychomotor retardation or agitation

Statistics and Trajectory: Stimulant Use Disorder

Statistics from the Substance Abuse and Mental Health Services Administration suggest that in 2017, about 1 percent of those aged 12 and over in the United States (2.2 million people) reported cocaine use; 774,00 used methamphetamines; and 1.8 million used prescription stimulants (SAMHSA 2018). This represents a stark increase from 2014. Cocaine/crack use was up 10 percent, methamphetamine use up 14 percent, and prescription stimulant use up 6 percent since 2014 (Brady et al. 2021).

CONCEPT CHECK 11.3

1. Like cocaine, methamphetamine also interacts with the neurotransmitter _____.
2. List three effects associated with cocaine use.
3. Which psychoactive substance is the most commonly used in the United States?

11.4 OPIOIDS AND OPIOID USE DISORDER

Opioids: psychoactive substances made from the opium poppy that relieve pain and reduce the activity of the nervous system.

When we are in pain, our bodies produce compounds to help reduce the discomfort, such as endorphins. This relief also can come from substances outside our bodies, called opioids, that operate in a similar manner. **Opioids** are psychoactive substances made from the opium poppy that relieve pain and reduce the activity of the nervous system. The sap from the poppy has been used for centuries for relief of acute pain. Opioids are also associated with symptoms of intoxication and withdrawal (Table 11.4).

Until some 30 years ago, physicians were encouraged to prescribe opioids for both acute and persistent pain because at the time there was little evidence for addiction (Berrettini 2017). However, researchers soon realized that opioid drugs are not only powerful pain killers; they are also some of the most addictive substances we have (Volkow et al. 2019). For a single prescription opioid, OxyContin, sales mushroomed from 47 million in the mid-1990s to nearly 1.1 billion in 2000, and in 2004 it became one of the most prescribed medications in the United States (Mendoza & Russell 2020). By 2020 more than 700,000 people in the United States had experienced an opioid overdose (Mendoza & Russell 2020; Volkow et al. 2019).

Table 11.4 Symptoms of opioid intoxication and withdrawal

Drug	Intoxication	Withdrawal
Opioids	Initial euphoria	Dysphoric mood
	Apathy	Nausea or vomiting
	Dysphoria	Muscle aches
	Impaired judgment	Dilated pupils
	Constricted pupils	Sweating
	Drowsiness	Diarrhea
	Slurred speech	Yawning
	Impaired attention	Fever
		Insomnia

Morphine, heroin, codeine, and methadone are all opioids. *Morphine* (named after Morpheus, the Greek god of sleep) was developed in the 1800s. Considered a safer alternative to opium at the time, it was commonly used for pain relief until its addictive nature was discovered. Later a new variety of opium called *heroin* was believed to be so safe that it was used in cough medicines. Soon it too was discovered to be highly addictive.

There are various ways to use opioids. They may be injected directly into veins, smoked, or inhaled through the nose (snorted). The first sensations people report are tingling and warmth. Some describe a flash of pleasure not unlike an orgasm, called a "thrill" or "flash," followed by sedation that may be accompanied by slurred speech. Heroin isn't always pure; it is often combined with other substances such as fentanyl, so it is difficult to predict its strength, which makes it easier to overdose or have unexpected side effects. Contaminated needles are also a concern when the drugs are injected, because they can spread blood-borne infections such as HIV, hepatitis, skin abscesses, and infections. Some users who trade sex for heroin put themselves at even greater risk for sexually transmitted diseases such as HIV. Up to 60 percent of chronic heroin users may be HIV-positive (Hodder et al. 2021).

Severe opioid intoxication is associated with suppression of the nervous system, loss of consciousness, seizures, and coma. The nervous system may be so suppressed that it can lead to death, especially if opioids are combined with other drugs that also suppress the nervous system, such as depressants.

Non-prescribed opioids are not the only such substance at risk for abuse. Prescription opioids such as Oxycodone and Vicodin can also be problematic. And there is evidence that pharmaceutical companies have encouraged the dispensing of prescriptions without regard to the possibility of patient dependence (Celentano 2020). In 2016, at least 11.5 million people over the age of 12 in the United States met the criteria for opioid use disorders.

Opioid withdrawal can increase pain sensitivity and spark a craving for more opioids. Nausea, sweating, fever, and gastrointestinal distress such as diarrhea and vomiting may also occur. Some withdrawal symptoms appear within eight hours after last use and can be at their worst between 36 and 72 hours. In heavy users the symptoms can last for five to seven days and may even persist for weeks and months. Opioid withdrawal can be unpleasant enough that some users will choose to continue their use of the drug despite a desire to stop.

Opioids decrease activity in the central nervous system, especially activity involved in emotions. They can thus decrease emotions such as sadness and fear and increase emotions such as pleasure. The molecules of opioids bind to receptors that typically connect where natural endorphins bind. When opioids bind to these sites, they produce a pleasurable calming, similar to the action of endorphins.

Symptoms and Description: Opioid Use Disorder

People with opioid use disorder experience problematic use of opioids along with at least two of the symptoms of substance use disorder (Diagnostic Overview 11.6 and Table 11.4).

Diagnostic Overview 11.6: Opioid Use Disorder

A problematic pattern of opioid use, manifested by at least two of the following:

- Drug often taken in larger amounts or over a longer period than was intended.
- A persistent desire or unsuccessful efforts to cut down or control opioid use.
- A great deal of time spent in activities necessary to obtain or use the opioid or recover from its effects.
- Craving, or a strong desire or urge to use opioids.
- Recurrent opioid use, resulting in a failure to fulfill major role obligations at work, school, or home.
- Continued opioid use despite persistent or recurrent social or interpersonal problems caused or exacerbated by the effects of use.
- Missed or reduced social, occupational, or recreational activities because of opioid use.
- Recurrent opioid use in situations in which it is physically hazardous.
- Continued opioid use despite knowledge of a persistent or recurrent physical or psychological problem that is likely to have been caused or exacerbated by the substance.
- Tolerance: a need for more opioid for intoxication or less of an effect when using the same amount of opioids.
- Withdrawal: Characteristics of withdrawal syndrome for opioids (see Table 11.4) or opioids' use to relieve or avoid withdrawal symptoms.

Severity is gauged by the number of symptoms:

- Mild: Presence of 2–3 symptoms.
- Moderate: Presence of 4–5 symptoms.
- Severe: Presence of 6 or more symptoms.

Impact: Symptoms must exceed cultural and contextual norms. Symptoms are related to clinically significant distress or create impairment in important areas of life such as with friends and family or at work or school.

Timeframe: 12 months.

Source: Information from APA (2022).

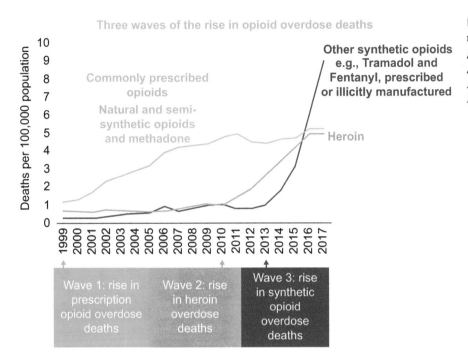

Figure 11.7 Three waves of the rise in opioid overdose deaths.

Source: National Vital Statistics System Mortality File, adapted from Mendoza & Russell (2020).

Statistics and Trajectory: Opioid Use Disorder

In 2019 in the United States, 5.7 million people (2.1 percent of those 12 or older) were estimated to have used heroin at some point in their lives (Strain 2021). Since 1999 there have been more than 700,000 overdoses of opioids, and opioid use disorder has been called a public health epidemic. Looking at deaths from all substances, two of three in some way involved an opioid (Mendoza & Russell 2020) such as heroin, commonly prescribed opioids, and synthetic opioids (see Figure 11.7). Some researchers suggested that the limits insurance companies have placed on reimbursement for behavioral treatments for pain, combined with the pharmaceutical industry's production and promotion of opioids, may in part be responsible for the proliferation of opioid prescriptions (Mendoza & Russell 2020).

Case Study: Opioid Use Disorder – Anthony Kiedis

Anthony Kiedis (Figure 11.8), a founding member of the Rock and Roll Hall of Fame band The Red Hot Chili Peppers, started experimenting with drugs in early childhood, beginning with marijuana at age 8, which he tried under his father's supervision. He continued using marijuana, prescription drugs, and alcohol through most of his teen years and first tried heroin at 14 with some of his father's friends.

By the time Kiedis was in college, heroin had begun to interfere with his ability to do well in school. He started skipping classes and was spending most of his time partying and going out with his friends instead of studying. By the age of 19 he had dropped out of UCLA and was working and doing drugs.

Eventually he recruited friends to start a band that eventually became The Red Hot Chili Peppers. With success came money, and money brought more access to heroin, which Kiedis would spend days at a time using or looking for. The only thing that stopped him was going on tour with the band. However, despite losing a close friend to an overdose of the drug, each time he returned from a tour he would immediately start using heroin again. Eventually, Kiedis' heroin intoxication caused problems with his performance, and withdrawal was so painful that he was incapacitated for days at a time. This finally led to his being fired from the band, a low point in his life. He went to rehab to try to recover and was allowed back into the band after he had been sober for 90 days. However, he relapsed and started using heroin again regularly.

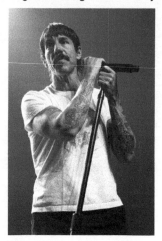

Figure 11.8 Anthony Kiedis. *Source: Scott Dudelson/Getty Images.*

We'll come back to Kiedis' story later in the chapter. To read more about Anthony Kiedis take a look at his memoir, *Scar tissue* (Kiedis & Sloman 2004).

CONCEPT CHECK 11.4

1. True or false: Your body contains natural opioids that reduce the sensation of pain.
2. Which of these substances are classified as opiates?

   Codeine
   Heroin
   Morphine
   Cocaine

3. True or false: Xavier is experiencing opioid withdrawal. He can expect to have an increased sensitivity to pain and to crave the substance.

11.5   CANNABIS AND CANNABIS-RELATED DISORDERS

Cannabis sativa: a plant that contains the psychoactive substance tetrahydrocannabinol (THC).

Cannabis sativa is also referred to as the hemp plant (Figure 11.9). It contains hundreds of chemicals, although tetrahydrocannabinol (THC) appears to be the ingredient responsible for many of its sought-after effects. The amount of THC present in the plant depends on a number of factors, including the climate where the plant was grown and the maturity of the buds and flowers when harvested, as well as how long the plant was stored. The more THC, the more powerful the effect; potent varieties such as hashish have more THC.

Cannabis has aspects of hallucinogens, depressants, and stimulant substances. Like other drugs, it can be taken orally in a pill or in foods, or as an inhalant when its vapors are breathed in (via smoking) to produce its effect.

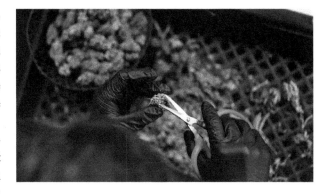

Figure 11.9 Employees pack and label jars of green buds at the Oakland, CA location of NUG, a cannabis dispensary.
Source: Marcos Borsatto/ EyeEm/Getty Images.

THC has both mild painkilling and stimulating effects on the nervous system. Although individual reactions can vary, symptoms of cannabis intoxication include changes in mood, dreamlike states, and heightened sensory experiences. Most effects can last up to six hours, with changes in mood persisting a bit longer. Low doses can lead to increased heart rate and altered perceptions, often making those who have taken it feel relaxed, sleepy, and content. They may spontaneously laugh, have disconnected rambling thoughts, and experience a distortion of time. Some become so groggy they fall asleep. Others can become anxious or irritable. Some also report increased sensory perceptions and become preoccupied by sights or sounds. Time slows and distances may feel magnified. Physical changes include red eyes, increased heartbeat, blood pressure, dry mouth, dizziness, and increased appetite.

With higher doses people may experience changes in the way they perceive their bodies or even have hallucinations. Some may feel paranoid and believe others are trying to hurt them. While some research suggests that marijuana can cause problems with long-term memory and motor coordination, other studies comparing nonusers and long-term users find only minor impairments in memory and learning (Grant et al. 2003).

Cannabis can cause problems with cognitive focus and tasks that require motor coordination. It can be difficult to drive under its influence, for example, but 4.7 percent of US adults say they have driven in this impaired state (Azofeifa et al. 2019). Cannabis can also impair concentration and creativity, leading to problems with work and school performance.

Although cannabis has been harvested for centuries, its use has only recently been tied to substance use conditions. Withdrawal effects can include insomnia, restlessness, irritability, flu-like symptoms, and gastrointestinal disturbances including nausea and loss of appetite. There is mixed evidence about the development of cannabis tolerance. Some chronic smokers report needing more of the drug to experience the euphoric highs of earlier use (Mason et al. 2021). Other longer-term users report experiencing more euphoria from smaller doses over time, called *reverse tolerance*

Diagnostic Overview 11.7: **Cannabis Use Disorder**

A problematic pattern of cannabis use as manifested by at least two of the following:

- Cannabis used in larger amounts or over longer periods of time than intended.
- Unsuccessful efforts to cut down or control cannabis use.
- A great deal of time spent in activities necessary to obtain or use cannabis or recover from its effects.
- Cravings.
- Cannabis use that results in missing obligations at work, school, or home.
- Continued cannabis use despite persistent or recurrent social or interpersonal problems caused or exacerbated by its effects.
- Continued cannabis use despite interpersonal problems caused by it.
- Cannabis use in situations in which it might be dangerous.
- Continued cannabis use despite physical or psychological problems caused by it.
- Tolerance: a need for more cannabis or less of an effect when using the same amount.
- Withdrawal: Characteristics of withdrawal syndrome for cannabis or cannabis use to relieve or avoid withdrawal symptoms.

Severity is gauged by the number of symptoms:

- Mild: Presence of 2–3 symptoms.
- Moderate: Presence of 4–5 symptoms.
- Severe: Presence of 6 or more symptoms.

Impact: Symptoms must exceed cultural and contextual norms. Symptoms are related to clinically significant distress or create impairment in important areas of life such as with friends and family or at work or school.

Timeframe: 12 months.

Source: Information from APA (2022).

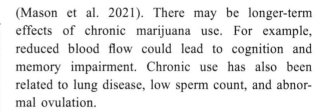

(Mason et al. 2021). There may be longer-term effects of chronic marijuana use. For example, reduced blood flow could lead to cognition and memory impairment. Chronic use has also been related to lung disease, low sperm count, and abnormal ovulation.

Symptoms and Description: Cannabis Use Disorder

People with cannabis use disorder display problematic use of cannabis (Diagnostic Overview 11.7).

Statistics and Trajectory: Cannabis Use Disorder

Cannabis was widely popular in the 1960s and 1970s; its popularity has since declined, but the drug remains one of the most commonly used psychoactive substances in the United States, where up to 15 percent of people over 12 (22 million) say they have used it in the last month. Some states now allow medical use of marijuana for benefits that include increased appetite and reduction of nausea, vomiting, tremors, and the number and severity of seizures. By 2020, more than 20 countries and more than 30 states in the United States had made at least some forms and amounts of marijuana legal for medical use or for personal consumption (Ferland & Hurd 2020). State laws aside, as of 2021 the federal government classifies cannabis as a Schedule I drug.

CONCEPT CHECK 11.5

1. _____ is the ingredient responsible for the psychoactive quality of cannabis.
2. True or false: Recent laws about cannabis have brought its use to an all-time high.

11.6 HALLUCINOGEN-RELATED DISORDERS

Hallucinogens are a class of psychoactive drugs that distort our conscious experiences and can produce changes in the way we perceive reality. While some drugs (such as alcohol) need to be taken in substantial amounts to produce such distortions, hallucinogens, also called psychedelics, easily create perceptual changes even in tiny doses. The term *psychedelic* was first used by psychiatrist Humphrey Osmond in 1956 and is derived from Greek *psyche* (soul or mind) and *delein* (to manifest or reveal), so the word translates to soul/mind revealing (Rucker et al. 2018).

People have used hallucinogenic agents for thousands of years in cultural and spiritual ceremonies to modify experience, often in surreal and inexpressible ways. Early use of plants with psychedelic properties can be traced back more than 5,700 years in Mexico (Rucker et al. 2018), pieces of peyote stored in caves in Texas have been dated to as early as 3780 BCE, and ancient Greek beverages may have contained traces of what we now call LSD (Johnson et al. 2019). The classic hallucinogens or psychedelics include mescaline, phencyclidine (PCP), lysergic acid diethylamide (LSD), peyote, and psilocybin mushrooms. Here we discuss the two most common, LSD and PCP.

In 1897 the Swiss chemist Dr. Albert Hoffman first discovered lysergic acid diethylamide or LSD quite by accident. The story goes that he unintentionally ingested a small quantity of it and had vivid visual hallucinations. A few days later he took more and reported its effects, and he also became an advocate for the substance. Hoffman convinced a company called Sandoz to produce a synthetical version of LSD under the brand name Delysid and began promoting it, at one time making it freely available to those who were interested in researching it.

LSD became a key substance in the consciousness-expanding movement of the 1960s. A potent but colorless and tasteless liquid, it can be taken in multiple forms such as powders or tablets or added to sugar cubes, gelatin squares, or even postage stamps or paper. The US government has used it as a "truth serum" as recently as 2003 but does not do so currently (Rosenberg 2018).

LSD acts on serotonin pathways, mostly by binding to serotonin receptor sites. Sometimes the drug will activate the receptor and sometimes it won't, however, which makes LSD unpredictable. Most hallucinogens, including LSD, will activate many parts of the brain including various sensory areas. The effects of LSD are usually felt within 30 to 60 minutes after the drug is taken. They include physiological changes such as dizziness and increases in heart rate, blood pressure, and body temperature. The psychoactive effects include a blending of sensory experiences and hallucinations affecting all five senses. LSD can also produce flashbacks to experiences with the drug months after it was taken (Jaffe 1990). People who use LSD experience a variety of symptoms of intoxication, including perceptual changes such as visual or aural hallucinations. Objects may undulate, flat things may look as if they have depth, and noises in the background may seem louder.

Hallucinogen: a psychoactive substance that distorts conscious experiences.

The way someone behaves while intoxicated, such as whether they are frightened by their hallucinations, depends on the setting and the individual's personality and mood at the time.

LSD is a synthetically produced hallucinogen but sometimes occurs naturally. For example, the fungus *Calaviceps purpurea* can grow on rye and is a source of LSD, and a related substance (lysergic acid amine) can be found in the Hawaiian baby wood rose and morning glory seeds (Jenkins & Gates 2020).

In its early years LSD had some medical uses and was given to treat alcohol problems, opioid addiction, and sexual disorders (Jenkins & Gates 2020). Before it was banned in 1967, it was intended to be marketed to help psychotherapy clients access repressed emotions and memory (Nutt 2019).

Phencyclidine (PCP) was first created in 1926. It has anesthetic qualities and was used for that purpose in the 1950s. Also known by the street names angel dust, killer weed, crystal, PeaCePill, hog, horse tracks, and busy bee, it is sometimes counterfeited or mixed with tobacco or marijuana, or with other plants such as mint or parsley.

PCP is typically injected, snorted, or smoked, and symptoms of intoxication begin shortly after. They include feelings of power, and with higher doses people experience flat moods, talkativeness, slow reaction time, high blood pressure, muscle weakness, amnesia, and hypothermia. Moderate doses may produce body distortion or an unreal or out-of-body feeling. PCP can also affect mood and sometimes produces violent behavior. Because symptoms can last for days, people with severe PCP intoxication can be misdiagnosed with psychotic disorders (more on those in Chapter 13). So it's vital to rule out substance use for those conditions. The longer PCP is used, the more likely that a person might experience unpredictable side effects from the substance.

Diagnostic Overview 11.8: Other Hallucinogen Use Disorder

A problematic pattern of hallucinogen use associated with at least two of the following:

- Use of more of the hallucinogen or over a longer period of time than intended.
- Unsuccessful efforts to cut down or control use.
- A great deal of time spent in activities necessary to obtain or use the hallucinogen or recover from its effects.
- Cravings for the substance.
- Hallucinogen use that results in missed obligations at work, school, or home.
- Continued hallucinogen use despite interpersonal problems caused by it.
- Hallucinogen use in situations in which it is dangerous.
- Tolerance: a need for more of the hallucinogen for intoxication or less of an effect when using the same amount of the hallucinogen.

Severity is gauged by the number of symptoms:

- Mild: Presence of 2–3 symptoms.
- Moderate: Presence of 4–5 symptoms.
- Severe: Presence of 6 or more symptoms.

Impact: Symptoms must exceed cultural and contextual norms. Symptoms are related to clinically significant distress or create impairment in important areas of life such as with friends and family or at work or school.

Timeframe: 12 months.

Source: Information from APA (2022).

Symptoms and Description: Other Hallucinogen Use Disorder

Despite hallucinogens' reputation for expanding consciousness, some health professionals worry that they can be problematic substances (Diagnostic Overview 11.8). Frequent users who develop aggressive behaviors can experience impairment in work, school, or social situations; they may use the substances when it is dangerous to do so, such as while driving; or they may encounter legal problems because possession of these substances is illegal.

Statistics and Trajectory: Other Hallucinogen Use Disorder

Fifteen percent of people in the United States have used LSD or another hallucinogen at some point in their lives (SAMHSA 2017), and as of 2017 over 1.4 million people over age 12 in the United States reported currently using hallucinogens (Jenkins & Gates 2020). LSD use has increased over 200 percent from 2002 to 2018 (Killion et al. 2021). The increase is much higher for those over 25 and among men (Yockey et al. 2019).

> ### CONCEPT CHECK 11.6
>
> 1. True or false: LSD has been researched for medical use.
> 2. True or false: PCP, now called angel dust, once had medical uses.
> 3. True or false: PCP, LSD, and other drugs in the class of hallucinogens are the only substances that can produce hallucinations.

11.7 OTHER DRUGS OF ABUSE

Just as new medicines are being developed, so too are illicit psychoactive substances. Sometimes new agents begin with medical uses and later are used as street drugs. Between 2009 and 2012, more than 160 new and undetected substances were found in a DNA analysis of illicit drugs confiscated in Europe alone (Herrmann et al. 2016). So far we've discussed many substances, but there are a few others that don't fit neatly into any particular category, such as inhalants, steroids, dissociative anesthetics, and GHB. We turn to those now.

Inhalants

Inhalants are substances, including spray paints and hairspray, that are breathed in, whether directly from the container or poured onto a cloth. Because they are solvents, they are absorbed rapidly into the bloodstream. People who try inhalants are drawn to the experiences produced by the substance, which can be similar to opioid or alcohol intoxication. Symptoms of inhalant intoxication include slurred speech, dizziness, lethargy and lack of coordination, and increases in aggressive behavior. Long-term use can lead to damage to the brain and nervous system as well as to the lungs, liver, and kidneys.

Steroids

Synthetic anabolic steroids are prescribed for conditions such as asthma or anemia, but they can also be abused by those who attempt to boost their physical stamina by increasing muscle mass. Steroids are similar to naturally occurring testosterone, and about 2–6 percent of males in the United States use the drugs illegally (Kanayama & Pope 2021). They may cycle steroids (using them on and off for several weeks at a time) or use them with other muscle-enhancing substances. While steroids don't produce a high, they can lead to dependence because continued use is necessary to maintain muscle gains or the disruptive emotions that may accompany them. The continued misuse despite negative effects is the reason dependence develops. Long-term effects of steroids include low mood, anxiety, increases in panic attacks, and the possibility of physical consequences such as blood clots, increased risk of heart attack and stroke, and liver and kidney damage from unsupervised use.

Dissociative Anesthetics

Dissociative anesthetics are substances that bring about sleepiness, decreased pain, and an out-of-body feeling. They have been called "designer drugs" and include methylenedioxymethamphetamine (MDMA) (ecstasy or molly) and 2C-B (known chemically as 4-Bromo-2,5-dimethoxypenethylamine) and also known as BDMPEA or nexus. People who use these substances often report increased perception or sensations, sometimes paired with intense sensory experiences of nightclubs, parties, and music (Schifano et al. 2021).

ECSTASY

Methylenedioxymethamphetamine (MDMA) or *ecstasy* is a stimulant-hallucinogenic drug that can induce euphoria and diminish anxiety. Under the influence of ecstasy, users report feelings of enhanced intimacy, increased sensitivity to sensory stimuli, and more emotional openness. Ecstasy produces its full effect about an hour after it is ingested, and this lasts about four to six hours. Long-term use is associated with dehydration, depression, and insomnia and can create long-term damage to serotonin neurons. Such use can also result in the need for more of the substance to maintain the person's typical mood. Some people experience heart, liver, or kidney failure from taking large doses.

Transport proteins are one of the cleanup mechanisms in the synapses. Molecules of ecstasy are attracted to the transport proteins and are taken into the axon terminal. This can create changes in the reuptake site, causing the transport proteins to work backward. Thus instead of recycling serotonin, the axon terminal pumps it out of the cell. Since there are then fewer ways to clean up the synaptic gap, serotonin floods the synapse, overstimulating the receptor sites. Because there's so much serotonin in the synapse, ecstasy affects the user's emotions, appetite, sleep, wakefulness, and consciousness. This overstimulation can produce permanent damage and reduce the amount of healthy serotonin in the brain.

KETAMINE

Ketamine (with street names K, special K, and Cat Valium) is a dissociative anesthetic that can reduce pain and is associated with a feeling of detachment. Its effect can be so strong that it can render a person unconscious and cause injury.

Ketamine can also produce perception distortion and emotional states like paranoia. Intoxication can last up to an hour but for as long as four to six hours. Large doses can lead to gastrointestinal distress and oxygen starvation in the lungs and brain. Unique to ketamine is its ability to improve mood long after the drug has worn off (Nutt 2019). Read section 6.4 to find out how ketamine is being used for treatment-resistant depression.

Gamma Hydroxybutyrate (GHB)

Originally used as a treatment for narcolepsy, *Gamma Hydroxybutyrate* (GHB) is a central nervous system depressant. Also used by athletes to enhance leanness, it decreases anxiety, and people who use it feel relaxed. High doses can lead to coma and death, however. In the late 1990s GHB was removed from stores and is now used only under medical supervision. Side effects of intoxication include sweating, headache, and impaired breathing. Because of its sedative and memory-impairing effects, GHB is one drug that can be used to facilitate sexual assault.

CONCEPT CHECK 11.7

Fill in the blanks with the substance that best describes the concept.
1. _____ are muscle-enhancing substances and don't produce a high but can be abused.
2. _____ is a stimulant hallucinogenic drug that can increase euphoria and diminish anxiety.
3. _____ can reduce pain because it is associated with feelings of detachment.
4. _____ is a central nervous system depressant originally used as a treatment for narcolepsy.

11.8 BEHAVIORAL ADDICTIONS

In addition to substance use disorders, the *DSM-5tr* also describes a category for behavioral addictions. Despite establishing the category, the *DSM* allows a diagnosis for only a single behavioral addiction, gambling disorder.

For most people, gambling is just a fun diversion, done responsibly with only slightly smaller bank accounts to show for their efforts. But there's a difference between a retiree at the penny slots and someone who gambles to the point of creating social and work impairment (Figure 11.10). People with a **gambling disorder** love

Gambling disorder: an addictive disorder that is associated with problematic gambling at the expense of the person's livelihood and wellbeing.

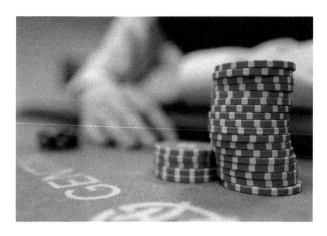

Figure 11.10 Those with gambling disorder are more likely to try to make up for lost winnings than people without gambling disorder.

Source: Sebastien Bozon/AFP via Getty Images.

risk and seek intense stimulation, excitement, and change, even at the expense of their livelihood and wellbeing (see Table 11.3).

Symptoms and Description: Gambling Disorder

Those with gambling disorder develop a preoccupation with gambling that can devastate their families' financial wellbeing. They focus on it so much that they put their personal relationships, occupational status, and financial stability at risk. They continue to gamble despite increasing family and financial distress, have difficulty controlling the urge to gamble, and are often unable to reduce the amount of time and money they spend gambling. Eventually they don't get the same thrill from gambling as before, so they have to increase their bets or the frequency of the activity to get the same effect. They often gamble to lift their mood, lie to hide how much money they spend, become irritable if they try to cut down their addiction, and rely on others to bail them out (Diagnostic Overview 11.9).

Diagnostic Overview 11.9: Gambling Disorder

Problematic gambling behavior as indicated by at least four of the following:

- Gambling with increasing amounts of money in order to achieve the desired excitement.
- Restlessness or irritability when trying to reduce or stop gambling.
- Unsuccessful efforts to reduce gambling.
- Preoccupation with gambling.
- Gambling when feeling emotional.
- Attempts to break even after losing.
- Lying to hide how much the person has been gambling.
- Negative impacts on work or relationships because of gambling.
- Need for others to provide money for gambling or to replace money lost from gambling.

Severity is based on the number of criteria that are met:

- Mild: 4–5 criteria.
- Moderate: 6–7 criteria.
- Severe: 8–9 criteria.

Impact: Symptoms must exceed cultural and contextual norms. Symptoms are related to clinically significant distress or create impairment in important areas of life such as with friends and family or at work or school.

Timeframe: 12 months.

Source: Information from APA (2022).

Statistics and Trajectory: Gambling Disorder

Gambling is fairly common. Up to 90 percent of the population has gambled in some form (Black & Shaw 2019), including in state lotteries and slot machines. However, the percentage of people who might meet the *DSM-5tr* criteria for gambling disorder is much smaller, with surveys suggesting that about 7 percent of the US population will do so (Black & Shaw 2019). Rates of gambling disorder are higher in the United States than in other countries but vary around the world based on access to gambling. For example, in New Zealand many forms of gambling are illegal and rates are relatively low at 1.9 percent (Black & Shaw 2019). Symptoms of gambling disorder are more common in both adolescents and college students (up to 14 percent of them gamble) and tend to decrease with age (Black & Shaw 2019). Gambling disorder is more often found in men and in those without college degrees (Dowling et al. 2018). When women meet the criteria for gambling disorder, their symptoms develop later in life than for men.

CONCEPT CHECK 11.8

1. True or false: The *DSM* lists several types of behavioral addiction including gambling disorder, sex addiction, and Internet addiction.
2. True or false: The availability of access to gambling is correlated with rates of gambling disorder.

11.9 MODELS AND TREATMENTS OF SUBSTANCE-RELATED DISORDERS

Demi, Buzz, and Anthony all sought treatment for their conditions. Demi has entered treatment since the documentary was made, and as of 2021 Buzz has been in recovery for more than 22 years. Anthony has been sober for more than 20 years at this point. Psychopathologists have created a number of theories about why people develop substance use and addictive disorders, including biological and psychological models.

Biological Models and Treatments of Substance Use Disorders

By their nature, psychoactive substances, and even gambling, have an impact on the brain and a rewarding effect. A number of biological factors influence both the use and abuse of psychoactive substances.

Genes can lend a biological predisposition to substance use disorders, as explained by both human and other animal models. For example, after identifying animals that desire alcohol over other drugs, researchers found they produced offspring that had the same preference (Hauser et al. 2020). Human twin research has produced similar evidence. Twin studies of alcohol use disorder show a concordance rate of around 50 percent in monozygotic twins and 30 percent in dizygotic twins. Adoption studies show that children whose biological parents had an alcohol use disorder had higher rates of the disorder even when adopted by parents who did not, which suggests that an environment free of alcohol misuse does not completely protect against the development of alcohol use disorder.

Many drugs create their intoxicating symptoms through their actions on neurotransmitters. Neurotransmitter systems may also be at play in creating the symptoms of tolerance, withdrawal, and ultimately substance use disorder. For example, as a drug increases the availability of certain neurotransmitters, the brain responds by decreasing the amount produced, leaving the person with a deficit over time. This means that to maintain balance the external substance is now needed, so eventually people come to desire more and more in order to feel comfortable, and suddenly stopping use could produce the telltale symptoms of withdrawal.

Reward circuits may also be at play in substance use disorders. The neurotransmitter dopamine plays a major role in many of the brain's reward systems. For some with substance use disorders, the substance will stimulate the reward circuit over and over and create sensitivity to the substance. This might be responsible for the feelings of craving that people experience, called the *incentive sensitization theory of addiction.* Another biological theory of substance abuse, the *reward deficiency syndrome theory*, suggests that people with substance use disorder have reward circuits that are not easily activated, so they turn to substances or behaviors such as gambling to stimulate their reward.

Detoxification is medically supervised withdrawal from a substance. It may occur in outpatient or residential programs and can include the use of medications along with group or individual therapy. Clients are helped to gradually decrease their dose of a substance in order to minimize the uncomfortable and sometimes dangerous side effects of withdrawal, or they are given medications to help alleviate the severe symptoms.

Just stopping use of a substance isn't enough. Prevention of reuse (relapse) is also an important goal. Medications can be helpful, such as *agonist drugs* that change or even block the effects of another drug. For example, disulfiram (Antabuse) can help those who are trying to reduce their alcohol use. When combined with alcohol it will lead to nausea, increases in heart rate, dizziness, and feelings of faintness. Because of the unpleasant symptoms, people who take Antabuse decrease their alcohol use and are less likely to relapse. However, the medication works only if people continue to take it.

Cognitive-Behavioral Models and Treatments of Substance Use Disorders

Learning theory suggests that operant conditioning (reinforcement and punishment) plays a major role in substance use and addictive disorders. Substances can reduce anxiety and boost pleasure, which may be reinforcing to those who use them. Some people look for increased doses of substances or behaviors in hopes of getting even more pleasure from the activity. But over time they may develop tolerances that make reinforcement less likely.

Several types of cognitive and behavioral treatments have been used to reduce the reinforcing aspects of substances, such as aversion therapy and acceptance and commitment therapy. *Aversion therapy* for substance and addictive disorders focuses on pairing unpleasant stimuli along with the substance. It can consist of medications such as disulfiram (Antabuse) to produce nausea with alcohol use or even pair frightening images (imagined or photographic) with the substance. Unfortunately, aversion therapy has limited use. It's helpful only for those who are motivated to take the medications or who are willing to expose themselves to the unpleasant stimuli over multiple treatments. Long-acting formulations of disulfiram that last for days can help to reduce to less than 20 percent the likelihood that clients will stop the medication on their own (De Sousa 2019).

Acceptance and commitment therapy (ACT) utilizes mindfulness techniques to help those with substance use and behavioral addictions become more aware of their own thoughts and cravings. Rather than actively suppressing or avoiding them, ACT encourages clients to confront them, thus becoming less distressed and reducing the likelihood that they might give in to them. Studies that examine the effectiveness of ACT indicate that it is as effective as other cognitive or behavioral approaches (Osaji et al. 2020).

Sociocultural Models and Treatments of Substance Use Disorders

Sociocultural models suggest that societal and cultural standards can inspire substance use and addictive disorders. People are at increased risk for developing substance use disorder when under persistent social or economic stress. This type of stress includes abusive relationships, unsupportive and chaotic family environments, poverty, and persistent racial discrimination. The effects of some substances can be even more rewarding as an escape from such continuing stressors.

Exposure to psychoactive substances can vary by culture and can occur through the media, family, or friends. Although many factors can influence the way a person is exposed to psychoactive substances, one study (Kuperman et al. 2013) showed that an important measure in predicting someone's alcohol use was the age at which that person's best friend had their first drink.

Sociocultural influences can include how much attention parents with substance use disorder give their children. Members of friendship networks may also use substances (Van Ryzin et al. 2012), leading to someone's having not only friends who use substances but caretakers as well.

Broader sociocultural factors can influence substance use. In the United States, for example, alcohol intoxication is often portrayed as funny, and being intoxicated in public is not considered offensive. In many cultures people are expected to drink alcohol, and in some environments like college and the military there is social pressure to engage in binge drinking.

Sociocultural treatments of substance use disorder focus on social settings. These programs can intervene on both the individual and community level. Methods include self-help and therapeutic communities such as Alcoholics Anonymous (see The Power of Evidence feature), and they often utilize those who are in recovery to help others.

Interventions can also occur at the community level, such as school or work environments (Olson et al. 2017). Most adolescents (75 percent) have reported having seen a substance use prevention message in the media or at school, and more than half (60 percent) have discussed substance use with a parent or another caretaker (SAMHSA 2017).

Multiperspective Models and Treatments of Substance Use Disorders

Multiperspective models of substance use disorders recognize the influence of biological, psychological, and social factors (Skewes & Gonzalez 2013) (see Figure 11.11). These models also suggest that multiple factors should be in play for the treatment of substance use disorders, combining interventions at the biological, psychological, and social levels.

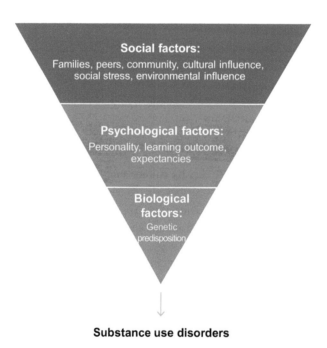

Figure 11.11 Multiperspective models of substance use disorders consider the effects of social, psychological, and biological contributing factors.

THE POWER OF EVIDENCE

Do 12-step programs really work?

For more than 80 years Alcoholics Anonymous (AA) has been a well-known intervention for people with alcohol use disorder. A peer-to-peer organization with members in more than 170 countries, it encourages abstinence from alcohol by using the 12-step philosophy (see Table 11.5). And it's popular. In North America alone, AA is the most commonly sought source of help with alcohol use disorder (Kelly et al. 2020). Today 2 million people around the world are active in AA and other 12-step facilitation (TSF) programs (Kelly et al. 2020). AA literature has been reproduced in dozens of languages.

Table 11.5 The 12 steps of 12-step programs

Steps	Description
Step 1: Honesty	After many years of denial, recovery can begin when with one simple admission of being powerless over alcohol – for alcoholics and their friends and family.
Step 2: Faith	It seems to be a spiritual truth, that before a higher power can begin to operate, you must first believe that it can.
Step 3: Surrender	A lifetime of self-will run riot can come to a screeching halt, and change forever, by making a simple decision to turn it all over to a higher power.
Step 4: Soul Searching	There is a saying in the 12-step programs that recovery is a process, not an event. The same can be said for this step – more will surely be revealed.
Step 5: Integrity	Probably the most difficult of all the steps to face, Step 5 is also the one that provides the greatest opportunity for growth.
Step 6: Acceptance	The key to Step 6 is acceptance – accepting character defects exactly as they are and becoming entirely willing to let them go.
Step 7: Humility	The spiritual focus of Step 7 is humility, asking a higher power to do something that cannot be done by self-will or mere determination.
Step 8: Willingness	Making a list of those harmed before coming into recovery may sound simple. Becoming willing to actually make those amends is the difficult part.
Step 9: Forgiveness	Making amends may seem like a bitter pill to swallow, but for those serious about recovery, it can be great medicine for the spirit and soul.
Step 10: Maintenance	Nobody likes to admit to being wrong. But it is absolutely necessary to maintain spiritual progress in recovery.
Step 11: Making Contact	The purpose of Step 11 is to discover the plan God (as you understand Him) has for your life.
Step 12: Service	For those in recovery programs, practicing Step 12 is simply "how it works."

Source: Alcoholics Anonymous World Services, Inc. (1989).

AA/TSF meetings take place weekly and last around 90 minutes, during which participants share experiences of their alcohol use and recovery and help each other practice the 12-step principles for coping with stress, improving relationships, and abstaining from alcohol use.

Despite their popularity, there have been questions about how effective AA/TSF programs are. A 2020 Cochrane Collaboration identified 27 studies with more than 10,000 participants that evaluated AA/TSF programs. The meta-analysis showed that AA/TSF programs were just as good as other treatments on all drinking-related outcomes, such as the number of days of not drinking alcohol, and better at helping people to abstain for longer periods of time. What's more, AA/TSF programs reduced the overall costs of health care for their participants (Kelly et al. 2020).

CONCEPT CHECK 11.9

1. The _____ theory suggests that people with substance use disorder have reward circuits that are not easily activated, so they turn to substances or behaviors such as gambling to stimulate their reward center.
2. _____ therapy for substance and addictive disorders focuses on pairing unpleasant stimuli with the substance.
3. _____ models suggest that societal and cultural standards, such as portrayals of intoxication as funny, can inspire substance use and addictive disorders.

PULLING IT TOGETHER

Psychoactive Drugs and Their Effects by Class

Table 11.6 Psychoactive substances and their effects by class

Type of drug	Description	Methods of ingestion	Principal medical uses	Desired effects	Known and potential short-term side effects
Stimulants					
Amphetamines	A class of stimulant drugs that activates the central nervous system	Oral	Narcolepsy	Alertness, elevated mood	Anxiety, headaches, blunted appetite, high blood pressure, psychosis
Cocaine	A stimulant drug made from the coca plant	Oral, sniffed, injected, smoked	Local anesthetic	Euphoria, confidence, energy, depressed appetite	Insomnia, sweating, anxiety, panic, depression, cardiovascular stress

Table 11.6 *(cont.)*

Type of drug	Description	Methods of ingestion	Principal medical uses	Desired effects	Known and potential short-term side effects
Nicotine	A type of drug that targets the nicotinic receptors. Found in tobacco	Smoked, gum, buccally (through the inside of the cheek).	Cessation of smoking habit	Euphoria, increased confidence, energy, decreased appetite	Heart disease, cancer, high blood pressure
Caffeine	A type of stimulant drug that is associated with increased central nervous system activity	Oral, drinking	Painkiller	Alertness, increased reaction time	Insomnia, high blood pressure
Methamphetamine	A stimulant drug associated with increased nervous system activity, elevated libido, and increased self esteem	Oral, smoked	None	Euphoria, alertness, energy	Irritability, insomnia, hypertension, seizures, nervousness, headaches, decreased appetite, psychosis
MDMA (ecstasy)	A stimulant-hallucinogenic drug that can induce euphoria and diminish anxiety	Oral	None	Increased mood, alertness and wakefulness, disinhibition	Anxiety, agitation, and insomnia in high doses; Dehydration, sweatiness, depressed mood, impaired cognitive and immune functioning
Depressants					
Alcohol	A type of depressant drug that is associated with reduced inhibition, slurred speech, and impairments in balance	Oral	Antiseptic	Relaxation and disinhibition	Depression, memory loss, liver damage, impaired reaction time
Barbiturates	A type of depressant drug that reduces stress induces sleep	Oral, injected	Sedative, sleeping pill	Reduced anxiety, reduced tension, sedation	Memory difficulties, withdrawal symptoms, convulsions
Hallucinogens					
Heroin	A psychoactive substance made from opium that relieves pain and reduces the activity of the nervous system	Injected, smoked, oral	None	Euphoria, pain relief	Reduced appetite, nausea, convulsions, coma

Table 11.6 *(cont.)*

Type of drug	Description	Methods of ingestion	Principal medical uses	Desired effects	Known and potential short-term side effects
LSD	A synthetic psychedelic hallucinogenic drug that produces altered states of consciousness	Oral	None	Hallucinations	Psychosis, paranoia, panic
Marijuana	A drug that has both painkilling as well as stimulating effects on the nervous system	Smoked, oral	Nausea associated with chemotherapy; treatment of nausea, insomnia, and lack of appetite	Enhanced sensation, relief of pain, distortion of time, relaxation,	Memory difficulties

11.10 CHAPTER REVIEW

SUMMARY

This chapter presented the following disorders:

- Alcohol use disorder
- Sedative-hypnotic-anxiolytic-related disorders
- Caffeine intoxication
- Tobacco use disorder
- Stimulant use disorder
- Opioid use disorder
- Cannabis use disorder
- Other hallucinogen use disorder
- Gambling disorder

Overview of Substance Use Disorders

- A psychoactive drug is a chemical used to alter mood, thoughts, or consciousness, such as tobacco, alcohol, and cannabis.

- The *DSM-5tr* describes substance-related disorders that result from a number of separate classes of drugs: depressants (such as alcohol and sedative hypnotics), stimulants, (such as tobacco, caffeine, and methamphetamines), opioids, cannabis, and hallucinogens. The DSM also describes a category of non-substance addictions that includes gambling disorder

Depressants

- Depressants work by reducing the level of activity in the nervous system.
- Alcohol is an ethanol-containing beverage that may be wine, beer, or a liquor such as vodka, gin, or whiskey.
- Those with alcohol use disorder have impaired control over the amount and frequency

with which they drink and often experience negative emotional states when they aren't drinking.

- The class of depressant substances also includes anxiolytic sedatives such as benzodiazepines (which are calming and can reduce anxiety) and tranquilizers such as hypnotics (which induce sleep), as well as barbiturates.
- Sedatives include the barbiturates and sedative hypnotics that are often prescribed for insomnia.
- Barbiturates are a type of depressant drug that reduces stress and induces sleep.
- Tranquilizers are medications often prescribed to treat muscle spasms and anxiety. The most common substances in this category are the benzodiazepines.
- Benzodiazepines are a group of central nervous system depressants for treating insomnia, anxiety, and seizures.
- Sedative, hypnotic, or anxiolytic use disorder involves a problematic pattern of sedative, hypnotic, or anxiolytic use leading to clinically significant impairment or distress.

Stimulants

- Stimulants are a group of psychoactive substances that increase activity in the central nervous system.
- Caffeine stimulates the cerebral cortex and boosts energy and alertness.
- The psychoactive substance in tobacco is a naturally occurring amount of nicotine, which reduces activity in many areas of the brain including the amygdala, hippocampus, and frontal lobes.
- Tobacco use disorder is a condition that involves problematic pattern of tobacco use.
- Cocaine is a stimulant that confers increased energy, decreased appetite, alertness, anxiety, and feelings of euphoria.
- Methamphetamine is a stimulant drug associated with increased nervous system activity and elevated libido and self-esteem.

- Stimulant use disorder is a disruptive pattern of using stimulants.

Opioids and Opioid Use Disorder

- Opiates are psychoactive substances made from opium that relieve pain and reduce the activity of the nervous system such as morphine, heroin, codeine, and methadone.
- Opioid use disorder is a problematic pattern of opioid use.

Cannabis and Cannabis-Related Disorders

- *Cannabis sativa* contains tetrahydrocannabinol (THC), which appears to be the ingredient responsible for many of its effects.
- Cannabis use disorder involves problematic pattern of cannabis use.

Hallucinogen-Related Disorders

- Hallucinogens are a class of psychoactive drugs that distort our conscious experiences and can produce changes in the way we perceive reality.
- Lysergic acid diethylamide (LSD) and phencyclidine (PCP) are both hallucinogens.

Other Drugs of Abuse

- Inhalants are substances, including spray paints and hairspray, that are breathed in, whether directly from the container or poured onto a cloth.
- Synthetic anabolic steroids are prescribed for conditions such as asthma or anemia, but they can also be abused by those who attempt to boost their physical stamina by increasing muscle mass.
- Dissociative anesthetics are substances that bring about sleepiness, decreased pain, and an out-of-body feeling.
- Ecstasy is a stimulant-hallucinogenic drug that can induce euphoria and diminish anxiety.

- Ketamine (with street names K, special K, and Cat Valium), is a dissociative anesthetic that can reduce pain and is associated with a feeling of detachment.

Behavioral Addictions

- People with a gambling disorder seek intense stimulation, excitement, and change, and they love risks.

Models and Treatments of Substance-Related Disorders

- Incentive sensitization theory of addiction suggests that substances will stimulate the reward circuit over and over and create sensitivity to the substance.
- Reward deficiency syndrome theory suggests that people with substance use disorder have reward circuits that are not easily activated, so they turn to substances or behaviors such as gambling to stimulate their reward.
- Learning theory suggests that operant conditioning (reinforcement and punishment) plays a major role in substance use and addictive disorders. Substances can reduce anxiety and boost pleasure, which may be reinforcing to those who use them.
- Aversion therapies for substance and addictive disorders focus on pairing unpleasant stimuli along with the substance.
- Acceptance and commitment therapy (ACT) utilizes mindfulness techniques to help those with substance use and behavioral addictions become more aware of their own thoughts and cravings.
- Sociocultural models suggest that societal and cultural standards can inspire substance use and addictive disorders.

DISCUSSION QUESTIONS

1. Some people are able to function despite their use of alcohol or other substances. Some function well on illegal substances. Should such people seek treatment? Why or why not?
2. How does the government treat illegal substances differently from other substances such as alcohol? Some people believe marijuana should not be illegal. Do you think addiction to it would be more likely or less likely if it were legal? Why?
3. *DSM-5* added a new category of behavioral addictions but allowed diagnosticians to diagnose only one: gambling disorder. Why do you think this is the case? What might happen if any behavior that met the criteria for gambling disorder could be diagnosed as a behavioral addiction?
4. Would you consider someone who drinks soda every day to be addicted to soda? Why or why not? What about shopping? Explain your answer.
5. In what ways has culture shaped your attitudes about psychoactive substances and substance use disorder?

ANSWERS TO CONCEPT CHECKS

Concept Check 11.1
1. Withdrawal
2. More use than intended
3. Use despite impairment
4. Activities given up

Concept Check 11.2
1. Recurrent alcohol use in situations in which it is physically hazardous
2. A persistent desire and unsuccessful efforts to cut down or control alcohol use
3. Craving or a strong desire or urge to use alcohol

4. False
5. True

Concept Check 11.3

1. Dopamine
2. Increased energy, decreased appetite, alertness, anxiety, and feelings of euphoria
3. Caffeine

Concept Check 11.4

1. True
2. Codeine [yes]
   Heroin [yes]
   Morphine [yes]

Cocaine [no]
3. True

Concept Check 11.5

1. THC
2. False

Concept Check 11.6

1. True
2. True
3. False

Concept Check 11.7

1. Steroids
2. Ecstasy

3. Ketamine
4. GHB

Concept Check 11.8

1. False
2. True

Concept Check 11.9

1. Reward deficiency syndrome
2. Aversion
3. Sociocultural

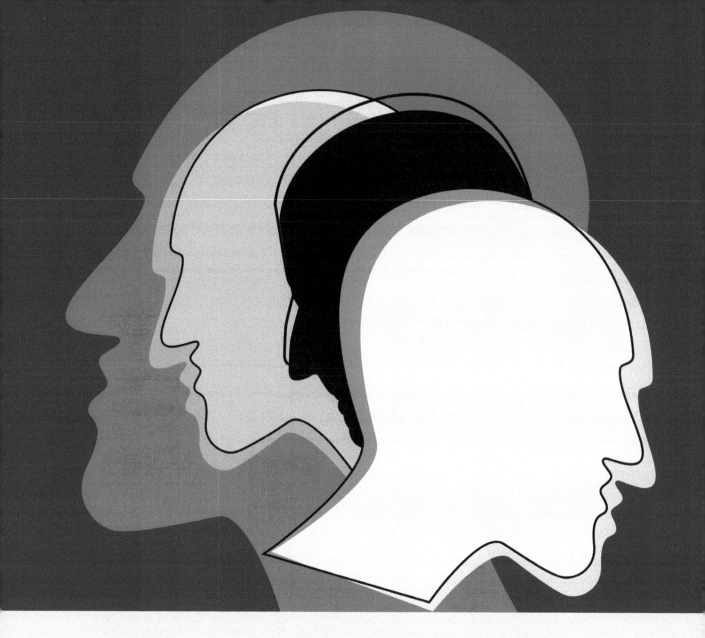

Kubkoo/DigitalVision Vectors/Getty Images Plus.

CHAPTER CONTENTS

12

Personality Disorders

CASE STUDY: Borderline Personality Disorder – Marsha Linehan

As a teenager growing up in Tulsa, Oklahoma, Marsha reported feeling increased tension and social withdrawal in addition to exhibiting self-destructive behaviors such as deliberately cutting her arm. Once she broke the lens from her eyeglasses and used it to start making small cuts on her left wrist. After a while her self-injurious behaviors become more serious, including slicing her arms and thighs and burning cigarettes on her body. Sometimes Marsha reported that it felt like someone else was performing these actions. "Looking back," she said, "it's as if it wasn't me doing all these things. It was someone else trying to harm me." Marsha's life was characterized by impulsivity, dissociative thinking, memory impairment, and a feeling of emptiness nearly all the time.

Growing up, Marsha had been surrounded by a talented artist mother, two good-looking brothers, and a "model daughter" (her sister). She never felt as if she belonged in the family. Her mother constantly tried to change Marsha's behavior and often failed; her sister remarked that Marsha simply could not please her mother no matter what she did. At school things were different. There Marsha was described as the thoughtful and popular person who usually took on leadership roles. These polarized opinions about her might have given Marsha a confused sense of self. She reported never having a serious long-term relationship, which she said severely interfered with her emotional stability. After high school, she isolated herself in her room at home, knowing her friends were all paired up with boys. She felt depressed, unaccepted, and unloved both inside and outside her house.

Marsha described herself as "totally out of control" to the extent that she felt like somebody else was harming her. She started developing an attachment to her psychiatrist and begged him not to leave. In a letter she said she thought she might kill herself without him. We'll return to Marsha's story later in the chapter.

Read more about Dr. Marsha Linehan in her memoir, *Building a life worth living: A memoir* (2020).

Learning Objectives

- Define the main features of personality disorders.
- Describe the three clusters of personality disorders.
- Describe the 10 personality disorders categorized in *DSM-5tr*.
- Identify models of and effective treatments for personality disorders.

12.1   OVERVIEW OF PERSONALITY DISORDERS

Personality is an individual's pattern of thinking, feeling, and behaving. Our personality characteristics can influence what we do, what we feel, the way we think, and the way we engage with those around us. However, while the pieces of our personality can help guide our behavior in predictable ways, our personalities are not fixed. They can change over time, and with experience we can change the way we react to people and events. It's this flexibility that helps us adapt to new people and the subtleties of new interactions. It's also something that people with personality disorders often lack.

Personality disorders:
psychological conditions
characterized by extremely
inflexible personality
characteristics that are persistent
and pervasive.

Personality disorders are psychological conditions characterized by extremely inflexible personality characteristics that are persistent and pervasive. These characteristics can sometimes be extreme and dysfunctional, and they can cause consistent problems with relationships or work or disrupt daily living. They usually become established during early adulthood, but often there are earlier signs of them.

Because personality is so intertwined with who we are and so ingrained, personality disorders can be difficult to treat. In fact, some individuals with personality disorders don't see the problems they have in life, despite the impairment their behaviors cause. For a behavior to be considered a personality disorder, it has to form a disruptive pattern that is both chronic and pervasive. *Chronic* means it doesn't come and go; it ends up being the main way the person interacts with other people all the time. In addition to being long-lasting, the disorder is pervasive, meaning that it creeps into every nook and cranny of a person's life.

You might think a person would dislike having a behavior pattern so disruptive and so impairing. Most of the time this is true, but sometimes people with personality disorders don't find their own behavior disagreeable. That is, some types of personality disorders are *ego syntonic*, meaning they do not bother the person who has them. Think of a friend of yours who has a shirt with a hole in it. You might find it unthinkable to leave the house wearing a garment with such an obvious problem, but your friend doesn't think twice about it. People can sometimes have the same response to their behaviors. When behaviors are ego *syn*tonic, they are compatible with the way people see themselves (think of the word *synonym*, meaning words that are similar). Most personality disorder behaviors, however, are **ego *dys*tonic**, meaning they are dissimilar to the way people see themselves. Ego dystonic disorders are easier to treat, since clients are usually more motivated to change aspects they don't like about themselves. If the behavior is ego syntonic, treatment can be difficult or even futile.

Ego dystonic: symptoms
dissimilar to the way people see
themselves.

DSM-5tr describes 10 personality disorders and divides them into three clusters – odd and eccentric, dramatic, and anxious (Figure 12.1) – which we discuss next. At any given time, about 12 percent of the United States population will meet the criteria for a personality disorder (Volkert et al. 2018).

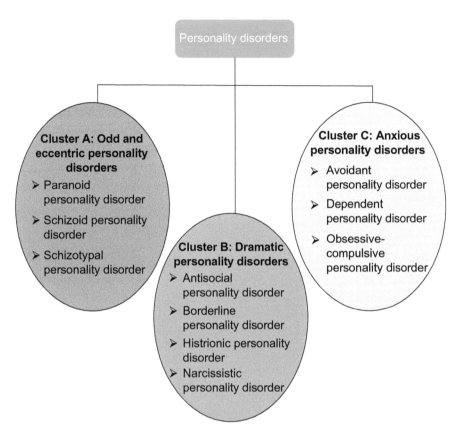

Some psychopathologists are calling for replacing the categorical personality disorders in the *DSM-5tr* (Figure 12.1) with a dimensional model. Such a model describes personality disorders using a severity gradient from high to low with a smaller number of traits, such as the Five-Factor Model of Personality. A dimensional model is a more evidence-based way to classify disordered personality than categorical types, which are plagued by notoriously low diagnostic reliability and both symptom similarity and high comorbidity with other conditions (see Table 12.4 in the Pulling It Together feature at the end of the chapter) (Hopwood et al. 2018).

CONCEPT CHECK 12.1

Indicate whether the following case examples describe a person who has ego dystonic or ego syntonic symptoms.

1. Roger has stolen money from his clients, friends, and family but doesn't seem stressed about these thefts.
2. Cassie doesn't have any friends because she is worried that if she says the wrong thing any friends she makes will abandon her.

> 3. Mara worries that her girlfriend will leave her. She has tried to be independent but is filled with doubt about her ability to make choices if left alone to take care of herself.
> 4. Sam has no friends and isn't close to his family. He doesn't feel that he needs anyone and wonders why other people seem so concerned about his lack of close relationships.

12.2   CLUSTER A: ODD AND ECCENTRIC PERSONALITY DISORDERS

DSM-5tr refers to the disorders in Cluster A as the "Odd and Eccentric Personality Disorders." The symptoms of these conditions include unusual or eccentric thinking or behavior, withdrawal from social activities due to unfounded suspicion about others' intentions, and unusual thoughts and perceptions. They may also include unusual ways of interacting with others that can lead to distress and impairment. Both social awkwardness and social withdrawal are common features in the odd personality disorders.

People with Cluster A personality disorders tend to have relationship struggles, due to the fact that others often see their behavior as peculiar, suspicious, or detached. Research suggests the prevalence of these disorders is about 2–3.6 percent of the worldwide population (Volkert et al. 2018) (see Figure 12.2). In the cluster of "odd" personality disorders are paranoid personality disorder, schizoid personality disorder, and schizotypal personality disorders.

Paranoid Personality Disorder

Paranoid personality disorder: a condition characterized by a long and unwavering history of attributing malicious intent to others that does not subside no matter how long the person may know these others.

Imagine you had a deep distrust of everyone and believed they all were out to do you harm, and this was the main assumption upon which you interacted with everyone you met. This distrust and suspicion is the central feature of **paranoid personality disorder**, a condition characterized by a long and unwavering history of attributing malicious intent to others that does not subside no matter how long the person may know these others. During role play to examine the relationships of those with paranoid personality disorder, they were more likely than those without the condition to infer hostile intentions in the acts of other participants and to react in anger (Lewis & Ridenour 2020). Those with paranoid personality disorder commonly question how trusting or loyal even their closest friends and family members are, and they will often keep them at a safe distance because they expect to be tricked by them (even without any evidence). They will also question how faithful their partners are.

SYMPTOMS AND DESCRIPTION

A diagnosis of paranoid personality disorder includes four symptoms that pervade every part of someone's life (Diagnostic Overview 12.1). The person expects to be

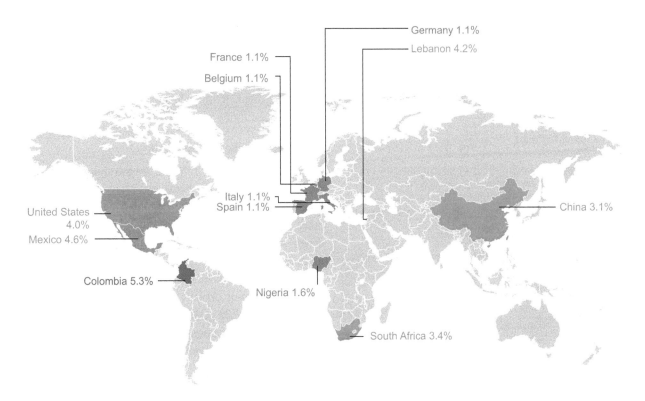

France 1.1%

Belgium 1.1%

Germany 1.1%

Lebanon 4.2%

Italy 1.1%
Spain 1.1%

United States
4.0%

Mexico 4.6%

Colombia 5.3%

Nigeria 1.6%

China 3.1%

South Africa 3.4%

exploited or harmed by others and is preoccupied with the trustworthiness of their friends. In addition, they think information they give about themselves will be used against them, and they misinterpret and read hidden meanings into harmless remarks. They are unforgiving of insults, are quick to counterattack, and often doubt the fidelity of their romantic partners. Their symptoms get worse when they are stressed. As you can imagine, they are always on guard, which causes significant impairment in their work lives and social lives. People with paranoid personality disorder tend to have a poor quality of life (Hopwood & Thomas 2012).

Figure 12.2 Lifetime prevalence of Cluster A personality disorders in selected countries, from the World Mental Health Surveys (2002–2017).
Source: Huang et al. 2009.

STATISTICS AND TRAJECTORY

Epidemiological research suggests that 1.5–1.8 percent of people in the general population worldwide will meet the criteria for paranoid personality disorder, and the condition is diagnosed equally often in women and men (Torgersen et al. 2012; Volkert et al. 2018).

Schizoid Personality Disorder

Most of us are connected to those around us. We acknowledge people in elevators and greet people we know at school or work when we pass them. We care, to some extent, about the opinions of our colleagues, teachers, and family. But what if you didn't perceive a connection to anyone, and you felt split off from everyone around you? **Schizoid personality disorder** is a personality disorder characterized by a

Schizoid personality disorder: a personality disorder characterized by a pervasive pattern of detachment from social relationships and limited emotional expression.

A suspiciousness of other people where their motives are interpreted as unkind, along with at least four of the following:

- Suspicion that others are exploiting, harming, or deceiving them.
- Doubts about the loyalty of others.
- Unwillingness to confide in other people due to belief that any information revealed will be used against them.
- Assumption that demeaning or threatening messages are behind everyday language.
- Persistent grudges.
- Misperception that ordinary interactions are attacks on character, with angry reaction.
- Suspicions about partner's fidelity.

Impact: Clinically significant distress or impairment in social, occupational, or other important areas of functioning. The pattern is inflexible and pervasive across a broad range of situations. Symptoms must exceed cultural and contextual norms.

Timeframe: Persistent and can be traced back at least to adolescence.

Source: Information from APA (2022).

pervasive pattern of detachment from social relationships and limited emotional expression. People with schizoid personality disorder may feel emotions, but they have a difficult time expressing them, and it may be hard for others to understand the emotional content of what they are trying to convey.

SYMPTOMS AND DESCRIPTION

Schiz means split, as in schism, and the split in schizoid personality disorder is between the person with the condition and their emotions, and between them and other people. Because those with the disorder neither desire nor enjoy social relationships, their condition tends to be ego syntonic, and they really prefer to be alone (Diagnostic Overview 12.2). The lack of desire for close relationships doesn't mean a lack of impairment. Those with schizoid personality disorder often also have occupational dysfunction, such as difficulty in relating to co-workers and customers or incorporating feedback from supervisors.

STATISTICS AND TRAJECTORY

Surveys estimates the prevalence of schizoid personality disorder to be about 1.2–1.8 percent worldwide. It is diagnosed slightly more often in men than in women (Torgersen et al. 2012; Volkert et al. 2018). There are some sociocultural theories for these differences (see sociocultural models and treatments for Cluster A personality disorders below for more information).

Schizotypal Personality Disorder

Schizotypal personality disorder: a personality disorder characterized by a pervasive pattern of discomfort in social relationships and by odd and eccentric behavior.

Schizotypal personality disorder is characterized by a pervasive pattern of discomfort in social relationships and by odd and eccentric behavior. Those with this disorder choose to be by themselves and don't have many close personal relationships other than first-degree relatives. This isn't to say they don't wish to have them; often they do.

SYMPTOMS AND DESCRIPTION

People with schizotypal personality disorder are suspicious and have beliefs that others may consider odd (Chemerinski et al. 2013; Rosell et al. 2014) (Diagnostic Overview 12.3). Some have psychotic-like symptoms such as delusions or hallucinations (Kwapil & Barrantes-Vidal 2012), and they dress, act, believe, and think in unusual ways. For example, they have *ideas of reference*, meaning they believe without any evidence that unconnected events like a song playing at a restaurant or national news events are about them (Rosell et al. 2014), though when pressed they will admit this is unlikely. Some people with schizotypal personality disorder will display *magical thinking*, which is the belief that their thoughts or actions can influence the world in irrational ways. For instance, they may believe they can change the weather or use symbols such as runes to change events in the past.

STATISTICS AND TRAJECTORY

Schizotypal personality disorder is one of the rarest of the personality disorders, found in only 0.7–1.1 percent of the general worldwide population. It is a little more common in men than in women (Torgersen et al. 2012; Volkert et al. 2018).

Models and Treatments of Cluster A Personality Disorders

Research evidence related to Cluster A personality disorders is rare; there is more evidence regarding models and treatment for schizotypal personality disorder (Kerns 2020). Despite the negative impact of personality disorders, not everyone with these conditions will be motivated to seek treatment. In fact, some of the aspects of various personality disorders may themselves create a less-than-ideal treatment environment. For example, although symptoms of paranoid personality disorder can lead to a fair amount of distress and impairment, those with the condition often have difficulty trusting therapists (Adshead & Sarkar 2012), and few therapists who treat people with this disorder think clients will stay in therapy long enough to see any improvement. In fact one in four people with a personality disorder will drop out of treatment (Berghuis et al. 2021). Similarly, most people with schizoid personality disorder don't experience significant distress with regard to their symptoms unless they are related to another condition such as depression (Feldman & Gitu 2021). As you can imagine, these clients are split off emotionally from their therapists and disengaged from treatment, and they may keep appointments only if brought by family members (Winarick 2020).

BIOLOGICAL MODELS AND TREATMENTS

From a biological viewpoint, people with schizotypal personality disorder are often relatives of those who might develop psychotic disorders such as schizophrenia. Because of this connection, you might also expect those diagnosed with schizophrenia to have relatives diagnosed with schizotypal personality disorder, and in fact there is research evidence that supports this claim. Some classic studies

---

Diagnostic Overview 12.2: Schizoid Personality Disorder

A long-lasting pattern of detachment from others, as indicated by at least four of the following symptoms:

- Lack of desire for close relationships, including being part of a family, and lack of enjoyment in them.
- Preference for solitary activities.
- Little if any interest in having sexual experiences with another person.
- Ability to take pleasure in few if any activities.
- Lack of close friends other than relatives.
- Indifference to the praise or criticism of others.
- Emotional coldness, detachment, or flattened affectivity.

Impact: Clinically significant distress or impairment in social, occupational, or other important areas of functioning. The pattern is inflexible and pervasive across a broad range of situations. Symptoms must exceed cultural and contextual norms.

Timeframe: Persistent and can be traced back at least to adolescence.

Source: Information from APA (2022).

Eccentric behavior and discomfort about close relationships, as well as cognitive or perceptual symptoms that result in at least five of the following:

- The false belief that events in the world directly relate to them.
- Odd beliefs.
- Odd, eccentric, or peculiar behavior.
- Peculiar perceptual experiences.
- Odd thinking and speech.
- Suspiciousness about others.
- Emotional expressions that are limited and sometimes unsuited to the situation.
- Difficulty forming and maintaining relationships.
- Excessive social anxiety.

Impact: Clinically significant distress or impairment in social, occupational, or other important areas of functioning. The pattern is inflexible and pervasive across a broad range of situations. Symptoms must exceed cultural and contextual norms.

Timeframe: Persistent and can be traced back at least to adolescence.

Source: Information from APA (2022).

have reported higher rates of diagnoses of schizotypal personality disorders in those *with* relatives diagnosed with schizophrenia than in those *without* such relatives (Kendler & Walsh 1995). And twin studies show increased rates of schizotypal personality disorder in families with members who have schizophrenia (Siever & Davis 2004).

Many of those with schizotypal personality disorder have some of the biological factors found in schizophrenia, such as variations in levels of dopamine, larger ventricles, and reduced gray matter (Kerns 2020; Rosell 2017) (see Chapter 13 for more on schizophrenia). And one recent study provided evidence that people diagnosed with schizotypal personality disorder were at increased risk of developing schizophrenia in the future. Of those initially diagnosed with schizotypal personality disorder, more than a third (33 percent) developed schizophrenia over the next 20 years (Hjorthøj et al. 2018).

Biological treatment options for Cluster A personality disorder are limited. Some clients with paranoid personality disorder are unwilling to take medications. For those who are willing, however, prescribers often opt for medications targeted at specific symptoms of anxiety (such as drugs typically prescribed for depression, or second-generation antipsychotics that may also reduce anxiety). Biological therapies for schizoid personality disorder have had limited success due to clients' reluctance to engage in their own treatment (Skodol 2017).

The biological perspective for schizotypal personality disorder focuses on medications. Antipsychotic medications are thought to be helpful due to the links the condition might have to schizophrenia. They have been effective for some clients in low doses. Also helpful are stimulant medications to assist with some of the cognitive symptoms, such as problems in thinking and concentrating that people with schizotypal personality disorder sometimes have (Kerns 2020).

PSYCHODYNAMIC MODELS AND TREATMENTS

Psychodynamic theories of paranoid personality disorder point to early family relationships, particularly rigid fathers and rejecting maternal figures. Such hostile and unstable social environments are often characterized by unreasonable and ever-shifting demands (Kellett & Hardy 2014). As a result, a person develops extreme hostility, feelings of persecution, and an expectation that others are untrustworthy (Cariola 2020; Koenigsberg et al. 2001).

Psychodynamic explanations for schizoid personality disorder suggest that the condition is a response to an unmet need for satisfactory relationships, particularly if parents have been unaccepting. To counter these early relationships, psychodynamic therapies focus on supporting the person's desire to create satisfying relationships (Caligor & Clarkin 2010).

COGNITIVE-BEHAVIORAL MODELS AND TREATMENTS

From the cognitive-behavioral standpoint, paranoid personality disorder is acquired through learning. That is, paranoid behaviors could once have been adaptive responses to stressful situations (Bradley et al. 2007). Vigilance and paranoia can act as an early warning system and get us prepared to fight. In this way paranoia can be part of healthy human psychology (Raihani & Bell 2019). The cognitive-behavioral theories suggest that symptoms of paranoid personality disorder are rooted in negative assumptions about people in general, such as "People are evil," or "People will attack you if they get the chance" (Beck & Weishaar 2019). These maladaptive cognitions around the intentions of others may have developed early in life and create a pattern of hypervigilance for deception in other people (Lobbestael & Arntz 2012; Triebwasser et al. 2013).

Cognitive-behavioral theories suggest that people with schizoid personality disorder have difficulty understanding the emotions of others (Chadwick 2014). Because they struggle to understand these emotions, they can't respond to them either. Cognitive theories suggest a schema of low self-confidence about being able to defend against attacks, combined with the conviction that people are generally bad and will try to deceive.

For schizotypal personality disorder, the cognitive-behavioral perspective suggests that people with the condition are more inclined to jump to conclusions and make confident but unusual decisions based on very limited evidence. These responses may be driven by feelings of isolation or paranoid thoughts they experience. Rather than sitting with the discomfort, they jump to unusual conclusions to fill in the gaps. This theory is consistent with the evidence that people with this disorder possess such a cognitive bias and are more likely to be influenced by their internal "gut" feelings (Kerns 2020).

Cognitive-behavioral therapy for paranoid personality focuses on reducing anxiety and helping to create realistic interpretations of the words and actions of other people (Kellett & Hardy 2014). Therapists will often try to increase trust in relationships (Beck et al. 2015).

While cognitive-behavioral theory for schizoid personality disorder emphasizes social skills training, especially teaching clients to become more curious about the feelings of others, the cognitive-behavioral approach for schizotypal personality disorder works on helping clients test the validity of their thoughts in an objective way (Matusiewicz et al. 2010). Social skills training can also be helpful (Skodol 2017).

SOCIOCULTURAL MODELS AND TREATMENTS

Sociocultural factors are also at play for Cluster A personality disorders. In the United States, for example, Black Americans are at greater risk for paranoid personality disorder symptoms, in part due to their increased exposure to prejudice, discrimination, and other events that may build the schemas that can contribute to

Table 12.1 Symptoms that may develop as a result of the COVID-19 pandemic in those with Cluster A personality disorders

Pandemic and quarantine psychological impact
Anxiety symptoms
Depressive symptoms
Avoidance behaviors such as minimizing direct contact
Delay in return to normality
Disruption of social networks

Source: Data from Preti et al. (2020).

the condition (Iacovino et al. 2014). Schizotypal personality disorder symptoms are higher in individuals, especially men, who have had a history of childhood maltreatment.

The COVID-19 pandemic may have had an especially negative impact on people with Cluster A personality disorders. Because of their symptoms (including suspiciousness, lack of interest in social relationships, and lack of close friends), the fear of getting COVID-19, along with the social impact of required isolation after exposure to the virus, can be risk factors for them to develop negative effects (Table 12.1).

MULTIPERSPECTIVE MODELS AND TREATMENTS

Some treatments for schizotypal personality disorder focus on preventing it from turning into schizophrenia. One approach proposed multiple treatments including medications, social skills training, and community interventions. These combination approaches delayed the onset of schizophrenia and reduced overall symptoms (Bateman et al. 2015).

CONCEPT CHECK 12.2

Match the case with the type of Cluster A personality disorder.
   A. Paranoid personality disorder
   B. Schizoid personality disorder
   C. Schizotypal personality disorders
   1. Brandon is a 22-year-old college graduate whose parents worry about his lack of interest in getting a job. He went to a few interviews at their urging, but with clear indifference as to the outcome. He didn't even tell his parents whether he got the job. He's never been close to anyone, talks to others only from necessity, and spends most of his time alone. He doesn't seem concerned about his lack of friends.
   2. Jerrod is convinced his roommate is trying to harm him. In fact, he finds the whole world threatening and doesn't trust anyone to be a close friend. An interview with a psychologist revealed that Jerrod doesn't have hallucinations or any other symptoms of psychosis.
   3. Kristin's parents have described her as "odd." She has trouble relating to her friends, feels anxious around them, and believes she doesn't fit in at college. The people she knows don't seem interested in the same things she finds fascinating, such as paranormal experiences, superstitions, and the evidence she has about the existence of ghosts in the college. These problems cause Kristin a great deal of distress.

12.3 CLUSTER B: DRAMATIC PERSONALITY DISORDERS

While Cluster A focuses on behaviors that are often seen as odd or eccentric, Cluster B of the *DSM-5tr* chapter on Personality Disorders identifies disorders that are more dramatic. Cluster B conditions have in common erratic, pronounced, and overly emotional behaviors that can cause distress and impairment in social and work functioning. They include antisocial personality disorder, borderline personality disorder, histrionic personality disorder, and narcissistic personality disorder. These conditions are rare; one epidemiological study that included people in Europe, North America, Australia, and New Zealand suggested that just 3.29 percent of the population shows evidence of any of the Cluster B personality disorders (Volkert et al. 2018) (Figure 12.6).

Antisocial Personality Disorder

Antisocial personality disorder is a condition in which a person breaks the rules of society and often with no remorse or anxiety. For a diagnosis of this disorder, we would expect to find conduct difficulties before the age of 15. We would also need to see three or more other symptoms including law breaking, frequent lying, impulsivity, aggressiveness, disregard for the safety of others, irresponsibility, or lack of remorse for having hurt others or even rationalizations for having done so (Figure 12.3).

Antisocial personality disorder: a personality disorder in which a person breaks the rules of society and often with no remorse or anxiety.

SYMPTOMS AND DESCRIPTION

People with antisocial personality disorder have trouble telling the truth, don't honor their obligations, and are impulsive, irritable, aggressive, and reckless with their own safety and that of others (Diagnostic Overview 12.4). They don't have much regard for the people they've tricked and see them as weak.

Unlike most personality disorders, which can be diagnosed only after the age of 18, antisocial personality disorder requires earlier evidence of symptoms of antisocial behavior for a diagnosis.

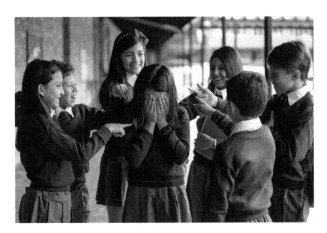

Figure 12.3 Bullying can be a key feature in antisocial personality disorder.
Source: andresr/E+/Getty Images.

Diagnostic Overview 12.4: Antisocial Personality Disorder

A pattern of disregard for and violation of the rights of others, as indicated by at least three of the following:

- Habit of breaking rules and laws.
- Deceitfulness.
- Impulsivity.
- Irritability and aggressiveness.
- Reckless disregard for safety of self or others.
- Consistent irresponsibility.
- Lack of remorse.

Timeframe: The person is at least 18 years and has shown prior evidence of a conduct disorder before age 15.

Impact: Clinically significant distress or impairment in social, occupational, or other important areas of functioning. The pattern is inflexible and pervasive across a broad range of situations. Symptoms must exceed cultural and contextual norms.

Source: Information from APA (2022).

STATISTICS AND TRAJECTORY

Surveys suggest that as much as 3.6 percent of the US population will have symptoms of antisocial personality disorder in any given year (Black 2019). Rates are similar worldwide at 3.13 percent (Volkert et al. 2018). Antisocial personality disorder is four times more common in men than in women; the prevalence in women is around 1 percent. Some research suggests that, for reasons not yet known, the symptoms start to decline after age 40, although the disorder may manifest itself differently in older adults in a way that is missed by the diagnostic criteria and also in women (Holzer et al. 2021).

Up to 80 percent of those with antisocial personality disorder have symptoms of substance use at some point (Black 2019). How are these two issues linked? Could it be that antisocial personality disorder and substance use disorder have the same roots in risk taking? We may need more research to know for sure. Consistent with this finding, however, is that 23 percent of people diagnosed with gambling disorder also have antisocial personality disorder (Black 2019; Grant et al. 2004).

THE POWER OF WORDS

ARE INTROVERTS ANTISOCIAL?

Some people don't like to go to parties or other gatherings and avoid large groups. We often call them antisocial, but are they? *Anti* means against, and people with antisocial personality disorder work against society. Sometimes, however, people who prefer to be in smaller groups are introverted rather than truly antisocial from a psychological perspective (Figure 12.4).

Some people think introverts are shy and keep to themselves while extroverts are outgoing, but there's more to it than that. Introverts do prefer their internal world of thoughts to the extrovert's external world of people, and some may be reserved when interacting socially. But the important dividing line between introversion and extroversion is actually *energy*.

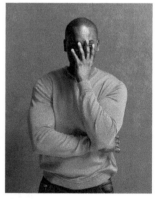

Figure 12.4 Are shy people antisocial?

Source: Digital Vision/ Photodisc/Getty Images.

Introverts recharge their internal energy by being by themselves, while extroverts tend to recharge by being around others. What do you find more interesting – what's inside your head or what's outside your head? Introverts find what's going on inside to be much more interesting. That's why they can distract themselves with their own thoughts and will retreat there for comfort and recharging. They can find others exhausting. Extroverts, on the other hand, prefer the world outside their head. They find others energizing and can get grumpy if they are alone too much.

In the United States the personality of extroverts is encouraged. Many self-help books, for example, encourage people to be charismatic and to reach out and connect with other people. It's easy for some to characterize those who are introverted as less interested in social interactions (Cain 2013). That's not necessarily the case. They certainly don't have a personality disorder that causes them to violate the rights of others, and while they might not want to participate in group activities, they typically aren't antisocial either, as someone with schizoid personality disorder is likely to be.

Source: Cain (2013).

Borderline Personality Disorder

Borderline personality disorder (BPD) is a condition marked by a long history of instability in a person's self-image, in their ability to control impulses, in their relationships, and in their moods. The instability exhibited by those with this condition can cause disruptions in relationships and frequent shifts in goals, work, and friends. It can leave someone feeling worried and with little sense of who they are as a person. This in turn can lead to a short temper, frequent fights, and fear of abandonment. Although borderline personality disorder is not very common, affecting less about 2 percent of the general population (Bayes & Parker 2017), the severity of its symptoms makes it overrepresented in treatment populations. About one in every ten people in outpatient mental health settings is diagnosed with borderline personality disorder, and about two in every ten people among psychiatric inpatients (Kessler & Wang 2008).

Borderline personality disorder: a personality disorder marked by a long history of instability in a person's self-image, in their ability to control impulses, in their relationships, and in their moods.

SYMPTOMS AND DESCRIPTION

The symptoms of borderline personality disorder can manifest in great deal of anger, self-harm, and a feeling of emptiness (Diagnostic Overview 12.5). The sense of identity is unstable, meaning the person is unable to pin down what they want to do, or their dreams for the future. They may even feel a sense of detachment or derealization from their own bodies or thoughts (Zanarini et al. 2016). Many people with borderline personality disorder describe feeling chronic and unspeakable distress that creates a need for numbing. Some use cutting and other self-injurious behavior to reduce the tension they feel, or "just to feel something" (McKenzie & Gross 2014). These symptoms result in their having unstable and intense relationships (Skodol 2017) in which they will idealize and then devalue the other person.

Diagnostic Overview 12.5: Borderline Personality Disorder

People with borderline personality disorder have an unstable view of themselves and their friends, and they experience rapidly shifting moods. Additional symptoms include:

- Attempts to prevent important others from abandoning them.
- Stormy relationships in which the other person is alternately idealized and condemned.
- Shallow understanding of self.
- Recklessness.
- Physical self-harm that may include cutting or suicide attempts.
- Feelings of emptiness.
- Intense anger.

Impact: Clinically significant distress or impairment in social, occupational, or other important areas of functioning. The pattern is inflexible and pervasive across a broad range of situations. Symptoms must exceed cultural and contextual norms.

Timeframe: Persistent and can be traced back at least to adolescence.

Source: Information from APA (2022).

They fear being abandoned but also take desperate measures, such as cutting themselves, to prevent it from happening (Skodol 2017).

Perhaps the most dramatic symptom among people with borderline personality disorder is suicidality (Amore et al. 2014). About 75 percent of people diagnosed with borderline personality disorder have attempted suicide at least once, and 10 percent will die by suicide (Hong 2016).

Although it is a complex condition by itself, borderline personality disorder is often comorbid with other disorders. Up to 85 percent of those with the condition will also have another psychological condition, such as depression or an anxiety disorder (Skodol 2017; Zanarini et al. 2016). They may engage in self-destructive behaviors such as substance use, self-harm, unsafe sex, or reckless driving. Sometimes people with this disorder use such self-destructive behaviors to distract themselves from a flood of negative emotions (Sadeh et al. 2014; Skodol 2017).

STATISTICS AND TRAJECTORY

Surveys suggest that as much as 1.6 percent of the US population will have symptoms of borderline personality disorder; rates are similar in women and men (Torgersen et al. 2012). Symptoms peak during young adulthood and often decrease as people get older (Skodol 2017). In fact, most people with borderline personality disorder (85 percent) show a reduction of symptoms within 10–15 years (Gunderson et al. 2011), although stress can trigger their return (Gunderson et al. 2011).

Histrionic Personality Disorder

Histrionic personality disorder: a personality disorder marked by a persistent pattern of attention seeking and excessive emotionality.

Histrionic personality disorder is marked by a persistent pattern of attention seeking and excessive emotionality. People with this disorder feel as if they don't exist when others don't pay attention to them. Because of this, they'll do almost anything for attention. This attention-seeking behavior can create problems in their social and occupational functioning.

SYMPTOMS AND DESCRIPTION

How would you behave if the attention of others was your life blood? How would you draw that attention toward yourself? People with histrionic personality disorder do so by changing their personalities, but their efforts can seem exhausting (see Chapter 7's The Power of Words box for more about the term hysteria, which is related to the term histrionic). They overreact to small things, appear to be self-focused, and will do nearly anything for attention even if it's negative

Source: *Information from APA (2022).*

Diagnostic Overview 12.6: Histrionic Personality Disorder

A pattern of excessive emotionality and attention seeking with at least five of the following symptoms:

- Discomfort when not the center of attention.
- Inappropriately provocative or seductive behavior.
- Shifting and shallow emotions.
- Physical appearance tailored to draw attention.
- Impressionistic and vague speech.
- Exaggerated emotional expressions.
- Suggestibility and susceptibility to the influence of others.
- Belief that relationships are more intimate than they actually are.

Impact: Clinically significant distress or impairment in social, occupational, or other important areas of functioning. The pattern is inflexible and pervasive across a broad range of situations. Symptoms must exceed cultural and contextual norms.

Timeframe: Persistent and can be traced back at least to adolescence.

(Diagnostic Overview 12.6). They will often dress in sexually provocative ways to draw attention to themselves, are overly concerned with the way people see them, consistently seek reassurance, become angry when they don't get it, and behave as if they are your best friend when you hardly know them (Figure 12.5).

STATISTICS AND TRAJECTORY

Surveys suggest that as much as 1.3 percent of the US population will have symptoms of histrionic personality disorder (Torgersen et al. 2012). The condition is only slightly more common in women than in men (Hartung & Lefler 2019).

Narcissistic Personality Disorder

Narcissistic personality disorder is marked by a persistent and excessive need to be admired and a lack of empathy. Histrionic personality disorder might seem similar to this condition, but it's quite different. People with histrionic personality disorder will do almost anything for attention because they feel they *need* it. People with narcissistic personality disorder, on the other hand, want attention and special treatment only from special people, and because they feel they *deserve* it.

Narcissistic personality disorder: a personality disorder marked by a persistent and excessive need to be admired and a lack of empathy.

SYMPTOMS AND DESCRIPTION

People with narcissistic personality disorder show pathological grandiosity and have difficulty with long-term relationships because they are demanding (Hardaker & Tsakanikos 2021). They believe they are special and should be appreciated only by other high-status special people, despite the fact that they have exaggerated their own importance (Diagnostic Overview 12.7). One of the problems they have in relating to others is that they don't have empathy and see other people only as sources of admiration.

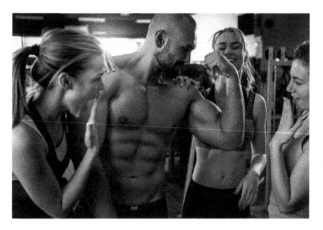

Figure 12.5 People with histrionic personality disorder have attention seeking behavior.

Source: hoozone/E+/Getty Images.

STATISTICS AND TRAJECTORY

Narcissistic personality disorder has the lowest incidence rates of any personality disorder (Dawood et al. 2020). Community samples have yielded rates between 0.5 percent and 5 percent in the US population (Ronningstam 2013). Rates of narcissistic personality disorder are similar around the world, with surveys suggesting that about 0.34 percent of people worldwide meet the criteria for the condition (Volkert et al. 2018) (see Figure 12.6). Rates may be low based on the lack of insight into their symptoms that people with the disorder have, and their unwillingness to discuss their difficulties or reveal their narcissistic attitudes (Dawood et al. 2020).

Models and Treatments of Cluster B Personality Disorders

Not only did Marsha's symptoms improve (see the chapter-opening story), but she went on to develop one of the most effective treatments for borderline personality disorder we have (more on that later).

Those with borderline personality disorder often seek help, for instance, but their symptoms can make treatment difficult. Risk of self-injury, constant impulsive behaviors, and shifting emotional states can be frustrating for many therapists and clients alike. In fact, the majority of people with borderline personality disorder (more than 97 percent) have seen an average of 6.1 therapists (Chapman et al. 2020).

People with histrionic personality disorder also tend to seek out therapy (French & Shrestha 2020), although again treatment is not easy because of the symptoms of the condition. Clients often will display seductiveness, tantrums, and other attention-seeking behaviors in the midst of treatment. Some will pretend to gain insights or experience improvements simply to please their therapists. Because of this manipulative response, therapists must be cautious and objective throughout treatment (French & Shrestha 2020).

Narcissistic personality disorder may be ego-syntonic, and therefore people with its symptoms may not see the condition as problematic even though it may cause significant disruptions in social and occupational functioning. Those with the condition may have difficulty recognizing the impact they have on other people. Sometimes they begin therapy because of a related condition (such as depression), but they will often try to pull the therapist into the role of admirer (Colli et al. 2014).

Diagnostic Overview 12.7: Narcissistic Personality Disorder

Grandiosity, a need to be admired, with a lack of empathy as indicated by at least five of the following:

- A sense of self-importance that doesn't match achievements.
- Preoccupation with success.
- Belief that they are special and unique.
- Need for excessive admiration.
- A sense of entitlement.
- Pattern of interpersonal exploitation.
- Lack of empathy.
- Envy of others.
- Arrogant behaviors and attitudes.

Impact: Clinically significant distress or impairment in social, occupational, or other important areas of functioning. The pattern is inflexible and pervasive across a broad range of situations. Symptoms must exceed cultural and contextual norms.

Timeframe: Persistent and can be traced back at least to adolescence.

Source: Information from APA (2022).

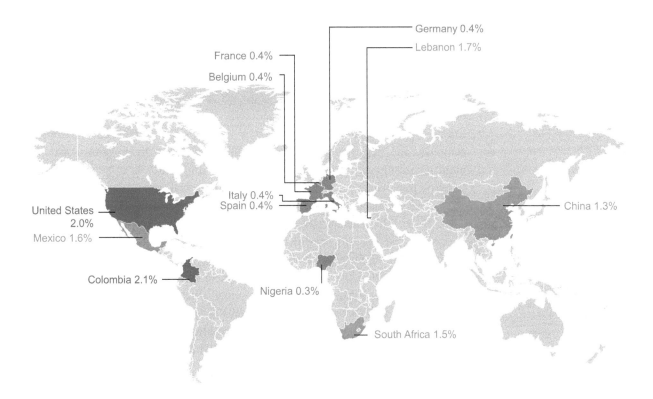

As with other conditions, there are biological as well as psychological models and treatments for the Cluster B personality disorders.

BIOLOGICAL MODELS AND TREATMENTS

Scientists have been trying to identify the cause or causes of antisocial behavior for some time. Is there a criminal mind? Are there really natural-born killers? Certainly, biology does play a role. Classic twin studies suggest that among monozygotic twins, in 67 percent of cases both siblings will have the condition if one does. There may be genes that influence the condition (Torgersen et al. 2012).

Some evidence suggests that those with antisocial personality disorder crave higher levels of sensation in order to maintain the normal feelings we all have. They are easily susceptible to boredom and pick activities that will give them a quick fix. The *underarousal hypothesis* for this disorder suggests that those with antisocial personality disorder have low levels of cortical arousal (Savage 2009) and seek more stimulation of all kinds in order to boost their arousal. The *fearlessness hypothesis*, on the other hand, suggests that people with antisocial personality disorder aren't that easy to frighten (Cardinale et al. 2021). Without fear, say of pain or embarrassment, the other symptoms come into play.

Specialized systems in the brain have evolved to reward some behaviors with pleasure while associating others with pain. These systems act like biological traffic lights. Potentially rewarding experiences (like food) get the green light and we want to approach them. Events that could be punished (like pain) or that won't bring a reward get the red light and we want to avoid them. In this way our

Figure 12.6 Lifetime prevalence of Cluster B personality disorders in selected countries, from the World Mental Health Surveys (2002–2017).

Source: Huang et al. (2009).

neural motivation systems regulate our sensitivity to rewards and punishments. The "green light" is the Behavioral Approach System (BAS), and the "red light" is the Behavioral Inhibition System (BIS).

The BAS is sensitive to reward and is activated when we sense something that could be rewarding. It controls our approach and approach-type behaviors. Our body makes potentially rewarding activities feel good. The BIS, in contrast, is sensitive to threat and non-reward. It is activated during punishment, boring activities, and negative events and regulates our sensitivity to punishment. It ultimately results in our avoiding these kinds of situations.

Some researchers suggest that people with antisocial personality disorder have lower BIS responses and overactive BAS reward responses (Hoppenbrouwers et al. 2015). This characteristic reduces any anxiety that people with antisocial personality disorder may have about the destructive things they are tempted to do, while also making the temptations more attractive.

Neurotransmitters may also be at play. People with antisocial behaviors, especially those who exhibit impulsive and aggressive behaviors, have lower levels of the neurotransmitter serotonin than do others (Thompson et al. 2014). Impulsivity and aggression have both been associated with lower levels of serotonin.

But neurotransmitters don't tell the entire story. Brain areas are also important. People with antisocial personality disorder show lower levels of activity in both their anterior cingulate cortex and their prefrontal cortex (Glenn et al. 2013). These areas are active in planning, execution, empathy, and judgment.

Other biologically oriented researchers have discovered that people with antisocial personality disorder respond differently to stress warnings. Their bodies just don't warn them of threats or danger in the same way. Because they are less aroused when other people might be stressed, for example, they experience slower EEG waves (Calzada-Reyes et al. 2012). This response allows them to filter out highly emotional or threatening external and internal cues and not learn that much from situations that others might find taxing. The brain circuit that might be tied to this response consists of the prefrontal cortex, anterior cingulate cortex, amygdala, hippocampus, and temporal cortex. A smaller number of interconnections in this circuit might be responsible for reduced stress reactions in both the sympathetic nervous system and the hypothalamic pituitary adrenal pathway. These all lead to the symptoms of antisocial personality disorder (Aghajani et al. 2017).

Researchers have identified biological models for borderline personality disorder as well. For example, studies of twins with this disorder provide evidence that it might have a genetic component (Fatimah et al. 2020). These studies have found that in 35 percent of cases, if someone who is an identical twin has the disorder, both twins will have it, while only 19 percent of DZ (fraternal) twins will both display symptoms (Skodol 2017). In fact, if a close relative has BPD, you are five times more likely to have it (Amad et al. 2014).

Studies have suggested that the differences in the amygdala, responsible for regulating emotions, could be a factor in borderline personality disorder. Neuroimaging theories of BPD say that the hippocampus and amygdala of those with the condition are smaller. In Chapter 2 (section 2.1) we discussed that the amygdala is an important brain structure for emotional regulation, and that the hippocampus is active in stress and memory regulation. In people with borderline personality disorder, the amygdala is overactive, and the areas responsible for controlling emotional responses are underactive (Young et al. 2021).

The frontal lobes in particular are implicated in our ability to plan, judge, decide, and regulate our emotions. Some theories suggest that poor communication among the structures in the frontal lobe and other structures may contribute to the constellation of symptoms of borderline personality disorder (Agha et al. 2017) and lead to problems with regulating emotions. Some evidence also suggests that people who display symptoms of BPD, especially clients with high amounts of impulsivity (such as suicidality or aggressiveness), display lower levels of the neurotransmitter serotonin.

While there are no FDA-approved medications for Cluster B personality disorders, medications can help reduce the symptoms of anxiety or depression that some people with these conditions experience (Cheli 2020). For example, drugs typically prescribed for depression, anxiety, and psychosis have been useful for reducing the symptoms of BPD (Bridler et al. 2015). However, prescribers must be cautious with these, given the frequency of suicide attempts among clients (Gunderson et al. 2011). These drugs are thus often prescribed along with psychotherapy (Skodol 2017).

THE POWER OF EVIDENCE

Can a brain scan reveal antisocial personality disorder?

Dr. James Fallon (Figure 12.7), a neuroscientist at the University of California, Irvine, discovered a specific area of the brain in the orbital cortex that he felt was involved in the lack of impulse control in people with antisocial personality disorder (Fallon 2006). After studying the brain scans of many people with the disorder, he was indeed able to identify low activity in this brain area.

This was exciting stuff – a potential lead to a test for antisocial personality disorder. Then came a twist. After being encouraged to check into his family background, Fallon discovered that one of his ancestors had allegedly murdered his own mother. In fact, there were seven alleged murders

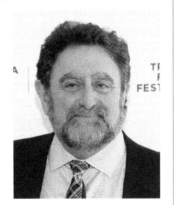

Figure 12.7 Dr. James Fallon.
Source: Ilya S. Savenok/Getty Images for the 2014 Tribeca Film Festival.

in that line of his family, including the case of Lizzie Borden, who in August 1892 was accused of killing her father and stepmother with an axe (she was later acquitted of the murder).

Fallon was shocked. He then studied the brain scans of all the members of his immediate family to see whether they too had the low activity he had observed in the orbital frontal cortex and had associated with antisocial personality disorder. None did, except for one – Fallon himself. He had exactly the orbital frontal profile shared by all the people he had been studying, who had antisocial personality disorder and were also murderers. He also shared with them all the known high-risk violence-related genes.

As you are no doubt well aware by now, biology doesn't determine everything – the environment plays a critical role, and many factors during childhood, such as lack of warmth, neglect, and harsh punishment, are also important for the development of antisocial personality disorder. Fallon's upbringing, however, had been filled with love and support from his entire extended family, and his discovery changed his thinking about the relationship between nature and nurture.

"I went into this with the bias of a scientist who believed, for many years, that genetics were very, very dominant in who people are – that your genes would tell you who were going to be. It's not that I do not think that biology, which includes genetics, is a major determinant; I just never knew how profoundly an early environment could affect somebody."

To read more about Fallon and his work, take a look at his book *The psychopath inside: A neuroscientist's personal journey into the dark side of the brain* (Fallon 2014).

Source: Ohikuare (2014).

PSYCHODYNAMIC MODELS AND TREATMENTS

Psychodynamic explanations of antisocial personality disorder suggest that a lack of love will lead to a lack of trust (Meloy & Yakeley 2010). Because of this lack, people with antisocial personality disorder cut themselves off emotionally and control others through power. There is some research that supports this. People with antisocial personality disorder are more likely to have loss in their lives, such as poverty, violence, abuse, or divorce (Torgersen et al. 2012).

One of the things that stops most of us from doing things that are against the rules is the anxiety we feel when we consider such behavior. Imagine that you never felt that anxiety. The psychoanalytic perspective for APD might suggest that you had a weak superego, while the behavioral perspective might say APD would make it more difficult to learn from punishment. One of the core components of antisocial personality disorder is the coldness and lack of empathy that allows people to break laws, mislead others, and fail to repay debts. If their bodies don't produce the anxiety response in reaction to negative experiences, then it makes sense they wouldn't feel any of the accompanying anxiety, including the cues we give others when they have broken even social rules (Blair et al. 2005; Torgersen et al. 2012).

Psychodynamic perspectives for borderline personality disorder suggest that early relationships, especially with parents, can lead to borderline personality disorder. If children feel rejected by their parents (because of lack of attention, for example) this may lead to lower self-esteem, greater dependence on other people, and problems separating from them.

Not every therapeutic approach is equally effective for borderline personality disorder. Some clients see the client–therapist interaction of classic psychoanalytic psychotherapy as a disinterested one and may view the therapist's interpretations as personal attacks. More contemporary psychodynamic approaches have been helpful. Some research suggests they can help reduce suicidality and self-harm and focus positively on the person's sense of self (Cristea et al. 2017).

Psychoanalytic theories of histrionic personality disorder were originally developed in the nineteenth century, in part to explain what was then called hysteria, and they did a better job than the state-of-the-art idea at the time (see Chapter 2, section 2.1). The core idea of the psychoanalytic theories was that controlling parents left clients with feelings of abandonment (Novais et al. 2015). The clients' solution? Staging dramatic crisis at every turn to keep the people around them engaged in their lives.

Psychodynamic theories suggest that early rejecting caregivers are the source of narcissistic personality disorder. Such caregivers lead people to overcompensate later by telling themselves (and the world) that they are perfect. In addition, rejecting caretakers are unable to model empathy (Schmidt 2019). There is some support for this claim. Children who are neglected are at greater risk of developing narcissistic personality disorder. It seems to be the case that people with narcissistic personality disorder more often feel shame and rejection than those without the condition, even early in their lives (Miller et al. 2017).

Psychodynamic therapists for narcissistic personality disorder aim to help clients to resolve insecurity (Crisp & Gabbard 2020). Although there is a wealth of psychodynamic models for personality disorders, especially in Cluster B, there isn't much data regarding their effectiveness as treatments. However, one meta-analysis of psychodynamic therapies for personality disorders discovered that although they were more helpful than no treatment, they didn't fare better than any other therapy in the treatment of personality disorders in general, except in the case of reducing suicidality in those with borderline personality disorder (Briggs et al. 2019).

COGNITIVE-BEHAVIORAL MODELS AND TREATMENTS

Cognitive-behavioral theories of antisocial personality disorder suggest that antisocial behavior may be learned in the same way everything is learned – through conditioning, and especially through modeling others' behaviors (Cabrera et al. 2017). Research suggests that some middle-school students are drawn to antisocial peers and may be more likely to engage in antisocial behaviors themselves in order to be liked (Juvonen & Ho 2008).

Most cognitive-behavioral theories of borderline personality disorder look at the way cognitions are related to regulation of emotions. People with borderline personality disorder have reported a greater daily variation in both the range and the intensity of emotions, particularly sadness, hostility, and fear (Houben et al. 2021), and a slower return to their baseline mood (Ebner-Priemer et al. 2015) than do people without the disorder. In addition, their memories of past events tend to be more negative than those of people without borderline personality disorder, based on their negative interpretations of what's occurring (Baer et al. 2012). Like many people, those with borderline personality disorder try to suppress their negative moods and interpretations, but they are generally less successful and respond impulsively to the way they feel in the moment (Selby et al. 2009). The result is that they end up feeling negative about relationships in general and cope poorly when unexpected events occur (Lazarus et al. 2014).

Cognitive-behavioral approaches for histrionic personality disorder often emphasize helping clients to problem-solve on their own and create new skills that let them feel comfortable when they aren't the center of attention (Beck & Weishaar 2019). Some cognitive-behavioral theorists take an opposite view, however, and suggest that people with narcissistic personality disorder have a history of being treated too positively. Feelings of grandiosity develop because they have learned to overvalue their own worth, but may not be as sensitive to positive information, and as a consequence they need rewards all the time (Hardaken & Tsakanikos 2021; Miller et al. 2017).

Cognitive-behavioral therapy has been found useful for reducing violence in people with antisocial personality disorder even five years after the treatment (Olver et al. 2013). Another approach targets the social environment, namely the young client's parents (Scott et al. 2014). This CBT approach teaches parents to reinforce prosocial behaviors and has been found to help some children. However, the more chaotic the family and the more stress it experiences, the less successful such early interventions appear to be (Kaminski et al. 2008).

Perhaps the treatment with the strongest research support is dialectical behavior therapy, developed by psychologist Marsha Linehan whom we met in this chapter's opening case. **Dialectical behavior therapy (DBT)** is a treatment for borderline personality disorder that aims to teach problem-solving skills, emotional regulation, and interpersonal skills (Linehan et al. 2015; Robins et al. 2004). It can be delivered in both individual and group sessions and emphasizes reducing self-harm by helping clients handle the stress that might be associated with it, including suicidal behaviors. Dialectical behavior therapy has been shown to reduce suicide attempts, treatment dropout rates, and hospitalizations (Linehan et al. 2015). Clients who receive DBT have been shown to be less angry and better adjusted, and amygdala reactivity often seems to be tempered. Reduced amygdala reactivity is associated with fewer emotional outbursts (Bertsch et al. 2019). A meta-analysis of DBT treatment in adolescents showed reductions of both self-harm and suicidal ideation (Kothgassner et al. 2021).

The cognitive-behavioral perspective suggests that people with histrionic personality disorder have distorted cognitions that they are helpless, and this leads them to look for other people to take care of them (Beck et al. 2015).

CBT helps clients with narcissistic personality disorder increase their empathy for others and interpret criticism without becoming defensive. However, these approaches have had limited success (King et al. 2020).

Dialectical behavior therapy (DBT): a treatment for borderline personality disorder that aims to teach problem-solving skills, emotional regulation, and interpersonal skills.

SOCIOCULTURAL MODELS AND TREATMENTS

Many factors during childhood, such as neglect, harsh punishment, and lack of warmth, play a role in the development of antisocial personality disorder (Johnson et al. 2006). People around those with the condition, especially their parents, often give in to their aggressive and manipulative tactics (Granic & Patterson 2006). People tend to grow out of APD, with symptoms starting to decline around age 40 (Hare et al. 1988). There is some evidence that the reduction of symptoms may be due to a bias of the diagnostic criteria that favors symptoms that are more likely to be endorsed in younger adults (Holzer et al. 2021; Holzer & Vaughn 2017).

Sociocultural factors can also influence borderline personality disorder. Many people with the disorder have reported significant abuse, neglect, instability, and psychopathology in their backgrounds. One study reported that up to 70 percent of people with borderline personality disorder had been sexually abused (Zanarini 2000), and there is evidence of harsh treatment from parents including neglect, rejection, verbal abuse, or other inappropriate behavior (Martín-Blanco et al. 2014; Skodol 2017). Those who endure these kinds of experiences are four times more likely to develop BPD than those who do not (Zelkowitz et al. 2001). Often these factors are reflected in their earliest memories (Bradley et al. 2007). Keep in mind, however, that most people who have a history of physical and psychological or sexual abuse or trauma do not develop BPD (Skodol 2017).

Sociocultural theories also suggest that in cultures that experience rapid changes, some members have difficulty understanding their new roles. They may struggle with feelings of confusion, emptiness, abandonment, and anxiety (Paris 2018).

The sociocultural perspective on histrionic personality disorder focuses on the idea that culture places some members of society in a more dependent role than others (Novais et al. 2015). In this view, histrionic personality disorder is simply an exaggeration of outdated societal expectations for women to be attention-seeking, especially those with exposure to trauma early in life (Cale & Lilienfeld 2002; Turner et al. 2020).

The sociocultural approach to narcissistic personality disorder emphasizes the role society has played by emphasizing individualism, which leads to too much self-expression and competition (Coldwell-Harris & Ayçiçegi 2006). This view points to high rates of narcissistic personality disorder in countries such as the United States (Foster et al. 2003), where society demands and rewards individualism. Thus treatment for the disorder centers on reducing sensitivity to criticism and increasing empathy (Campbell & Miller 2011).

The COVID-19 pandemic has been a risk factor for a number of negative symptoms in those with Cluster B personality disorders. People with Cluster B personality disorders often have symptoms of fear of abandonment, relationship instability, and impulsivity. Required isolation during the peak of the COVID-19 pandemic, along with isolation after exposure to the virus, have been risk factors for worsening symptoms of the condition (see Table 12.2).

Table 12.2 Symptoms that may develop as a result of the COVID-19 pandemic in those with Cluster B personality disorders

Pandemic and quarantine psychological impact
Anxiety symptoms
Depressive symptoms
Impulsivity
Anger
Suicidality (intense suicidal ideation and suicide)
Extreme fear
Emotion dysregulation
Emotional exhaustion
Alcohol abuse or dependency symptoms
Irritability
Numbness
Worsening of eating disorders symptomatology
Emotional eating

Source: Data from Preti et al. (2020).

CONCEPT CHECK 12.3

Indicate the most likely Cluster B personality disorder described in the case below.
  A. Antisocial personality disorder
  B. Borderline personality disorder
  C. Histrionic personality disorder
  D. Narcissistic personality disorder
  1. James has a long history of unstable connections with other people, including in his romantic relationships and friendships. This instability extends to nearly every area of his life. He is indecisive about his career and experiences rapid shifts in his mood. He is also filled with fear of being alone.
  2. As a child, Erin was caught damaging property and lying to get out of class and was suspended after fights with other students. Now, at 30, she steals money from her friend and family, has been caught lying to get what she wants, and has been arrested multiple times. She has no remorse for any of her actions.
  3. Teresa is often late for work but tries to convince her supervisor she needs the extra sleep to come up with the brilliant ideas she provides. In reality she exploits her colleagues and steals their work, but she thinks she is special and deserves the best of everything, including the wealth and fame she daydreams about. Her behavior causes problems at work and with the few friends she has.
  4. Dom craves attention. He's been known to flirt with everyone, uses showy vocabulary, and dresses in a way that draws attention to his body. Despite getting as much attention as he does, Dom has few friends, and his attention-seeking behavior creates problems at work.

Case Study: Antisocial Personality Disorder – Ian Brady

Born in Scotland in 1938, Ian Brady (Figure 12.8) didn't always follow the rules. When he was as young as 9 years old, he reported breaking into a house "just to look around." He enjoyed the feeling of being inside someone's home without their permission. Soon he went from just looking to taking things, and by the time he was 13 he had been arrested for burglary – twice. As a young child he displayed what some called a "sadistic streak." Growing up in a neighborhood of greater Manchester (in northern England), he wore a long trench coat and acquired the nickname "the Undertaker" due to his love of watching horror movies and torturing animals. At 17, he spent three months in a local jail and then two years in prison. Years afterward he said that some of his later criminal tendencies were influenced by his fellow inmates.

Brady's father died before Ian was born, so his mother had to support him by herself, working through much of his early childhood. However, he eventually moved in with his aunt and uncle, and his mother visited weekly on Sundays.

Brady transferred to a private school for above-average students when he was 11 years old. While he was intelligent and received good grades, he was known for misbehaving and getting into arguments with other students. He didn't have any close friends as a child and considered himself a loner. Later he expressed a bitter hatred of society and became obsessed with Hitler and Nazism, even buying audio recordings of Nazi speeches. Brady grew to love the idea of being

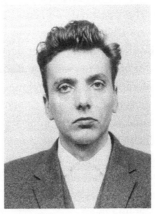

Figure 12.8 Ian Brady.
Source: Evening Standard/ *Getty Images.*

worshiped and firmly believed there was nothing wrong with committing a justifiable crime.

Over time, things got worse for Brady and those who encountered him. Eventually he was jailed for life after being found guilty, with his partner Myra Hindley, of the murders of five children in the case that became known as the Moors Murders. Even after he was arrested, Brady was oppositional and resistant and showed no remorse for the killings. He was violent in prison, refused medication and therapy, and even challenged his incarceration. He died in prison in 2017.

To read more about Ian Brady, take a look at *Ian Brady: The untold story of the Moors murders*, by Alan Keightley (2017).

12.4 CLUSTER C: ANXIOUS PERSONALITY DISORDERS

People with one of the "anxious" personality disorders in Cluster C show symptoms of anxiety and fear. The disorders include avoidant personality disorder, dependent personality disorder, and obsessive-compulsive personality disorder. They are some of the most common personality disorders; about 3.03 percent of people worldwide meet the criteria for one of them (Volkert et al. 2018) (see Figure 12.9).

Avoidant Personality Disorder

People who are allergic to cats have heightened sensitivity to a protein in cat saliva that dries on the fur when cats clean themselves (which they do a lot). While most people are not affected by the flakes of dried saliva on cats, someone with a high level of sensitivity will have a serious histamine reaction to even a slight exposure. In somewhat the same way, we can say that people with avoidant personality disorder are allergic to criticism.

Avoidant personality disorder: a personality disorder marked by a pervasive pattern of social inhibition, a sense of inadequacy, and hypersensitivity to the criticism of others.

Avoidant personality disorder is a personality disorder marked by a pervasive pattern of social inhibition, a sense of inadequacy, and hypersensitivity to the criticism of others (see Diagnostic Overview 12.8). Because they feel inadequate, people with this disorder are extremely reactive to any negative evaluation and believe they can sense it anywhere. They are uncomfortable in settings in which they might encounter criticism and live in a constant state of fear, doing all they can to prevent others from rejecting them. The walls they erect around themselves work both ways, however; they prevent anyone from either attacking *or* accepting them.

SYMPTOMS AND DESCRIPTION

Figure 12.9 Lifetime prevalence of Cluster C personality disorders in selected countries, from the World Mental Health Surveys (2002–2017).
Source: Data from Huang et al. (2009).

People with avoidant personality disorder bypass social activities for fear of criticism. They don't get too close to others because they are concerned that close friends will use against them any information they acquire. Because they hold back so much and have few social interactions, they don't have much practice being around other people. Their poor social skills then reinforce their conviction that they are unlovable and unappealing, starting a vicious circle that can force them away from other people despite the fact that they desperately want friends. This

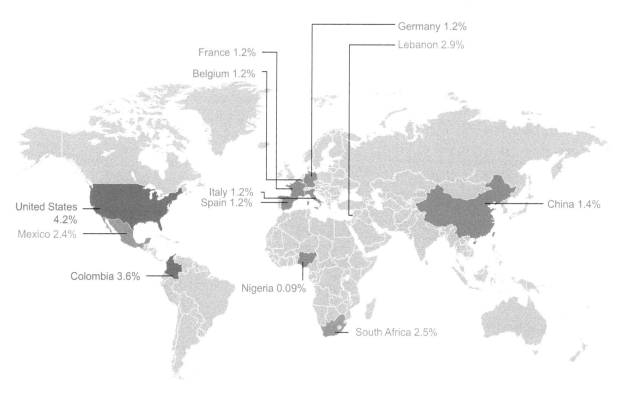

Germany 1.2%
Lebanon 2.9%
France 1.2%
Belgium 1.2%
Italy 1.2%
Spain 1.2%
China 1.4%
United States 4.2%
Mexico 2.4%
Colombia 3.6%
Nigeria 0.09%
South Africa 2.5%

result leaves them feeling not only anxious but often very depressed. Unlike those with schizoid personality disorder, those with avoidant personality disorder long for interpersonal connection.

STATISTICS AND TRAJECTORY

Worldwide, 2.4 percent of adults meet the criteria for avoidant personality disorder, and men experience the condition as often as women. This estimate may be low because avoidant personality disorder is considered an underrecognized and poorly understood disorder (Kvarstein et al. 2021). Symptoms are diagnosed only in adulthood, but they have been found in children (Lampe & Malhi 2018).

Dependent Personality Disorder

Imagine that you didn't trust yourself to make even the smallest decision, such as what to eat or what to wear, much less what career to pursue, because you were afraid to make the wrong choice. In order to get along in the world, you might then reach out to others to make those decisions for you. You might even cling to them for fear they will leave you to fend for yourself. Individuals with **dependent personality disorder** have a pervasive pattern of excessive need to be taken care of and a dependent, clinging pattern of behavior.

Diagnostic Overview 12.8: Avoidant Personality Disorder

Feelings of inadequacy and an extreme response to negative evaluation indicated by at least four of the following:

- Avoidance of work that requires significant interpersonal contact.
- Unwillingness to engage with others unless certain of being accepted.
- Restrained intimate relationships.
- Preoccupation with criticism.
- Inhibition in interpersonal situations.
- View of the self as inept and inferior.
- Reluctance to take risks.

Impact:	Clinically significant distress or impairment in social, occupational, or other important areas of functioning. The pattern is inflexible and pervasive across a broad range of situations. Symptoms must exceed cultural and contextual norms.
Timeframe:	Persistent and can be traced back at least to adolescence.

Source: Information from APA (2022).

Dependent personality disorder: a personality disorder marked by a pervasive pattern of excessive need to be taken care of and a dependent, clinging pattern of behavior.

SYMPTOMS AND DESCRIPTION

People diagnosed with dependent personality disorder have an excessive need to be taken care of, despite the fact that there is no real necessity for them to depend on other people (Diagnostic Overview 12.9). They feel that even the smallest decision should be made by others, to whom they cling for fear of being left alone. Their need to be taken care of leads them to be overly passive, obedient, and even submissive to others. For example, they will appear to agree with others even when they don't, because they fear abandonment (Bornstein 2012). If one relationship ends, they will seek another one.

STATISTICS AND TRAJECTORY

Dependent personality disorder is diagnosed in less than 1 percent of the US population (Sansone & Sansone 2011). The condition is equally common in men and women.

Diagnostic Overview 12.9: Dependent Personality Disorder

An excessive need to be taken care of that leads to submissive and clinging behavior and fear of separation, as indicated by at least five of the following:

- Difficulty making everyday decisions alone.
- Need for others to take responsibility.
- Suppression of differences of opinion, out of fear of losing approval.
- Difficulty initiating projects or doing things on their own.
- Willingness to perform unpleasant tasks in order to obtain support from others.
- Fear of being unable to care for themselves.
- Urgent need to replace relationships.
- Preoccupation with fear of being left alone.

Impact: Clinically significant distress or impairment in social, occupational, or other important areas of functioning. The pattern is inflexible and pervasive across a broad range of situations. Symptoms must exceed cultural and contextual norms.

Timeframe: Persistent and can be traced back at least to adolescence.

Source: Information from APA (2022).

Obsessive-Compulsive Personality Disorder

Obsessive-compulsive personality disorder (OCPD): a personality disorder marked by a pervasive pattern of orderliness and control at the expense of efficiency.

There are certainly correct ways to do certain things. But those with **obsessive-compulsive personality disorder (OCPD)** are so focused on doing things correctly, or what they see as correctly, that they don't get much accomplished.

SYMPTOMS AND DESCRIPTION

Obsessive-compulsive personality disorder is very different from obsessive-compulsive disorder (OCD). In Chapter 4 we discussed OCD as an ego-dystonic condition. People with this disorder wish they didn't experience the obsessions or compulsions they do, and they actively seek treatment. OCPD symptoms, on the other hand, are often ego-syntonic. People with this Cluster C condition usually don't realize how much social and work dysfunction their symptoms cause. Because of their preoccupation with maintaining control, they aren't at all flexible or efficient (Diagnostic Overview 12.10). They are hyper-focused on doing things the way they think they should be done and believe their way is the right and best way to do things, despite never feeling satisfied with the outcome. They are late finishing work tasks because they can never feel the work is perfect, and they will pass on socializing with friends because they need to catch up with work. Although they don't meet the criteria for hoarding disorder (see Chapter 4), they often see objects as things that should be hoarded against future problems (such as mailed credit card offers or tools), although their collections of these objects aren't relevant to real-life solutions (Diedrick & Voderholzer 2015).

STATISTICS AND TRAJECTORY

About 7.9 percent of adults in the United States meet the criteria for OCPD (Diedrich & Voderholzer 2015) (Figure 12.9). Men are twice as likely as women to receive the diagnosis (Burkauskas & Fineberg 2020).

Models and Treatments of Cluster C Personality Disorders

There isn't much recent research on the Cluster C personality disorders, and many therapists adopt a supportive approach and work in a multiperspective mode. However, they often face some challenges. Although people with avoidant personality disorder do seek treatment for their condition, they are often doubtful of their own ability to change. They are also concerned about being abandoned by the therapist. Many practitioners spend time building and maintaining trust with the client (Skodol 2017).

Treatment for dependent personality disorder can be difficult as well. The main goal is to help clients increase responsibility for themselves while not becoming dependent on the therapist. Since people with OCPD rarely seek treatment, they often will present in treatment settings for associated conditions such as anxiety or depression. In other cases, a friend, family member, or co-worker will suggest counseling or therapy. Despite their reluctance to seek treatment on their own, many people with OCPD respond well to it, especially psychodynamically based and CBT-based therapy (Kikkert et al. 2016; Smith et al. 2017).

Diagnostic Overview 12.10: Obsessive-Compulsive Personality Disorder

Preoccupation with orderliness and control, at the expense of efficiency, as indicated by at least four of the following:

- Preoccupation with details and rules.
- Perfectionism that interferes with finishing tasks.
- Excessive devotion to productivity, to the exclusion of anything else.
- Inflexible morality.
- Inability to discard worthless objects.
- Reluctance to delegate.
- Miserly spending style.
- Unwillingness to compromise.

Impact: Clinically significant distress or impairment in social, occupational, or other important areas of functioning. The pattern is inflexible and pervasive across a broad range of situations. Symptoms must exceed cultural and contextual norms.

Timeframe: Persistent and can be traced back at least to adolescence.

Source: Information from APA (2022).

BIOLOGICAL MODELS AND TREATMENTS

Treatment with medications for Cluster C personality disorders tends to focus on specific symptoms and associated psychological concerns such as anxiety or depression. For example, prescribers will often use medications typically prescribed for anxiety or depression, such as SSRI, for those with Cluster C conditions (Rao 2020).

PSYCHODYNAMIC MODELS AND TREATMENTS

Psychodynamic theories of avoidant personality disorder point to the development of the superego as the beginning of avoidant personality disorder. In this phase of development some parents are overly critical, and some children develop a negative sense of self that can become internalized. Children become distrusting and overly self-critical (Keefe et al. 2020).

Psychodynamic theories for dependent personality disorder suggest that people who are diagnosed with dependent personality disorder have an excessive need for nurturance (Bornstein 2012). Some theories explain this as resulting from early loss or early rejection experiences that turn into a longstanding obsession with rejection.

COGNITIVE-BEHAVIORAL MODELS AND TREATMENTS

The cognitive-behavioral theories suggest that individuals with avoidant personality disorder develop internal cognitive schemas that assume rejection and criticism. They see any interaction through that lens and at the same time filter out positive interactions. These cognitions lead those with the disorder to see themselves as inferior. CBT for avoidant personality disorder works to build social skills (Lampe & Malhi 2018). Some of the same treatments used for social phobia can be helpful for this disorder, such as exposure treatments, social skills training, and anxiety management, in order to increase social contacts and confront uncomfortable social situations as a way of building the skills to handle them smoothly.

The cognitive-behavioral approach for dependent personality disorder views the condition as a result of early reinforcement for clinging behavior, in which children are rewarded for being needy and punished for being independent. They then develop cognitions that support and maintain their dependance (Beck et al. 2015), and they end up believing they are needy and weak. CBT for dependent personality disorder focuses on helping clients challenge their own assumptions about their dependence on others and building confidence about making their own decisions (Beck et al. 2015). Therapy can focus on skills training, such as for assertiveness, and can challenge the client's assumption that they must rely on other people to be safe. Exposure techniques in which clients must confront situations on their own can also increase independence (Lampe & Malhi 2018).

CBT for obsessive-compulsive personality disorder focuses on cognitions that may maintain perfectionist thinking and the belief that flaws are not to be tolerated. Treatment can help clients challenge their own perfectionism and build skills to combat procrastination and worry (Bhukhari et al. 2018).

SOCIOCULTURAL MODELS AND TREATMENTS

Early studies of people with avoidant personality disorder found that they remembered their parents as more rejecting and less affectionate than did people without the disorder (Eikenaes et al. 2015). Early rejection by parents may lead to low self-esteem: "If my parents don't like me, how can anyone?" (Carr & Francis 2010). Group-based therapy formats for avoidant personality disorder can help combat these feelings and facilitate practicing social interactions (Weinbrecht et al. 2016).

Like people with other personality disorders, those with Cluster C personality disorders have also experienced negative symptoms as a response to COVID-19 and the associated isolation. People with Cluster C personality disorders often have difficulty with social situations. Along with their typical inhibition and lack of self-confidence, required isolation during the peak of the pandemic and isolation after exposure to the virus have been risk factors for worsening symptoms (Table 12.3).

Table 12.3 Symptoms that may develop as a result of the COVID-19 pandemic in those with Cluster C personality disorders.

Pandemic and quarantine psychological impact
Post-traumatic stress symptoms
Anxiety symptoms
Depressive symptoms
Insomnia
Serious worries about physical health
Compulsive symptoms
Extreme fear
Acute stress disorder
Avoidance behaviors such as minimizing direct contact
Delay in return to normality
Disruption of social networks

Source: Data from Preti et al. (2020).

CONCEPT CHECK 12.4

Identify the Cluster C personality disorder most likely described in the cases below.
  A. Avoidant personality disorder
  B. Dependent personality disorder
  C. Obsessive-compulsive personality disorder
  1. Harvey is viewed by all his friends as a workaholic and not at all social. He's at his desk every morning by 6:00am and takes few breaks, but always at exactly the same time. Despite his efforts Harvey never gets much accomplished, because most of his time is spent making sure all his work is absolutely perfect.
  2. Bima is extremely sensitive to the criticism of other people, so much so that she fears the rejection of her close friends and family nearly all the time. She doesn't try new things for fear of embarrassment and rejection, and because of this hesitation she has been held back from promotion at work and from close relationships with her friends.
  3. Azad lives with his parents and agrees with everything they say. In fact, he tries to agree with everything his friends say and suggest as well. He is afraid that if he doesn't, they will abandon him as a friend. He doesn't trust himself to make even small decisions and relies on his friends and family to make decisions for him.

PULLING IT TOGETHER

Key Themes of Personality Disorders

Table 12.4 Key themes of personality disorders

Disorder	Cluster	Key themes	Conditions with similar symptoms	Common comorbid conditions
Paranoid personality disorder	A	Distrust and suspiciousness	Schizophrenia delusional disorder	Major depressive disorder Substance use disorders Agoraphobia Obsessive-compulsive disorder
Schizoid personality disorder	A	Apathy and detachment from others, including family members	Schizophrenia delusional disorder	Major depressive disorder Anxiety disorders Schizophrenia Delusional disorder

Table 12.4 *(cont.)*

Disorder	Cluster	Key themes	Conditions with similar symptoms	Common comorbid conditions
Schizotypal personality disorder	A	Discomfort in social relationships and odd and eccentric behavior	Schizophrenia delusional disorder	Bipolar I disorder Bipolar II disorder Social phobia Specific phobia Post-traumatic stress disorder Schizophrenia
Antisocial personality disorder	B	Breaking rules and harming others without remorse	Conduct disorder	Social phobia Generalized anxiety disorder Substance use disorder
Borderline personality disorder	B	Instability in relationships, mood, and ever-changing view of self	Major depressive disorder; bipolar disorder	Major depressive disorder Substance use disorder Anxiety disorders
Histrionic personality disorder	B	Always needs attention from others	Major depressive disorder; somatic symptom disorder	Substance use disorders
Narcissistic personality disorder	B	Inflated sense of self-importance and extreme preoccupation with themselves		Bipolar I disorder Substance use disorder Anxiety disorder
Avoidant personality disorder	C	Extreme reaction to the criticism of others	Social anxiety disorder	Depressive disorders Social phobia Obsessive-compulsive disorder Eating disorders

Table 12.4 (*cont.*)

Disorder	Cluster	Key themes	Conditions with similar symptoms	Common comorbid conditions
Dependent personality disorder	C	Insatiable need for care from others		Substance use disorders
Obsessive-compulsive personality disorder	C	Fixation with rules and lists that interferes with them getting things done		Anxiety disorders Anorexia nervosa

Source: Adapted from Eynan et al. (2016).

12.5   CHAPTER REVIEW

SUMMARY

This chapter presented the following disorders:

- Paranoid personality disorder
- Schizoid personality disorder
- Schizotypal personality disorder
- Antisocial personality disorder
- Borderline personality disorder
- Histrionic personality disorder
- Narcissistic personality disorder
- Avoidant personality disorder
- Dependent personality disorder
- Obsessive-compulsive personality disorder

Overview of Personality Disorders

- Personality is an individual's pattern of thinking, feeling, and behaving.
- Personality disorders are psychological conditions characterized by extreme inflexible personality characteristics that are persistent and pervasive.
- The *DSM-5tr* divides personality disorders into three clusters, odd, dramatic, and anxious.
- Personality disorders can be either ego-dystonic or ego-syntonic.

Cluster A: Odd and Eccentric Personality Disorders

- Paranoid personality disorder, schizoid personality disorder, and schizotypal personality disorder are characterized by odd or eccentric thinking, suspicious withdrawal, and unusual thoughts and perceptions.

Cluster B: Dramatic Personality Disorders

- Antisocial personality disorder, borderline personality disorder, histrionic personality disorder, and narcissistic personality disorder are characterized by erratic, dramatic, and overly emotional behavior.

Cluster C: Anxious Personality Disorders

- Those with avoidant personality disorder, dependent personality disorder, or obsessive-compulsive personality disorder display symptoms of anxiety and fear.

DISCUSSION QUESTIONS

1. Some personality disorders cause impairment but no distress, such that people never feel the need to seek treatment for them. What are the advantages and disadvantages of classifying these conditions as psychological disorders?
2. What are some of the ways that certain personality disorders can make treatment more difficult?
3. Unlike most diagnostic categories in *DSM-5tr*, personality disorders haven't been updated in several decades. What changes might you expect to be made in the future? Why?
4. Is there or could there be a personality disorder likely to be diagnosed in one gender more than the other? What might influence these diagnoses?
5. Imagine that a child has a genetic vulnerability to antisocial personality disorder. How might this child's environment shape the likelihood of developing the disorder?

ANSWERS TO CONCEPT CHECKS

Concept Check 12.1

1. Ego syntonic
2. Ego dystonic
3. Ego dystonic
4. Ego syntonic

Concept Check 12.2

1. Schizoid personality disorder
2. Paranoid personality disorder
3. Schizotypal personality disorder

Concept Check 12.3

1. Borderline personality disorder
2. Antisocial personality disorder
3. Narcissistic personality disorder
4. Histrionic personality disorder

Concept Check 12.4

1. Obsessive-compulsive personality disorder
2. Avoidant personality disorder
3. Dependent personality disorder

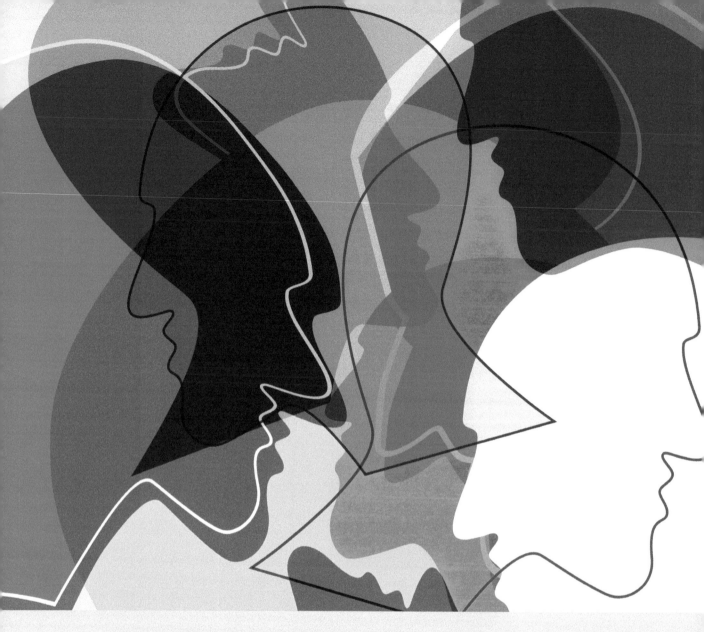

CHAPTER CONTENTS

Kubkoo/iStock/Getty Images Plus.

13

Schizophrenia and Psychotic Disorders

CASE STUDY: Schizophrenia – Elyn Saks

Elyn's first episode of psychosis happened in her first semester at Yale Law School. She was meeting some friends to study, but when she spoke to them, the words that came out made no sense. "'Memos are visitations, they make certain points. The point is on your head. Pat used to say that. 'Have you killed anyone? I think someone's infiltrated my copies of the cases,' she said. 'We've got to case the joint. I don't believe in joints, but they do hold your body together.'" Later she went up to the roof of the school and started to jump around and sing, finding that she couldn't seem to slow herself down. At one point she was hospitalized.

Things got worse after law school when Elyn discovered that her long-term therapist was closing his practice. She was found by her best friend in her apartment, incoherent. "Tell the clocks to stop. Time is. Time has come." "White is leaving," Elyn said somberly. "I'm being pushed into a grave. The situation is grave." "Gravity is pulling me down. I'm scared. Tell them to get away."

Elyn started to believe that she had killed hundreds of thousands of people simply with her thoughts and worried that nuclear explosions were about to be set off in her brain. She couldn't seem to shake the idea, and it haunted her. Occasionally she would see things that weren't there, like a man with a raised knife. She said the experience was like a waking nightmare.

We'll come back to Elyn's story later in the chapter.

If you'd like to learn more about Elyn Saks, take a look at her memoir, *The center cannot hold: My journey through madness* (2007), or watch her TED talk.

Learning Objectives

- Describe the symptoms associated with psychotic disorders.
- Compare the positive and negative symptoms of psychosis.
- Summarize the epidemiology, diagnostic criteria, and clinical features of the psychotic disorders.
- Discuss current theories of the etiology of psychotic disorders.
- Describe common side effects of antipsychotic medications.
- Discuss the psychosocial treatments of psychotic disorders.

13.1   OVERVIEW OF PSYCHOSIS

Right now you are reading these words. You are holding the textbook (or an electronic version of it) in your hands. Maybe you have a glass of ice water nearby. Perhaps in the background you are listening to music, or a friend is talking, or you are outside and you hear people. You know the words are real, your drink is real, the people are real, all the things around you are real. But your perceptions of the words, the chill of the ice water, and all the sounds around you are just that, perceptions. Your five senses bring you this information, your brain processes it, and you pull all the sensations into a coherent story, the story of what's happening around you. But what if your brain creates sensations of things that aren't around you, and the story you perceive is disconnected from true experiences, a split between your senses, your perceptions, and reality? What if you heard voices of people who aren't actually there? What if you believed that your electronic textbook was absorbing the thoughts from your brain and broadcasting them to the world? These kinds of breaks from reality characterize psychosis.

Psychosis: a condition in which a person has lost some contact with reality.

The word **psychosis** describes a condition in which a person has lost some contact with reality. During a period of psychosis, the individual's thoughts and perceptions are out of sync with reality, and understandably they may have difficulty knowing what is real and what isn't. Much like Elyn, who experienced false beliefs that she was responsible for hundreds of murders and false sensory perceptions that included the sight of a man with a raised knife, people with the symptoms of psychosis can find them disconcerting and even terrifying.

Psychotic symptoms can appear in a number of psychological disorders like anxiety and mood disorders, and they can even occur with substance use (see Chapter 11). However, when psychotic symptoms appear as the central feature of a psychological disorder, a psychopathologist might categorize them as signs of a **psychotic disorder** such as schizophrenia. In this chapter we'll examine the symptoms of psychosis, the psychological conditions that feature psychosis, and the theories and various treatment approaches.

Psychotic disorder: a psychological condition defined by the presence of significant symptoms of psychosis.

Let's start with some of the central symptoms of psychosis that are characteristic of all the disorders in this chapter. There are two general types of symptoms in psychotic disorders: positive symptoms and negative symptoms.

Positive Symptoms of Psychosis

Positive symptoms: a set of symptoms of psychosis that are in addition to what is expected in the human experience, such as delusions, hallucinations, and disorganized thoughts, speech, and behavior.

There are five domains of **positive symptoms**: delusions, hallucinations, and disorganized thoughts, speech, and behavior. They are referred to as positive not because they are good, but because they occur in addition to typical behavior. They are symptoms that people with psychosis exhibit that other people do not and are additions to the human experience. For example, most people do not have hallucinations as Elyn did, so hallucinations are an addition to expected behavior.

DELUSIONS

Delusions are fixed false beliefs that are not amenable to change in the light of conflicting evidence, though most people would understand them to be untrue. Delusions occur in two general types: bizarre and non-bizarre. *Bizarre delusions* are beliefs that are totally impossible. *Non-bizarre delusions* are unlikely but possible. For example, if someone believed the nightly local newscast was a way to communicate their daily whereabouts to a government agency, although this is unlikely, it's possible (perhaps by some means involving microphones and cameras). On the other hand, if a person believed their organs were turning into straw, that would be a bizarre delusion since it is impossible.

The content of delusions may include a variety of themes, as you can see in Table 13.1.

Delusions: a positive symptom of psychosis in which a person experiences fixed false beliefs that are not amenable to change in the light of conflicting evidence, though most people would understand them to be untrue.

HALLUCINATIONS

While delusions represent beliefs, **hallucinations** are sensory perceptions with no corresponding sensory input. People who experience hallucinations may see things that aren't there or hear things that no one else hears. Their perceptions of hallucinations are as vivid as if they are actually occurring, however.

Although many people may consider hallucinations to be a hallmark of psychosis, they can also occur outside the context of psychotic disorders. About 5 percent of people without a psychological condition report hearing voices, and occasional hallucinations can occur when people are under the influence of substances, stressed, or tired without necessarily causing an impact in their everyday lives (McGrath et al. 2015). The hallucinations associated with psychosis are different, however. These can be more recurrent, persistent, and disturbing. They may affect a person's ability to sleep or to function at work, and they can even increase substance use if the person tries to create a buffer or self-soothe after a disturbing hallucination. Hallucinations can arrive through all five senses. Most, however, are auditory or visual.

Hallucinations: a positive symptom of psychosis in which a person experiences sensory perceptions with no corresponding sensory input.

Table 13.1 Types of delusions

Type of delusions	Definition	Example
Persecutory	The person's belief that others are acting against them.	"My food is being poisoned by the government."
Grandiose	Belief of having made some important discovery, or having a great power.	"I can control the weather with my thoughts."
Somatic	Experience of unusual bodily sensations or body functions.	"Small bugs that no one can see are under my skin."
Erotomanic type	Belief that another person is in love with the individual.	"A famous movie star signals their love and devotion for me through codes in television interviews."
Jealous type	Belief that a spouse or partner is unfaithful despite evidence to the contrary.	"My partner is cheating on me."

DISORGANIZED THOUGHTS AND SPEECH

The way we speak is often a sign of the way we think. Therefore, the disorganized speech often found in people with psychosis is a clue to the disordered thoughts these individuals have. Disorganized speaking patterns can range from rapid switches from one unrelated topic to the next, called *loose associations*, to totally incomprehensible word patterns, called *incoherence*. The sentences that Elyn said in the opening case were examples of disorganized thought and speech.

DISORGANIZED BEHAVIOR

Disorganized or abnormal motor behavior may manifest itself in a variety of ways including *catatonia*, a problem with movement. In *agitated catatonia*, the person has uncontrollable movements and may flap their arms or spin in circles. A person with *stuporous catatonia* is immobile and nonreactive. People with catatonia may also exhibit *waxy flexibility* (you can move their arms and they will stay in that position). Disorganized motor behaviors can present themselves in several ways such as a resistance to instructions (negativism), as rigid postures, or as staring. Catatonia can also occur with other mental conditions such as mood disorders.

Negative Symptoms of Psychosis

Negative symptoms: a symptom of psychosis in which a person has deficits in expected behaviors.

Negative symptoms of psychosis are deficits in expected behaviors. These are things you'd expect everyone to have, but that people with psychosis lack. They are subtractions from the human experience. Although less noticeable than positive symptoms, they can account for significant impairment. The negative symptoms of psychosis include flat affect, avolition, alogia, and anhedonia.

FLAT OR RESTRICTED AFFECT

Flat or *restricted affect*, also known as *diminished emotional expression*, is the lack of expressed emotions in the face, seen as reduced levels of eye contact, speech intonation, and movements of the hand, head, and face that might typically give an emotional emphasis to speech.

AVOLITION

Avolition is a lack of will, usually seen as a decrease in purposeful activities. The individual may sit aimlessly for long periods of time and show little interest in participating in work or social activities.

ALOGIA

Alogia is reduced elaboration in speech. A person with alogia may talk very little, if at all. This diminished speech output can lead to withdrawal from social interactions and exacerbate other negative symptoms of psychosis.

ANHEDONIA

Anhedonia is the decreased ability to experience pleasure from positive stimuli; it may lead to lack of interest in social interactions.

The presence of psychotic experiences doesn't necessarily mean that a person has a psychotic disorder. Psychotic experiences are not uncommon, even in people without psychotic disorders. In a study of more than 34,000 people over 18 years of age, a little more than a quarter (26.9 percent) reported experiencing at least one type of psychotic experience, such as delusions of persecution in which they think someone intends them harm, or perceptual abnormalities, which make things around them seem unreal (similar to hallucinations) (Bourgin et al. 2020). In some cultures, such symptoms, sometimes called voice hearing, are celebrated experiences, for example, hearing the voice of a loved one after they have died (Vermeiden et al. 2019).

CONCEPT CHECK 13.1

Identify whether each is a positive or negative symptom of psychosis.
1. Enrico remains still for hours and is unreactive to outside noises.
2. Nathaniel's mood is flat and is not changed by outside circumstances.
3. Reina believes, without evidence, their roommate is trying to kill them by adding something to their coffee.
4. Jacqueline speaks using as few words as possible.
5. Rosanna hears someone whispering to her, but no one is there.
6. Anastasia spends all day in bed and does not have the will to do anything.

13.2   SCHIZOPHRENIA AND PSYCHOTIC DISORDERS

We've seen that there are a number of conditions under which symptoms of psychosis may emerge. However, when these symptoms are prominent, psychopathologists will often diagnose one of the conditions listed in the Schizophrenia Spectrum and Other Psychotic Disorders chapter of *DSM-5tr*. In this section we'll discuss four: schizophrenia, brief psychotic disorder, schizophreniform disorder, and schizoaffective disorder.

Schizophrenia

Schizophrenia is a psychological condition characterized by disordered thinking, delusions, hallucination, and disordered behavior and emotions. The experience of these symptoms can be terrifying and disruptive, and the devastating impact of schizophrenia is clear.

Schizophrenia has more than just a devastating emotional impact; it also has a very significant financial cost. Because of the nature and intensity of the

Schizophrenia: a psychological condition characterized by disordered thinking, delusions, hallucination, and disordered behavior and emotions.

symptoms, this disorder can be a very resource-intensive condition. The dollar costs of treating schizophrenia make up around 3 percent of the entire US health care budget and nearly 75 percent of all US mental health care expenses (Knapp et al. 2004). Schizophrenia cost the United States an estimated $281.6 billion in 2020, based on the costs of health care, incarceration, and housing support (Canady 2021). For each person diagnosed at 25, the cost of support is $92,000 each year. The expense can be extremely difficult for families trying to care for their loved ones; in fact many people go without the care they need because the costs can be overwhelming.

In addition, people with schizophrenia are at increased risk for many co-occurring conditions, including higher rates of suicide and physical illnesses such as cardiovascular disease, diabetes, and obesity (Mizuki et al. 2021; Smith et al. 2013). As a result, their life expectancy is 10–20 years shorter than for people without schizophrenia (Laursen 2019).

SYMPTOMS AND DESCRIPTION

Diagnosing schizophrenia is more complicated than merely identifying psychosis. For this disorder to be diagnosed, the symptoms must be present for a minimum amount of time and cause distress and impairment. Yet people with schizophrenia don't always exhibit these symptoms of psychosis, and they often experience long stretches of time with no symptoms whatsoever.

This waxing and waning of symptoms can occur with other conditions. Think back to the last time you had a cold. At first you were probably sneezing and coughing and feeling horrible. Then you started to feel better, but you still had some leftover sluggishness. You could consider the time during which the symptoms were at their worst to be the *active phase* of your illness. The other period is a *residual* (leftover) phase (Figure 13.1).

A diagnosis of schizophrenia works in much the same way (Diagnostic Overview 13.1). Continuous signs of the disorder must last for at least six months, and at least one month must be an active phase. At this point the person will show two or more of the symptoms of psychosis most of the day for nearly every day.

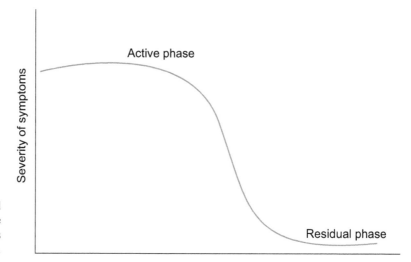

Figure 13.1 In the residual phase, people still have symptoms but they aren't as intense as in the active phase.

This is often followed by several months of a residual phase, in which the person sometimes exhibits two or more positive symptoms with less severe impact, or perhaps only negative symptoms. Some people may experience an active phase for several months.

STATISTICS AND TRAJECTORY

Surveys suggest that around 1–2 percent of the US population will have symptoms of schizophrenia at some point in their lives (Erlich et al. 2014). It's estimated that 20 million people in the world had schizophrenia in 2017 (Figure 13.2), with rates about equal for women and men. Twenty is the most common age of onset for schizophrenia (Solmi et al. 2021), and about 90 percent of people with the disorder will seek treatment at some point (Anderson et al. 2010; Narrow et al. 1993). However, the median time between the symptoms' first emergence and a person's seeking treatment can be as long as 74 weeks (Marder 2021).

Other Psychotic Disorders

Other psychotic disorders described in the *DSM-5tr* are delusional disorder, brief psychotic disorder, schizophreniform disorder, and schizoaffective disorder.

Diagnostic Overview 13.1: Schizophrenia

At least two of the following categories of symptoms from the table below. At least one must be delusions, hallucinations, or disorganized speech.

Must include one of the following	Can also include any of the following
Delusions Hallucinations Disorganized thought and speech	Disorganized behavior Negative symptoms
Impact:	Symptoms must exceed cultural and contextual norms. Symptoms are related to clinically significant distress or create impairment in important areas of life such as with friends and family or at work or school.
Timeframe:	At least six months total (at least one month of active phase symptoms and may include periods of residual symptoms).

Source: Information from APA (2022).

Figure 13.2 Share of population diagnosed with schizophrenia 2019.

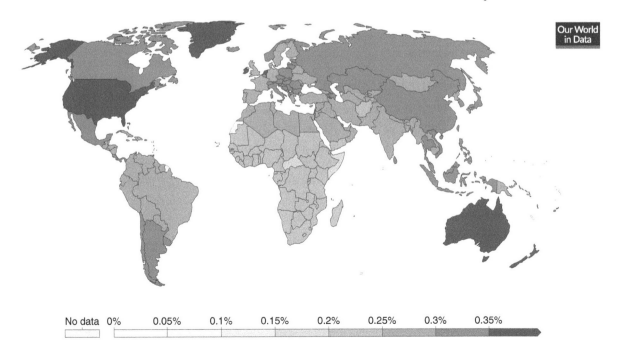

No data 0%   0.05%   0.1%   0.15%   0.2%   0.25%   0.3%   0.35%

THE POWER OF WORDS

"CRAZY"

Suppose someone drives faster than you are comfortable with and switches lanes all the time. That's "crazy." A person accuses their partner of being unfaithful and looks through their cellphone for evidence of an affair. "Crazy." Some people are protesting in support of a cause you aren't the least interested in. All "crazy." *Crazy* can be an especially troublesome word when we use it as a catchall for negative behavior. Let's examine the power of crazy.

The word *crazy* dates back to the 1570s when it meant "diseased, sickly," and later "broken, impaired, full of cracks or flaws." Concrete crazing is the development of random cracks in the surface of concrete. The more common way we use the word now, however, seems to date back to the 1610s, when it came to mean "deranged, demented, of unsound mind or behaving as so," except during the 1920s when it also meant "cool, exciting" in the new jazz scene.

It's typical that we encounter behaviors from other people that make little sense to us. For some people that can be an uncomfortable feeling. Calling such behavior "crazy" can be a shortcut to describing what we ourselves wouldn't do, but it also can prevent us from trying to understand the behavior or viewpoints of others. Dismissing it as "crazy" jumbles all behavior into one unacceptable category.

But using the word "crazy" in this way also draws us deeper into the habit of stigmatizing mental health conditions. The word creates a gap between "normal" and "crazy" behavior, and it signals that the people who act in a "crazy" way are to be marginalized. If you have "normal" feelings, on the other hand, your behaviors are understood. Thus, using the word "crazy" as a shortcut for actions we want to dismiss as irresponsible or inexplicable can be a mental health microaggression, both patronizing and dismissive.

DELUSIONAL DISORDER

Delusional disorder: a psychotic disorder in which a person experiences only delusions and no other symptoms of psychosis.

In **delusional disorder**, a person experiences only delusions and no other symptoms of psychosis (Diagnostic Overview 13.2). People with delusional disorder may believe others want to harm them, or that celebrities are secretly in love with them. Surveys suggest that the lifetime prevalence of delusional disorders is between 0.02% and 0.1% in the United States (Joseph & Siddiqui 2020). The condition affects women slightly more often than men (55 percent vs 45 percent).

Diagnostic Overview 13.2: Delusional Disorder

The presence of one (or more) delusions.	
Impact:	Functioning is not impaired beyond the impact of the delusion. Symptoms must exceed cultural and contextual norms.
Timeframe:	One month or longer. No prior diagnosis of schizophrenia.

Source: Information from APA (2022).

BRIEF PSYCHOTIC DISORDER

In **brief psychotic disorder**, a person shows sudden positive symptoms of psychosis in response to a stressor (Diagnostic Overview 13.3). These symptoms last at least a day but no longer than 30 days. After 30 days, the person's behaviors typically return to the way they were before (although symptoms may return after the experience of another stressor). Eighteen is the most common age of onset for brief psychotic disorder (Solmi et al. 2021). A diagnosis of brief psychotic disorder is often made retroactively, after the symptoms have improved. However, there is evidence that populations known to be under high stress, such as immigrants, refugees, and earthquake victims, have higher rates of brief psychotic disorder than do those without those stressors (Fusar-Poli et al. 2022).

The COVID-19 pandemic has also been associated with brief psychotic symptoms in some people. For example, a 30-year-old man in Qatar with no prior history of psychosis became severely anxious about his health after a positive COVID-19 test. Although his COVID symptoms were mild, he was admitted to a quarantine facility. He became highly anxious, and about a week later, he started to develop paranoid delusions and auditory hallucinations (Haddad et al. 2020).

Brief psychotic disorder: a psychotic disorder in which a person shows sudden positive symptoms of psychosis in response to a stressor.

SCHIZOPHRENIFORM DISORDER

Individuals with **schizophreniform disorder** meet the main criteria for schizophrenia but show symptoms that last only one to six months (rather than at least six months, as required for schizophrenia) (Diagnostic Overview 13.4). They are not necessarily as impaired as those with schizophrenia. Surveys suggest that lifetime prevalence in the United States may be about 0.2 percent (Erlich et al. 2014).

Schizophreniform disorder: a psychotic disorder in which the person meets the main criteria for schizophrenia with less impairment and for a shorter time period.

Diagnostic Overview 13.3: Brief Psychotic Disorder

Symptoms of psychosis as indicated by at least one of the following categories of symptoms. One of the symptoms must include either delusions, hallucinations, or disorganized speech.

Must include one of the following	Can also include any of the following
Delusions Hallucinations Disorganized thought and speech	Disorganized behavior Negative symptoms
Impact:	Symptoms must exceed cultural and contextual norms. Symptoms are related to clinically significant distress or create impairment in important areas of life such as with friends and family or at work or school.
Timeframe:	At least one day but less than one month. Afterwards, behavior returns to earlier pattern.

Source: Information from APA (2022).

Diagnostic Overview 13.4: Schizophreniform Disorder

Symptoms of psychosis as indicated by at least two symptoms of psychosis. One of the symptoms must include either delusions, hallucinations, or disorganized speech.

Must include one of the following	Can also include any of the following
Delusions Hallucinations Disorganized thought and speech	Disorganized behavior Negative symptoms
Impact:	Symptoms must exceed cultural and contextual norms. Symptoms are related to clinically significant distress or create impairment in important areas of life such as with friends and family or at work or school.
Timeframe:	An episode of the disorder lasts at least one month but less than six months.

Source: Information from APA (2022).

SCHIZOAFFECTIVE DISORDER

Schizoaffective disorder: a psychotic disorder in which an individual experiences a mix of the symptoms of mood disorder and schizophrenia.

In **schizoaffective disorder**, an individual experiences a mix of the symptoms of mood disorder and schizophrenia (Diagnostic Overview 13.5). They may exhibit positive symptoms of psychosis, such as the hallucinations or delusions associated with schizophrenia, along with the manic or depressive episodes associated with bipolar disorder or depression.

Diagnostic Overview 13.5: Schizoaffective Disorder

Symptoms of psychosis as indicated by at least two symptoms of psychosis. One of the symptoms must include either delusions, hallucinations, or disorganized speech.

Must include one of the following	Can also include any of the following
Delusions Hallucinations Disorganized thought and speech	Disorganized behavior Negative symptoms

Along with the symptoms of psychosis people also experience symptoms of a depressive or manic episode.

At some point delusions or hallucinations are present when the person's mood is not depressed or manic. The mood symptoms are present for the majority of the time during the condition.

Impact:	Symptoms must exceed cultural and contextual norms. Symptoms are related to clinically significant distress or create impairment in important areas of life such as with friends and family or at work or school.

Source: Information from APA (2022).

Schizoaffective disorder

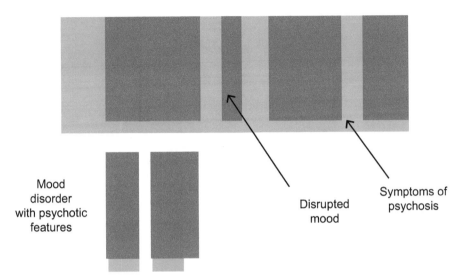

Mood disorder with psychotic features

Disrupted mood

Symptoms of psychosis

Figure 13.3 Schizoaffective disorder differs from a mood disorder with psychotic features in that, in mood disorder, the person has psychotic symptoms only during a depressive or manic episode, rather than continuously.

The person's mood is affected, and the psychotic symptoms remain even when the mood disorder improves. In fact, the diagnosis of schizoaffective disorders requires at least two weeks of hallucinations and/or delusions in the absence of mood symptoms.

Schizoaffective disorder is distinct from a bipolar disorder with psychotic features or a depressive disorder with psychotic features. In those conditions (often called mood disorder with psychotic features), a person has symptoms of psychosis, such as hallucinations or delusions, that occur only while also having symptoms of the depressive or manic episodes. For example, the person hears a voice only when they are depressed (Figure 13.3).

Case Study: Schizoaffective Disorder – Lori Schiller

In her late twenties, Lori said she had been hearing voices in her head for the better part of the last 12 years. "The Voices," as she called them, were often threatening and demeaning, telling her she was worthless and that she should "Go to hell!" Lori likened the effect of the Voices to being "possessed" by demonic spirits. Despite the psychological toll, she hid her symptoms from her friends and family for fear of being labeled "crazy." In addition to having auditory hallucinations, she occasionally had visual ones too, usually manifesting as horrifying and disturbing images. She claimed to see body parts hanging from tree branches and fences, and the faces of the people around her melting like wax.

In conjunction with hearing the Voices, Lori reported feeling paranoid about many electronic devices, including televisions, radios, and telephones, because she thought they were speaking directly to her and sending her threatening messages. When she was near active electronic devices, she felt frightened and apprehensive. As her symptoms worsened, Lori also became more detached from her family. Once

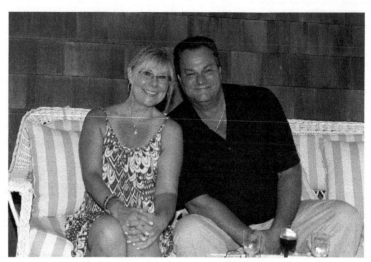

Figure 13.4 Lori Schiller.
Source: Patrick McMullan/Patrick McMullan via Getty Images.

a free and outgoing spirit, she eventually had diminished social interactions and adopted an asocial personality.

Lori described her moods during that time as being "up and down." During her high periods, she reported having increased energy despite a lack of sleep. She woke up early to take long, meaningless drives because she felt it relaxed her and dulled the Voices in her head. She also admitted to making a number of questionable decisions during her high moods, including impulsive business investments and excessive alcohol consumption. During her down periods, Lori reported feeling an extremely depressive mood. She slept for most of the day and found herself unable to summon the will to get out of bed to go to class, socialize, or do any of the things she would normally do. She felt fatigued and lacked energy for the majority of the day. It was during these periods that she felt her strongest urges to give in to the Voices' demands, due to increased feelings of worthlessness and a lowered self-image, but the Voices were there even when her mood was more upbeat.

To find out more about Lori (Figure 13.4), read her memoir *The quiet room: A journey out of the torment of madness* (Schiller & Bennett 2008).

CONCEPT CHECK 13.2

Identify the likely condition in each case.
1. Torrey, a 45-year-old man, presents with a belief of many years' duration that someone is following him and using the events from his life to create a blockbuster movie. Although he feels frustrated at being taken advantage of, he denies any significant depressive symptoms and is often able to enjoy playing cards with his friends. He also denies having any other symptoms.

2. Raymundo is a 35-year-old man who presents at his primary care physician's office complaining of auditory hallucinations that have worsened over the past six months. He notes that the devil has been telling him he is "no good," and that he "will not amount to anything." During the last several months, Raymundo says, he has been feeling "depressed" and sleeping poorly. He has no desire to get out of bed and has lost interest in even watching sports (normally one of his favorite activities). Even when his mood improves, he says, he still cannot "get the voices out of my head."

THE POWER OF EVIDENCE

Effective treatment for schizophrenia

Many people believe schizophrenia is such a devastating disorder that those who have the condition can't live productive and fulfilling lives. But what does the evidence say?

Schizophrenia can be a difficult disorder, and it's true that some people who have it struggle. For example, research suggests that schizophrenia and other psychotic disorders often lead to homelessness. But not everyone with schizophrenia has persistent symptoms, and the severity of symptoms can vary greatly, along with people's circumstances and life situations.

In fact, many individuals with schizophrenia thrive. They have jobs, families, and fulfilling hobbies. What makes the difference is the severity of their symptoms and their access to effective treatments. Most don't need to stay in a hospital, and they fare best by attending outpatient treatment and living at home. The key to living well with schizophrenia, or any chronic illness, is to find the right treatment and stick with it. A 16-year follow-up study found that, with treatment, people with schizophrenia and substance use disorders experienced improvements in symptoms and quality of life. They also tended to live independently, work, and have social support.

Nearly half of those diagnosed with schizophrenia have improved to the point that they can work and live on their own. About a quarter need support, and only 15 percent have persistent struggles with their symptoms to the point where they need frequent hospitalization and become homeless.

Sources: Drake et al. (2020); Lilienfeld & Arkowitz (2010).

13.3 MODELS AND TREATMENTS OF PSYCHOTIC DISORDERS

Despite spending time in many hospitals during and after law school, Elyn, whom we met in the chapter-opening case, has been out of the hospital for nearly four decades. She currently holds an endowed chair of Law, Psychology, and Psychiatry at the University of Southern California School of Law. She attributes her improvement to her treatment and the support of her friends and family. Things are much improved for Lori as well. She now teaches courses on psychotic disorders to mental health professionals.

Psychotic disorders are the result of many factors. Like most other psychological disorders, they've been shown to have both a biological underpinning and non-biological influences. For example, a recent meta-analysis suggested that the stress of the COVID-19 pandemic may also impact the likelihood of having symptoms of psychosis (Brown et al. 2020). While medications can be helpful to reduce the symptoms of psychosis, as we'll see in this section, these drugs can also bring significant long-term side effects (Murray et al. 2016). Psychological mechanisms can also be related to the symptoms of psychosis, so many psychological treatments have been developed to augment medications and help people cope with their symptoms, improve their wellbeing, and lower the possibility of relapse.

Biological Models and Treatments of Psychotic Disorders

As you'll see in the next section, there is clear evidence of the biological origin of psychotic disorders, including differences in genetic vulnerability, brain structures, neurodevelopment, and neurochemical pathways.

GENETIC VULNERABILITY

Genes play a significant role in schizophrenia. The more closely a person is related to someone with schizophrenia, the greater their likelihood of having the disorder. There is a 1 in 100 chance of a person's being diagnosed with schizophrenia. This risk rises to 1 in 10 for a person whose parent or sibling has the disorder, and it reaches 1 in 2 if the sibling with the disorder is an identical twin (Figure 13.5). These numbers hold whether the individuals grow up in the same household or apart (Gottesman 1991; Plomin et al. 2000).

NEURODEVELOPMENT IN THE UTERUS

Neurodevelopment refers to the growth and maturation of the nervous system. The neurodevelopmental hypothesis of schizophrenia proposes that the nervous system differences found in those with schizophrenia are due, in part, to factors that occur during the growth of the nervous system before birth (McGrath et al. 2003). These factors can be genetic (like having a family member with schizophrenia), environmental (like maternal malnutrition, infection, or incompatible blood types), or both (Fatemi & Folsom 2009).

BRAIN STRUCTURES

There are several differences in the brains of individuals diagnosed with schizophrenia. Brain scans reveal that people with schizophrenia have larger ventricles –

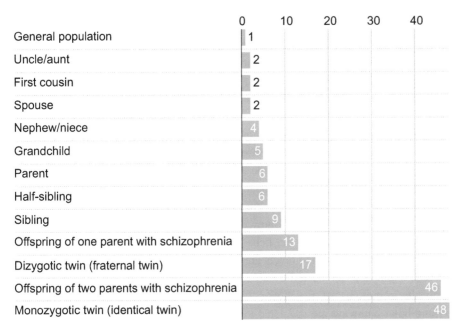

	0	10	20	30	40	
General population	1					
Uncle/aunt	2					
First cousin	2					
Spouse	2					
Nephew/niece	4					
Grandchild	5					
Parent	6					
Half-sibling	6					
Sibling	9					
Offspring of one parent with schizophrenia	13					
Dizygotic twin (fraternal twin)	17					
Offspring of two parents with schizophrenia					46	
Monozygotic twin (identical twin)					48	

■ Percentage of risk

Figure 13.5 Heritability of schizophrenia (percentage of risk). A person's percentage of risk of developing schizophrenia varies based on their relationship to another person with the disorder.

fluid-filled cavities – in their brain than do people without this disorder (Galderisi 2000) (see Figure 13.6). Other researchers found that the hippocampus and areas within the cerebral cortex were a bit smaller than would be expected (Lui et al. 2009). These structural differences are not enough, however, to explain the vast behavioral and emotional differences in those with schizophrenia.

Brains of identical twins

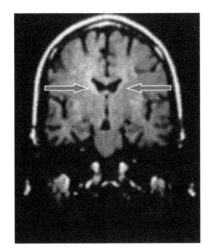

Without schizophrenia

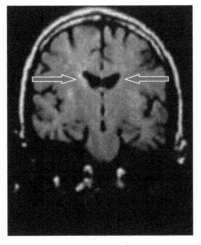

With schizophrenia

Figure 13.6 MRI scans of a twin without schizophrenia (left) and a twin with schizophrenia (right) show differences in the size of the ventricles (the dark areas in the middle).
Source: Adapted from image by Dr. Daniel Weinberger, NIMH, Clinical Brain Disorders Branch.

NEUROCHEMICAL PATHWAYS

Dopamine hypothesis of schizophrenia: a biological model of psychosis that suggests the neurotransmitter dopamine plays a key role in the disorder.

The **dopamine hypothesis of schizophrenia** suggests that the neurotransmitter dopamine plays a key role in the disorder. The four major dopamine pathways in the brain are the mesolimbic pathway, the mesocortical pathway, the nigrostriatal pathway, and the tubero-infundibular pathway. Current theories suggest that a complex imbalance of dopamine in two of these pathways might lead to the symptoms of schizophrenia, as well as to the side effects of medications used to balance out dopamine in the brain (Conklin & Iacono 2002). For example, there may be too much dopamine in the mesolimbic system, which is involved in emotion and thinking. Too much dopamine in this area could explain the delusions, hallucinations, and distorted thinking often found in people with psychosis (Table 13.2). On the other hand, low dopamine levels in the prefrontal area have been implicated in managing our behavior, attention, and motivation (Stahl 2017). For example, low dopamine levels are associated with low motivation, depressed moods, inability to focus, and tremors. Not all dopamine pathways are associated with the symptoms of psychosis; for example, the nigrostriatal and tubero-infundibular pathways are unrelated to symptoms of psychosis.

Antipsychotic medication: a type of drug used to reduce the symptoms of psychosis.

Antipsychotic medications are a type of drug used to reduce the symptoms of psychosis as seen in schizophrenia (Table 13.3). These medications diminish psychosis in about 70 percent of patients (Sadock & Sadock 2010) in just a few weeks (Emsley et al. 2006).

By blocking dopamine, these medications reduced dopamine activity in brain areas in which it was thought to be overactive. Since they were used so regularly, medications such as haloperidol (Haldol) were known as typical antipsychotics.

Typical antipsychotics: also known as first-generation antipsychotics, are beneficial in targeting the positive symptoms of psychosis, like hallucinations and delusions.

Typical antipsychotics, also known as first-generation antipsychotics, are beneficial in targeting the positive symptoms of psychosis, like hallucinations and delusions. The impact of these drugs on the lives of people experiencing the symptoms is powerful. Many have seen dramatic improvement in just a few weeks of treatment (Huhn et al. 2019).

While they reduce dopamine levels in places in which its concentration may be too high, typical antipsychotics may also reduce it in places in which it is in the

Table 13.2 Key dopamine pathways involved in psychosis

Pathway	Mesolimbic pathway	Mesocortical pathway to the prefrontal cortex	Nigrostriatal pathway	Tubero-infundibular pathway
Level of dopamine for those experiencing symptoms of psychosis	High	Low	Normal	Normal
Effect	Positive symptoms of psychosis	Negative symptoms of psychosis	Unrelated to the symptoms of psychosis	Unrelated to the symptoms of psychosis

Source: Information from Stahl (2017).

Table 13.3 Some medications used in the treatment of schizophrenia

Generic name	Trade name	Generation (first or second generation)	Risk for extrapyramidal side effects (1 is the lowest)
chlorpromazine	Thorazine	First	2
perphenazine	Trilafon	First	5
haloperidol	Haldol	First	5
pimozide	Orap	First	5
risperidone	Risperdal	Second	1
clozapine	Clozaril	Second	1
olanzapine	Zyprexa	Second	1
quetiapine	Seroquel	Second	1
ziprasidone	Geodon	Second	1
aripiprazole	Abilify	Second	2
iloperidone	Fanapt	Second	1
lurasidone	Latuda	Second	1
paliperidone	Invega	Second	1
asenapine	Saphris	Second	1
brexpiprazole	Rexulti	Second	1
cariprazine	Vraylar	Second	1

Source: Information from Stahl (2017).

normal range such as the nigrostriatal pathway, resulting in adverse effects such as tardive dyskinesia. **Tardive dyskinesia** is a neurological condition characterized by involuntary repetitive movements. The name of this condition literally means "late to arrive" (tardy) "abnormal" (dysfunction) "movements" (kinetics), because it is associated with abnormal movements like lip smacking, blinking, puckering, and grimacing. Tardive dyskinesia is estimated to occur in one in five people who take the typical antipsychotics (Miyamoto et al. 2003). Although it can be controlled with medication, the condition is considered permanent.

Tardive dyskinesia: a neurological condition characterized by involuntary repetitive movements.

Another disadvantage of typical antipsychotics is that the treatment effects seem to focus only on the positive symptoms of psychosis. Although those are important symptoms, the negative symptoms, including flat affect, avolition, and alogia, also have a great impact on the lives of people who experience them.

More recently, newer medications have been discovered that reduce both the positive and negative symptoms of psychosis. Since these new medications were not the ones normally given, they are called atypical antipsychotics. **Atypical antipsychotics**, also called second-generation antipsychotics, target dopamine as well as other neurotransmitters (Table 13.3). They have the additional benefit of producing lower rates than do typical antipsychotics of *extrapyramidal side effects*, medication-induced movement side effects such as tardive dyskinesia (Stahl 2017). They do cause weight gain and higher rates of diabetes than the earlier medications, however (Stahl 2017).

Atypical antipsychotics: also called second-generation antipsychotics, medications that target dopamine as well as other neurotransmitters to reduce the symptoms of psychosis.

A recent trend in psychopharmacology is the use of long-acting injectable antipsychotics (LAIs). These medicines suspend second-generation antipsychotic medications in an oil-based formulation that is injected into the muscle. A benefit to these medications is that clients don't have to remember to take them and thus increases the likelihood that clients will have a consistent dose of the medication in their system. This can result in positive benefits for reduction of symptoms. In one study for example (C. Y. Huang et al. 2021), LAIs were found to reduce suicide risk by half in those with schizophrenia, compared to rates for those who took oral antipsychotics. The same study found that those who switched to LAIs from oral antipsychotics had a lower mortality rate in general.

Cognitive-Behavioral Models and Treatments of Psychotic Disorders

The cognitive-behavioral perspective recognizes the biological underpinning of psychosis, but it also suggests that cognitive and behavioral factors may exacerbate the condition, and thus that it may be helpful to focus on them in treatment. From a cognitive-behavioral perspective, people with psychotic disorders have limited cognitive resources due to the demands of their symptoms. They may therefore have difficulty inhibiting negative behaviors and paying attention to social cues. They may also struggle to follow the rules and norms of communication, using shortcuts to streamline the informational and sensory overload in their brain. Delusions, for example, may be attempts to explain the perceptions they experience. Negative symptoms may also arise from the need to conserve emotional and cognitive resources.

Cognitive-behavioral therapy for psychosis (CBTp) focuses on helping those with psychosis improve their functioning and decrease the stress that is often associated with the symptoms. CBTp also can be helpful in countering delusions and hallucinations.

Behavioral interventions can combat the negative symptoms of psychosis, helping clients to be more active, to recognize possible negative reactions toward their symptoms, and to seek help when they need to.

One strategy of CBTp relies on *hallucination reinterpretation and acceptance.* This technique uses some of the hallmark interventions of CBT (such as cognitive restructuring) to help clients explore their beliefs about their hallucinations and reduce their distress. For example, a client may have an auditory hallucination of a threatening voice. To make sense of it, they may create a misinterpretation of the situation (a delusion), such as the belief that "I'm not safe" when they hear the voice. This interpretation may lead the client to isolate from others and to feel scared and anxious. However, reinterpreting the hallucination with an alternate thought, such as "This is an auditory hallucination," may reduce problematic behaviors and emotions (Figure 13.7). CBTp can also be useful for educating clients with details about the biological theory behind their delusions and hallucinations, and to discover triggers for and challenge their beliefs about their symptom.

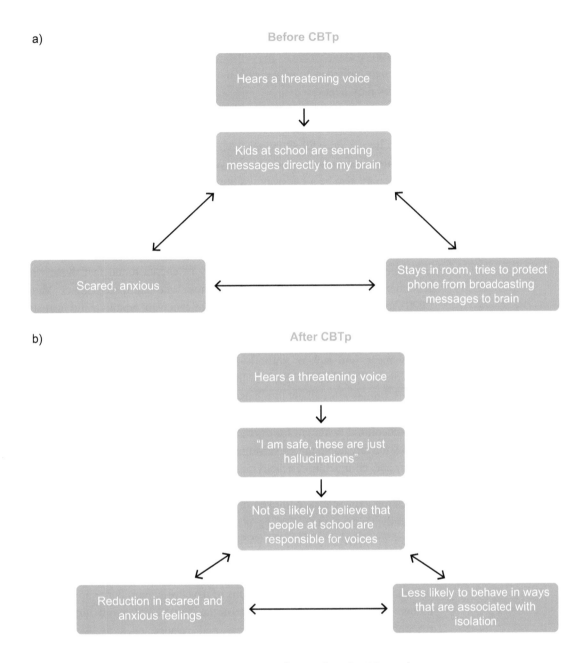

a) Before CBTp

Hears a threatening voice

↓

Kids at school are sending messages directly to my brain

Scared, anxious ⟷ Stays in room, tries to protect phone from broadcasting messages to brain

b) After CBTp

Hears a threatening voice

↓

"I am safe, these are just hallucinations"

↓

Not as likely to believe that people at school are responsible for voices

Reduction in scared and anxious feelings ⟷ Less likely to behave in ways that are associated with isolation

Sociocultural Models and Treatments of Psychotic Disorders

Figure 13.7 a) and b) Cognitive-behavioral therapy for psychosis aims to reduce the distress associated with hallucinations.

Cultures can vary in how accepting they are of the symptoms of psychosis because their willingness to accept the experience of psychosis varies. Some even welcome the experience. For example, up to 52 percent of people with auditory hallucin-ations report positive and pleasurable experiences associated with voices they hear (Armstrong et al. 2021). Those whose cultures value mediums, healers, shamans, and spirituality have more positive experiences with auditory hallucinations (sometimes referred to as voice hearing) (Armstrong et al. 2021). However, few of the diagnostic assessments commonly administered in the United States capture these positive experiences of psychosis (Armstrong et al. 2021), which may leave practitioners baffled as to why clients may decide not to take medications to reduce the voices they hear.

Sociocultural issues and structural inequities may also be related to symptoms of psychosis because they can increase stressors. People with psychosis are more likely to live in stressful situations such as poverty, for example. Stress may be a factor in triggering new episodes of psychosis.

There may also be a two-way relationship between symptoms of psychosis and stress. That is, symptoms of psychosis may interfere with the ability to complete an education and create problems with obtaining or holding a job, all pushing the person into poverty and thus creating a stress factor.

Stress isn't the only factor involved in symptoms of psychosis. Another is differences in family dynamics. One study of clients found that those who had less contact with relatives did better than those who had more contact (Yuni et al. 2020). Those who experienced high levels of criticism, hostility, and intrusiveness from their families tended to have more frequent relapses of psychotic symptoms (Izon et al. 2021). Exposure to high *expressed emotion* – criticism, emotional over-involvement, and lack of warmth – is related to more frequent returns of the symptoms of psychosis, especially in those with a persistent disorder. An individual is 3.7 times more likely to relapse in this case than if exposed to a family with low expressed emotion (Gandhi et al. 2020).

Sociocultural treatment for psychosis includes social skills training that may be helpful for engaging in conversations, getting assistance from health care providers, and completing the activities of daily living. It may also be helpful for clients to become members of self-help groups that discuss problem-solving, share medication experiences, and even role-play difficult situations.

Family therapy may also be effective (Li & Arthur 2005). This treatment focuses on educating families about the symptoms of psychosis, medications, stigma reduction, and communication skills. It may assist with reducing high expressed emotion if family members learn to adjust their expectations and become more tolerant of the symptoms of psychosis. Family therapy can also help reduce the pressures of being part of the family and avoid highly emotional reactions. It can help reduce stress and relapse rates as well as hospital readmissions.

Multiperspective Models and Treatments of Psychotic Disorders

Most therapists agree that a multiperspective approach to treating psychosis is helpful (APA 2020). This approach consists of using medication to help with the core symptoms of psychosis and folding in other treatments to help with the

Table 13.4 Current American Psychiatric Association treatment guidelines for schizophrenia

Recommendation	Strength of supporting research
Patients with schizophrenia should be treated with an antipsychotic medication and monitored for side effects	High
Patients with schizophrenia whose symptoms have improved with an antipsychotic medication continue to be treated with an antipsychotic medication	High
Patients with treatment-resistant schizophrenia are treated with clozapine	Moderate
Patients with schizophrenia who are experiencing a first episode of psychosis are treated in a coordinated special care program	Moderate
Patients with schizophrenia are treated with Cognitive-behavioral therapy for psychosis (CBTp)	Moderate
Patients with schizophrenia receive psychoeducation	Moderate
Patients with schizophrenia receive assertive community therapy if there is a history of poor engagement with services leading to frequent relapse or social disruption (homelessness, legal difficulties)	Moderate

Source: APA (2020).

behavioral, cognitive, and social symptoms. The recommendations listed in Table 13.4 are treatments in which the APA has the highest confidence, meaning their likely benefits outweigh any potential harm.

Assertive community therapy is a multiperspective, team-based, multidisciplinary approach that can help those with psychosis. It's often used when clients have transitioned out of inpatient settings but might benefit from more independence. Assertive community therapy focuses on helping clients manage their housing, employment, and social support as well as aspects of their psychotherapy and medication.

Assertive community therapy: a multiperspective, team-based, multidisciplinary approach that can help those with psychosis.

CONCEPT CHECK 13.3

Name the treatment modality in each case.
1. Granger was taking a medication that reduced his hallucinations but that didn't appear to have an impact on his lack of pleasure.
2. Manny experienced auditory hallucinations along with a lack of will to do anything. He recently started taking a medication that his doctor of nursing practice says may help both these types of symptoms.
3. May was diagnosed with schizophrenia last year. She's currently being helped by a team of people who help to manage her medication and housing, as well as provide psychotherapy.
4. Ron is enrolled in a type of therapy that helps him interpret his hallucinations in order to decrease his stress.

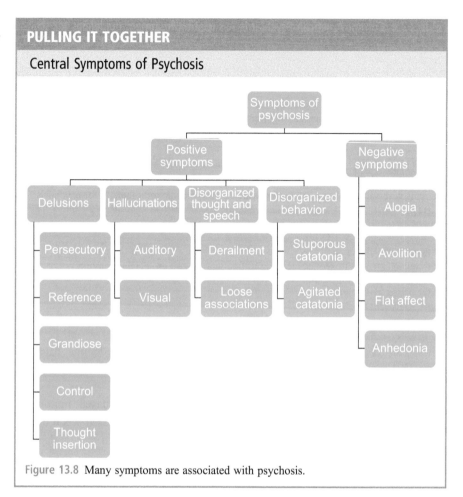

Figure 13.8 Many symptoms are associated with psychosis.

SUMMARY

This chapter presented the following disorders:

- Schizophrenia
- Delusional disorder
- Brief psychotic disorder
- Schizophreniform disorder
- Schizoaffective disorder

Overview of Psychosis

- Psychosis is a condition in which a person has lost some contact with reality.
- The two general types of symptoms for psychotic disorders are positive symptoms and negative symptoms.
- The five domains of positive symptoms are delusions, hallucinations, and disorganized thoughts, speech, and behavior.
- Delusions are fixed false beliefs that are not amenable to change in light of conflicting evidence.
- Hallucinations are sensory perceptions with no sensory input.
- Disorganized or abnormal motor behavior may manifest itself in a variety of ways including catatonia, a problem with movement.
- Negative symptoms are deficits in behavior – things that are expected but are sometimes absent in psychosis.
- The negative symptoms of psychosis include flat affect, avolition, alogia, and anhedonia.
- Positive symptoms of psychosis include delusions, hallucinations, disorganized thought and speech, and disorganized behavior.

Schizophrenia and Psychotic Disorders

- Schizophrenia is a psychotic disorder characterized by delusions, hallucination, and disordered thinking, behavior, and emotions. Continuous signs of the disorder must last for at least six months. At least one month must be an active phase.
- In brief psychotic disorder a person shows sudden positive symptoms of psychosis that last between 1 and 30 days.
- A diagnosis of schizophreniform disorder must meet the main criteria for schizophrenia but show symptoms that last only one to six months.
- In schizoaffective disorder an individual experiences a mix of the symptoms of a mood disorder and schizophrenia.

Models and Treatments of Psychotic Disorders

- The dopamine hypothesis of schizophrenia suggests that imbalances in the neurotransmitter dopamine plays a key role in the disorder.
- The neurodevelopmental hypothesis proposes that the nervous system differences found in schizophrenia are due, in part, to factors that occur during the growth of the nervous system before birth.
- There is strong evidence that psychosocial influences may interact with genetic vulnerability in psychosis.
- Antipsychotic medications reduce the symptoms of psychotic disorders such as schizophrenia.
- Older medication such as the typical antipsychotic improve the positive symptoms of psychosis but have limited impact on the negative symptoms.
- Newer atypical antipsychotics have a lower rate of side effects like tardive dyskinesia and offer relief of both positive and negative symptoms of psychosis, but they are associated with higher rates of weight gain and diabetes.
- In addition to medications, psychological intervention can improve symptoms of psychosis.

DISCUSSION QUESTIONS

1. Why are media images about mental illnesses, such as in the movies, so negative?

2. What factors could influence the difficulty that people with symptoms of psychosis have in staying on medication?
3. What factors have contributed to changing public attitudes about schizophrenia?

ANSWERS TO CONCEPT CHECKS

Concept Check 13.1

1. Positive symptom
2. Negative symptom
3. Positive symptom
4. Negative symptom
5. Positive symptom
6. Negative symptom

Concept Check 13.2

1. Delusional disorder
2. Schizoaffective disorder

Concept Check 13.3

First-generation antipsychotic

Second-generation antipsychotic
Assertive community therapy

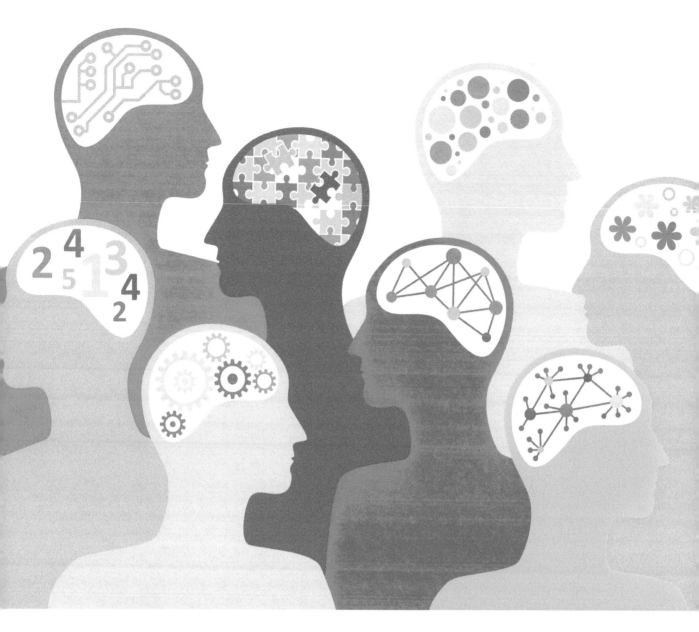

CHAPTER CONTENTS

14

Neurodevelopmental and Neurocognitive Disorders

CASE STUDY: Attention Deficit Hyperactivity Disorder – Jessica McCabe

Jessica was known as a "smart kid." By the age of 18 months she was speaking in full sentences, and by third grade she was reportedly scoring beyond a high school level on standardized tests. But she struggled, too; she had few friends, spaced out in class, and lost things all the time. In middle school she would constantly forget to bring in her homework. By the time she was 21, Jessica had dropped out of college, moved back home, and been fired from or quit more than 15 jobs. Her credit history was poor because she kept forgetting to pay her bills, and when she married, she was divorced within a year. She had problems focusing and felt overwhelmed all the time. All this was occurring despite Jessica's feeling she worked so much harder than everyone she knew. By the time she was 32, she had no idea what to do with her life, nor why she was finding it so difficult to succeed. We'll come back to Jessica's story later.

To learn more about Jessica McCabe (Figure 14.1), take a look at her TEDx talk (www.ted.com/talks/jessica_mccabe_this_is_what_it_s_really_like_to_live_with_adhd_jan_2017?language=en) or her popular YouTube series How to ADHD (www.youtube.com/channel/UC-nPM1_kSZf91ZGkcgy_95Q).

Learning Objectives

- Distinguish between neurodevelopmental and neurocognitive disorders.
- Summarize the diagnostic criteria, etiology, and treatment of autism spectrum disorder.
- Summarize the diagnostic criteria and severity levels of intellectual developmental disorder.
- Describe the models and treatment of intellectual developmental disorder.
- Describe the main features and treatment of delirium.
- Distinguish between major and mild neurocognitive disorder.
- Discuss the main causes and treatments of major and mild neurocognitive disorder.

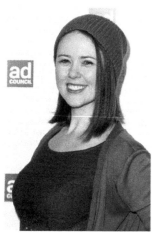

Figure 14.1 Jessica McCabe.
Source: Tommaso Boddi/Getty Images.

Neurodevelopmental disorders: a group of psychological disorders that show symptoms during the developing years and can slow neurological growth or interfere with the achievement of certain cognitive or social milestones.

Neurocognitive disorders: psychological disorders characterized by cognitive decline that often arises from a medical condition or from substance withdrawal or intoxication.

14.1 OVERVIEW OF NEURODEVELOPMENTAL DISORDERS AND NEUROCOGNITIVE DISORDERS

The human brain changes over time during our growth and development, affecting the way we manage information and apply the knowledge we have gained. This brain growth also leads to the achievement of certain cognitive and social abilities, for which society sets milestones. For example, by a certain age, children are expected to be able to take turns at games, and to be comfortable being away from their parents for a time. Most of the conditions we've discussed in the other chapters of this book are developmental in some respect. That is, they tend to begin at a certain age, and there may even be differences between the way their symptoms present in younger people and in older ones.

Some conditions that are thought to be neurologically based begin to be evidenced during the developing years. Psychopathologists categorize these conditions as **neurodevelopmental disorders**. Neurodevelopmental disorders show symptoms during the developing years and can slow neurological growth or interfere with the achievement of certain cognitive or social milestones. They tend to persist throughout the lifespan.

While neurodevelopmental disorders begin early in life, neurocognitive disorders typically first show symptoms much later. **Neurocognitive disorders** are characterized by cognitive decline that often arises from a medical condition or from substance withdrawal or intoxication. They lead to impairments in cognition such as language difficulties, problems with memory, perceptual disturbances, and problems in planning and organizing. *DSM-5tr* organizes the neurocognitive disorders by severity (major or mild) and by cause.

In this chapter we will examine these two sets of conditions linked with brain development. The neurodevelopmental disorders, which we look at first, include attention deficit hyperactivity disorder, autism spectrum disorder, and intellectual developmental disorder, and the neurocognitive disorders include delirium, major neurocognitive disorder, and mild neurocognitive disorder.

CONCEPT CHECK 14.1

Indicate whether the condition described is likely to be a neurodevelopmental or a neurocognitive disorder.
1. Edward is 60 years old and has trouble focusing on a project to the point that it has interfered with his work. He's had this problem since he was 7.
2. Emilia is 75 years old and has had symptoms of intellectual developmental disorder since she was 2.

3. Gary is in the hospital. He is 60 and often forgets who he is. These symptoms developed during the last year.
4. Christel appears disinterested in people around her and gets upset if someone interrupts her repetitive behaviors. These behaviors have been noticeable since she was 3 years old.

14.2 ATTENTION DEFICIT HYPERACTIVITY DISORDER

Reading a novel takes considerable focus. You have to pay attention to the context and meaning of the story, the plot, and the characters, but at the same time it's likely that other things are going on around you. Music might be playing in the background, you could have distracting thoughts, and notifications might pop up on your phone. You might feel an impulse to get up, check your phone, or pay attention to those distractions around you. To be successful in your reading, you must be able to bring it to the foreground of your attention and activity, and to put in the background those things that don't require your immediate attention.

Maintaining focus in this way is an important part of doing well in school, and even of building relationships with your family and friends (such as by waiting your turn to speak). To get along well in society, we need to hold back or inhibit our impulses. At its most severe, when people have trouble focusing on tasks or inhibiting their impulses in a way that impairs their ability to function and thrive, their difficulty may meet the diagnostic criteria for attention deficit hyperactivity disorder. **Attention deficit hyperactivity disorder (ADHD)** is a neurodevelopmental condition in which a person has a pattern of inattention or disruptive hyperactivity/impulsivity.

Attention deficit hyperactivity disorder (ADHD): a neurodevelopmental condition in which a person has a pattern of inattention or disruptive hyperactivity/impulsivity.

Symptoms and Description: Attention Deficit Hyperactivity Disorder

Because ADHD is a neurodevelopmental disorder, its symptoms begin in childhood (although the diagnosis might not be made until they are adults). There are two categories, symptoms of inattention and symptoms of hyperactivity/impulsivity. Symptoms of inattention may manifest themselves as careless mistakes or the loss of items or tools important to finishing your work. Symptoms of hyperactivity and impulsivity include behaviors such as fidgeting, excessive talking, and having difficulty waiting your turn.

To receive a diagnosis of ADHD, a person must display six or more symptoms of inattention or six or more symptoms of hyperactivity/impulsivity in a variety of

Diagnostic Overview 14.1: Attention Deficit Hyperactivity Disorder

A persistent pattern of inattention and/or hyperactivity-impulsivity in a variety of situations as described below:

Inattention: At least six of the following symptoms:

- Careless mistakes or failure to give close attention to details.
- Difficulty sustaining attention.
- Failure to listen when spoken to directly.
- Failure to follow through on instructions or to finish tasks.
- Difficulty organizing tasks.
- Reluctance to engage in tasks that require sustained mental effort.
- Loss of items important for completing tasks.
- Tendency to be easily distracted by extraneous stimuli.
- Forgetfulness in daily activities.

Hyperactivity and impulsivity: Six (or more) of the following symptoms:

- Tendency to fidget.
- Tendency to get up when expected to remain seated.
- Running when it's inappropriate.
- Inability to play quietly.
- State of being often "on the go," acting as if "driven by a motor."
- Excessive talking.
- Inappropriate blurting out of answers.
- Difficulty waiting for turn.
- Tendency to interrupt others.

Impact: There is clear evidence that the symptoms interfere with, or reduce the quality of, social, academic, or occupational functioning. Symptoms must exceed cultural and contextual norms.

Timeframe: Several inattentive or hyperactive-impulsive symptoms were present for at least six months prior to age 12 years.

Source: Information from APA (2022).

settings, to the point that the behaviors interfere with or reduce the quality of social, academic, or work functioning (Diagnostic Overview 14.1).

Without the proper supports, such as medications, changes in the environment to limit distractions, and organizational tools, ADHD can reduce a person's performance, and many children with ADHD underperform in school (Arnold et al. 2020; Langberg & Becker 2012). However, the disorder affects more than just school; it can also disrupt relationships. Children with ADHD can seem demanding, intrusive, and irritable to their friends and family. In addition, between 45 percent and 60 percent have behavioral symptoms and meet the criteria for conduct disorder diagnosis (see Chapter 10 for more about conduct disorders) (Ahmad & Hinshaw 2016).

There are several presentations of ADHD. In the *combined presentation*, a person experiences six or more symptoms of inattention along with six or more symptoms of hyperactivity and impulsivity. In the *predominantly inattentive presentation*, a person has six or more symptoms of inattention but fewer than six symptoms of hyperactivity/impulsivity. In the *predominantly hyperactive/impulsivity presentation*, a person has six or more symptoms of hyperactivity/impulsivity but fewer than six of inattention (see Figure 14.2).

Presentations of ADHD can change over time. For about half of those with the disorder, symptoms will persist into adulthood (Hinshaw 2018). In adults, severe ADHD is often associated with substance use, mood and anxiety disorders, marital problems, and deficient job performance.

Statistics and Trajectory: Attention Deficit Hyperactivity Disorder

Symptoms of ADHD appear early, before the age of 12. ADHD diagnoses for children in lower-income countries (0.6 percent) are significantly lower than in upper- and middle-income countries (2.2 percent) and in high-income countries (3.3 percent) (Fayyad et al. 2017). These variations may be due to differences not in rates of ADHD, but rather in identifications of the disorder. Surveys suggest that as many as 8 percent of children in the United States will have indications of the disorder in any given year (Fayyad et al. 2017). Rates in the

United States are some of the highest in the world (Figure 14.3) and may be influenced by high awareness of the disorder.

Sociocultural factors may influence who is diagnosed with ADHD. For example, one study has shown that people from minoritized populations are less likely to be diagnosed with ADHD (Zuckerman & Pachter 2019). This is an important consideration because having a diagnosis of ADHD serves as a gateway to specific learning plans and accommodations.

Boys are twice as likely to show symptoms of ADHD, and the gender difference in diagnosis rates is more pronounced in younger people than in adults (Hinshaw 2018). Girls who show symptoms of ADHD are more likely to present with symptoms of inattention and therefore have fewer disruptive behavior symptoms than boys, which may make their symptoms easier for parents and teachers to miss (Biederman et al. 2002).

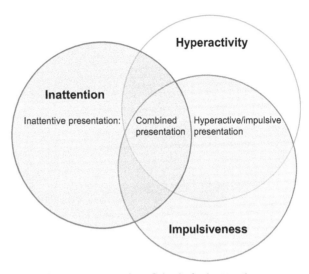

- Combined presentation: Criteria for inattentive and hyperactivity-impulsivity are both met;
- Predominantly inattentive presentation: Criteria are met for inattention but not for hyperactivity-impulsivity;
- Predominantly hyperactive/impulsive presentation: Criteria are met for hyperactivity-impulsivity but not for inattention.

Figure 14.2 Presentations of ADHD include combined presentation, predominantly inattentive, and predominantly hyperactive/impulsive presentation.

Models and Treatments of Attention Deficit Hyperactivity Disorder

Jessica from the chapter's opening case started taking medication for her ADHD after being diagnosed with the disorder as a child. She said that before she started taking medication, "trying to get my brain to focus on anything I wasn't excited about was like trying to nail Jello to the wall." Medication was part of her treatment, and she described the experience as "putting on glasses and realizing you could see without squinting." She's happier and more successful than ever, and after starting treatment and reading more research about ADHD, she started her own business and now has a team of volunteers helping her with an ADHD YouTube channel.

Although ADHD is a neurodevelopmental condition, meaning it has biological bases that are clearly identifiable, there are behavioral and sociocultural aspects to the disorder as well. Medication wasn't enough for Jessica, for example; to overcome her symptoms she also needed behavioral strategies like keeping lists and using timers to keep herself on task. With reasonable accommodations and supportive environments, people with ADHD do well at work and in school settings (Geyer 2021).

BIOLOGICAL MODELS AND TREATMENTS

Biological factors associated with ADHD include differences in heritability, size of certain brain areas, and levels of neurotransmitters. Siblings of children with

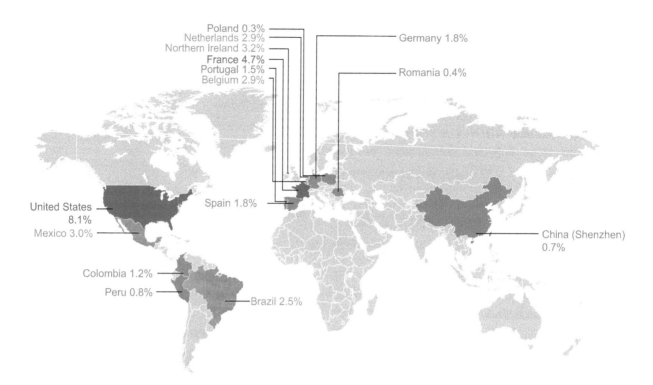

Poland 0.3%
Netherlands 2.9%
Northern Ireland 3.2%
France 4.7%
Portugal 1.5%
Belgium 2.9%
Germany 1.8%
Romania 0.4%
United States 8.1%
Mexico 3.0%
Spain 1.8%
China (Shenzhen) 0.7%
Colombia 1.2%
Peru 0.8%
Brazil 2.5%

Figure 14.3 Lifetime prevalence of ADHD in selected countries, from the World Mental Health Surveys (2002–2017). *Source: Scott, De Jonge, et al. (2018).*

ADHD are up to four times more likely to be diagnosed than those without a sibling who has ADHD. Twin studies of people with ADHD also support the idea that the disorder has a genetic component.

Differences in the size and structure of brain areas in ADHD (see Figure 14.4) include variations in the prefrontal cortex (key in cognition, motivation, and behavior), the striatum (active in working memory and planning), and the cerebellum (involved in motor behaviors). The cerebral cortex is smaller, for instance,

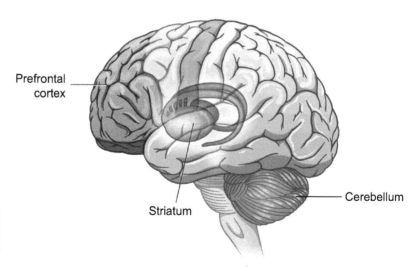

Prefrontal cortex

Striatum

Cerebellum

Figure 14.4 The prefrontal cortex, striatum, and cerebellum are key brain areas associated with ADHD.

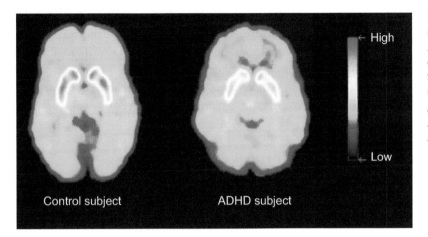

Figure 14.5 This PET scan shows that subjects with ADHD have lower levels of dopamine transporters in the nucleus accumbens than control subjects.
Source: Brookhaven National Laboratory / Science Photo Library.

with less connectivity between the frontal areas of the cortex and the parts of the brain that influence memory, attention, motor behavior, and emotional reactions. Because the cortex continues to develop over time, however, the presentation of ADHD can change, and sometimes the symptoms associated with hyperactivity will decline (resolve) as people get older (Hoogman et al. 2017).

Neurotransmitters are also important in the development of ADHD. Weak norepinephrine and dopamine signals in the prefrontal cortex are associated with the disorder (Figure 14.5). These neurotransmitters play an important role in sustaining attention, controlling impulsivity, and managing error processing. Many medications useful in the treatment of ADHD are aimed at manipulating the levels of these neurotransmitters.

Stimulant medications that increase levels of dopamine in attentional areas of the brain have been useful in treating symptoms of ADHD, especially those such as Ritalin, Dexedrine, and Adderall that work by increasing the availability of dopamine and norepinephrine (see Table 14.1). A recent meta-analysis that included data for more than 10,000 children showed that these medications reduced core symptoms and also increased overall quality of life (Cortese et al. 2018). The majority of children with ADHD (70–85 percent) responded positively to them, experiencing decreases in demanding, disruptive, and non-compliant behavior and increases in positive moods and goal-directed behavior, with high-quality interpersonal interactions.

Table 14.1 Some FDA-approved medications for ADHD

Generic name	Brand name	Class of medication
atomoxetine	Strattera	Selective norepinephrine reuptake inhibitor
amphetamine	Adderall	Stimulant
methylphenidate	Concerta, Ritalin, Quillivant, Daytrana	Stimulant

Source: Information from Stahl (2017).

The medications can have side effects, including insomnia and gastrointestinal effects. They can also decrease appetite, increase sleep disturbances, and create irritability and stomach pain. Some stimulants carry a risk of abuse. Prescription of stimulant medications has increased dramatically since 2003, growing 344 percent between 2003 and 2015 (Anderson et al. 2018), and some people are concerned about inappropriate overuse in children without ADHD who merely display disruptive behaviors.

COGNITIVE-BEHAVIORAL MODELS AND TREATMENTS

Behavioral therapies can also be used to treat ADHD. These treatments help parents, teachers, and other caretakers to reinforce attentive and prosocial behaviors. By using reinforcement, behavioral therapy allows children to begin to anticipate the consequences of their own behavior, which can decrease their impulsivity. Recently the United States FDA approved a new behavioral tool to help treat ADHD that was developed in the form of a game. The prescription-only game, called EndeavorRx, is meant for those with ADHD between 8 and 12 years old. In it, children navigate through a course and collect targets while avoiding bumping into obstacles. Doing well requires focusing and managing multiple tasks at the same time. Children who played the game 25 minutes a day, 5 days a week, for 4 weeks showed improvements in ADHD symptoms (Kollins et al. 2020).

SOCIOCULTURAL MODELS AND TREATMENTS

Some evidence suggests that children with ADHD are more likely to be members of families with parents who have encountered frequent disruptions such as missed deadlines, or difficulty with planning dinners or other household tasks. These disruptions may be associated with the genetic influence of ADHD, meaning children with ADHD may grow up in an environment that could be disorganized because they may have parents with ADHD (Ahmad & Hinshaw 2016).

Those who study the sociocultural models are understandably concerned about the cultural, linguistic, and racial biases that may influence diagnosis. For example, a child from a marginalized population may have behaviors (such as directness, physical movement during communication, and high outward displays of emotion) that are unfairly characterized as problematic and atypical (Slobodin & Masalha 2020).

Sociocultural factors and structural inequities can have an impact on the treatment of ADHD as well. Medication prescriptions and duration of medication use is lower in people with limited access to prescribers and to high-quality health insurance coverage (Slobodin & Masalha 2020). Researchers also point out that underutilization of ADHD treatment may be due to limited access to mental health care providers with cultural competency or diverse ethnic backgrounds. Other practitioners may, for example, overemphasize independence and separation from parents as a goal of treatment and underemphasize religious or culturally specific goals of treatment (Slobodin & Masalha 2020).

MULTIPERSPECTIVE MODELS AND TREATMENTS

Many people, like Jessica in the chapter-opening case, find that medication alone isn't enough. Pharmacological interventions are typically one part of a multimodal treatment approach that also includes behavioral interventions (Mechler et al. 2021).

CONCEPT CHECK 14.2

Indicate whether each case represents a symptom of inattention or hyperactivity.
1. Alaya constantly fidgets in her chair and is unable to sit still.
2. Rati has trouble concentrating on tasks.
3. Jankin has a habit of interrupting other people and almost never waits his turn when playing games.
4. Gwen is easily distracted and because of this makes careless mistakes in her schoolwork.

THE POWER OF WORDS

NEURODIVERSITY

Everyone's brain works a little differently. According to the neurodiversity paradigm, this isn't necessarily a bad thing. *Neurodiversity* refers to the idea that neurological differences like those seen in ADHD, autism spectrum disorder, and other neurological and neurodevelopmental differences are typical variations in the development of humans. Celebrating these examples of difference runs in stark contrast to many models of psychopathology that categorize such conditions as psychological disorders.

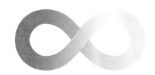
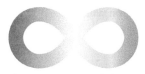

Figure 14.6 This rainbow infinity image is one of the symbols for autism spectrum disorder and neurodiversity pride.
Source: Sudowoodo/ iStock/Getty Images Plus.

The word *neurodiversity* combines the two words *neurological* and *diverse* and was first used by Judy Singer, an author and neurodiversity advocate (herself diagnosed with autism spectrum disorder). Recognition of neurodiversity aims to celebrate the differences among people that have no doubt been around throughout history. This recognition helps reduce stigma and allows people of all kinds to tap into their talents.

In his blog, social psychologist and diversity advocate Dr. Nick Walker describes several principles of neurodiversity. For example, neurodiversity is a natural and valuable form of human diversity, the idea of having just one kind of healthy or normal brain is culturally constructed, and there are social dynamics such as power inequity at play in the way neurodiverse individuals are described and diagnosed.

Critics of the term suggest that it minimizes the challenges caretakers and people with severe conditions face. After all, many people with severe autism spectrum disorder and intellectual disabilities simply cannot care for themselves, while many of those who advocate using the term *neurodiverse* are able to live independently.

Throughout this book we have emphasized that most conditions we describe exist on a continuum. At the extremes, differences can become disorders. The point of transition can vary from person to person and is also based on the availability of sociocultural support or hindrances imposed by society.

Source: Singer (2017).

14.3   AUTISM SPECTRUM DISORDER

Autism spectrum disorder: a neurodevelopmental disorder characterized by deficits in social communication and interaction, along with restricted and repetitive behaviors, interests, and activities.

Autism spectrum disorder is a neurodevelopmental disorder characterized by deficits in social communication and interaction, along with restricted and repetitive behaviors, interests, and activities. Autism spectrum disorder can affect the way those with the symptoms connect with other people, limiting their ability to communicate and interact with them.

The term *autism spectrum disorder* reflects the scientific consensus that several previously separate disorders – autism disorder, Asperger's disorder, and childhood disintegrative disorder – are most likely a single condition instead, with different levels of severity. When *DSM-IVtr* was current, the then-separate disorders were diagnosed differently in different parts of the United States, often based on what services were available for clients with a given diagnosis. Now that the condition is diagnosed on a spectrum, this is no longer the case.

Symptoms and Description: Autism Spectrum Disorder

Autism spectrum disorder is characterized by two main categories of symptoms: deficits in social communication and social interaction, and restricted, repetitive behaviors, interests, and activities. Both components are required for a diagnosis, although specific symptoms may not be consistently present in everyone (Diagnostic Overview 14.2).

Deficits in social communication and social interaction include problems with both verbal and nonverbal communication as well as deficits in developing and maintaining relationships. People with autism spectrum disorder might struggle to understand speech or have repetitive speech patterns such as *echolalia*, the tendency to echo the phrases they hear. Some will have slowed language development, and only half will develop the capacity to speak. The nonverbal behaviors of those with autism spectrum disorder can also show impairment. They may lack the facial expressions or gestures typical in social interaction, such as smiles, and have difficulty using and understanding nonverbal communication cues like facial expressions in others. They may struggle with the back-and-forth of social communication, such as sharing and receiving interests or emotions and initiating and responding to social interactions from other people. Some also struggle to experience or express empathy for others' views or interests.

In addition to social and communication difficulties, people with autism spectrum disorder also show *restricted, repetitive behaviors, interests, and activities.* They may line up toys precisely, insist on following routines, eat the same food every day, display an over-attachment to or preoccupation with objects (such as cars), and respond differently than others to environmental stimulation. For example, some will be indifferent to temperature or even pain, while others will have adverse responses to certain sounds, textures, or smells. This symptom may manifest itself as a preoccupation with or aversion to certain textures or tastes, or an extreme sensitivity to certain types of touch. For example, some people show an aversion to certain clothing based on the way it feels on their skin. Others may become preoccupied with sensations and grow fascinated with certain sensory aspects of the environment (such as edges and shiny surfaces). An insistence on sameness may manifest itself as difficulty making transitions from one place or activity to another, or the need to eat particular foods and in a certain order. Adults with autism spectrum disorder may consistently drive the same route as a self-soothing behavior, without actually needing to go anywhere.

Those with autism spectrum disorder may also have repetitive motor behaviors. These include hand or finger flapping, rocking, swinging, and walking on their toes. Some individuals' repetitive behaviors can cause injuries, such as banging their head against a wall.

Like all neurodevelopmental disorders, autism spectrum disorder produces symptoms early in a person's life, typically before the third birthday, and many with the condition will have symptoms that persist into adulthood. Because of their symptoms, adults with autism spectrum disorder may have problems keeping jobs and managing the daily tasks of living. Those with moderate forms of the disorder may have difficulty understanding the views of other people, struggle to maintain friendships, and experience cognitive and language difficulties as well as challenges with social and behavioral functioning. This cluster of symptoms leads to

---

Diagnostic Overview 14.2: Autism Spectrum Disorder

Deficits in social communication and social interaction, as shown by deficits in social interchange, nonverbal communication, and relationships.

Restricted, repetitive patterns of behavior, interests, in at least two of the following ways:

- Stereotyped or repetitive motor movements, use of objects, or speech.
- Insistence on sameness, inflexible adherence to routines, or ritualized patterns of verbal or nonverbal behavior.
- Highly restricted, fixated interests that are abnormal in intensity or focus.
- Over- or under-sensitivity to sensory aspects of the environment.

Impact: Symptoms must exceed cultural and contextual norms. Symptoms are persistent and present in multiple contexts and cause significant impairment.

Timeframe: Symptoms must be present in the early developmental period.

Source: Information from APA (2022).

Table 14.2 Severity of autism spectrum disorder

Level	Deficits in social communication and social interaction	Restricted, repetitive patterns of behavior, interests, or activities
Level 3: Requiring very substantial support	Severe deficits in social communication and social interaction lead to very limited and rare social interactions.	Extreme difficulty in coping with change. Restricted/repetitive behaviors and activities impair functioning in all areas of a person's life.
Level 2: Requiring substantial support	Even with supports, deficits in social communication lead to social impairments. Limited initiation of social interaction and may speak in short sentences or only discuss certain topics.	Difficulty coping with change. May respond to changes with significant distress. Restricted/repetitive behaviors and activities cause problems with function in more than one area.
Level 1: Requiring support	Without support, deficits in social communication cause impairments. May have difficulty starting and maintaining social interactions.	May have difficulty changing from one activity to another. May require some help with organization and planning.

Source: Information from APA (2022).

problems in many aspects of life and can make it difficult for the individuals to live on their own. This is not to say that those with autism spectrum disorder can't find useful work or successful relationships; in fact, they often excel in these aspects of their lives. Reality shows such as *Love on the Spectrum* help to dispel the stereotype that people with autism spectrum disorder are disinterested in romantic relationships.

Individuals are evaluated in terms of the amount of support they might need to function well, their level of social interaction and communication, and the extent of their restricted interests and repetitive behaviors (see Table 14.2).

Statistics and Trajectory: Autism Spectrum Disorder

In the 1990s, autism spectrum disorder reportedly affected 1 in 2,000 children, but current rates put the incidence at about 1 in every 60 children in the United States (Maenner et al. 2020). Most of this increase is a result of changes in the diagnostic criteria over time and an increase in awareness of the condition. Instead of being a single disorder, it is now seen as a spectrum encompassing what used to be considered three different disorders (Genovese & Butler 2020) (see The Power of Evidence box). World prevalence rates for autism spectrum disorder vary, in part due to the different ways countries assess and track the condition (Chiarotti & Venerosi 2020) (see Figure 14.7).

The first signs of autism spectrum disorder are typically seen in infants. Females with the disorder show more severe symptoms, but in the United States around 80 percent of all cases occur in males. However, there is evidence that girls with autism spectrum disorder may show different symptoms than boys and their symptoms may be overlooked (de Giambattista et al. 2021). About 90 percent of

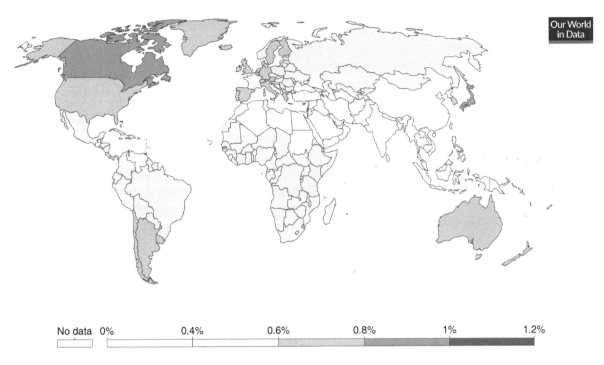

No data 0% 0.4% 0.6% 0.8% 1% 1.2%

those with the disorder will continue to show symptoms into adulthood (AlSalehi & Alhifthy 2020). Despite this prevalence and our increased awareness of autism spectrum disorder, the nature of the condition in adulthood is little understood, since only about 2 percent of the research funds allocated to studying the disorder is earmarked for investigating lifespan issues. The bulk of the research is focused on understanding the nature of autism spectrum disorder in children and working to improve early identification of the condition (Harris et al. 2021).

Figure 14.7 Prevalence of autism spectrum disorder worldwide, 2017.
Source: Roth (2018).

Models and Treatments of Autism Spectrum Disorder

Like many neurodevelopmental disorders, autism spectrum disorder has biological roots. The goal of treatment is to help those with the disorder more effectively interact with the environment. Practitioners use a variety of biological and psychological interventions to promote healthy behaviors while reducing emotional and behavioral problems such as impulsivity, inattention, and aggression (Howes et al. 2018; Rosen et al. 2018).

BIOLOGICAL MODELS AND TREATMENTS

Biological models of autism spectrum disorder investigate the role of genes, brain structures, and brain circuits in the condition. Genetic studies have revealed that siblings of children with autism spectrum disorder are 50 times more likely to have

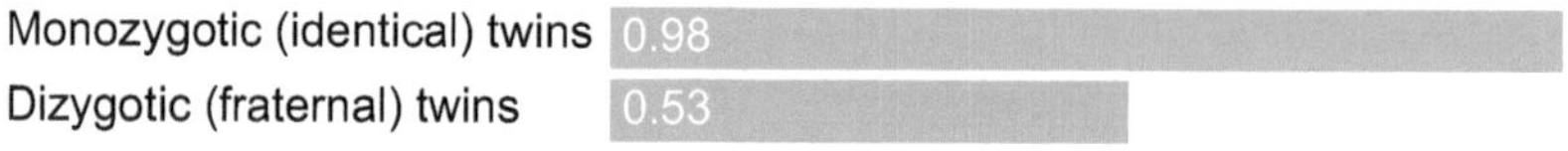

Figure 14.8 The prevalence of autism spectrum disorder is higher for those who are more closely related.

Source: Data from Tick et al. (2016).

| Monozygotic (identical) twins | 0.98 |
| Dizygotic (fraternal) twins | 0.53 |

the condition than are siblings of children without it (Figure 14.8) (Sigman et al. 2006). However, there is no one gene that explains the condition. Some studies suggest that more than 100 genes may be involved to different degrees (AlSalehi & Alhifthy 2020).

Neuroimaging studies reveal differences in the brains of those with autism spectrum disorder, including in the amygdala, orbital frontal cortex, insula, temporoparietal cortex, and cerebellum. These are areas of the brain that typically help us use our own facial expression and apply empathy and reasoning to social situations, and they show less activation than in individuals without autism spectrum disorder (Weston 2019). For example, in addition to its role in maintaining balance, the cerebellum is an important area of the nervous system that helps manage a person's ability to shift attention.

Research has also focused on the role that brain circuits may play in autism spectrum disorder, revealing that there is sometimes too much and sometimes too little stimulation in these brain circuits in those with the disorder. For example, under-stimulation of one circuit (between the amygdala and prefrontal cortex) may be responsible for communication difficulties, while under-stimulation of another (connecting the stratum, thalamus, and orbital frontal cortex) may be related to the severe repetitive and restrictive behaviors and interests of person with autism (Ibrahim et al. 2019).

In the United States, about half the children with autism spectrum disorder have been prescribed medication to target specific symptoms of their condition (see Table 14.3) (Madden et al. 2017). Drugs are used that reduce overactivity, calm stereotyped movement behaviors (such as hand flapping), and ease sleep problems. However, it's unclear how helpful these medications actually are (Madden et al. 2017). They may make it easier for those with autism spectrum disorder to become engaged in structured programs such as school or to participate in behavioral treatments. But they can have adverse side effects, and those with autism spectrum disorder experience greater side effects from their medications (perhaps related to sensory sensitivity) than do those without it (Accordino et al. 2016; Persico et al. 2021).

COGNITIVE-BEHAVIORAL MODELS AND TREATMENTS

Although behavioral models don't suggest a behavioral origin for autism spectrum disorder, techniques such as operant conditioning can be used in highly structured settings to reduce the impact of ritualistic behaviors and disruptive tantrums, and parents can use similar techniques at home. Behavioral and educational interventions can also be effective in helping improve school performance. Since 30 percent

Table 14.3 Indications for medications for autism spectrum disorder

Symptoms	Medication
Hyperactivity, impulsivity, distractibility	Stimulants and non-stimulant medications
Aggression	Antipsychotic drugs, mood stabilizers
Self-injurious behavior	Mood stabilizers, antipsychotic drugs
Extreme difficulty with transitions	SSRI antidepressants
Extreme compulsive behaviors	SSRI antidepressants
Irritability	Antidepressants
Mood swings	Mood stabilizers
Anxious and phobic symptoms	Antidepressants

of those with autism spectrum disorder have impaired communication skills, intervention can teach them to use assistive communication boards, which are pictorial devices with which they can express themselves (Figure 14.9). In fact, as many as 25 percent of diagnosed children make such significant progress with early interventions that in time they no longer meet the criteria for autism spectrum disorder (AlSalehi & Alhifthy 2020).

SOCIOCULTURAL MODELS AND TREATMENTS

Early sociocultural theorists believed that having intelligent but disconnected parents during the critical developmental period were at fault in the development of autism spectrum disorder. Research doesn't support the idea that rigid or rejecting parenting is related to the disorder (Sicile-Kira 2014). Despite the fact that the social environment isn't the cause of autism spectrum disorder, improving the social interactions in which parents engage with their children or with other support people can be helpful. School-based programs can also be

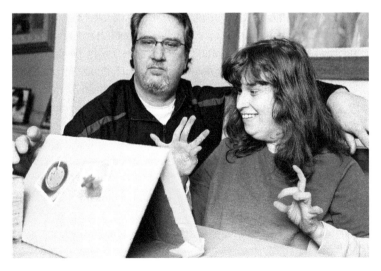

Figure 14.9 For those requiring very substantial support, communication boards may be helpful. This father of a child with autistic spectrum disorder and other developmental disorders holds up a picture card for his nonverbal daughter while homeschooling during the coronavirus pandemic.
Source: ktaylorg,/E+/Getty Images.

beneficial and can assist in providing work and social living skills and improving communication.

There is a surprising lack of cross-cultural research on autism spectrum disorder, part of which is due to the "90–10" divide. That is, 90 percent of the world's children live in low- and middle-income countries, yet only 10 percent of research is performed among or about those populations (Franz et al. 2017). In higher-income countries there is a range of options for intervention, from medication to social skills training. In lower-income populations, however, both treatment options and research are more limited (Franz et al. 2017). There is also evidence of gender imbalance in research in autism spectrum disorder, with only one woman studied for every six men studied (Sohn 2021).

MULTIPERSPECTIVE MODELS AND TREATMENTS

Multiple treatments can support the health of those with autism spectrum disorder. Medication can target specific symptoms, and a meta-analysis of non-pharmacological interventions found four different types of these interventions to be the most useful for adults with autism, namely those that focus on social functioning and language skills, vocational skills, cognitive training, and skills for independent living (Speyer et al. 2021).

THE POWER OF EVIDENCE

Vaccines and autism

In 1998 a British researcher published a paper that examined 12 children, all diagnosed with autism (as it was then called). In the paper he stated that the measles-mumps-rubella vaccine caused the disorder. People were looking for an explanation for the sudden rise in diagnoses of the disorder, which was being called an autism epidemic, and many latched on to the researcher's idea. Later, however, the paper was formally retracted after ethical lapses and other flaws were found in the research, and it was also discovered that sponsors had paid the researcher more than half a million dollars to publish the study. But it was too late: The idea was already circulating that vaccines might be dangerous and lead to autism (Figure 14.10). What does other research about vaccines say?

More than a dozen follow-up studies have been done since 1998. Some examined vaccinations in general, others the measles-mumps-rubella (MMR) vaccine specifically, and yet others combinations of vaccines and even certain substances in the vaccines, such as thimerosal. All the studies failed to find differences in the rates of autism between vaccinated and unvaccinated children. More recently, in 2014, a meta-analysis of five studies with data for more than 1.2 million children failed to find any association between the development of autism and vaccines (Taylor et al. 2014), and in 2019, a study of more than 660,000 children over 11 years of age again found no link between the two.

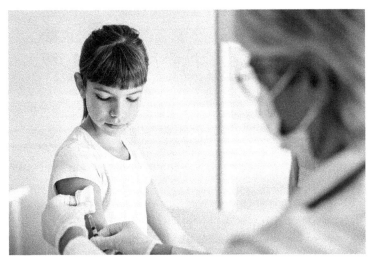

Figure 14.10 Are vaccines related to autism?
Source: Morsa Image/DigitalVision/Getty Images.

First, let's look at the way the Centers for Disease Control and Prevention (CDC) measures the autism rate. Since there is no blood test or scan for autism, the CDC relies on behavior checklists. Researchers collect records for 8-year-old children who live in specific counties around the country, and every two years they ask clinicians to read these records for mentions of specific behaviors that might be related to autism spectrum disorder, such as evidence of repetitive behaviors or social problems. From the results they decide whether a given child might meet the criteria for the disorder, and they use that information to calculate the prevalence rates for the county and then extrapolate for the state and the country.

But why the sudden increase in diagnoses of autism, and later in autism spectrum disorder? Although the condition now known as autism spectrum disorder was first described back in the 1940s, the diagnostic criteria have changed dramatically since that time. For example, in 1987 the *DSM* required that 8 of 16 criteria be present to meet the diagnosis. Now, an individual may meet the current criteria with as few as five symptoms. Increased awareness, screening, and treatment of autism spectrum disorder may also affect the reporting of incidence. All these factors combined have led to an increase in the number of children diagnosed with the disorder, but it is not clear that the disorder itself is more widespread than it was in the past.

Scientists are hard at work at trying to find the etiology of autism spectrum disorder. "We know that autism has a genetic cause and that there are environmental factors that we don't understand yet," says Margaret Spoelstra, executive director of Autism Ontario (Eggertson 2010). It appears, however, that the MMR vaccine isn't one of those environmental factors.

Sources: Eggertson (2010); Taylor et al. (2014).

CONCEPT CHECK 14.3

Indicate whether each case is an example of impairment in social communication/ social interaction, or an example of restricted, repetitive behavior, interests, or activity.

1. Monika lines up her toys and realigns them every few minutes. She becomes very upset if anyone tries to interfere with her activity.
2. When Barbara comes into a room, she disregards the people there and focuses only on objects, especially shiny ones. She sees any overtures from people as intrusions.
3. Myron never maintains eye contact with other children. In addition, he doesn't participate in social play, shared interests, or activities with others.
4. Idris spins the wheels of a toy train for hours. All his activities center on trains.

14.4 INTELLECTUAL DEVELOPMENTAL DISORDER

Intellectual developmental disorder (IDD): a neurodevelopmental disorder that consists of deficits in general mental abilities across a wide variety of domains.

Intellectual developmental disorder (IDD), formerly referred to as intellectual disability, is a neurodevelopmental disorder that consists of deficits in general mental abilities across a wide variety of domains. These deficits affect both intellectual and adaptive functioning and are severe enough to interfere with daily activities; many individuals with intellectual developmental disorder may require assistance. The diagnostic criteria base the severity of the disorder on the extent of the deficits and the amount of assistance required.

Symptoms and Description: Intellectual Developmental Disorder

A diagnosis of intellectual developmental disorder requires assessment of both intellectual functioning and adaptive functioning, based on individually administered tests that should be normed, and on standardized measures (Diagnostic Overview 14.3) (for more regarding tests and measurements, see Chapter 3).

Intellectual functioning: the ability to think, learn, solve problems, and adapt and learn from new situations.

   Intellectual functioning is the ability to think, learn, solve problems, and adapt and learn from new situations. Deficits in intellectual functioning include difficulties with reasoning, planning, problem solving, academic learning, abstract thinking, judgment, and learning from experience.

   Formal intelligence tests calculate an individual's intelligence quotient (IQ) and measure processing speed and abilities in verbal comprehension, working memory, perception, and abstract thought and often have a mean IQ of 100. Measures of IQ are only an approximation of an individual's intellectual function as measured by the specific test, however, and they do not predict a person's ability to function well in life.

The *DSM-5tr* doesn't rely only on IQ to identify IDD for a number of reasons. For one thing, a number of factors including cultural influences can affect a person's IQ scores while having little to do with their intellectual functioning. Many people with IQs below 70 are able to manage their lives and function independently. Thus, to be diagnosed with IDD, individuals with low IQ must also have deficits in adaptive functioning. **Adaptive functioning** is the ability to perform the activities of daily living. It includes a certain level of conceptual (language and reasoning) skills, social skills, and everyday practical skills such as the ability to take care of yourself or keep a job (see Table 14.4). Someone's level of adaptive functioning can also be affected by their ability to communicate, opportunity to obtain a formal education, personal motivation, personality, vocational opportunity, and access to family and community support.

The severity of IDD is based on the level of deficits in intellectual and adaptive functioning and is divided into four categories: mild, moderate, severe, and profound (see Table 14.5). The vast majority of people of those affected (80–85 percent) have mild IDD, and they can live independently and support themselves. Often the deficits in their language and social skills aren't identified until school age, when these register in standardized tests (often administered around 6 years of age). With support, people with mild IDD are able to develop basic skills in reading, writing, and mathematics, as well as skills for daily living such as driving, using public transportation, and managing self-care. They can learn important job-related skills such as arriving at work on time. But they may have limitations in completing tasks that require short-term memory. They also have difficulty

Diagnostic Overview 14.3: Intellectual Developmental Disorder (Intellectual Disability)

Intellectual developmental disorder is a disorder that includes both intellectual and adaptive functioning deficits in conceptual, social, and practical domains.

Impact: Associated with failure to meet developmental and sociocultural standards for personal independence and social responsibility.

Timeframe: Onset during the developmental period.

Source: Information from APA (2022).

Adaptive functioning: the ability to perform the activities of daily living.

Table 14.4 Domains of adaptive functioning

Domain	Examples
Conceptual skills (allow us to think through abstract ideas and complex issues and problem solve)	Language, reading, writing, math, reasoning, knowledge, memory and problem solving, reasoning, acquisition of practical knowledge, judgment in unfamiliar situations
Social skills (make us aware of others)	Making and keeping friends, social judgment, recognizing own actions
Practical skills (allow us to undertake personal care and work)	Self-care (including hygiene, grocery shopping, cooking), completion of job responsibilities, money management, recreation, self-management of behavior

Table 14.5 Intellectual developmental disorder has four levels of severity

Mild:	Moderate:
• Has some functional limitations • Is overly concrete in thinking • Has limited social judgment • Can care for themselves • Can hold jobs requiring limited conceptual skills	• Has delayed language development • Has trouble dressing and feeding themselves • Exhibits limited academic skills • May require assistance • With training may feed self and provide self-hygiene
Severe:	Profound:
• Has limited vocabulary (two- or three-word sentences) • Can dress in uncomplicated clothes and feed self with spoon • Cannot travel or shop alone • Requires supportive living conditions	• May not be able to understand verbal communication • Is fully dependent on others

learning and understanding complex language, and because of this deficit they may be overly literal (concrete) in their thinking. They may require support for more complex tasks such as making legal and health care decisions.

About 10 percent of those with intellectual developmental disorder function at the level of moderate IDD and usually have IQs that range between 35 and 55. Since impairments in function are more apparent in moderate IDD, they are often identified earlier in life, often by 3–5 years of age. By the age of 3, people with moderate IDD may have difficulty with language and may have learned only a handful of words. With support, however, in adulthood they can care for themselves.

Those with severe IDD have IQs in the range of 20–40. Symptoms may start to become evident during infancy. Because of their impairment, individuals with severe IDD may require supervision and structured environments. With these supports in place, they can perform simple tasks such as feeding themselves with a spoon, but they cannot travel, shop, or cook without supervision, and they may speak in only three-word sentences. Over time they come to require regular care to accomplish their daily activities.

About 1–2 percent of those with IDD function at the profound level of the disorder and have IQs below 25. They require structured environments and considerable help, which leaves them dependent on caretakers. Some may have only nonverbal communication skills and will respond only to familiar people.

Statistics and Trajectory: Intellectual Developmental Disorder

Between 1 percent and 3 percent of people in the general population are estimated to have some degree of intellectual developmental disorder (Patel et al. 2020). The reported prevalence of IDD is 1 percent globally, with a male to female incidence ratio of 2:1. Prevalence varies by country (see Figure 14.11), with the highest rates reported in low- to middle-income countries. However, reported rates can be affected by inaccurate reporting due to the stigma that some associate with IDD.

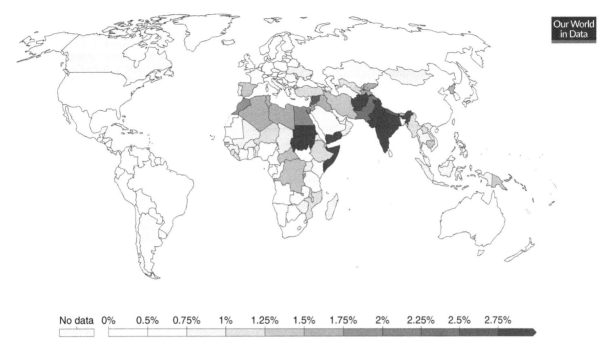

Models and Treatments of Intellectual Developmental Disorder

Many biological and environmental factors can lead to IDD. The majority of cases of mild IDD tend to be environmental, while cases of moderate, severe, and profound IDD tend to be biological (Patel et al. 2020).

BIOLOGICAL MODELS AND TREATMENTS

Many biological factors may lead to IDD, including chromosomal disorders, exposure to toxins, infections, brain injuries, and nutritional deficits. Hundreds of genes can be implicated in IDD (Ellison et al. 2013), and for 25 percent of cases there is no specific genetic cause (Marrus & Hall 2017). However, the two most common types of chromosomal influences that produce IDD are Down syndrome and Fragile X syndrome.

Down syndrome (identified by Langdon Down in 1866) is the most common form of chromosomal IDD. In this disorder an individual has an extra 21st chromosome (that is, three instead of two), which is why the condition is sometimes referred to as trisomy 21. The incidence of Down syndrome tends to be correlated with maternal and paternal age. Women in their twenties have a 1 in 2,000 possibility of having a baby with Down syndrome, increasing to 1 chance in 500 for women who are 35 to 45, and 1 in 18 for women aged 45 and older (MacLennan 2020).

Figure 14.11 Share of world population with intellectual developmental disorder, 2018. *Source: Roth (2018).*

Down syndrome: a neurodevelopmental disorder in which an individual has an extra 21st chromosome.

Although the reason for the connection between Down syndrome and maternal age is unclear, one theory has to do with the age of the ova. Since all ova are produced 20 weeks after the fetus is formed, the likelihood they will be exposed to toxins or radiation increases over time, which could affect the typical division of the chromosomes and create the extra 21st related to Down syndrome (Pueschel & Goldstein 1991). Another theory suggests that as women age, normal hormonal changes may be involved in the development of Down syndrome (Pandya et al. 2013). Older fathers may also influence the risk for Down syndrome. Men over age 40 were twice as likely to have a Down syndrome child than men younger than 20 years old (Daud et al. 2021).

Medical practitioners can detect Down syndrome in a fetus by examining a sample of amniotic fluid, which surrounds the developing fetus in the uterus until birth. In the procedure called *amniocentesis*, a health care provider uses ultrasound to show the baby's position and then uses a needle to remove a sample of this fluid for testing. Another procedure, called *chorionic villus sampling* (CVS), uses a needle that is inserted into the uterus or guided through the cervix to remove a small sample of the placenta to be tested. Because these tests are invasive, some medical professionals opt for screening tests of the pregnant person's blood, which can detect possible markers for Down syndrome fairly early in pregnancy. However, such screening is not a replacement for diagnostic tests (Abele et al. 2015; Samura 2020).

The majority of those with Down syndrome will have an IQ between 35 and 55. However, the disorder affects more than just IQ. Those with Down syndrome have characteristic facial features including folds in the corners of their eyes, a flat nose, and a small mouth, which may affect the way they pronounce certain words. They also tend to have congenital heart malformations and are at increased risk of early-onset dementia of the Alzheimer's type (more about Alzheimer's in section 14.6). Despite these factors, most people with Down syndrome will lead typical lives, and many excel.

The second most common chromosome condition responsible for IDD is **Fragile X syndrome**, which is related to a mutation that makes the X chromosome look as if it's hanging and fragile (see Figure 14.12). Those with Fragile X are mostly men; women with the syndrome exhibit milder symptoms.

Fragile X syndrome: a condition related to a mutation that makes the X chromosome look as if it is hanging and fragile.

Fragile X syndrome

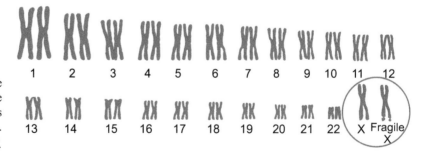

Figure 14.12 In Fragile X syndrome, the X chromosome looks as if it is hanging by a fragile thread.
Source: TBC.

Men with Fragile X have moderate or severe IDD, along with behavioral symptoms such as social anxiety and increased aggression, including self-injurious behavior. Physical characteristics associated with Fragile X include larger ears and wider head circumferences. One of every 4,000 males and 1 of every 8,000 females is born with Fragile X.

Metabolic conditions that disrupt the body's ability to break down or produce chemicals can also lead to IDD. Phenylketonuria (PKU) is one of the most common of these metabolic disorders and highlights the reciprocal-gene environment model (take a look at Chapter 2, section 2.7 for more on the reciprocal gene environment model). PKU is a rare genetic condition with a prevalence of around 0.006 percent of births worldwide (Mojibi et al. 2021). There are no symptoms at birth, but those with the condition cannot break down the amino acid phenylalanine (PHE), found in foods that are high in protein such as nuts, soy, and dairy. The phenylalanine builds up and damages the nerves in the brain, resulting in severe intellectual dysfunction. People can be tested for PKU, and screening tests are typically performed within 72 hours after birth. In the United States all newborns are required to get a PKU test, and if the test is positive, the child is started on a special diet to avoid any impact on the nervous system (Chen et al. 2021).

Environmental influences during pregnancy and other critical developmental periods may also be related to IDD. These include birth complications and exposure to toxins, infections, and diseases. Exposure *in utero* to substances such as opioids, cocaine, and some teratogenic medications may also lead to IDD. Perhaps the most common substance related to IDD is alcohol. Fetal exposure to even small amounts of alcohol during critical periods can inhibit the production of retinol acid, which aids in development of the nervous system. Maternal and paternal alcohol use can lead to fetal alcohol spectrum disorder. *Fetal alcohol spectrum disorder* (FASD) is a condition in a child that results from prenatal alcohol exposure and that can manifest in a mix of physical and intellectual deficits (see the list below) (Kaminen-Ahola 2020; May et al. 2021). Maternal infections and diseases during pregnancy, such as rubella and HIV, untreated hypertension, asthma, and urinary tract infection can also increase the risk of intellectual disability in the newborn. The Centers for Disease Control (2021) lists the following signs and symptoms of fetal alcohol spectrum disorders:

- Low body weight.
- Poor coordination.
- Hyperactive behavior.
- Difficulty with attention.
- Poor memory.
- Learning disabilities.
- Speech and language delays.
- Intellectual disability.
- Poor reasoning and judgment skills.
- Sleep and sucking problems as a baby.

- Vision or hearing problems.
- Problems with the heart, kidneys, or bones.
- Shorter-than-average height.
- Small head size.
- Abnormal facial features, such as a smooth ridge between the nose and upper lip.

IDD can also be the result of damage that occurs after birth, during the early developmental period when the brain is growing rapidly. Infections such as encephalitis and meningitis, head trauma (whether caused by accidents or abuse), intracranial tumors, malnutrition, and exposure to toxic substances such as lead-based paints, mercury, radiation, pesticides, and excessive X-rays can all be damaging to the developing child.

While medications currently don't treat the underlying causes of IDD, they can be useful in reducing associated symptoms such as seizures, controlling self-injuries and aggressive behavior, and improving mood. Atypical antipsychotics can be particularly helpful for managing aggressive behavior (Unwin & Deb 2011), and antidepressants can help improve mood and encourage sleep.

PSYCHOLOGICAL MODELS AND TREATMENTS

Although biological models may best explain IDD, behavioral, educational, and sociocultural factors can offer important interventions. For example, parents and teachers can use behavioral strategies to reduce potentially harmful negative behaviors in those with IDD.

SOCIOCULTURAL MODELS AND TREATMENTS

The sociocultural model examines the role of society and the environment construct of IDD. For example, one of the diagnostic criteria for IDD relies on assessment of intellectual functioning and impairment, but social factors such as the person's age, their cultural background, and examiner bias may influence the way IQ tests are administered and interpreted (see the list below) (Reynolds et al. 2021). Patel et al. (2020) list the factors that may influence administration and interpretation of tests of intellectual and adaptive functioning as follows:

Test factors
　　Cultural bias of the tests
Subject factors
　　Age
　　Sociocultural background
　　Motor impairments
　　Ability to communicate
　　Other medical or mental conditions
Other factors
　　Examiner factors
　　Testing environment

Social factors may also influence the assessment and interpretation of adaptive functioning. Society sets expectations for having a job and living independently, yet the environment often offers unique challenges such as the need to drive a car or navigate public transportation to get to work. All these factors can limit a person's ability to engage in expected individual and societal obligations.

People with intellectual developmental disorder are more likely to come from lower socioeconomic backgrounds (Emerson et al. 2010), which means they may have experienced social disadvantages that can contribute to the disorder. For example, mothers may be less likely to receive good prenatal care, and babies may be at increased risk for premature birth and damaging early exposure to teratogens such as lead. Young children may have access to fewer learning opportunities at school, and their parents might work multiple jobs at nonstandard hours, making them less available to become involved with school. All these factors may interact with biological conditions that could create IDD.

Sociocultural and structural factors make the difference in the ability of those with IDD to succeed. Intervention programs provide them with what we all need – comfortable places to live, proper education, and social and economic opportunities. However, people with IDD can also be subject to prejudice, discrimination, and exclusion. For example, in the United Kingdom they are sometimes not offered the same treatments for medical care as those without IDD (Allison & Strydom 2009).

Special education programs offer a variety of interventions and services specifically for those with IDD, while mainstreaming places them in the regular classroom with their fellow students. Both models have advantages and disadvantages. Specialized education can provide intensive training to improve certain skills deficits, but it can also increase stigma and isolation, and for some students it may be less intellectually challenging. There are also disadvantages to mainstreaming children with IDD in classrooms without specialized education. They may still be viewed negatively by their peers, and they may not receive special skills training. In some school systems, children with IDD spend some of their time in specialized education classes and the rest in classrooms with children without IDD.

Some adults with IDD reside in group homes where they can obtain help with daily tasks (such as cleaning and cooking) while learning social skills and gaining vocational training. These group homes can be helpful for increasing independence and the ability to find work.

CONCEPT CHECK 14.4

Indicate the level of severity of intellectual developmental disorder in each case below.

1. Allison has a limited vocabulary and speaks only in two- or three-word sentences. She can feed herself with a spoon but can't travel or shop alone.

> 2. Ronan can care for himself and is able to hold jobs that require limited conceptual skills.
> 3. Theo has trouble dressing and feeding himself and exhibits limited academic skills. Because he has attended classes, he can feed himself and provide self-hygiene.
> 4. Lynette is fully dependent on others for her care.

14.5 DELIRIUM

Delirium is a sudden confused mental state caused by an underlying medical illness or substance use. It can affect a person's arousal, attention, and orientation, and it is often accompanied by disruptions in sensory perception and emotion. When in a state of delirium, a person is distracted and disoriented and may have difficulty thinking clearly.

Symptoms and Description: Delirium

Delirium is not a persisting condition; rather it is acute, which means its onset is sudden and it will subside quickly (Diagnostic Overview 14.4) (see also Table 14.9 in the Pulling It Together feature at the end of this chapter). Someone experiencing delirium may behave as if they are intoxicated, leaving them unable to recognize their children, partners, or close friends. Because of their symptoms they can't focus on even the simplest tasks. They may also show impairment in memory and language. Symptoms of delirium can become more severe during the evening, a condition known as *sundowning*. However, delirium can become chronic in certain cases where there is a persistent etiology (such as medication that might produce it as a side effect).

There are two types of delirium. In *hyperactive delirium* the person becomes overactive, agitated, or restless. They may have disrupted flow of speech and thought, hallucinate, and experience severe disorientation and anxiety. They also may experience changes in their emotions, such as by becoming easily agitated or angry.

In *hypoactive delirium* patients are underactive, sleepy, and slow to respond. Hypoactive delirium is more common than hyperactive and affects about 75 percent of those with delirium. They may appear apathetic, have decreased responses to outside stimuli, exhibit a flat and unresponsive emotional demeanor, and withdraw into themselves. Health care providers often misdiagnose hypoactive delirium as depression. However, proper assessment, including for attention and memory, may be able to distinguish delirium from other conditions.

Diagnostic Overview 14.4: Delirium

- A disturbance in attention and awareness.
- An additional disturbance in cognition.

Timeframe: Develops over a short period of time and may fluctuate in severity during the course of a day.

Source: Information from APA (2022).

Some people will even move quickly between hyperactive and hypoactive delirium in a condition called *mixed delirium*, becoming overly alert and then a few moments later sleepy and listless. Since delirium may have multiple causes, it's difficult to be certain what triggers the various types of delirium; however, nutritional deficiencies and older age are associated with mixed delirium (Morandi et al. 2020).

Statistics and Trajectory: Delirium

It is difficult to estimate the prevalence of delirium, since it is such an acute (that is, short-lived) condition and can vary based on population, age, and setting. Researchers have estimated, however, that up to 30 percent of hospitalized adults experience it, especially those who have had surgeries, experience dehydration, are prescribed certain medications, and are isolated from a familiar environment. More than two million people a year in the United States experience it (Ospina et al. 2018). Delirium is more common in those who are older, have cognitive conditions, or have severe medical conditions (see Figure 14.13). It is uncommon in outpatient settings; however, among those who have had surgery, post-operative delirium can affect up to 50 percent of patients (Ospina et al. 2018).

Symptoms of delirium can have an impact on overall health and mortality. People with delirium have twice the mortality rate as the rest of the population, have hospital stays up to 2.4 times longer and a higher chance of needing long-term care, and are 12 times more likely to develop dementia later on (Bates & Alici 2014; Thom et al. 2019). In addition, they are more likely to experience major neurocognitive disorder (we'll discuss that in section 14.6).

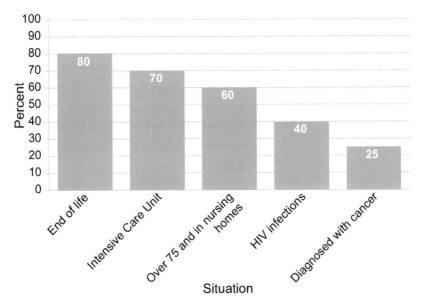

Figure 14.13 Percentage of people who have experienced symptoms of delirium.

Source: Data from Cleveland Clinic (n.d.).

Despite the impact of delirium, more than 60 percent of people who presented with its symptoms were not properly diagnosed by health care professionals. The confusional state of delirium is a sign that something is wrong. Multiple factors that can lead to delirium can also bring on further problems and cognitive decline. Delirium itself can be dangerous (leading to falls, for example), and the longer someone is in the state of delirium, the more likely it will cause damage to the brain.

Models and Treatments of Delirium

Prompt treatment of delirium is essential to prevent further cognitive decline and associated problems such as injuries from falls. While treatment options are limited, however, 40 percent of cases of delirium can be prevented (see Table 14.6) (Inouye et al. 2014).

BIOLOGICAL MODELS AND TREATMENTS

There are several known causes of delirium, including alcohol use, infections such as pneumonia, dehydration, medications such as antihistamines, hospitalization or surgery, organ failure (such as kidney or liver failure), lack of oxygen, lack of sleep, and pain.

Treatments for delirium will vary depending on the cause. While there are no FDA-approved medications for delirium, commonly prescribed treatments include antibiotics for infections, fluids and electrolytes for dehydration and intoxication, and even antipsychotic medications to treat agitation and hallucinations, such as haloperidol (Haldol), risperidone (Risperdal), and quetiapine (Seroquel) (Ospina et al. 2018). Prevention of delirium is also important and includes monitoring the use of prescription drugs often associated with the condition. This can be difficult in outpatient settings, especially for people who are prescribed multiple medications for multiple conditions by multiple providers. Proper coordination of care can be important.

Table 14.6 Tips to help prevent and treat delirium in hospital patients

Promote good sleep habits	During the day, help to keep the patient awake and avoid naps. Daytime sunlight and nighttime darkness can be helpful.
Provide reassurance	Explain surroundings, help the patient to understand what is happening in the hospital.
Provide familiar objects	Items from home such as blankets, bedside clocks, or photos and familiar music can increase comfort.
Encourage movement	Encourage physical activity and movement for those who can participate.
Provide mental stimulation	Discussions about current events and family news can be helpful in keeping patients alert.

Source: Data from Cleveland Clinic (n.d.).

PSYCHOLOGICAL MODELS AND TREATMENTS

The main goal of psychological treatment of delirium is to provide reassurance and reduce the agitation and anxiety that might accompany the condition. Having family members or friends present can be helpful. Behavioral and environmental interventions can also be beneficial to improve sleep and encourage physical activity. There are several reasons that physical activity can help treat delirium, including the fact that it stimulates brain activity (Gual et al. 2020). Regular physical activity can lower the risk of developing delirium by 28 percent. The activity doesn't have to be strenuous; people who knitted, sang, or played bingo six to seven days a week had a 73 percent lower chance of experiencing post-operative delirium than those who didn't participate in any regular activity (Lee et al. 2020).

Psychological interventions can also be helpful in preventing or reducing the impact of delirium. Most focus on increasing the person's safety and restoring a sense of control, and they may also include paying careful attention to hospital patients with delirium to prevent them from removing intravenous or feeding tubes or fleeing from the facility. Surrounding the patient with familiar soothing sounds or belongings like photos and clothing can also reduce anxiety. In a study of more than 800 patients, rates of delirium were much lower (9 percent vs 15 percent) for those who received psychological and behavioral interventions such as mental stimulation, sleep promotion, and encouragement of physical activity (Bates & Alici 2014).

CONCEPT CHECK 14.5

1. Which of the following best describe a diagnosis of delirium?
A. An 80-year-old man has begun progressively forgetting the faces of important people in his life.
B. A 70-year-old woman in an inpatient setting suddenly forgets where she is, and the symptoms seem more intense in the evening.
C. A 75-year-old woman has been forgetful for years, but her memory has gotten worse lately.
2. Which of the following symptoms might support a diagnosis of delirium?
A. Slurred speech
B. Tremors
C. Gradual onset of forgetfulness
D. Confusion and visual hallucinations

14.6 MAJOR AND MILD NEUROCOGNITIVE DISORDERS

So much of getting along well and smoothly in the world depends on our constantly recalling a stream of information. To send a simple text, for instance,

Diagnostic Overview 14.5: Mild Neurocognitive Disorder

Mild decline in cognitive functioning as evidenced by:

- Concern of a clinician, someone close to the person or the person themselves.
- Neuropsychological testing.

Impact: Does not interfere with capacity for independence in everyday activities.

Rule out: Symptoms do not occur exclusively in the context of a delirium.

Source: Information from APA (2022).

you have to find your phone, open the app, and remember the name of the person and the message you want to send. In some cases you'll need a password. You may have occasionally picked up your phone and forgotten whom you meant to text. But imagine gradually becoming unable to recognize the people in your photos or even the people around you. Imagine being in a place where you don't recognize anyone or anything around you, and you don't have the ability to do the basic things necessary to care for yourself.

Like nearly every other part of your body, your brain changes as you age. As it does, its speed of processing information slows, along with your ability to remember information. These declines in processing speed, memory, and learning are natural parts of aging. However, when they interfere with everyday life, something more than typical cognitive aging may be the cause.

Mild Neurocognitive Disorder

Mild neurocognitive disorder: a neurocognitive disorder (NCD) in which individuals have memory and cognitive deficits that are noticeable but not yet significant enough to create problems with everyday activities.

Mild neurocognitive disorder is a neurocognitive disorder (NCD) in which individuals have memory and cognitive deficits that are noticeable but not yet significant enough to create problems with everyday activities. Symptoms include forgetting appointments or recent events, having difficulty making decisions, and experiencing problems with executive functioning (Diagnostic Overview 14.5).

Mild neurocognitive disorder is an intermediate state that occurs prior to the onset of more severe neurocognitive disorder. The purpose of adding the condition in the *DSM-5* was to recognize the early presentation before more severe symptoms set in. Mild NCD symptoms include some cognitive decline that may make everyday life difficult, but at this stage people are still relatively independent.

Major Cognitive Disorder

Major neurocognitive disorder: a neurocognitive disorder (NCD) marked by a decline in areas of cognitive functioning that results in impairment.

Formerly referred to as *dementia*, **major neurocognitive disorder** is marked by a decline in areas of cognitive functioning that results in impairment. The impairment may affect attention, memory, visual perception, and the ability to manage decision making, language, and awareness. It can also alter behavior and personality (Diagnostic Overview 14.6). Impairments may be minor at first and can be helped with memory tools; however, over time they become so severe that people can't function independently. They may become lost in familiar places and forget important biographical information, such as the names of their close friends, partner, or even themselves.

Many factors can lead to symptoms of neurocognitive disorders, including substance use, medical conditions, and mental health conditions such as depression. Psychopathologists categorize neurocognitive disorders both by severity (major or mild) and by cause, such as the following:

- Alzheimer's disease.
- Another medical condition.
- Frontotemporal lobar degeneration.
- HIV infection.
- Huntington's disease.
- Lewy body disease.
- Parkinson's disease.
- Prion disease.
- Substance/medication use.
- Traumatic brain injury (TBI).
- Vascular disease.
- Multiple etiologies.

Diagnostic Overview 14.6: Major Neurocognitive Disorder

Significant decline in cognitive functioning as evidenced by:

- Concern of a clinician, someone close to the person or the person themselves.
- Neuropsychological testing.

Impact:	Symptoms must exceed cultural and contextual norms. Symptoms interfere with independence.
Rule out:	Symptoms do not occur exclusively in the context of a delirium.

Source: Information from APA (2022).

In this chapter we will cover the main criteria for neurocognitive disorder and focus on neurocognitive disorder due to Alzheimer's, because of the prevalence of this condition.

There are individual differences in the progression of symptoms of neurocognitive disorder, but several areas of cognitive functioning are typically affected as the condition progresses, and they include more than just memory. Some people with the disorder have difficulty distinguishing between previously familiar items such as telephones and tables, a condition called *agnosia*, which explains why they also have difficulty understanding other people. In *facial agnosia*, a person may not remember faces that should be familiar to them.

Neurocognitive disorder can also affect executive functioning, causing difficulty in completing tasks that require specific steps and timing. The emotional symptoms that accompany neurocognitive disorder can include depressed mood, agitation, and apathy. It is not yet known whether these result from changes in the brain or from the individual's frustration at recognizing their cognitive decline.

As of 2017 there were 47 million people with neurocognitive disorders around the world (Keene et al. 2017), a number that is expected to reach 135 million by 2050. Among people 65 years of age and older the prevalence is around 1–2 percent, increasing to as much as 50 percent for those over 85 (Alzheimer's Association 2020). There is a positive correlation between age and neurocognitive disorder (see Figure 14.14).

Figure 14.14 The percentage of people with Alzheimer's disease increases with age.

Source: Data from Alzheimer's Association (2020).

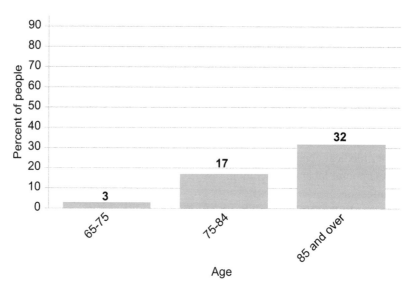

Neurocognitive Disorder Due to Alzheimer's Disease

In the early 1900s, Dr. Alois Alzheimer noticed differences in the brain tissue of a woman in her early fifties who had died after several years of increasing cognitive impairment, disorientation, and disruptive behavior. During the autopsy, Alzheimer discovered abnormal clumps, now called *amyloid plaques*, and bundles of tangled fibers, called *tau tangles*, in her brain. Later the condition became known as Alzheimer's disease.

Neurocognitive disorder due to Alzheimer's disease: a neurocognitive disorder marked by loss of thinking and language ability, and changes in personality and mood.

SYMPTOMS AND DESCRIPTION

Neurocognitive disorder due to Alzheimer's disease is a neurocognitive disorder that manifests gradually but can progress quickly and become difficult to manage in later stages as the brain deteriorates. Symptoms include memory loss, loss of thinking and language ability, and changes in personality and mood. For a diagnosis (Diagnostic Overview 14.7), the criteria for either major or mild neurocognitive disorder should be met (look back at Diagnostic Overviews 14.5 and 14.6), along with the criteria for Alzheimer's disease.

Specific brain changes have been associated with Alzheimer's disease. Most notably, over time the brain shrinks dramatically leading to nerve death and tissue loss. It is believed that plaques and tangles are responsible for these changes (see Figure 14.15). Beta-amyloid plaques are abnormal clusters of proteins that build up between the nerve cells of the brain when a protein called beta-amyloid begins to collect there. As the plaques accumulate, they damage the parts of

Diagnostic Overview 14.7: Major or Mild Neurocognitive Disorder Due to Alzheimer's Disease

- Criteria are met for major or mild neurocognitive disorder.
- Gradual progression of impairment in one or more cognitive domains.
- Criteria are met for Alzheimer's disease as follows:
  1. Evidence of Alzheimer's disease from family history or genetic testing.
  2. Clear evidence of decline in memory and learning and steadily progressive, gradual decline in cognition, without extended plateaus.

Source: Information from APA (2022).

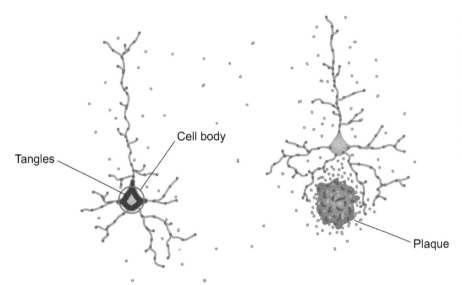

Tangles

Cell body

Plaque

Figure 14.15 Specific brain changes associated with Alzheimer's disease. Neurofibrillary tangles within neurons (dark brown), beta amyloid molecules (small purple dots), and amyloid plaques (large purple sphere). *Source: Adapted from Spires-Jones & Hyman (2014).*

the brain responsible for memory and cognition, including the cerebral cortex, hippocampus, and amygdala (Villemagne et al. 2018). The dying and dead nerve cells do not get cleared away; rather, they form neurofibrillary tangles, also called tau tangles, which are twisted strands of another protein. The tangles prevent nutrients and other important molecules from entering the remaining cells (Alzheimer's Association 2020). The plaques and tangles thus result in cell death and enlargement of the ventricles.

STATISTICS AND TRAJECTORY

Alzheimer's disease is the most common form of neurocognitive disorder, representing 60–80 percent of cases (Alzheimer's Association 2020) and affecting more than 5.3 million people in the United States and even more worldwide. Black Americans are two to three times more likely than the general population to be diagnosed with Alzheimer's disease, and two in three people with Alzheimer's are women. The death rate from Alzheimer's disease and other forms of neurocognitive disorders is substantial: 38.45 per 100,000 people died in 2017 in the United States from Alzheimer's disease and other forms of neurocognitive disorders (see Figure 14.16).

While the reported rates of Alzheimer's disease in low- and middle-income countries tend to be lower, these data may reflect the stigma and lack of assistance surrounding the condition rather than its actual incidence.

The average time from diagnosis to mortality is four to eight years (although some people live for more than 20 years after diagnosis). In those with *early-onset Alzheimer's*, symptoms appear in their forties or fifties.

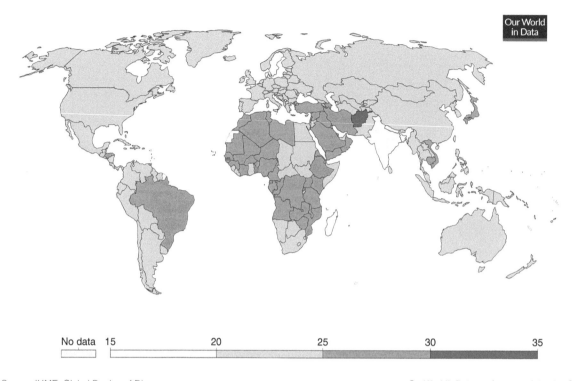

No data   15   20   25   30   35

Source: IHME, Global Burden of Disease   OurWorldInData.org/causes-of-death • CC BY
Note: To allow comparisons between countries and over time this metric is age-standardized.

Figure 14.16 Worldwide death rate of Alzheimer's disease and other dementias, 2019.

Source: IHME, Global Burden of Disease. https:// ourworldindata.org/grapher/ dementia-death-rates? country=~RUS

Case Study: Alzheimer's – Barbara ("B") Smith

Barbara Smith (Figures 14.17 and 14.18), known to the world as "B," was a supermodel, celebrity chef, TV host, author, and more. When she was about 64, however, B began to have problems remembering things. She started experiencing personality changes and poor judgment, forgot things, and asked the same questions repeatedly. One day, on a routine bus trip from Manhattan to her home in Sag Harbor, New York, B mistakenly got off at the wrong stop and failed to meet her husband as planned. For 17 hours she walked up and down the streets of Manhattan in 35-degree weather with sleet and snow. That night she took a ferry to Staten Island, simply following the other passengers. The next morning, a family friend happened to spot her at a diner back in Manhattan. Three years later, B couldn't recognize her family.

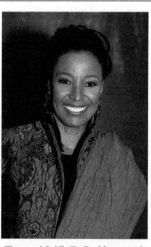

Figure 14.17 B. Smith poses in the lobby during Mercedes-Benz Fashion Week Fall 2007 February 2, 2007 in New York City.

Source: Katy Winn/Getty Images for IMG.

To learn more about B, take a look at *Before I forget: Love, hope, help, and acceptance in our fight against Alzheimer's* (Smith et al. 2016).

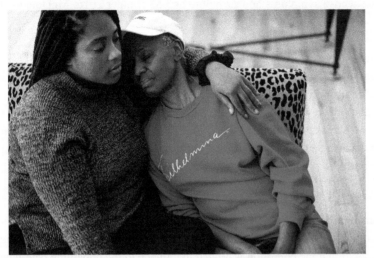

Figure 14.18 Three years later, B. Smith napped on the shoulder of her daughter, Dana Gasby, as she and her family grappled with Alzheimer's disease.

Source: Karsten Moran for The Washington Post *via Getty Images.*

Other Neurocognitive Disorders

In addition to the causes we discuss below, many other conditions can lead to mild or major neurocognitive disorder, including brain tumors, endocrine conditions, nutritional deficiencies, and the use of substances such as alcohol, inhalants, and sedatives.

VASCULAR NEUROCOGNITIVE DISORDER

In **vascular neurocognitive disorder**, the blood vesicles in the brain become damaged or blocked, resulting in a decreased flow of oxygen to those parts of the brain. Unlike the gradual symptoms and overall decline of Alzheimer's disease, sudden cognitive dysfunction in specific functions can sometimes occur. In most cases, however, the lack of oxygen leads to decreases in attention, processing speed, or executive functioning. Damage to the vesicles can be caused by a stroke (bringing about a sudden blocked flow of blood or bleeding in the brain), high blood pressure, fat deposits in the blood, or even traumatic brain injuries (more on that a little later). About 25 percent of people who have had strokes will develop symptoms of neurocognitive disorder (Aamodt et al. 2021); this percentage increases with age.

FRONTOTEMPORAL NEUROCOGNITIVE DISORDER

Also known as *Pick's disease*, **frontotemporal neurocognitive disorder** is characterized by selective degeneration of the nerves in the frontal and temporal lobes

Vascular neurocognitive disorder: a neurocognitive disorder in which the blood vesicles in the brain become damaged or blocked, resulting in a decreased flow of oxygen to those parts of the brain.

Frontotemporal neurocognitive disorder: a neurocognitive disorder characterized by selective degeneration of the nerves in the frontal and temporal lobes of the cerebral cortex, creating deficits in executive functioning, language, and behavior.

of the cerebral cortex, creating deficits in executive functioning, language, and behavior. Frontotemporal neurocognitive disorder is the fourth most common neurocognitive disorder with early-onset symptoms, representing up to 70 percent of those whose symptoms appear before age 65 (Finger 2016; McDonald 2017).

HUNTINGTON'S DISEASE

Huntington's disease: a genetic condition associated with personality changes and memory and mood problems that become progressively more disruptive over time.

Huntington's disease is a genetic condition with early onset (typically between the ages of 20 and 55) that is associated with personality changes (including lack of inhibition) and memory and mood problems that become progressively more disruptive over time. People with Huntington's disease may have outbursts of screaming and irritable mood and may slam doors. Characteristic of the disease are motor conditions such as involuntary twitching and spasms of the limbs.

PARKINSON'S DISEASE

Parkinson's disease: a neurological disorder that results in tremors, rigidity, difficulty initiating movements, and, over time, difficulty controlling the muscles.

Parkinson's disease is a neurological disorder that results in tremors, rigidity, difficulty initiating movements, and, over time, difficulty controlling the muscles. It is thought that the condition is related to damage to the dopamine pathways. The vast majority of people with Parkinson's disease (75 percent) will develop symptoms of neurocognitive disorder.

LEWY BODY DISEASE

Lewy body disease: a neurocognitive disorder caused by microscopic abnormal protein deposits that develop in the brain and damage the neurons.

Nearly 20 percent of all cases of neurocognitive disorder are related to **Lewy body disease**, the second most common type of NCD. Lewy bodies are microscopic round, abnormal protein deposits that develop in the brain and damage the neurons. Like Alzheimer's, Lewy body disease progresses slowly over time and includes problems with movement and alertness, as well as hallucinations.

HIV

The human immunodeficiency virus, HIV, can also lead to neurocognitive disorders by affecting cognition, attention, and memory. Those with symptoms may also display tremors and weakness and become withdrawn over time. They may have difficulty following conversations and can be slow to organize their thoughts.

HEAD TRAUMA

Chronic traumatic encephalopathy (CTE): a condition caused by blows to the head from accidents, gunshots, or repetitive sports injuries.

Chronic traumatic encephalopathy (CTE) is a condition caused by blows to the head from accidents, gunshots, or repetitive sports injuries. Symptoms of CTE can be physical, cognitive (such as difficulty thinking or remembering), social/emotional, and sleep-related (Table 14.7).

While it's important to reach out to your health care provider, there are some steps you can take that may help your recovery from this disorder. The following steps and recommendations for recovery from concussion are reproduced from the

Table 14.7 Symptoms of a mild traumatic brain injury and concussion

Physical	Cognitive	Social or emotional	Sleep-related
Bothered by light or noise	Attention or concentration problems	Anxiety or nervousness	Sleeping less than usual
Dizziness or balance problems	Feeling slowed down	Irritability or easily angered	Sleeping more than usual
Feeling tired, no energy	Foggy or groggy	Feeling more emotional	Trouble falling asleep
Headaches	Problems with short- or long-term memory	Sadness	
Nausea or vomiting (early on)			
Vision problems			

Source: Reproduced from Centers for Disease Control and Prevention, National Center for Injury Prevention and Control. www.cdc. gov/traumaticbraininjury/concussion/symptoms.html

Centers for Disease Control and Prevention, National Center for Injury Prevention and Control (www.cdc.gov/traumaticbraininjury/concussion/getting-better.html):

Start your recovery by taking it easy
As symptoms improve, you may gradually return to regular activities. Recovery from a mild TBI or concussion means you can do your regular activities without experiencing symptoms. Recovery from a mild TBI or concussion may be slower among:

- Older adults
- Young children
- Teens
- People who have had a concussion or other TBI in the past

The first few days
- Take it easy the first few days after a mild TBI or concussion when symptoms are more severe.
- You may need to take a short time off from work or school, although usually no more than 2 to 3 days.
- Ask your health-care provider for written instructions about when you can safely return to work, school, or other activities, such as driving a car.

As you start to feel better
- As you start to feel better after the first few days of your injury, you can gradually return to regular (non-strenuous) activities, such as taking a short walk.
- Avoid activities that make your symptoms come back or get worse.

When symptoms are nearly gone
- When your symptoms are mild and nearly gone, you can return to most of your regular activities.

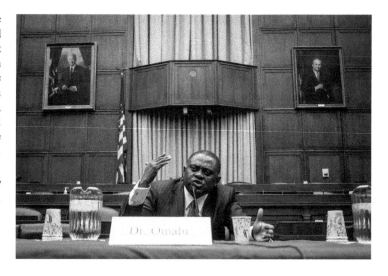

Figure 14.19 Forensic pathologist and neuropathologist Dr. Bennet Omalu, credited with discovering chronic traumatic encephalopathy (CTE) in former NFL players, participates in a 2016 Capitol Hill briefing about the condition, sponsored by Rep. Jackie Speier (D-CA).
Source: Pete Marovich/Getty Images.

- If your symptoms do not get worse during an activity, then that activity is OK for you. If your symptoms get worse, you should cut back on that activity.

It is only recently that the National Football League (NFL) recognized that concussion can lead to neurocognitive disorders like CTE in professional football players (Figure 14.19). The condition is characterized by memory loss, confusion, impulse control problems, anxiety, and depression. As a result of this realization, the NFL has allocated up to $1 billion toward a fund to compensate players who have retired and have CTE, and it is working on safety technology and rule changes to prevent head trauma on the field.

PRION DISEASE

Prion disease: a neurocognitive disorder caused by slow-acting virus-like proteins that can damage brain cells.

Prion disease, also called *Creutzfeldt–Jakob disease*, is a neurocognitive disorder caused by prions, slow-acting virus-like proteins that can live for years before they reproduce and damage brain cells. When symptoms emerge, however, the course of the condition is rapid. Characteristic symptoms include body spasms, hallucinations, difficulty speaking, and fatigue.

Models and Treatments of Neurocognitive Disorders

B Smith passed away in 2020, but not before she made an impact on the treatment of those with Alzheimer's disease. She helped to create the Brain Health Registry, which offers free online cognitive screenings for those who might have the disorder. Many who do, may not be aware of it. In fact, a report by the Alzheimer's Association found that only 45 percent of people with Alzheimer's are given a diagnosis by their doctor (Alzheimer's Association 2020).

BIOLOGICAL MODELS AND TREATMENTS

Alzheimer's disease and the other neurocognitive disorders are neurological conditions, which means they are mostly biological in origin.

Genetic conditions may be a risk factor for developing Alzheimer's disease. For example, between a quarter and a half of first-degree relatives of those with the disorder will also develop it. In addition to the brain differences described earlier, differences in neurotransmitter levels have been found in those affected by the disease. For example, acetylcholine, a neurotransmitter important in memory, is deficient, and the deficiency is in proportion to the level of cognitive decline (Bodur et al. 2021).

Scientists are working hard to find new treatments and preventions for Alzheimer's disease. In one technique, a researcher created a molecule that was able to inhibit the buildup of amyloid plaques in the hippocampus of mice. This early research may help to prevent Alzheimer's in the future. Currently, however, there is no cure for the disease, and no treatment will slow its progression. Medications have been used to alleviate the cognitive and behavioral symptoms.

Two classes of medications are prescribed for the cognitive symptoms of neurocognitive disorders including Alzheimer's (see Table 14.8). Cholinesterase inhibitors such as donepezil (Aricept), rivastigmine (Exelon), and galantamine (Reminyl) help by preventing the breakdown of acetylcholine in the brain. They do have adverse effects, however, including weight loss, liver damage, and gastrointestinal symptoms such as diarrhea and nausea.

Medications in the second category, such as memantine (Namenda), boost glutamate, a neurotransmitter active in learning and memory. These drugs do not help in the long term, however, and the improvements are not permanent. That is, once patients stop using them (which three in four do because of side effects like gastrointestinal distress), they lose the benefit gained from the medication.

Recently, the FDA approved a new medication called aducanumab (Aduhelm) as the first that attempts to target the cause of Alzheimer's disease. Aducanumab is reported to help clear the amyloid plaques, which was the basis for its approval,

Table 14.8 Some FDA-approved medications for Alzheimer's disease

Generic name	Brand name	Class of medication
donepezil	Aricept	Cholinesterase inhibitor
rivastigmine	Exelon	Cholinesterase inhibitor
galantamine	Razadyne	Cholinesterase inhibitor
memantine	Namenda	Glutamate regulators
donepezil and memantine	Namzaric	Dual cholinesterase inhibitor and glutamate regulator

Source: Information from Stahl (2017).

although the research trials did not demonstrate that the medication slows cognitive decline. Aducanumab is also expensive, with an expected annual price of over $55,000 per patient (Crosson et al. 2021).

Prescribers have also used medications to alleviate the emotional symptoms that often accompany neurocognitive disorders. These include antidepressants and antianxiety and antipsychotic drugs, which can decrease agitation, delusions, and hallucinations.

PSYCHOLOGICAL MODELS AND TREATMENTS

Treatments exist to alleviate the symptoms of neurocognitive disorder that don't rely on medication. The goal of these interventions is to improve cognitive functioning and overall quality of life by actively managing the condition, encouraging physical activity, using cognitive stimulation, and providing help for caretakers.

Active management of the symptoms of neurocognitive disorders can improve quality of life. Techniques include reducing behaviors that can be distressing to both the person with the condition and their family, such as nighttime wandering, demands for attention, and insufficient personal care. Smart homes and other technologies can help achieve these goals as well. For example, smart homes can "learn" a person's typical patterns and alert caregivers when something may be wrong, such as the person's not getting up or eating at their usual time or leaving appliances such as stoves on (Figure 14.20). Devices can also help a person continue a task. If, for example, someone forgets what they are doing halfway through a task (such as making a cup of tea), the device can remind them of the steps to continue. Cameras with emotional

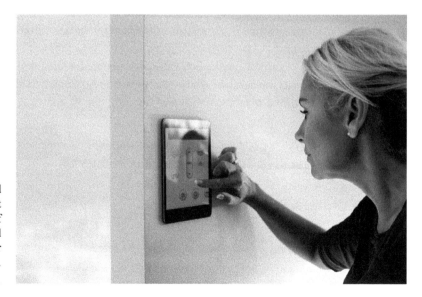

Figure 14.20 Smart homes and other technologies can assist people with symptoms of neurocognitive disorders and help them stay in their homes longer.
Source: Maskot/Getty Images.

recognition software can also adjust the lights and temperature to help encourage better moods. If people with neurocognitive disorders become disoriented and wander from home, smart watches can raise an alert if they travel outside a certain area.

A recent meta-analysis suggested that physical activity, including exercise video games, can improve quality of life by increasing the individual's ability to perform the activities of daily living, even in the case of major neurocognitive disorder (Swinnen et al. 2020). Especially during the early phase of an NCD (or before), cognitive stimulation such as mentally challenging work or leisure activities can also help those with these disorders. Some researchers believe that such early stimulation provides a cognitive reserve and helps to delay the early phase of the condition.

About 90 percent of those with Alzheimer's disease are cared for by a family member. Playing this role can be very challenging, and caregivers give better care when they too have support. Some caregivers frequently feel overwhelmed, and over time caretaking can exact a toll on both their physical and mental health. Those who care for people with Alzheimer's disease can benefit from having friends and family members who stay in touch, are patient, and help with meals and errands. Without this kind of help, stress can increase. For example, during the COVID-19 pandemic, caregivers of people with neurocognitive disorders reported higher levels of depression and anxiety due to the isolation they experienced (Altieri & Santangelo 2021).

SOCIOCULTURAL MODELS AND TREATMENTS

Sociocultural factors influence the diagnosis and treatment of neurocognitive disorders. For instance, women may be at greater risk of age-related conditions because of their generally longer lifespan. We also know that Black Americans are more likely to be diagnosed with neurocognitive disorders, perhaps because they have higher rates of cardiovascular diseases such as hypertension, which is related to vascular neurocognitive disorder (Jones 2021). Other factors may also be at play. A study of more than 60,000 Black American women that examined the relationship between experiences of racism and subjective cognitive function revealed that the more drastic the racism experienced, the greater the impact on subjective cognitive functioning (Coogan et al. 2020).

Sometimes the sociocultural factor of discrimination is much more evident. The NFL announced in the summer of 2021 that it would end its policy of using race-based cognitive norms when evaluating the severity of injury a player may have suffered from playing in the League (Possin et al. 2021). In essence the League had historically suggested that Black players (who make up about half its team rosters) started with lower cognitive ability, making it more difficult for them to qualify for compensatory payments and ensuring they received lower payments than white players. As of 2021, more than 2,000 League players had submitted claims of neurocognitive disorder related to playing football. Awards were granted to 379 with mild neurocognitive disorder and 207 with moderate disorder.

Sociocultural aspects are also at play in the treatment and management of neurocognitive disorders. Caretaking depends more heavily on family members in those families with fewer socioeconomic resources.

MULTIPERSPECTIVE MODELS AND TREATMENTS

Treatments for neurocognitive disorders are only moderately helpful. A number of approaches can be of some use, such as medication and psychological interventions including support for caregivers. The goals are to maintain quality of life, maximize function in everyday activity, and enhance mood while promoting social engagement and fostering a safe environment. However, none of these interventions can stop the progression of neurocognitive disorder.

CONCEPT CHECK 14.6

Indicate the most probable type of neurocognitive disorder in each case.
1. Scott has a neurocognitive disorder that is thought to be caused by amyloid plaques and neurofibrillary tangles that accumulate in parts of his brain.
2. Dana has symptoms of neurocognitive disorder that appear to be due to damage to her brain's dopamine pathways.
3. Vito recently experienced a stroke and is now showing symptoms of neurocognitive disorder.

PULLING IT TOGETHER

Differentiating Delirium from Neurocognitive Disorder

Table 14.9 The symptoms of delirium are different from the symptoms of a neurocognitive disorder

Characteristic	Delirium	Neurocognitive disorder
Onset	Acute	Gradual
Course	Fluctuates	Gradually becomes worse
Awareness	Impaired	Often clear until advanced stages
Memory	Poor working memory and immediate recall	Poor short-term memory
Delusions	Often short-lived and changing	Fixed

14.7 CHAPTER REVIEW

SUMMARY

This chapter presented the following disorders:

Neurodevelopmental disorders

- Attention deficit hyperactivity disorder
- Autism spectrum disorder
- Intellectual developmental disorder

Neurocognitive disorders
- Delirium
- Major and mild neurocognitive disorders
- Other neurocognitive disorders

Overview of Neurodevelopmental Disorders and Neurocognitive Disorders

- Symptoms of neurodevelopmental disorders appear during the developing years and tend to persist throughout the lifespan.
- Neurocognitive disorders are characterized by cognitive decline that often arises from medical conditions or from substance withdrawal or intoxication.

Attention Deficit Hyperactivity Disorder

- Attention deficit hyperactivity disorder is a neurodevelopmental condition in which a person has a pattern of inattention or disruptive hyperactivity/impulsivity.
- In a combined presentation, criteria for inattention and hyperactivity-impulsivity are both met.
- In those with a predominantly inattentive presentation, only criteria for inattention are met.
- In those with a predominantly hyperactive/impulsive presentation, only criteria for hyperactivity-impulsivity are met.
- Treatments for ADHD include both psychological counseling and medications.

Autism Spectrum Disorder

- Autism spectrum disorder is a neurodevelopmental disorder characterized by deficits in social communication and interaction along with restricted, repetitive behaviors, interests, and activities.
- Deficits in social communication and interaction include problems with both verbal and nonverbal communication and with developing and maintaining relationships.
- People with autism spectrum disorder also show restricted, repetitive behaviors, interests, and activities.
- Autism spectrum disorder is rated for severity based on the amount of support the person requires.

Intellectual Developmental Disorder

- Intellectual developmental disorder is a neurodevelopmental disorder that consists of deficits in general mental abilities.
- Intellectual functioning is the ability to think, learn, solve problems, and adapt and learn from new situations.
- Adaptive functioning is the ability to perform the activities of daily living.
- The severity of intellectual developmental disorder is based on its impact on intellectual and adaptive functioning and is divided into four levels, mild, moderate, severe, and profound.
- Many biological factors may lead to intellectual developmental disorder, including chromosomal disorders, exposure to toxins, infections, brain injuries, and nutritional deficits.

Delirium

- Delirium is a sudden confused mental state.
- In hyperactive delirium the person becomes overactive, agitated, or restless.

- In hypoactive delirium patients are underactive, sleepy, and slow to respond.
- Symptoms of delirium can have an impact on overall health and mortality.

Major and Mild Neurocognitive Disorders

- Mild neurocognitive disorder brings a decline in cognitive functioning that does not result in impairment.
- Major neurocognitive disorder brings a decline in cognitive functioning that does result in impairment.
- Alzheimer's disease is the most common cause of neurocognitive disorders.
- Several conditions can lead to major and mild neurocognitive disorder, including brain tumors, endocrine conditions, nutritional deficiencies, and the use of substances such as alcohol, inhalants, and sedatives.
- Although there are no cures for neurocognitive disorders, medications and psychological interventions can improve quality of life.

DISCUSSION QUESTIONS

1. Although there is evidence of a biological connection for ADHD, there are many myths to what might create it, from "bad" parenting to the ingestion of certain foods. What are some ADHD myths you have heard, and what are some ways to increase evidence-based knowledge about this disorder?
2. What cultural factors and expectations might decrease adaptive functioning in those with mild to moderately severe IDD? How might our cultural expectations of independent living rather than group living influence diagnoses of these disorders?
3. Treatment of major neurocognitive disorder can improve symptoms if they are found early. What are some ways we can promote early detection?
4. Research has not produced a link between autism and vaccines, although many people believe there is one. What evidence or information might you provide someone to help them critically examine this claim?

ANSWERS TO CONCEPT CHECKS

Concept Check 14.1

1. Neurodevelopmental
2. Neurodevelopmental
3. Neurocognitive
4. Neurodevelopmental

Concept Check 14.2

1. Hyperactivity
2. Inattention
3. Hyperactivity
4. Inattention

Concept Check 14.3

1. Restricted, repetitive behavior, interests, or activity

2. Impairment in social communication/social interaction
3. Impairment in social communication/social interaction
4. Restricted, repetitive behavior, interests, or activity

Concept Check 14.4

1. Severe
2. Mild
3. Moderate
4. Profound

Concept Check 14.5

1. B
2. D

Concept Check 14.6

1. Alzheimer's disease
2. Parkinson's disease
3. Vascular neurocognitive disorder

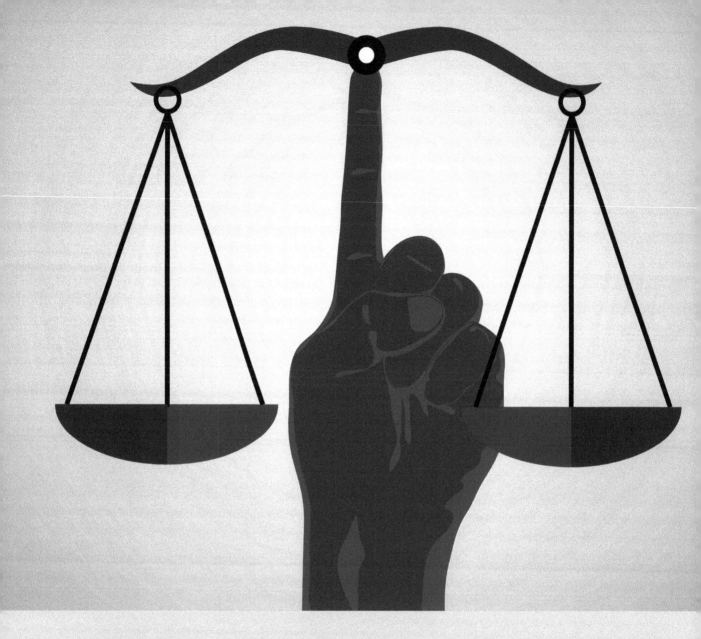

CHAPTER CONTENTS

15

Legal and Ethical Issues

CASE STUDY: Daniel M'Naghten

Daniel M'Naghten (Figure 15.1) had had a rough couple of months, but in the last few weeks things had gotten worse. He told his family and friends that spies and crews of people followed him when he was alone. It's most likely M'Naghten experienced symptoms of a delusional disorder, persecutory type. That is, he was troubled by false beliefs that someone was out to harm him. Most of his delusions centered around a British political party, the Tories. "They follow me and persecute me wherever I go, and have entirely destroyed my peace of mind. I can get no rest from them night or day . . . in fact they wish to murder me." M'Naghten started carrying a gun to protect himself. This behavior was quite different from the way he normally behaved. Although he was sometimes described as awkward, most people who knew him described him as "serious, mild, inoffensive, and humane."

Around 3:40pm on Friday January 20, 1843, M'Naghten spotted Edward Drummond, who really did work for the Tories. He took out his pistol and shot Edward point-blank in the left side of the back, just below the shoulder blade. M'Naghten was tackled by the police before he could take another shot at Edward. But it made no difference: Edward Drummond died five days later from his injuries.

"I was driven to desperation by persecution," M'Naghten said, claiming that Edward was one of the "crew" that had been following him and was out to kill him.

Should M'Naghten be punished for the injuries he caused? How should the legal system handle cases where someone does not have control over their actions? What does justice look like? We return to M'Naghten's case later in this chapter.

Throughout this book, you've learned a great deal about psychopathology. We know that some psychological conditions produce symptoms that make it difficult for people to control their behavior. In fact, some disorders are so disruptive that it may be impossible, in the midst of a delusion for example, for an individual to distinguish what's right from what's wrong. You've also learned that many of these conditions have effective treatments.

Learning Objectives

- Describe the process of civil commitment.
- Define competence to stand trial.
- Compare the laws regarding the "insanity defense."
- Explain how mental health practitioners protect patients' rights, including the right to treatment and the right to refuse treatment.

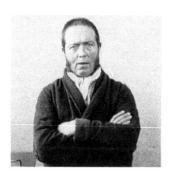

Figure 15.1 Daniel M'Naghten was at the center of the 1843 case that set standards for the insanity defense in what came to be known as the M'Naghten Rule.

Source: Photo by Henry Hering, photographer (c.1856) – Bethlem hospital museum archives. Public domain: https://en. wikipedia.org/wiki/Daniel_M% 27Naghten#/media/File:Daniel_ McNaughton_c_1856.jpg.

Civil commitment: a process by which individuals may be forcibly treated if they are found to be dangerous to themselves or to others.

This raises some important questions. Should we hold individuals with psychological conditions responsible for criminal behaviors that arise from their conditions? Should we punish people whose conditions lead to the injury of others? Should they be forced into treatment? What rights do patients have? What should we do about people who don't *want* treatment? Under what circumstances can we restrict an individual's freedom or force someone into a treatment facility?

In this chapter, we address some ongoing legal and ethical issues in psychopathology. We'll see that the way that society views psychopathology affects the way these conditions are treated. Over the years, society's views have tried to address the balance between the rights of the individual and the rights of society, and the legal cases and laws we use to maintain that balance reflect the ever-changing ways in which a society views psychopathology and those who experience it.

15.1 CIVIL COMMITMENT

Under ideal situations and most of the time, people seek treatment for serious psychological concerns on their own by finding their way into therapy or by receiving medication from medical professionals. However, there are times when a person might refuse treatment altogether or might accept only partial treatment. People refuse treatment for many reasons: discomfort with the treatment options, inability to afford treatment, and even cultural prohibitions against certain types of treatments. What should happen when a person needs treatment but refuses it? On such occasions, individuals may be forced into treatment through **civil commitment**, a process by which individuals may be forcibly treated if they are found to be dangerous to themselves or to others.

Criteria for and Prevalence of Civil Commitment

Civil commitment laws date back to the nineteenth century. By the 2000s, up to 25 percent of admissions to inpatient mental hospital facilities in the United States were involuntary (Manahan 2004). A recent meta-analysis examined 35 studies of over 130,000 patients diagnosed with schizophrenia and found that more than 59 percent of the resulting hospitalizations were involuntary (Yang et al. 2020), although the involuntary hospitalization rates for schizophrenia vary by country (Figure 15.2).

Civil commitment doesn't always mean involuntary hospitalization, however. As of 2019, 47 US states had outpatient civil commitment programs in which individuals may be compelled to attend outpatient psychotherapy programs (McDermott, Ventura, et al. 2020).

The legal system uses civil commitment when people need treatment and pose a danger to themselves or to other people. If Daniel M'Naghten, for example, had

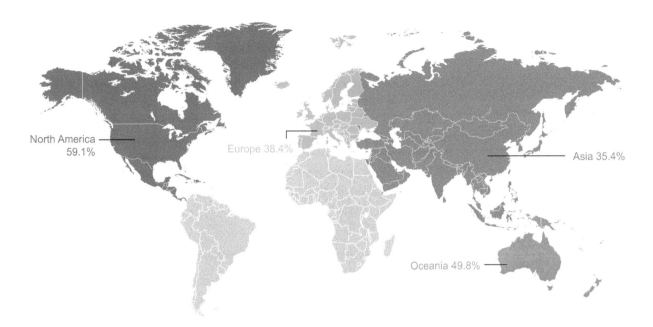

North America
59.1%

Europe 38.4%

Asia 35.4%

Oceania 49.8%

let someone know about his plot to hurt members of the Tory party, it's possible that he could have been forced into treatment to prevent him from causing harm.

Typically, three conditions might lead to a civil commitment:

- The person has a mental condition in need of treatment.
- The person is in danger of hurting themselves or others.
- The person is unable to care for themselves.

Figure 15.2 Involuntary hospitalization rates for schizophrenia around the world. *Source: Yang et al. (2020).*

Legal Definition of Mental Illness

The legal definition of mental illness is not the same as the definition of a psychological disorder. An individual who meets the *DSM-5tr* criteria for a psychological disorder does not necessarily meet a state's definition of mental illness. While each state has its own legal definition of mental illness, it generally refers to a severe emotional or cognitive disturbance that creates problems for the individual's health and safety. This may include abnormal thoughts, behaviors, or feelings that lead to clinically significant distress or impairment in important functions.

Grave Disability

What do you do when a person is so impaired by a mental disorder that they can't provide for their basic needs? What's the humane thing to do?

Parens patriae is Latin for "parent of the nation," and it is a government policy by which the government may act as a legal protector of people who cannot protect themselves. That is, the state acts to protect an individual who needs help. This was the idea behind Project Help, a New York City program created in the late 1980s by then Mayor Ed Koch. Project Help's goal was to remove people with mental conditions from the streets and commit them to treatment because they had a grave disability. **Grave disability** is a criterion for involuntary commitment that is met when a person cannot provide for their own basic needs.

One of the first people to be committed under Project Help was Joyce Brown, who had become homeless in 1986 after leaving her sister's care. Brown lived on the streets near 2nd Avenue for at least a year. She was committed in October 1987 after a series of incidents in which she made threats, tore up money, exposed herself, and urinated in public. You'll learn later in this chapter how Brown responded to her commitment.

Dangerousness to Self and Others

Some people falsely believe that those with psychological conditions are dangerous by definition (Setlack et al. 2020). They are seen to behave unpredictably and it is believed that they might do other, possibly dangerous, unpredictable things. The public often believes, incorrectly, that people with psychological disorders are more prone to violence than those without mental conditions. Even judges tend to perceive those with psychological conditions to be more likely to be a risk for violence (Simonsson et al. 2020).

The perception that psychological disorders are related to violence is particularly related to marginalized populations. For example, Black Americans are perceived as more dangerous even when they don't exhibit violent behavior. What's more, they are also more likely to be involuntarily committed (Lindsey et al. 2010).

Evidence of dangerousness doesn't seem to support this assertion, however. Although there is evidence of a slight increase in violence among people with psychological disorders (Elbogen & Johnson 2009) the story is complicated. Nearly all (90 percent) of people with psychological disorders are not violent or dangerous (Glied & Frank 2014). Instead, specific *symptoms* (rather than specific disorders) are more likely to lead to violence. Hallucinations and delusions, in particular, seem to be related to perceptions of violence. Substance abuse and severe psychopathology seem to be the conditions most associated with violence (Nichtová et al. 2020).

Process of Civil Commitment

To compel someone into treatment there must be clear and convincing evidence before the commitment can take place. What counts as evidence varies from state to state. Prior to the twentieth century, simply having the need for treatment was enough to hospitalize individuals against their will (Meyer & Weaver 2006). Critics were concerned, however, that people could be denied freedom for nothing more than holding to alternative lifestyles or moral values because anyone could

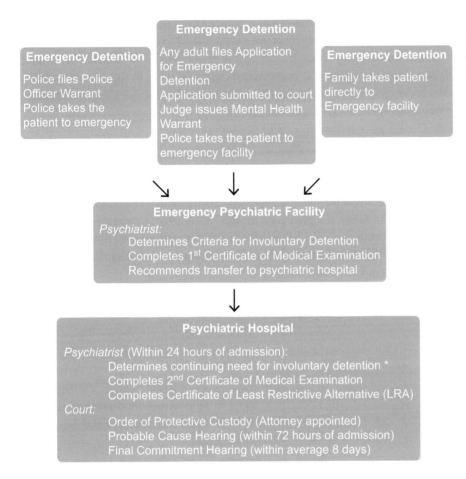

Figure 15.3 Process of civil commitment.

Source: Adapted from Hashmi et al. (2014).

define the need for treatment – a doctor, a law enforcement officer, or even a family member. Indeed, many individuals were committed for reasons such as homosexuality and for racial and social control purposes that had nothing to do with psychological disorders. Due to concerns about patients' rights and personal liberties, however, views began to change in the early 1900s and laws were enacted to improve the process of civil commitment.

The process has several steps, each of which seeks to maximize the likelihood that the use of commitment isn't abused (Figure 15.3). It's a good idea to first try to persuade people to enter treatment of their own volition. In many cases, clients will voluntarily commit themselves if the person understands the seriousness of their condition and that treatment options are available. If they refuse, the prosecuting attorney may seek an involuntary commitment order. The person must be notified, often by the police, of the commitment order, which states the reasons for the commitment and any recommendations for treatment. In addition, the individual has the right to legal representation and must be granted an independent psychological and physical evaluation by a qualified mental health clinician. The client will have an opportunity to contest the commitment with a lawyer to represent them.

If commitment proceeds, the length of stay varies from state to state; the average time is about three days. This gives clinicians an opportunity to fully evaluate an individual.

In some emergency cases, it's simply not possible to go through all these steps. If, for example, a client is in immediate danger of hurting themselves or someone else, states give certain clinicians the right to certify that the client needs emergency temporary commitment and treatment. These clinicians must declare that the individual is an imminent danger to themselves or others.

One criticism of the civil commitment process is that despite being called to do so, mental health practitioners aren't always very good at predicting violent behavior in the distant future (Monahan 2018). They can make reliable predictions about dangerousness only in the short term (between 2 and 20 days ahead). The farther into the future the prediction is, the less reliable. Critics of civil commitment also question its value because involuntary treatment isn't always effective: Clients may not be honest during the evaluation process, and it's difficult to force a person to participate in psychotherapy.

CONCEPT CHECK 15.1

For each case presented below, indicate the criterion for hospitalization.
1. Dylan has been depressed for the last few months, so much so that he has stopped eating and has been thinking about killing himself. His therapist recommended that Dylan have inpatient treatment for his depression, but he refused. His therapist decided to have Dylan involuntarily hospitalized to prevent him from being a danger to himself. _____
2. Since Noah first developed symptoms of psychosis a year ago, his mental health has slowly deteriorated. Currently he spends most of his time in bed and is unable to care for his basic needs. His mental health care practitioner has decided to have him involuntarily committed. _____

15.2   COMPETENCE TO STAND TRIAL

Competence to stand trial: a legal construct that says in order to be tried, a defendant must understand the charges brought against them and be able to assist in their own defense.

Competence to stand trial is the legal construct that says in order to be tried, a defendant must understand the charges brought against them and be able to assist in their own defense (Murrie et al. 2020). To substantiate this determination, a person must go through a competency evaluation meant to ensure they understand the charges against them and can work with their defense attorneys to conduct an adequate defense. It's usually the defense attorney's responsibility to make sure clients are competent to stand trial (Figure 15.4). However, questions of competence can also be raised by judges or even arresting officers. The abilities of a defendant to understand information, think rationally, make good choices, and understand the gravity of the situation are all factors in making the determination of competency (Murrie et al. 2020). Defendants typically demonstrate the necessary capacity for competency nearly 60 percent of the time (Murrie et al. 2020).

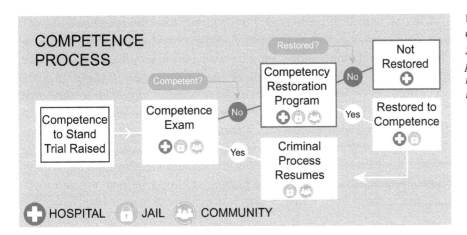

Figure 15.4 An example of the competence process.

Source: Adapted from www. prainc.com/competency-restoration-thoughts-from-the-field/.

Many psychological factors could impede a person's ability to understand charges and assist in defense. Defendants who hear voices in their head may be so distracted by the voices that they may not recall the timeline of the incident, and problems with short-term memory or depression may make it difficult to work with an attorney to prepare a legal defense. While many defendants may have impaired competence, only a small handful are evaluated. Around 60,000 competency evaluations are conducted each year in the United States and the numbers have been increasing (Warburton et al. 2020). From these, around 20 percent of defendants are found incompetent to stand trial.

Who gets referred for competency evaluations? Defendants referred for competency evaluations typically have less education and less money than those who are not referred, and they tend to be unemployed and unmarried. Further, members of racially marginalized groups are more likely to be judged incompetent to stand trial (McDermott, Warburton, & Auletta-Young 2020).

What happens when a person is found incompetent to stand trial as is true in up to 40 percent of cases? They will most likely lose authority to make decisions for themselves, and many will face commitment until such time as they are competent to stand trial. Under this system, it's possible that an innocent person who is not competent to stand trial could spend years in a mental health facility with no way to show their innocence. The Supreme Court didn't enact the decision on its own; there was a challenge to the existing laws that led people to be treated poorly. In *Jackson v Indiana* (1972), the Court ruled that defendants could not be indefinitely committed: they had to either be found competent and tried or be released and treated under civil commitment procedures (Kaufman et al. 2012).

In some US states, defendants may be forcibly medicated to *create* competence to stand trial. In other states, defendants are held until they *become* competent to stand trial. Critics of forced treatment are concerned about the consequences of forcibly medicating a person to make them competent to stand trial. The side effects of the medications, such as sluggishness, may be distracting to jurors, who might attribute those side effects to the state the defendant was in at the time the alleged crime was committed.

When an individual's competence to stand trial has been questioned, the next step is a competence exam. If the exam finds the individual able to stand trial, the criminal process resumes. If the person is instead found incompetent to stand trial, an order for *restoration of competence* is issued, which sets aside a period during which someone waits to develop the abilities necessary for them to stand trial. Competency restoration programs are treatments that might help the person meet the criteria for competence and may include jail-based programs or medications. From this point, the person may either be restored to competency or not. If they are restored, the criminal process resumes. If it is decided that they have not yet been restored to competence, the criminal process stays on hold until competency to stand trial is found to be restored.

CONCEPT CHECK 15.2

For each case indicate whether the person meets the criteria for competency to stand trial.

1. Last night Jayden drank so much that he really can't remember what he did. His friends say he crashed his car and injured a pedestrian who was walking near Jayden's residence hall. Is Jayden competent to stand trial?
2. Grace has been depressed for the last three months and hasn't felt like her typical self. Because of her depression she finds she is sleepy all the time. During her last babysitting job she fell asleep and the 3-year-old she was watching was injured. The parents of the child want to press charges. Would Grace be considered competent to stand trial?
3. Six months ago Bryce was assaulted. Shortly after the assault, he started to have symptoms of PTSD as well as auditory hallucinations. The voices he heard told him to break into the house of the person who assaulted him. Bryce knew this was wrong but he broke into the house anyway. Is Bryce competent to stand trial?
4. While walking home last week, Sam heard voices in his head that told him the person walking behind him wanted to attack him. To prevent the attack Sam struck first. Sam is still having auditory hallucinations and his attorney can't seem to get him to answer any questions because he is distracted by the voices he hears. Is Sam competent to stand trial?

15.3   THE INSANITY DEFENSE AND CRIMINAL COMMITMENT

The criminal justice system's intended function is to protect society. You can argue that there are two main reasons for the justice system to punish individuals for criminal behavior: first, to discipline them for what they did so they won't do it again, and second, to deter others from committing similar crimes. However, not all people are punished for their criminal behavior because in some situations, such as when circumstances are beyond the defendant's control, it would be ineffective and unfair to do so.

Think about the case at the start of the chapter: Daniel was driven by persecutory delusions and protected himself in the only way he knew from what he thought would be his own murder. Daniel and those they hurt all deserve our compassion. It might make more sense to identify people who could be at risk for hurting others and provide treatment to prevent such incidents from happening. If Daniel, for example, had had treatment for his delusions, it's possible that Edward Drummond would never have been shot.

If an individual is accused of a crime and the legal system determines that a mental condition may have been the cause of the crime, instead of being punished the defendant may be sent to an institution for treatment. This step is called criminal commitment. The mental disorder may be present at the time of the trial or may have existed only intermittently around the time of the crime. (Recall that some mental conditions have acute symptoms, while some others may be persistent.)

To identify an appropriate punishment, courts need to decide whether a person is criminally responsible for the crime of which they are accused and whether they are able to defend themselves in a court of law. The **insanity defense**, also called being **not guilty by reason of insanity (NGRI)**, is a legal plea that suggests a defendant is not responsible for a criminal act because they were experiencing a psychological condition at the time of the act was committed. If an individual has a condition that caused them to act in a way that led them to commit a crime and if, at the time of the crime, they could not tell the difference between right and wrong or could not control their behavior, then the individual's lawyer will enter a plea of not guilty by reason of insanity.

Not guilty by reason of insanity (NGRI): a legal plea that suggests a defendant is not responsible for a criminal act because they were experiencing a psychological condition at the time the act was committed.

If you watch a lot of criminal justice shows, you might think that most cases of criminal commitment come from NGRI pleas. In fact, however, most cases of criminal commitment arise because the court determines that the defendant is incompetent to stand trial. By some estimates, for every person found NGRI, 45 are committed to a mental health facility after a competency evaluation (Butler 2006). Most defendants (around 75 percent) are restored to competency after six months, a smaller percentage (19 percent) within a year, and a very small proportion (4 percent) have an average treatment length of more than a year (Beltrani & Zapf 2020).

Of those found NGRI, only 1 percent are sent home. The rest are put under some kind of supervision (called conditional release), most likely in prison or sometimes in mental hospitals or in outpatient settings. The average length of stay in a mental hospital is six years for those accused of murder; for those accused of lesser crimes, it is three years (Kirchebner et al. 2020; Silver et al. 1994). Studies indicate that defendants found NGRI are a low risk for committing additional crimes (Kapoor et al. 2020; Novosad et al. 2016).

Rules of the Insanity Defense

Many rules have been used to define insanity. They include the M'Naghten Rule, the Irresistible Impulse Test, the Durham Test, the American Law Institute Test, and the American Psychiatric Association Rule.

M'NAGHTEN RULE (1843)

Contemporary views of the insanity defense originated from the 1843 case you learned about at the start of this chapter, in which Edward Drummond died from his injuries after being shot by Daniel M'Naghten. In this landmark British case, the court ruled that M'Naghten was not criminally responsible for his actions because he was delusional due to a mental disorder and unable to determine right from wrong. This reasoning became known as the **M'Naghten Rule** (O'Donnell 2020).

At the core of the M'Naghten Rule is the doctrine of *mens rea* or a "guilty mind," which says an individual must have an intention to break the law to be responsible for breaking that law. For example, Jeffrey Dahmer, who killed 17 people between 1978 and 1991, failed in his attempt to use the NGRI defense because he tried to hide his crimes, an action that suggested he knew they were against the law. Critics of the M'Naghten Rule suggest that it requires the jury and judge to know whether the defendant could tell right from wrong at the time of the crime (Meyer & Weaver 2006), which may be difficult to judge.

M'Naghten Rule: a legal principle that suggests individuals are not responsible for their actions if, because of a mental condition, they did not know what they were doing or did not know it was wrong.

IRRESISTIBLE IMPULSE TEST (1834)

Irresistible impulse test: a legal principle that suggests an individual should not he held legally responsible if driven by an uncontrollable impulse or a diminished capacity to resist the impulse.

The **irresistible impulse test** (first used in Ohio in 1834) suggests that an individual should not be held legally responsible for an action if driven by an uncontrollable impulse or experiencing diminished capacity to resist a "fit of passion" or the impulse to commit the crime (Meyer & Weaver 2006).

Critics of this defense have suggested that it can be easily abused. Pejoratively called the "Twinkie Defense," it was used unsuccessfully in the 1979 trial of Dan White for the murders of Harvey Milk and George Muscone. White claimed that he suffered from diminished capacity due to depression brought on by eating unhealthy junk foods (such as Twinkies). Diminished capacity is a legal defense that requires a defendant's mental functions to have been impaired during the commission of the crime. The "gay panic defense" is another irresistible impulse test. This claims that heterosexual defendants find same-sex sexual advances so offensive and frightening that they induce a psychotic state. Many US states have banned irresistible impulse defenses.

DURHAM TEST (1954)

In 1954 in Washington DC, Monte Durham was convicted of housebreaking. Durham's defense at the trial was that he was of "unsound mind" at the time of the offense. However, his insanity defense plea was rejected on the grounds that it had not been proven that Durham didn't know the difference between right and wrong.

On appeal, Durham's attorney argued that a new standard of criminal responsibility should be used. The attorney suggested that the ability to know right from wrong wasn't enough, that more evidence from mental health experts was needed, and that experts should determine whether a mental disorder created a "meaningful contribution" to the criminal act. The judge agreed and the decision was reversed.

The central argument of the **Durham Test** is that the "accused is not criminally responsible if his unlawful act was the product of a mental disease or mental defect."

The Durham Test offered more flexibility but ended up being too vague, partly because the *DSM* wasn't as precise in its disorder descriptions in the 1950s as it is today. Furthermore, because the Durham Test didn't require defendants to show incapacitation or lack of understanding that the act was wrong, critics were concerned about the test's reliance on expert witnesses to decide whether the criminal act was a direct product of some mental condition. While the Durham Test isn't currently used, some US states like New Hampshire place a high burden of proof on the defendant to show evidence of the meaningful contribution of mental illness to the commission of the crime.

Durham Test: a legal principle that suggests a jury may find a defendant is not guilty by reason of insanity because the act in question was committed due to a psychological condition.

AMERICAN LAW INSTITUTE TEST (1955)

In the late 1950s, a group of attorneys, judges, and legal scholars assembled to reconsider the insanity defense. They recognized that the threat of punishment was unlikely to deter those with mental illness, and that treatment and compassion were more important than punishment. The group worked to create a better definition of insanity, which became known as the **American Law Institute Test** (also known as the ALI Rule). This rule holds that "a person is not responsible for criminal conduct if at the time of such conduct as the result of mental disease or defect he lacks substantial capacity either to appreciate the criminality (wrongfulness) of his conduct or to conform his conduct to the requirements of the law." This means that if a mental condition creates a situation in which a person doesn't know the difference between right and wrong and can't control their behavior, they should not be held responsible for the act. The ALI Rule also restricted the types of mental conditions that qualified for a verdict of NGRI, suggesting that a long history of criminal acts in and of itself is not evidence of a mental condition.

American Law Institute Test: the legal principle of criminal responsibility that suggests a person is not criminally responsible for their conduct if they lack the capacity to understand that their behavior was wrong, or if they are not able to conform their conduct to the requirements of the law.

Increased challenges to the ALI Rule may have resulted from its successful use in the John Hinckley Jr. trial (Walker et al. 2020). In 1981, John Hinckley Jr. (Figure 15.5) attempted to assassinate then-President Ronald Reagan to get the attention of actress Jodie Foster. He thought that by getting a place in history he would become her equal (an idea he may have drawn from the movie *Taxi Driver*, in which the main character tries to assassinate a US senator). Hinckley was found not guilty by reason of insanity under the ALI Rule, but there was public outrage that he used the defense to get away with the crime. In September 2021, some 40 years later, he was granted unconditional release.

AMERICAN PSYCHIATRIC ASSOCIATION (1983)

After the Hinckley trial, the American Psychiatric Association Insanity Defense Work Group recommended that the insanity defense should be used only if the individual did not know right from wrong at the time. The *Insanity Defense Reform Act* was signed into law in 1984 and made pleading not guilty by reason of insanity defense more difficult. It was a return to M'Naghten Rule. The APA Rule is used in federal courts and about one-half of state courts, while the ALI Rule is used in the remaining states except three: Idaho, Montana, and Utah do not allow an insanity defense to be mounted and have done away with the insanity defense altogether. In 2020 the Supreme Court of the United States upheld the Kansas law that eliminated the insanity defense (Roytman 2020).

INSANITY DEFENSE CONCERNS

The insanity defense is rarely used, and it fails more often than it succeeds. However, there are some common misconceptions about it. For example, most people think the insanity defense is used much more often than it really is. In one study of college students, the students estimated that the insanity defense is used in 30 percent of criminal cases and is successful 30 percent of the time. In actuality it is used in fewer than 1 percent of cases and is successful in only about 15 percent of those cases (see Figure 15.6). What's more, those who overestimate the number of insanity defense pleas are more negative in their thoughts about the insanity defense (Adjorlolo et al. 2019).

Also, some think the insanity defense is used to escape responsibility for criminal behavior. The fact is that, except in the most infrequent of cases, people found not guilty by reason of insanity are committed to a mental institution for

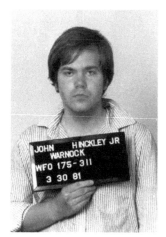

Figure 15.5 John Hinckley, Jr. spent 35 years in a mental institution after he was found not guilty by reason of insanity for shooting President Ronald Reagan.

Source: Pete Marovich/Getty Images.

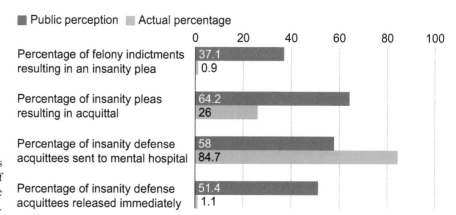

■ Public perception ■ Actual percentage

Percentage of felony indictments resulting in an insanity plea	37.1 / 0.9
Percentage of insanity pleas resulting in acquittal	64.2 / 26
Percentage of insanity defense acquittees sent to mental hospital	58 / 84.7
Percentage of insanity defense acquittees released immediately	51.4 / 1.1

Figure 15.6 The public's perception of the prevalence of the insanity defense is not the same as the actual occurrence.

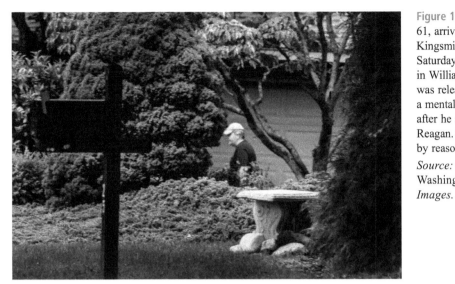

Figure 15.7 John Hinckley, Jr., 61, arrives home in the gated Kingsmill community on Saturday, September 10, 2016, in Williamsburg, VA. Hinckley was released permanently from a mental institution – 35 years after he shot President Ronald Reagan. He was ruled not guilty by reason of insanity.
*Source: Jahi Chikwendiu/*The Washington Post *via Getty Images.*

much longer than they would have been, had they simply been found guilty. Outcomes are not any better for those found not guilty by reason of insanity for non-violent crimes. They are committed for periods more than eight times longer than those found guilty and put in prison (Perlin 2000). Race and type of mental disorder can affect the jurors' decision making. In a study of mock trials, when participants read a fictional account, they were more likely to vote guilty for a Black defendant with schizophrenia than for a Black defendant with depression. However, there were no significant differences for white defendants (Maeder et al. 2020).

John Hinckley, Jr., for example, was found not guilty of shooting President Reagan by reason of insanity, and many were concerned that he got away with his crime. But did he? He was sent to a mental institution in 1981, and according to hospital records by 1984 his most dangerous symptoms were in remission. His condition (narcissistic personality disorder, schizoid personality disorder, and what would now be called persistent depressive disorder) was in full remission. Despite this, he wasn't released for another 35 years (Figure 15.7). In 2016 a federal district court judge ordered Hinckley to be released. Today he works for a church and sells books through an anonymous Amazon profile. Though he is described as a "recluse," the Secret Service still watches over him.

Guilty But Mentally Ill

Because of concerns about the Hinckley verdict, 20 states eventually abandoned the NGRI defense or made it more difficult to obtain. Some states instituted a new plea: **Guilty But Mentally Ill (GBMI)**, which requires that

Guilty But Mentally Ill (GBMI): a plea which requires that an individual both serve a sentence for their crime and receive treatment for the condition that was present at the time of the crime.

an individual both serve a sentence for their crime and receive treatment for the condition that was present at the time of the crime. Thus, a guilty but mentally ill verdict ensures that the individual is both punished and treated. US states that still have the insanity defense allow pleas of either NGRI or GBMI, but not both.

GBMI individuals are more likely to get longer sentences than in states with NGRI defenses (Callahan et al. 1992). However, prisoners found GBMI are no more likely to receive treatment than other guilty prisoners, so a GBMI verdict is essentially the same as a guilty verdict (van Es et al. 2020).

THE POWER OF EVIDENCE

Do people found not guilty by reason of insanity "get away" with their crime?

Public perception of the insanity defense suggests that many people feel it is overused, and that it has become a way to escape punishment (Gamache et al. 2021). However, many who were found not guilty by reason of insanity ended up regretting their plea. Typically, a person found not guilty is free to go home. But nearly all US states demand that those found not guilty by reason of insanity must be automatically committed to a psychiatric facility, usually with no limit on the length of time they are to spend there. Many states fail to release data about the amount of time spent in confinement by those found to be NGRI (Wendzel 2020). However, a 2014 study estimated that the average length of stay for all NGRI pleas was five to seven years. For those civilly committed with similar diagnoses, the average was three days (Fitch 2014).

This is true even though it is unlikely that people found NGRI will interact with the criminal justice system in the future. While the national rate of recidivism (repeating and being convicted of the same crime) is about 60 percent, in Maryland, for example, it was half that for those released after being found NGRI.

Gender can also be a factor in the insanity defense. We've learned in this chapter that it's relatively rare to have a successful insanity defense. As in many areas, however, gender can play a role in this determination. Researchers (Yourstone et al. 2008) presented homicide cases to judges, clinicians, and psychology students and asked them to indicate whether the defendant would meet the definition of insanity given the circumstances. The cases were all the same except that some had a female defendant while others had a male defendant. More often than not, the female defendants were rated as meeting the criteria for insanity, paralleling what we see in actual decisions. A 1995 study (Cirincione et al. 1995) examined insanity defense acquittals (the defendant is found not guilty) in seven US states and discovered that in every state the acquittal rate for women was greater than that for men. Similar statistics are found in other countries as well (Kirchebner et al. 2020). Because of biases, women are also

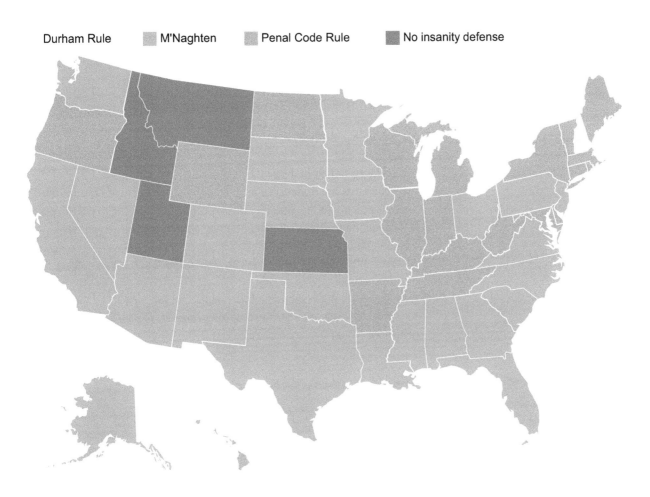

Durham Rule   M'Naghten   Penal Code Rule   No insanity defense

Figure 15.8 The insanity defense among the states.
Source: Data from The Insanity Defense Among the States, created by FindLaw's team of legal writers and editors – last updated January 23, 2019: www.findlaw.com/criminal/criminal-procedure/the-insanity-defense-among-the-states.html

more likely to be diagnosed with a psychological disorder, to require hospitalization pending trial, and to be found incompetent to stand trial (Dirks-Linhorst et al. 2019).

States that allow the insanity defense generally follow one of four legal standards for accepting insanity as a defense, but they often combine these standards or follow their own modified interpretation (Figure 15.8). Table 15.1 lists the four standards.

Table 15.1 The insanity defense: state laws

Laws and rules	Standard
The M'Naghten Rule	Defendant unable to distinguish between right and wrong or otherwise didn't understand actions because of a "disease of the mind."
The Irresistible Impulse Test	Defendant unable to control impulses due to a mental disorder, leading to the commission of a criminal act.
The Model Penal Code Test	Defendant unable to act within legal constraints or failed to understand the criminality of acts due to a mental defect.
The Durham Rule	Defendant's mental defect led to the commission of a criminal act, regardless of clinical diagnosis.

CONCEPT CHECK 15.3

Match each rule with the description.
- A. American Law Institute Test
- B. Durham Test
- C. Irresistible Impulse Test
- D. M'Naghten Rule
- E. Not guilty by reason of insanity
1. A defendant is not responsible for a criminal act if experiencing a psycho-logical condition at the time the act was committed.
2. A defendant must have an intention to break the law to be responsible for breaking that law.
3. A defendant should not be held legally responsible for an action if driven by a fit of passion.
4. A defendant is not responsible for criminal conduct who lacks the ability to appreciate the wrongfulness of the conduct or can't control their behavior.

15.4 PATIENTS' RIGHTS

When receiving a treatment from a medical professional you have a set of patient rights that must be adhered to throughout your treatment. In this section we outline some of these rights and offer some examples of when things can go wrong.

Informed Consent

Imagine you have a terrible stomach ache, so bad that you decide to go to the doctor about it. The doctor examines you, leaves the room, and returns with a hypodermic. Then, without asking, he injects the needle's contents into your arm. Afterward your stomach feels a little better, but you now have a headache, a fever, and no appetite.

In this scenario, you probably would have liked to be consulted about whether you wanted the shot, and to make this decision you'd have wanted to know the advantages, disadvantages, and side effects of the treatment. The same is true for treatment of psychological conditions. **Informed consent** is the principle that those who participate in research or treatment deserve to understand the proced-ures, risks, and benefits of the treatment and have the right to refuse to participate. Being able to give informed consent includes knowing as much as possible about the treatment, its advantages and disadvantages, and what alternatives might be

Informed consent: the principle that those who participate in research or treatment deserve to understand the procedures, risks, and benefits of the treatment and have the right to refuse to participate.

available. In addition, knowledge about confidentiality and its limits is key to giving an informed consent.

Confidentiality

Imagine you are a psychologist in private practice. You are working with a new client and in the middle of his first session he confesses "I feel terrible." He explains his discomfort: "The main reason I'm here is that three years ago, I was involved in a hit and run accident. I was using my phone while I was driving, and I hit someone in the crosswalk. I wasn't paying attention. I panicked and fled the scene. I learned later that the person died. I feel terrible. I've come here to handle my grief." Would you report your client to the police?

Clients entrust their mental health practitioners with private information, and the principle of **confidentiality** means that information obtained from a client by a mental health professional should not be revealed to others. The law says that the communication between clients and therapists is "privileged," which means that it must remain private. There are, however, some limits to that privilege, and it's important that therapists let their clients know under what circumstances their information will be shared.

Confidentiality: the provision that information obtained from a client by a mental health professional should not be revealed to others.

Duty to Warn

In the 1960s the dehospitalization movement along with more effective medications, and focus on patients' rights increased the number of previously hospitalized patients being treated in outpatient settings. Because of this movement it became harder for mental health care practitioners to initiate involuntary hospitalizations. This created an increased burden on mental health care practitioners to protect the public from people who might cause harm to others. To protect mental health practitioners some US states enacted laws to provide protection for practitioners who did not hospitalize clients who subsequently harmed another person (Felthous et al. 2020). That changed in 1976.

The 1976 case of *Tarasoff v Regents of the University of California* established that a therapist not only has a duty to warn but also a duty to attempt to protect the potential victim (Wortzel et al. 2020). A client named Prosenjit Poddar had let his therapist know that he wanted to harm Tatiana Tarasoff. The campus police were notified, but the therapist never attempted to contact Tarasoff. The campus police interviewed Poddar, who denied making any threats and was released after being questioned. He then found Tatiana Tarasoff and stabbed her to death.

The Tarasoff case and others helped to clarify the role of mental health professionals in their duty to protect others. If a client tells their therapist they will harm someone, the therapist has a duty to warn that person. **Duty to warn** is the

Duty to warn: the principle that a mental health professional is compelled to break confidentiality in order to notify an individual whom their client has threatened.

principle that a mental health professional is compelled to break confidentiality in order to notify an individual whom their client has threatened. The California Supreme Court ruled that the duty to warn wasn't enough; the therapist also had a duty to protect. The **duty to protect** is the principle that a mental health professional is compelled to break confidentiality to safeguard a potential victim of their client. Duty to protect bills (Walker et al. 2020) allow mental health practitioners to break confidentiality in order to "protect the client or others from imminent danger or harm." With the duty to protect, the therapist has the legal obligation to protect a third party from danger through other methods of intervention, such as inpatient treatment or more rigorous outpatient therapy. For many states, the threats from a client must be specific and about specific individuals. However, for some states (such as Colorado), the threats may extend to buildings or specific locations (Figure 15.9).

Duty to protect: the principle that a mental health professional is compelled to break confidentiality to safeguard a potential victim of their client.

Right to Treatment

Right to treatment is the legal right of an involuntarily committed individual to receive active care for their condition. This right includes expectations about the proper treatment of people who are undergoing psychiatric treatment. In certain situations, especially if the client cannot care for themselves, there should be minimal expectations for the person's safety, comfort, and treatment. In the past, and sometimes even today, these expectations were not met. Until the 1970s some mental institutions didn't provide much treatment and were merely storehouses for people with mental conditions. Such abuses led to legal actions. For example, *Wyatt v Stickney* (1972) ruled that the state had an obligation to provide "adequate treatment" to everyone who has been committed involuntarily (Dvoskin et al. 2020).

Right to treatment: the legal right of an involuntarily committed individual to receive active care for their condition.

From that court case came what are known as the **Wyatt Standards**. These guidelines state that a mental institution must provide patients with a humane psychological and physical environment, qualified and sufficient staff, individual treatment plans, and minimal patient restrictions (West 2020). Since the Wyatt Standards were instituted, additional regulations have been put in place to help ensure adequate treatment of patients. For example, since *O'Connor v Donaldson* (1975), institutions have been required to periodically review the cases of those involuntarily committed. Commitment must be ended if the patient is no longer dangerous. The Protection and Advocacy for Mentally Ill Individuals Act (1988) set up protection systems in all states to investigate possible abuse and neglect (Fentiman 2020; Geller 2012).

Wyatt Standards: guidelines which state that a mental institution must provide patients with a humane psychological and physical environment, qualified and sufficient staff, individual treatment plans, and minimal patient restrictions.

Right to Refuse Treatment

The right to treatment ensures that people who are involuntarily committed receive treatment, but what if they don't want the treatment? After all, 75 percent of people

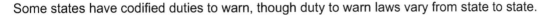

Some states have codified duties to warn, though duty to warn laws vary from state to state.

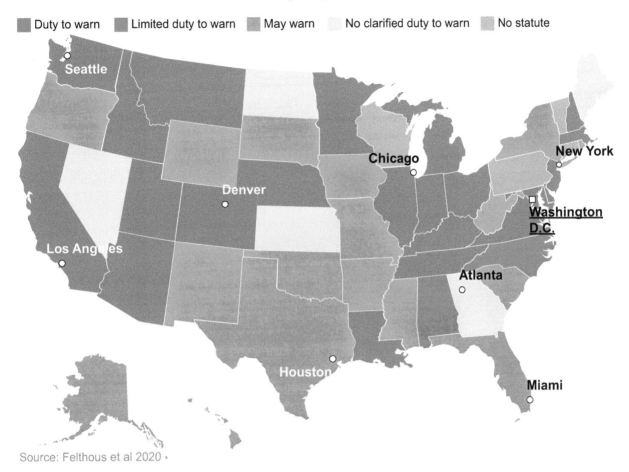

Source: Felthous et al 2020 ·

with schizophrenia and 90 percent with depression have adequate decision-making capacity (Grisso & Appelbaum 1995). A recent meta-analysis of 49 studies showed that over 70 percent of people who were hospitalized with severe psychological conditions such as schizoaffective disorder and schizophrenia had the insight to understand their treatment options (Pons et al. 2020). What happens if the person decides to refuse the recommended treatment?

Remember the case of Joyce Brown who was involuntarily committed in New York with Project Help? The courts ruled that the state had no right to commit her if she had no intention of getting treatment, and she was ordered released after having been committed for more than 11 weeks. Further rulings supported this order. For example, *O'Connor v Donaldson* (1975) suggested that "a state cannot constitutionally confine ... a non-dangerous individual, who is capable of surviving safely in freedom by himself or with the help of willing and responsible family and friends" (Bernard 1977).

Figure 15.9 Some states have codified duties to warn, though duty to warn laws vary from state to state. Some states have permissive warning that allows mental health professionals to ease confidentiality discretionarily, but do not mandate it, and do not impose liability to failing to warn. Other states have not established any kind of statutory duty to warn, though it may be imposed by case law. Twenty-two states have mandatory duty to warn statutes.
Source: Data from Felthous et al. (2020).

Right to refuse treatment: the legal principle that an individual can decline care.

The **right to refuse treatment** is the legal principle that an individual can decline care. It requires that people must be fully informed about the treatment and must give written consent. Patients can refuse treatment, but that decision can be overruled if the patient is found to be dangerous or is not legally able to make decisions for themselves. In those cases, the treatment may commence without the patient's consent.

Critics of the right to refuse treatment are concerned that clients may be deprived of useful treatments and suffer needlessly (Bloch & Green 2021). The right to refuse treatment is not recognized in all US states, but in many cases courts can decide that the patient does not have to be treated against their will.

CONCEPT CHECK 15.4

Indicate which patient right might be violated in each case.
1. Leo has been concerned that his wife, Sarah, has become increasingly depressed over the last few months. Fortunately, Sarah's psychiatrist prescribed medication that seemed to reduce her symptoms. Sarah hates this medication, however, because it makes her nauseated. Sarah's psychiatrist suggests that Leo sneak the medicine into Sarah's food.
2. Ousmane has suffered from severe obsessive-compulsive disorder for the last few years. It has become so debilitating that he has checked himself into a hospital for help. However, since his admission to the hospital, Ousmane has not received any active care for his condition.
3. Dimitri has become absent-minded because of his anxiety. In fact, he recently forgot when his next appointment with his psychologist was scheduled. His sister decided to call Dimitri's psychologist to find out, and although she had never communicated with the psychologist before, he was more than happy to let her know the time and date of Dimitri's next appointment.

PULLING IT TOGETHER

Criteria for Insanity

1853   M'Naghten Rule:

A legal principle that suggests individuals are not responsible for their actions if, because of a mental condition, they did not know what they were doing or did not know it was wrong.

Irresistible Impulse Test: **1834**

A legal principle that suggests an individual should not be held legally responsible if driven by an uncontrollable impulse or has a diminished capacity to resist the impulse.

1954   Durham Test:

A legal principle that suggests a jury may find a defendant is not guilty by reason of insanity because the act in question was committed due to a psychological condition.

American Law Institute Test: **1955**

The legal principle of criminal responsibility that suggests a person is not criminally responsible for their conduct if they lack the capacity to understand that their behavior was wrong, or if they are not able to conform their conduct to the requirements of the law.

Figure 15.10 The criteria for the insanity defense have changed over time.

15.5   CHAPTER REVIEW

SUMMARY

Civil Commitment

- A person with a psychological disorder may be forced into treatment if they are found to be dangerous to themselves or to others.
- The legal definition of a mental disorder may be different from the *DSM-5tr* criteria for a psychological disorder.
- *Parens patriae* is the policy that means the government may act as a legal protector for people who cannot protect themselves.
- While people with psychological disorders are not dangerous by definition, the state governments may use police power to protect society from people who are dangerous.
- The process of civil commitment has several steps to ensure that it is not abused.

Competence to Stand Trial

- Competence to stand trial is the legal construct that says a person must understand the charges brought against them and be able to assist in their own defense.

The Insanity Defense and Criminal Commitment

- Many rules have been used to define insanity, including the M'Naghten Rule, the Irresistible Impulse Test, the Durham Test, the American Law Institute Test, and the American Psychiatric Association Rule.
- Criminal commitment is the principle that people whose mental condition may have caused them to commit a crime may be ordered into treatment (either to an institution or an outpatient clinic).

Patients' Rights

- Patients' rights are intended to protect those who are receiving treatment for mental health conditions. The rights include informed consent, confidentiality, a duty to warn, and the right to refuse or to receive adequate treatment.

DISCUSSION QUESTIONS

1. Thinking about legal pleas such as NGRI or GBMI, what do you believe are some of the factors that drive the way society treats those with psychological disorders who commit crimes?
2. Now that you know more about the insanity defense, what do you think should happen to the man who had the seizure at the beginning of the chapter? Would he meet the criteria for insanity at the time of the injuries? Should he be punished for the death and injuries he created, if so how?
3. What should therapists do with clients who refuse to take medicines that might help them?
4. There are strict ethics guidelines about confidentiality and psychotherapy. What do you believe would occur if therapists could decide for themselves what information to share about their clients? Why are the ethics guidelines so strict about the circumstances in which therapists may reveal information about their clients?
5. What are the ethical implications for therapists who monitor their clients' social media posts without telling their clients they are doing so?

ANSWERS TO CONCEPT CHECKS

Concept Check 15.1

1. Dangerous to himself
2. Grave disability

Concept Check 15.2

1. Yes
2. Yes

Concept Check 15.3

3. Yes
4. No

Concept Check 15.3

1. B
2. D
3. C
4. E

Concept Check 15.4

1. Right to refuse treatment
2. Right to treatment
3. Confidentiality

Glossary

Abnormal behavior: conduct that differs from typical developmental, cultural, or societal norms and creates distress or impairment in functioning.

Abnormal psychology: the scientific study of psychological disorders.

Acute stress disorder (ASD): a trauma and stressor-related disorder in which people have symptoms of PTSD lasting up to 30 days.

Adaptive functioning: the ability to perform the activities of daily living.

Adjustment disorder: a trauma and stressor-related disorder in which a person has experienced a stressor and is having a greater than expected emotional or behavioral response due to the difficulty of coping with it.

Agoraphobia: an anxiety disorder characterized by fear of having a panic attack, which causes a person to avoid places and situations where having such an attack would be particularly embarrassing or dangerous.

Alcohol use disorder: a substance-related disorder associated with impaired control over the amount and frequency with which they drink and often experience negative emotional states when they aren't drinking.

American Law Institute Test: the legal principle of criminal responsibility that suggests a person is not criminally responsible for their conduct if they lack the capacity to understand that their behavior was wrong, or if they are not able to conform their conduct to the requirements of the law.

Anorexia nervosa: an eating disorder characterized by a disturbed body image and an intense fear of weight gain.

Anorexia nervosa, binge-eating/purging type: a type of anorexia nervosa characterized by compensatory behaviors to limit weight gain.

Anorexia nervosa, restricting type: a type of anorexia nervosa characterized by limiting food intake in order to control weight.

Antipsychotic medication: a type of drug used to reduce the symptoms of psychosis.

Antisocial personality disorder: a personality disorder in which a person breaks the rules of society and often with no remorse or anxiety.

Anxiety: a mood state characterized by concern over an uncertain outcome.

Anxiety sensitivity: a tendency to interpret bodily sensations as evidence of harmful symptoms.

Assertive community therapy: a multiperspective, team-based, multidisciplinary approach that can help those with psychosis.

Asylums: inpatient institutions created to provide care for people with psychological disorders.

Attention deficit hyperactivity disorder (ADHD): a neurodevelopmental condition in which a person has a pattern of inattention or disruptive hyperactivity/impulsivity.

Atypical antipsychotics: also called second-generation antipsychotics, medications that target dopamine as well as other neurotransmitters to reduce the symptoms of psychosis.

Autism spectrum disorder: a neurodevelopmental disorder characterized by deficits in social communication and interaction, along with restricted and repetitive behaviors, interests, and activities.

Avoidant personality disorder: a personality disorder marked by a pervasive pattern of social inhibition, a sense of inadequacy, and hypersensitivity to the criticism of others.

Behavioral exposure: a behavioral technique that involves repeated presentation of anxiety-producing stimuli when the client is unable to react in their typical maladaptive manner.

Behavioral medicine: an interdisciplinary field concerned with health and illness that combines knowledge of the social and medical sciences to improve health and combat illness.

Behavioral perspective: a theory of psychopathology that uses learning theory to understand problematic behaviors and change them to more constructive ones.

Binge-eating disorder (BED): an eating disorder in which a person experiences episodes of uncontrolled eating with distress, but without any compensating behaviors (such as purges) to counteract the binges.

Biofeedback: a technique in which a person is trained to become aware of physiological functions, such as heartbeat or breathing, and attempts to influence those functions.

Biological psychology: also known as *neuropsychology*, is the branch of psychology that examines the connection between bodily systems and behavior.

Biological theories: an explanation of psychopathology that suggests that psychological disorders are caused by human physiology.

Biomedical therapies: a family of therapies that use surgery, medication, or other physiological interventions for the treatment of psychological conditions.

Bipolar disorders: mood disorders in which a person may alternate between a sad, depressive mood and elevated, irritable, or manic episodes.

Bipolar I disorder: a bipolar mood disorder in which a person cycles between mania and the other mood episodes.

Bipolar II disorder: a mood disorder in which a person alternates between depressive and hypomanic episodes.

Body dysmorphic disorder (BDD): an obsessive-compulsive and related disorder associated with an imagined defect in appearance and compensatory behaviors.

Body mass index (BMI): a ratio of height and weight that includes comparison to others.

Borderline personality disorder (BPD): a personality disorder marked by a long history of instability in a person's self-image, in their ability to control impulses, in their relationships, and in their moods.

Brief psychotic disorder: a psychotic disorder in which a person shows sudden positive symptoms of psychosis in response to a stressor.

Bulimia nervosa: an eating disorder characterized by recurrent episodes of binge eating and by compensatory behaviors.

Callous-unemotional type of conduct disorder: a specifier for conduct disorder associated with children who are insensitive to the feelings of others, have shallow emotions, and don't feel guilty or have empathy for the things they might do to others.

Cannabis sativa: a plant that contains the psychoactive substance tetrahydrocannabinol (THC).

Case study: an extensive examination of the experience of a single individual or group that allows researchers a deep look at the subject.

Central nervous system: a division of the nervous system that comprises the brain and spinal cord.

Chronic traumatic encephalopathy (CTE): a condition caused by blows to the head from accidents, gunshots, or repetitive sports injuries.

Circadian rhythm sleep-wake disorder: a sleep disorder characterized by misalignment between internal and external influences on sleep and wakefulness.

Civil commitment: a process by which individuals may be forcibly treated if they are found to be dangerous to themselves or to others.

Classical categorical approach: a diagnostic system in which the categories are distinct.

Classical conditioning: a type of learning in which a response typically associated with one stimulus becomes associated with a new stimulus.

Classification system: an attempt to create a set of groups or categories and to sort or assign people or objects to those categories based on their attributes or relationships.

Client-centered therapy: a psychotherapy based on humanistic personality theory that works to create a nondirective and accepting environment and leads the client toward personality change.

Clinical assessment: the process of systematically gathering information for diagnosis and treatment planning.

Clinical interviews: a procedure used to collect a detailed history of a person's life, including current and past symptoms.

Clinical psychologists: mental health professionals who research, evaluate, and treat psychological conditions.

Clinical research model: a clinical psychology training program that emphasizes clinical psychology research over direct work with clients.

Cognitive behavior therapy (CBT): a psychotherapeutic technique where the goal is to identify any negative self-talk and examine it fully.

Cognitive perspective: a theory in psychology that emphasizes the internal processes of thought, or cognition, that help us make sense of the world.

Cognitive therapy (CBT): a type of treatment that emphasizes the link between thoughts and emotions.

Comorbid: the presence of more than one diagnosis.

Compensatory behaviors: behaviors intended to prevent weight gain or feelings of guilt from eating.

Competence to stand trial: a legal construct that says in order to be tried, a defendant must understand the charges brought against them and be able to assist in their own defense.

Compulsions: behaviors or mental actions that a person feels they must do as a response to an obsession.

Computerized tomography scans (CT scans): a neuroimaging technique that uses computer-enhanced X-rays in order to examine structures.

Conduct disorder: a condition associated with children and adolescents where they exhibit physically violent behavior toward others.

Confidentiality: the provision that information obtained from a client by a mental health professional should not be revealed to others.

Confounding variables: outside factors that might account for differences in the dependent variable.

Continuous positive airway pressure (CPAP): a treatment for sleep apnea in which a small machine and mask keep the airway open by sending a constant stream of compressed air.

Continuum: a range of severity from mild to disruptive.

Control group: in an experiment, the participants who do not receive a treatment or experience.

Correlation coefficient: a numerical description of the direction and strength of relationship between two variables.

Correlational method: a research design that explains how two or more conditions vary in relation to each other.

Counseling psychologist: a mental health professional who helps those with difficulty adjusting to life stressors to achieve greater wellbeing.

Cultural relativism: the idea that our understanding of psychopathology should be based on a person's culture rather than on one universal definition of the term.

Culture: the shared customs, institutions, values, and habits that distinguish a group.

Cyclothymic disorder: a milder but persistent bipolar mood disorder characterized by periods of hypomanic symptoms and mild depressive episodes.

Danger: a tendency towards violence.

Defense mechanisms: these are unconscious arrangements that the ego uses to satisfy id instincts indirectly.

Deinstitutionalization: the replacement of inpatient psychiatric care with community outpatient services.

Delayed ejaculation disorder: a sexual dysfunction characterized by delayed or absent ejaculation.

Delirium: a sudden confused mental state caused by an underlying medical illness or substance use.

Delusional disorder: a psychotic disorder in which a person experiences only delusions and no other symptoms of psychosis.

Delusions: a positive symptom of psychosis in which a person experiences fixed false beliefs that are not amenable to change in the light of conflicting evidence, though most people would understand them to be untrue.

Dependent personality disorder: a personality disorder marked by a pervasive pattern of excessive need to be taken care of and a dependent, clinging pattern of behavior.

Dependent variables: in an experiment, the measurement collected to determine if there was any effect of the independent variable.

Depersonalization-derealization disorder (DPDRD): a dissociative disorder in which people feel cut off from their own body, as if they are watching their own body from above.

Depressant: a psychoactive substance that reduces activity in the nervous system.

Depressive disorders: a category of mood disorder characterized by sad moods or lack of pleasure.

Derealization: a sense of unreality and detachment from the world, like being in a fog or a dream in which the world around you feels unreal.

Deviate: a departure from typical or accepted standards.

Diagnosis: a label applied to a disorder whose symptoms tend to occur together.

Dialectical behavior therapy (DBT): a treatment for borderline personality disorder that aims to teach problem-solving skills, emotional regulation, and interpersonal skills.

Diathesis-stress model: a multiperspective approach that implicates stressors are involved in the development of psychological symptoms.

Dimensional approach: a diagnostic classification system which rates the degree to which certain characteristics are exhibited in an individual.

Disruptive impulse and conduct disorders: a chapter in the *DSM-5tr* that contains conditions that reflect behaviors that might violate the rights of others or break societal norms.

Disruptive mood dysregulation disorder (DMDD): a depressive mood disorder found in children aged 6 to 18 that is characterized by severe temper outbursts and a persistent irritable or angry mood.

Dissociation: a split of your consciousness or attention into separate streams.

Dissociative amnesia: a condition in which people forget important personal information much more than you would expect with normal forgetfulness.

Dissociative disorders: disorders characterized by a sudden loss of the integration of consciousness, identity, or memory.

Dissociative fugue: a specifier for dissociative amnesia where in addition to experiencing amnesia, people may drive away from home and start a new life in a new location.

Dissociative identity disorder (DID): a dissociative disorder in which two or more distinct identities, sometimes called *alters*, exist inside one person, each with its own unique characteristics.

Distress: a feeling of anxiety or pain.

Dopamine hypothesis of schizophrenia: a biological model of psychosis that suggests the neurotransmitter dopamine plays a key role in the disorder.

Double-blind: an experimental procedure in which neither the subject nor the experimenter knows to which experimental conditions that subject is assigned.

Down syndrome: a neurodevelopmental disorder in which an individual has an extra 21st chromosome.

Durham Test: a legal principle that suggests a jury may find a defendant is not guilty by reason of insanity because the act in question was committed due to a psychological condition.

Duty to protect: the principle that a mental health professional is compelled to break confidentiality to safeguard a potential victim of their client.

Duty to warn: the principle that a mental health professional is compelled to break confidentiality in order to notify an individual whom their client has threatened.

Dysfunction: behaviors, emotions, or thoughts that are outside the ordinary and that result in a person's being impaired or distressed.

Dyssomnias: conditions that can affect the quantity, quality, or timing of sleep, like insomnia, sleep apnea, and narcolepsy.

Dysthymic episode: a mild depressive episode that doesn't meet the full criteria for a major depressive episode.

Eating disorder: a psychological condition characterized by severe disturbances in eating behavior.

Ego dystonic: symptoms dissimilar to the way people see themselves.

Electroconvulsive therapy (ECT): a biological treatment that uses electricity to induce seizures in anesthetized patients.

Electroencephalogram (EEG): a device that uses electrodes on the scalp to record the electrical activity or brain waves produced by the neurons.

Emotional processing theory: a theory which suggests that traumatic events can lead to problems if they are not processed adequately.

Empathy: the willingness and ability to understand another person's inner world.

Etiology: the presumed cause of a disorder.

Excoriation disorder: an obsessive-compulsive and related disorder in which an individual picks at their own skin and causes skin lesions or wounds.

Exhibitionistic disorder: a condition in which a person experiences a sustained, focused pattern of sexual arousal, persistent sexual thoughts, fantasies, urges, or behaviors related to exposing their genitals to an unsuspecting person.

Exorcism: a religious ritual that treated abnormality by coaxing spirits such as demons from the body.

Experiment: a method by which one or more independent variables is manipulated by researchers and the result is measured through one or more dependent variables.

Experimental group: in an experiment, the group that receives some treatment or experience.

Experimenter bias: inaccurate measurements due to the researcher's expectations.

Exposure therapy: a therapeutic approach which repeatedly presents the client with a distressing object to reduce associated anxiety and the fear response over time.

Factitious disorder: a somatic symptom disorder in which a person will either fake, exaggerate, or intentionally produce symptoms of an illness in order to play the sick role.

Fear: an emotion that is associated with a threat, danger, or pain.

Female orgasmic disorder: a condition associated with persistent delay or absence of orgasm following a typical arousal phase.

Female sexual interest/arousal disorder: a condition characterized by a lack of interest in sexual activity or a significantly and persistently low level of sexual arousal.

Fetishistic disorder: a paraphilic disorder in which fantasies, urges, or behaviors related to nonliving objects or nongenital body parts serve for sexual arousal.

Fight, flee, or freeze response: a reaction to danger or stressful situations that prepares your body for vigorous activity and to handle stress.

Fragile X syndrome: a condition related to a mutation that makes the X chromosome look as if it is hanging and fragile.

Frontotemporal neurocognitive disorder: a neurocognitive disorder characterized by selective degeneration of the nerves in the frontal and temporal lobes of the cerebral cortex, creating deficits in executive functioning, language, and behavior.

Frotteuristic disorder: a condition in which a person experiences sexual urges to touch or rub against an unsuspecting and nonconsenting person and becomes aroused by doing so.

Functional magnetic resonance imaging (fMRI): an assessment that examines brain activity over time by detecting the differences in blood oxygen between brain areas that are more and less active.

Functional neurological symptom disorder (conversion disorder): a somatic symptom disorder where a person's psychological worry or concern is transformed into a physical symptom.

Gambling disorder: an addictive disorder that is associated with problematic gambling at the expense of the person's livelihood and wellbeing.

Gender dysphoria: a condition in which a person experiences distress and/or impairment associated with their gender identity being different from the gender assigned at birth.

Gender expression: the way a person behaves and interacts with others, including dress, appearance, and behaviors.

Gender identity: a range of characteristics that characterize the way you think about the biological features that inform who you are.

Generalized anxiety disorder (GAD): an anxiety disorder marked by unexplained, excessive worry that's not linked to anything in particular.

Genito-pelvic pain/penetration disorder: a condition in which the muscles in the outer third of the vagina contract involuntarily and painfully, which prevents sexual intercourse.

Grave disability: a criterion for involuntary commitment that is met when a person cannot provide for their own basic needs.

Group therapy: a psychotherapy treatment technique that treats multiple clients in a collective setting.

Guilty But Mentally Ill (GBMI): a plea which requires that an individual both serve a sentence for their crime and receive treatment for the condition that was present at the time of the crime.

Hallucinations: a positive symptom of psychosis in which a person experiences sensory perceptions with no corresponding sensory input.

Hallucinogen: a psychoactive substance that distorts conscious experiences.

Health psychology: a general branch of psychology concerned with the way psychological factors affect wellness, illness, and medical treatments.

Histrionic personality disorder: a personality disorder marked by a persistent pattern of attention seeking and excessive emotionality.

Hoarding disorder: an obsessive-compulsive and related disorder associated with difficulty discarding unneeded possessions.

Humors: bodily fluids that were thought to influence mental functioning.

Huntington's disease: a genetic condition associated with personality changes and memory and mood problems that become progressively more disruptive over time.

Hypersomnolence disorders: sleep disorders characterized by excessive (hyper) sleepiness (somnolence) or difficulty maintaining wakefulness.

Hypomanic episode: a mood episode in which a person has symptoms of mania but they do not impair the person's ability to function effectively.

Illness anxiety disorder: a somatic symptom disorder characterized by excessive fear of having an illness despite evidence to the contrary.

Impulse-control disorders: a condition in which people feel overwhelming urges to engage in behaviors that may violate the rights of others or conflict with societal norms.

Impulses: strong urges to behave in certain ways.

Independent variables: the factor that an experimenter manipulates to create different experiences for participants.

Informed consent: the principle that those who participate in research or treatment deserve to understand the procedures, risks, and benefits of the treatment and have the right to refuse to participate.

Insomnia: a condition characterized by having difficulty falling asleep or staying asleep, waking up too early, or having non-refreshing sleep.

Intake report: document that summarizes the patient's relevant history, symptoms, and next steps for the client such as diagnosis, goal setting, and a treatment plan.

Intellectual developmental disorder: a neurodevelopmental disorder that consists of deficits in general mental abilities across a wide variety of domains.

Intellectual functioning: the ability to think, learn, solve problems, and adapt to and learn from new situations.

Intermittent explosive disorder: a condition in which people have sudden episodes of angry verbal outbursts or aggressive, violent behavior that are significantly out of proportion to the situation.

Interpersonal and social rhythm therapy (IPSRT): treatment for bipolar disorders that helps clients manage relationships and daily rhythms.

Interpersonal psychotherapy: a treatment that examines the changes, reactions, and deficits in an individual's relationships and emphasizes the resolution of relationship stressors as a way to address mood disorders.

Intersexuality: a condition in which a person is born with sexual anatomy that doesn't fit into the categories of male or female.

Irresistible impulse test: a legal principle that suggests an individual should not be held legally responsible if driven by an uncontrollable impulse or a diminished capacity to resist the impulse.

Kleptomania: a condition in which people can't resist the impulse to take items, usually of nominal value like cosmetics, even when they don't really need them.

Lewy body disease: a neurocognitive disorder caused by microscopic abnormal protein deposits that develop in the brain and damage the neurons.

M'Naghten Rule: a legal principle that suggests individuals are not responsible for their actions if, because of a mental condition, they did not know what they were doing or did not know it was wrong.

Magnetic resonance imaging (MRI): a non-invasive imaging technique that uses magnets and radio equipment to produce detailed images, particularly of soft tissue.

Major depressive disorder: a depressive disorder characterized by two or more weeks of low mood or anhedonia and at least four other symptoms of a major depressive episode.

Major depressive episode: a mood episode that often includes lack of interest and sad moods along with cognitive and behavioral symptoms that lasts at least two weeks.

Major neurocognitive disorder: a neurocognitive disorder (NCD) marked by a decline in areas of cognitive functioning that results in impairment.

Male hypoactive sexual desire disorder: a condition associated with a reduced interest in sex but may have typical physical responses to sex.

Malingering: the intentional production or faking of symptoms for external gain.

Managed care: a health care system in which the insurance companies control and coordinate medical and psychological services.

Mania: an emotional and behavioral condition associated with an elevated, expansive, sometimes irritable mood and abnormally increased energy or activity.

Manic episode: a type of mood episode where a person's moods are abnormally elevated, and their emotions, thinking, and reactions might be so elevated that they do things that get them into trouble or put them in danger.

Meal support: a service that helps patients change the way they think about meals and eating.

Mechanism of action (MOA): a description of the way a drug functions.

Melatonin: a hormone that promotes sleepiness, in the morning, and in the afternoon decreasing light causes it to increase melatonin.

Mental hygiene movement: a theory of psychopathology that proposed that psychological disorders were a result of people's being separated from nature.

Mental status examination (MSE): an assessment of cognitive functioning that looks for the presence and sometimes the absence of symptoms.

Meta-analysis: a research technique in which many studies on a single topic are considered together and conclusions drawn about our current knowledge.

Methylation: a process by which a gene may be switched off by the body.

Mild neurocognitive disorder: a neurocognitive disorder (NCD) in which individuals have memory and cognitive deficits that are noticeable but not yet significant enough to create problems with everyday activities.

Monoamine hypothesis of depression: a biological theory of depression that suggests that symptoms of depression are brought on by malfunction of a class of neurotransmitters called monoamines.

Monoamine oxidase inhibitors (MAOIs): a class of antidepressant drugs whose purpose is to keep the family of monoamine neurotransmitters (serotonin, norepinephrine, and dopamine) in the synaptic gaps in the brain long enough for the monoamines to bind to the receptor sites in order to deliver their message.

Mood disorders: psychological conditions marked by tumultuous emotional states that can result in problematic social functioning and thinking behaviors, and in physical symptoms.

Moral treatment: a treatment that emphasized moral discipline and humane care and included prayers, rest, and a serene, beautiful environment.

Multiperspective approach: a perspective that assumes the psychological symptoms we develop (or fail to develop) are likely the result of multiple factors.

Narcissistic personality disorder: a personality disorder marked by a persistent and excessive need to be admired and a lack of empathy.

Narcolepsy: a condition characterized by daytime sleepiness and sudden lapses into sleep, called sleep attacks, during the day.

Nasogastric feeding tube: a temporary flexible tube that passes through the nose to deliver liquid food to the stomach.

Negative correlation: occurs where increasing scores on one variable are matched with decreasing scores on the other.

Negative symptoms: a symptom of psychosis in which a person has deficits in expected behaviors.

Neurocognitive disorder due to Alzheimer's disease: a neurocognitive disorder marked by loss of thinking and language ability, and changes in personality and mood.

Neurocognitive disorders: psychological disorders characterized by cognitive decline that often arises from a medical condition or from substance withdrawal or intoxication.

Neurodevelopmental disorders: a group of psychological disorders that show symptoms during the developing years and can slow neurological growth or interfere with the achievement of certain cognitive or social milestones.

Neurogenesis: new nerve growth.

Neuron: a standard cell of the nervous system.

Neuropsychological tests: an assessment that measures the physiological responses that might be indicators of psychological events.

Neurotransmitters: molecules that communicate, or transmit, messages from one neuron to the next, including neurons in particular areas of the brain.

Nightmare disorder: a sleep-wake disorder in which a person experiences frequent disturbing dreams.

Not guilty by reason of insanity (NGRI): a legal plea that suggests a defendant is not responsible for a criminal act because they were suffering from a psychological condition at the time the act was committed.

Obsession: an unwanted thought that a person finds disturbing.

Obsessive compulsive disorder (OCD): a psychological disorder associated with obsessions, or obsessions linked to compulsions.

Obsessive-compulsive personality disorder (OCPD): a personality disorder marked by a pervasive pattern of orderliness and control at the expense of efficiency.

Operant conditioning: a type of learning that uses training to make desirable behaviors more likely to occur again and reduce the occurrence of others.

Opioids: psychoactive substances made from the opium poppy that relieve pain and reduce the activity of the nervous system.

Oppositional defiant disorder: a childhood disorder marked by repeatedly irritable, angry, defiant, argumentative, and often vindictive behavior.

Panic attack: a period of intense fear or discomfort that is linked with specific physical and psychological symptoms.

Panic disorder: an anxiety disorder characterized by the presence of frequent, recurrent panic attacks, along with the fear of panic attacks.

Paranoid personality disorder: a condition characterized by a long and unwavering history of attributing malicious intent to others that does not subside no matter how long the person may know these others.

Paraphilias: repeated intense sexual urges or fantasies about situations or objects outside societal sexual norms.

Paraphilic disorders: a condition in which an individual expresses problematic or inappropriate sexual fantasies, urges, or behaviors.

Parasomnias: sleep disorders characterized by problematic movements and dreams during sleep, or problems with sleep and wake patterns.

Parent management training (PMT): a behavioral treatment that aims to help parents learn successful discipline techniques, increase structure and predictability, and manage their child's behavior more effectively to promote desired behavior.

Parkinson's disease: a neurological disorder that results in tremors, rigidity, difficulty initiating movements, and, over time, difficulty controlling the muscles.

Pedophilic disorder: a paraphilic disorder where a person experiences sexually arousing fantasies or behaviors involving activity with a prepubescent child and accompanying distress or impairment.

Peripheral nervous system: a division of the nervous system that joins the rest of the body to the central nervous system.

Persistent depressive disorder (PDD): a depressive disorder characterized by a chronic low mood and other symptoms of depressive mood episodes.

Personality disorders: psychological conditions characterized by extremely inflexible personality characteristics that are persistent and pervasive.

Personality inventory: a test used to measure an individual's pattern of thinking, feeling, and behaving.

Phobia: a psychological symptom in which fear is unreasonably great or interferes with a person's life.

Placebos: medications without active ingredients.

Positive correlation: an association between two variables where both variables move in the same direction.

Positive symptoms: a set of symptoms of psychosis that are in addition to what is expected in the human experience, such as delusions, hallucinations, and disorganized thoughts, speech, and behavior.

Positron emission tomography (PET scan): a neuroscience imaging technique that uses radioactive glucose to indicate areas of activity.

Post-traumatic stress disorder (PTSD): a trauma and stressor-related disorder associated with experiencing a traumatic event, re-experiencing the trauma, and exhibiting symptoms of negative changes in mood and chronic arousal.

Practitioner-scholar model: a clinical psychology program that emphasizes clinical practice.

Premature ejaculation: a condition where a person has a persistent history of early ejaculation, poor control over ejaculation, and feelings of dissatisfaction and distress.

Premenstrual dysphoric disorder (PMDD): a depressive disorder in which a person shows symptoms of depression in most of their menstrual cycles during the weeks around menstruation.

Presenting problem: the reason a person has come in for treatment.

Prevalence: the proportion of a population who have a disease or health condition at a specific period of time.

Prion disease: a neurocognitive disorder caused by slow-acting virus-like proteins that can damage brain cells.

Projective tests: a kind of personality test that uses the interpretation of ambiguous stimuli to uncover unconscious conflicts.

Prolonged grief disorder: a depressive disorder in which a person experiences persistent grief that both exceeds cultural norms and causes significant distress and impairment.

Prosocial emotions: feelings such as responsibility, remorse or guilt for hurting someone, and empathy.

Prototypical approach: a diagnostic classification system in which the essential characteristics of disorders are identified, and which allows the identification of non-essential variations as well.

Psychiatry: a branch of medicine that treats mental and behavioral conditions.

Psychoactive drug: a chemical used to alter behavior, mood, thoughts, or consciousness, such as tobacco, alcohol, and cannabis.

Psychoanalysis: a psychodynamic treatment rooted in Freud's approach to psychotherapy.

Psychodynamic theories: a family of theories that focus on unconscious motivation.

Psychodynamic therapies: a family of treatments that have at their core the exploration of unconscious internal conflict.

Psychological disorders: psychological conditions that depart from the norm, are usually maladaptive, and may cause personal distress.

Psychological factors affecting other medical conditions: a condition diagnosed when physical illnesses are created or exacerbated by the interaction of biological, psychological, and emotional and social conditions.

Psychological theories: theories of psychopathology that explain psychopathology as influenced by environmental factors such as stress, trauma, or family situations.

Psychoneuroimmunology: a field that examines the relationship between the immune system and the stress response.

Psychopathology: the science of diagnosing and understanding all psychological disorders, including their causes, descriptions, and treatments.

Psychopharmacologists: researchers and practitioners who study and often prescribe medications for psychological disorders.

Psychopharmacology: the treatment of psychological conditions using medication.

Psychosis: a condition in which a person has lost some contact with reality.

Psychotic disorder: a psychological condition defined by the presence of significant symptoms of psychosis.

Pyromania: an impulse-control disorder associated with an irresistible drive toward deliberate and purposeful fire-setting that recurs on multiple occasions.

Random assignment: assigning participants to the experimental group and the control group entirely by chance, so that each person has an equal likelihood of appearing in each group.

Rapid eye movement (REM) sleep: a period of sleep characterized by darting eye movements and dreams.

Reciprocal-gene environment model: a multiperspective approach that suggests that with biological predispositions for certain conditions, patients themselves can increase the stress that makes symptoms worse.

Reliability: the consistency of a measurement.

REM sleep behavior disorder: a type of REM parasomnia in which a person will act out their dreams.

Right to refuse treatment: the legal principle that an individual can decline care.

Right to treatment: the legal right of an involuntarily committed individual to receive active care for their condition.

Schizoaffective disorder: a psychotic disorder in which an individual experiences a mix of the symptoms of mood disorder and schizophrenia.

Schizoid personality disorder: a personality disorder characterized by a pervasive pattern of detachment from social relationships and limited emotional expression.

Schizophrenia: a psychological condition characterized by disordered thinking, delusions, hallucination, and disordered behavior and emotions.

Schizophreniform disorder: a psychotic disorder in which the person meets the main criteria for schizophrenia with less impairment and for a shorter time period.

Schizotypal personality disorder: a personality disorder characterized by a pervasive pattern of discomfort in social relationships and by odd and eccentric behavior.

Scientist-practitioner model: a balanced clinical psychology program in which students learn both clinical skills and research skills.

Sedative, hypnotic, or anxiolytic use disorder: a substance-related disorder associated with impaired control over the amount and frequency of sedatives, hypnotics, or anxiolytics use and the experience of negative emotional states when not using those substances.

Selective serotonin reuptake inhibitors (SSRIs): a class of medications that increase the efficiency with which serotonin binds to postsynaptic neurons in the nervous system by blocking its reabsorption into the presynaptic neurons.

Serotonin-norepinephrine reuptake inhibitors (SNRIs): a class of medications that aim to keep both serotonin and norepinephrine in the synapse longer.

Sex: a set of various biological characteristics, such as hormones, chromosomes, and reproductive organs, that distinguish males and females.

Sexual arousal disorder: a condition where a person has an aversion to sexual contact, which can be experienced in a variety of ways.

Sexual desire disorders: conditions characterized by decreased sexual desire or a total lack of sexual interest or sexual fantasy.

Sexual dysfunctions: conditions in which a person has a concern with one or more areas of the sexual response cycle.

Sexual masochism disorder: a paraphilic disorder where a person experiences recurrent and intense sexually arousing fantasies, urges, or behaviors stemming from the act of being humiliated, beaten, bound, or otherwise made to suffer.

Sexual orientation: the nature of a person's emotional and physical attractions to others.

Sexual response cycle: a pattern of biological and psychological events that occurs in response to sexual stimulation.

Sexual sadism disorder: a paraphilic disorder where a person is aroused by the suffering of others and may inflict pain on them.

Sleep: a state of minimal consciousness associated with reduced motor and sensory activity.

Sleep apnea: a sleep disorder in which breathing stops.

Sleep terrors: also known as night terrors, are a sleep condition in which people experience sudden episodes of panic during Stage 4 sleep.

Social anxiety disorder: also known as *social phobia*, is an anxiety disorder characterized by performance anxiety in social situations.

Sociocultural perspective: a theoretical perspective that emphasizes the way social and cultural elements in the environment might interact with the person.

Somatic symptom disorder: a psychological condition where a person experiences significant physical symptoms that cause distress and/or impairment in the absence of a diagnosable condition.

Somatic symptom disorders: psychological conditions characterized by excessive focus on physical symptoms or health despite the absence of health concerns.

Specific phobias: an anxiety disorder characterized by fears of certain objects or certain situations.

Specifiers: in the *DSM* an extension to the diagnosis that is used to further clarify a diagnosis and allow more precision and information about a certain condition.

Standardized: a common set of steps is used to administer and score a measurement.

Stimulants: psychoactive substances that increase activity in the nervous system.

Substance use disorders: psychological conditions associated with compulsive use or craving of a drug that leads to impairment in social, work, or school functioning.

Supernatural theories: a theory that suggests that psychopathology is caused by demons or sin.

Suprachiasmatic nucleus: a part of the hypothalamus which is involved in sleep and wakefulness.

Symptom questionnaires: tests that measure the presence or absence of certain symptoms.

Tardive dyskinesia: a neurological condition characterized by involuntary repetitive movements.

Transgender or gender nonconforming (TGNC): people who are TGNC have a gender identity that is different from the gender that was assigned to them at birth.

Transvestic disorder: a condition where a person will dress in clothing of another gender and associate it with recurrent and intense sexual fantasies, urges, or behaviors.

Trephination: a procedure which entailed drilling holes in the skull, presumably to release demons or evil spirits from within.

Trichotillomania: an obsessive-compulsive and related disorder in which an individual repeatedly pulls out their hair.

Tricyclic antidepressants: a class of antidepressant drugs that have three rings in their molecular structure.

Typical antipsychotics: also known as first-generation antipsychotics, are beneficial in targeting the positive symptoms of psychosis, like hallucinations and delusions.

Vagus nerve stimulation (VNS): a treatment for depressive disorders in which an implanted pulse generator sends regular mild pulses of electrical energy to the vagus nerve to stimulate the brain.

Validity: the degree to which an assessment measures what it claims to measure.

Variables: the characteristics of behavior or experiences, such as exposure to trauma, that can be described and measured.

Vascular neurocognitive disorder: a neurocognitive disorder in which the blood vesicles in the brain become damaged or blocked, resulting in a decreased flow of oxygen to those parts of the brain.

Voyeuristic disorder: a paraphilic disorder in which a person has intense sexually arousing fantasies, urges, or behaviors that involve watching an unsuspecting person naked or engaged in sexual activity.

Worry: uneasiness about the past or even the future.

Wyatt Standards: guidelines which state that a mental institution must provide patients with a humane psychological and physical environment, qualified and sufficient staff, individual treatment plans, and minimal patient restrictions.

References

Aamodt, E. B., Schellhorn, T., Stage, E., Sanjay, A. B., Logan, P. E., Svaldi, D. O., . . . Beyer, M. K. (2021). Predicting the emergence of major neurocognitive disorder within three months after a stroke. *Frontiers in Aging Neuroscience*, *542*.

Abbott, S. M., Reid, K. J., & Zee, P. C. (2015). Circadian rhythm sleep-wake disorders. *Psychiatric Clinics*, *38*(4), 805–823.

Abdel-Hamid, I. A., & Ali, O. I. (2018). Delayed ejaculation: Pathophysiology, diagnosis, and treatment. *The World Journal of Men's Health*, *36*(1), 22–40.

Abele, H., Wagner, P., Sonek, J., Hoopmann, M., Brucker, S., Artunc, . . . Kagan, K. O. (2015). First trimester ultrasound screening for Down syndrome based on maternal age, fetal nuchal translucency and different combinations of the additional markers nasal bone, tricuspid and ductus venosus flow. *Prenatal Diagnosis*, *35*(12), 1182–1186.

Abramson, L. Y., Alloy, L. B., Hankin, B. L., Haeffel, G. J., MacCoon, D. G., & Gibb, B. E. (2002). Cognitive vulnerability-stress models of depression in a self-regulatory and psychobiological context. In I. H. Gotlib & C. L. Hammen (Eds.), *Handbook of depression* (pp. 268–294). New York, NY: Guilford Press.

Accordino, R. E., Kidd, C., Politte, L. C., Henry, C. A., & McDougle, C. J. (2016). Psychopharmacological interventions in autism spectrum disorder. *Expert Opinion on Pharmacotherapy*, *17*(7), 937–952.

Adjorlolo, S., Chan, H. C. O., & DeLisi, M. (2019). Mentally disordered offenders and the law: Research update on the insanity defense, 2004–2019. *International Journal of Law and Psychiatry*, *67*, 101507.

Adler, D. A., Irish, J., McLaughlin, T. J., Perissinotto, C., Chang, H., Hood, M., . . . Lerner, D. (2004). The work impact of dysthymia in a primary care population. *General Hospital Psychiatry*, *26*(4), 269–276. http://doi.org/10.1016/j.genhosppsych.2004.04.004

Adshead, G., & Sarkar, J. (2012). The nature of personality disorder. *Advances in Psychiatric Treatment*, *18*(3), 162–172. doi:10.1192/apt.bp.109.006981

Aftab, A., & Rashed, M. A. (2021). Mental disorder and social deviance. *International Review of Psychiatry*, *33*(5), 478–485.

Agha, M., Nisar, A., Liaqat, H., Choudry, U. K., Choudry, A. K., & Shoaib, M. (2017). Neurophysiological perspectives of borderline personality disorders. *Acta Psychopathologica*, *3*, 3.

Aghajani, M., Klapwijk, E. T., van der Wee, N. J., Veer, I. M., Rombouts, S. A., Boon, A. E., . . . Colins, O. F. (2017). Disorganized amygdala networks in conduct-disordered juvenile offenders with callous-unemotional traits. *Biological Psychiatry*, *82*(4), 283–293.

Agras, W. S., Fitzsimmons-Craft, E. E., & Wilfley, D. E. (2017). Evolution of cognitive-behavioral therapy for eating disorders. *Behaviour Research and Therapy*, *88*, 26–36.

Ahlgrim, C. (2018). *Amanda Bynes "went into a deep depression" because she disliked how she looked as a boy in "She's the Man."* Insider. Retrieved September 12, 2021, from www.insider.com/amanda-bynes-paper-magazine-interview-depression-shes-the-man-2018-11

Ahmad, S. I., & Hinshaw, S. P. (2016). Attention-deficit/hyperactivity disorder: Similarities to and differences from other externalizing disorders. In T. P. Beauchaine & S. P. Hinshaw (Eds.), *The Oxford handbook of externalizing spectrum disorders* (pp. 19–37). New York, NY: Oxford University Press.

Ahmed, I., & Thorpy, M. (2010). Clinical features, diagnosis and treatment of narcolepsy. *Clinics in Chest Medicine*, *31*(2), 371–381. https://doi.org/10.1016/j.ccm.2010.02.014

Aiton, F., & Silverman, R. (2021). Understanding and improving sleep for children with FASD. In R. A. S. Mukherjee & N. Aiton (Eds.), *Prevention, recognition and management of fetal alcohol spectrum disorders* (pp. 305–318). Cham: Springer.

Akın, O., Yeşilkaya, E., Sari, E., Akar, Ç., Başbozkurt, G., Macit, E., . . . Gül, H. (2016). A rare reason of hyperinsulinism: Munchausen syndrome by proxy.

Hormone Research in Paediatrics, *86*(6), 416–419. https://doi.org/10.1159/000446497

Akinhanmi, M. O., Biernacka, J. M., Strakowski, S. M., McElroy, S. L., Balls Berry, J. E., Merikangas, K. R., . . . Tamminga, C. (2018). Racial disparities in bipolar disorder treatment and research: A call to action. *Bipolar Disorders*, *20*(6), 506–514.

Alcoholics Anonymous World Services, Inc. (1989). *Twelve steps and twelve traditions*. Alcoholics Anonymous World Services.

Alda, M. (2021). The moving target of psychiatric diagnosis. *Journal of Psychiatry & Neuroscience: JPN*, *46*(3), E415–E417.

Aldao, A., Mennin, D. S., Linardatos, E., & Fresco, D. M. (2010). Differential patterns of physical symptoms and subjective processes in generalized anxiety disorder and unipolar depression. *Journal of Anxiety Disorders*, *24*, 250–259.

Alderfer, J., Hansen, R. A., & Mattingly, T. J. (2021). Understanding authorized generics: A review of the published clinical data. *Journal of Clinical Pharmacy and Therapeutics*, *46*(6), 1489–1497.

Aldrin, B., & Abraham, K. (2009). *Magnificent desolation: The long journey home from the moon*. New York, NY: Harmony Books.

Alim, T. N., Charney, D. S., & Mellman, T. A. (2006). An overview of posttraumatic stress disorder in African Americans. *Journal of Clinical Psychology*, *62*(7), 801–813.

Alipour, F., & Ahmadi, S. (2020). Social support and posttraumatic stress disorder (PTSD) in earthquake survivors: A systematic review. *Social Work in Mental Health*, *18*(5), 501–514.

Allen, J. B., & Iacono, W. G. (2001). Assessing the validity of amnesia in dissociative identity disorder: A dilemma for the DSM and the courts. *Psychology, Public Policy, & Law*, *7*, 311–344.

Allen, M. S., & Walter, E. E. (2019). Erectile dysfunction: An umbrella review of meta-analyses of risk-factors, treatment, and prevalence outcomes. *The Journal of Sexual Medicine*, *16*(4), 531–541.

Allison, L., & Strydom, A. (2009). Intellectual disability across cultures. *Psychiatry*, *8*, 355–357.

Alloy, L. B., & Abramson, L. Y. (2010). The role of the behavioral approach system (BAS) in bipolar spectrum disorders. *Current Directions in Psychological Science*, *19*(3), 189–194.

Alloy, L. B., Bender, R. E., Whitehouse, W. G., Wagner, C. A., Liu, R. T., Grant, D. A., . . . Abramson, L. Y.

(2012). High behavioral approach system (BAS) sensitivity, reward responsiveness, and goal-striving predict first onset of bipolar spectrum disorders: A prospective behavioral high-risk design. *Journal of Abnormal Psychology*, *121*(2), 339–351. http://doi.org/10.1037/a0025877

Alonso, J., Liu, Z., Evans-Lacko, S., Sadikova, E., Sampson, N., Chatterji, S., . . . WHO World Mental Health Survey Collaborators (2018). Treatment gap for anxiety disorders is global: Results of the World Mental Health Surveys in 21 countries. *Depression and Anxiety*, *35*(3), 195–208.

Alozai, U., & McPherson, P. K. (2020). Malingering. [Updated June 27, 2020]. *StatPearls* [Internet]. Treasure Island (FL): StatPearls Publishing. www.ncbi.nlm.nih.gov/books/NBK507837/

AlSalehi, S. M., & Alhifthy, E. H. (2020). Autism spectrum disorder. In M. A. M. Salih (Ed.), *Clinical child neurology* (pp. 275–292). Cham: Springer.

Alström, J. E., Nordlund, C. L., Persson, G., Harding, M., & Ljungqvist, C. (1984). Effects of four treatment methods on social phobic patients not suitable for insight-oriented psychotherapy. *Acta Psychiatrica Scandinavica*, *70*(2), 97–110.

Althof, S. E., & Needle, R. B. (2017). Treating low sexual desire in men. In Z. D. Peterson (Ed.), *The Wiley handbook of sex therapy* (pp. 32–39). Chichester: John Wiley & Sons.

Altieri, M., & Santangelo, G. (2021). The psychological impact of COVID-19 pandemic and lockdown on caregivers of people with dementia. *The American Journal of Geriatric Psychiatry*, *29*(1), 27–34.

Alzheimer's Association (2020). 2020 Alzheimer's disease facts and figures. *Alzheimer's & Dementia*, *16*(3), 391–460. https://doi.org/10.1002/alz.12068

Amad, A., Ramoz, N., Thomas, P., Jardri, R., & Gorwood, P. (2014). Genetics of borderline personality disorder: Systematic review and proposal of an integrative model. *Neuroscience & Biobehavioral Reviews*, *40*, 6–19.

American Psychiatric Association (1994). *Diagnostic and statistical manual of mental disorders* (4th ed.). Arlington, VA: Author.

American Psychiatric Association (2000). *Diagnostic and statistical manual of mental disorders* (4th ed. text rev.). Arlington, VA: Author.

American Psychiatric Association (2013). *Diagnostic and statistical manual of mental disorders* (5th ed.). Arlington, VA: Author.

American Psychiatric Association (2020). *The American psychiatric association practice guideline for the treatment of patients with schizophrenia.* Arlington, VA: Author.

American Psychiatric Association (2022). *Diagnostic and statistical manual of mental disorders* (5th ed., text rev.). Arlington, VA: Author.

American Psychological Association (2015). Guidelines for psychological practice with transgender and gender nonconforming people. *American Psychologist, 70*(9), 832–864.

Amore, M., Innamorati, M., Vittorio, C. D., Weinberg, I., Turecki, G., Sher, L., ... Pompili, M. (2014). Suicide attempts in major depressed patients with personality disorder. *Suicide and Life-Threatening Behavior, 44*(2), 155–166.

Anastas, T. M., Miller, M. M., Hollingshead, N. A., Stewart, J. C., Rand, K. L., & Hirsh, A. T. (2020). The unique and interactive effects of patient race, patient socioeconomic status, and provider attitudes on chronic pain care decisions. *Annals of Behavioral Medicine, 54*(10), 771–782. https://doi.org/10.1093/ABM/KAAA016

Anderson, K. K., Fuhrer, R., & Malla, A. K. (2010). The pathways to mental health care of first-episode psychosis patients: A systematic review. *Psychological Medicine, 40*(10), 1585–1597.

Anderson, K. N., Ailes, E. C., Danielson, M., Lind, J. N., Farr, S. L., Broussard, C. S., & Tinker, S. C. (2018). Attention-deficit/hyperactivity disorder medication prescription claims among privately insured women aged 15–44 years – United States, 2003–2015. *Morbidity and Mortality Weekly Report, 67*(2), 66.

Anderson, L. M., Berg, H., Brown, T. A., Menzel, J., & Reilly, E. E. (2021). The role of disgust in eating disorders. *Current Psychiatry Reports, 23*(2), 1–12.

Andrews, G., Hobbs, M. J., Borkovec, T. D., Beesdo, K., Craske, M. G., Heimberg, R. G., & Stanley, M. A. (2010). Generalized worry disorder: A review of DSM-IV generalized anxiety disorder and options for DSM-V. *Depression and Anxiety, 27*(2), 134–147. doi:10.1002/da.20658

Antal, H., Hossain, M. J., Hassink, S., Henry, S., Fuzzell, L., Taylor, A., & Wysocki, T. (2015). Audio-video recording of health care encounters for pediatric chronic conditions: Observational reactivity and its correlates. *Journal of Pediatric Psychology, 40*(1), 144–153.

Antelmi, E., Lippolis, M., Biscarini, F., Tinazzi, M., & Plazzi, G. (2021). REM sleep behavior disorder: Mimics and variants. *Sleep Medicine Reviews,* 101515. doi:10.1016/j.smrv.2021.101515

Antony, M. M. (2014). Behavior therapy. In D. Wedding & R. J. Corsini (Eds.), *Current psychotherapies* (10th ed., pp. 193–230). Independence, KY: Cengage Publications.

Armstrong, L. V., Hogg, L., & Jacobsen, P. (2021). Do voice-hearing assessment measures capture the positive experiences of individuals, and to what extent? A systematic review of published assessment measures. *Psychosis,* 1–14. https://doi.org/10.1080/17522439.2021.1924242

Armstrong, S. C. (2009). *Not all black girls know how to eat: A story of bulimia.* Chicago, IL: Chicago Review Press.

Arnold, L. E., Hodgkins, P., Kahle, J., Madhoo, M., & Kewley, G. (2020). Long-term outcomes of ADHD: Academic achievement and performance. *Journal of Attention Disorders, 24*(1), 73–85.

Arroll, B., Macgillivray, S., Ogston, S., Reid, I., Sullivan, F., Williams, B., & Crombie, I. (2005). Efficacy and tolerability of tricyclic antidepressants and SSRIs compared with placebo for treatment of depression in primary care: A meta-analysis. *Annals of Family Medicine, 3*(5), 449–456. https://doi.org/10.1370/afm.349

Atuk, E., & Richardson, T. (2021). Relationship between dysfunctional beliefs, self-esteem, extreme appraisals, and symptoms of mania and depression over time in bipolar disorder. *Psychology and Psychotherapy: Theory, Research and Practice, 94,* 212–222.

Atwood, M. E., & Friedman, A. (2020). A systematic review of enhanced cognitive behavioral therapy (CBT-E) for eating disorders. *International Journal of Eating Disorders, 53*(3), 311–330.

Avidan, A. Y., & Kaplish, N. (2010, June). The parasomnias: Epidemiology, clinical features, and diagnostic approach. *Clinics in Chest Medicine.* https://doi.org/10.1016/j.ccm.2010.02.015

Axelrod, M. I., & Santagata, M. L. (2021). Behavioral parent training. In A. Maragakis, C. Drossel, & T. J. Waltz (Eds.), *Applications of behavior analysis in healthcare and beyond* (pp. 135–154). Cham: Springer.

Aybek, S., Nicholson, T. R., Zelaya, F., O'Daly, O. G., Craig, T. J., David, A. S., & Kanaan, R. A. (2014). Neural correlates of recall of life events in conversion disorder. *JAMA Psychiatry, 71*(1), 52–60.

Ayearst, L. E., & Bagby, R. M. (2010). Evaluating the psychometric properties of psychological measures. In M. M. Antony & D. H. Barlow (Eds.), *Handbook of assessment and treatment planning for psychological disorders* (pp. 23–61). New York, NY: Guilford Press.

Ayers, C. R., Saxena, S., Golshan, S., & Wetherell, J. L. (2009). Age at onset and clinical features of late life compulsive hoarding. *International Journal of Geriatric Psychiatry, 25*, 142–149.

Azofeifa, A., Rexach-Guzmán, B. D., Hagemeyer, A. N., Rudd, R. A., & Sauber-Schatz, E. K. (2019). Driving under the influence of marijuana and illicit drugs among persons aged ≥ 16 years – United States, 2018. *Morbidity and Mortality Weekly Report, 68*(50), 1153.

Badawi, H. F., & El Saddik, A. (2019). Biofeedback in healthcare: State of the art and meta review. In A. El Saddik, M. S. Hossain, & B. Kantarci (Eds.), *Connected health in smart cities* (pp. 113–142). Cham: Springer.

Baer, R. A., Peters, J. R., Eisenlohr-Moul, T. A., Geiger, P. J., & Sauer, S. E. (2012). Emotion-related cognitive processes in borderline personality disorder: A review of the empirical literature. *Clinical Psychology Review, 32*(5), 359–369.

Baglivio, M. T., Wolff, K. T., Piquero, A. R., Greenwald, M. A., & Epps, N. (2017). Racial/ethnic disproportionality in psychiatric diagnoses and treatment in a sample of serious juvenile offenders. *Journal of Youth and Adolescence, 46*(7), 1424–1451.

Bala, A., Nguyen, H. M. T., & Hellstrom, W. J. (2018). Post-SSRI sexual dysfunction: A literature review. *Sexual Medicine Reviews, 6*(1), 29–34.

Ballentine, K. L. (2019). Understanding racial differences in diagnosing ODD versus ADHD using critical race theory. *Families in Society, 100*(3), 282–292.

Bandelow, B., & Michaelis, S. (2015). Epidemiology of anxiety disorders in the 21st century. *Dialogues in Clinical Neuroscience, 17*(3), 327–335.

Barateau, L., Lopez, R., Franchi, J. A. M., & Dauvilliers, Y. (2017). Hypersomnolence, hypersomnia, and mood disorders. *Current Psychiatry Reports, 19*(2), 13. https://doi.org/10.1007/s11920–017-0763-0

Barber, J. P., Milrod, B., Gallop, R., Solomonov, N., Rudden, M. G., McCarthy, K. S., & Chambless, D. L. (2020). Processes of therapeutic change: Results from the Cornell-Penn Study of Psychotherapies for Panic Disorder. *Journal of Counseling Psychology, 67*(2), 222–231. https://doi-org.proxy.library.emory.edu/10.1037/cou0000417

Barbui, C., Motterlini, N., & Garattini, L. (2006). Health status, resource consumption, and costs of dysthymia. A multi-center two-year longitudinal study. *Journal of Affective Disorders, 90*(2–3), 181–186.

Barkowski, S., Schwartze, D., Strauss, B., Burlingame, G. M., & Rosendahl, J. (2020). Efficacy of group psychotherapy for anxiety disorders: A systematic review and meta-analysis. *Psychotherapy Research, 30*(8), 965–982.

Barlow, D. H., Gorman, J. M., Shear, M. K., & Woods, S. W. (2000). Cognitive-behavioral therapy, imipramine, or their combination for panic disorder: A randomized controlled trial. *Journal of the American Medical Association, 283*, 2529–2536.

Basco, M. R., & Rush, A. J. (2005). *Cognitive-behavioral therapy for bipolar disorder*. New York, NY: Guilford Press.

Bass, C., & Halligan, P. (2014). Factitious disorders and malingering: Challenges for clinical assessment and management. *The Lancet, 383*(9926), 1422–1432.

Bateman, A. W., Gunderson, J., & Mulder, R. (2015). Treatment of personality disorder. *The Lancet, 385*(9969), 735–743.

Bates, A. T., & Alici, Y. (2014). Understanding and treating delirium. *Psychiatric Times, 31*(12), 41.

Bayes, A., & Parker, G. (2017). Borderline personality disorder in men: A literature review and illustrative case vignettes. *Psychiatry Research, 257*, 197–202.

Bayramova, A. (2018). Erectile dysfunction: Causes and diagnosis. *Clinical Case Reports Open Access, 1*(1), 101.

Beaulieu, J. M., & Gainetdinov, R. R. (2011). The physiology, signaling, and pharmacology of dopamine receptors. *Pharmacological Reviews, 63*(1), 182–217.

Bech, P. (2009). Clinical features of mood disorders and mania. In M. G. Gelder, N. C. Andreasen, J. J. Lopez-Ibor, Jr., & J. R. Geddes (Eds.). *The new Oxford textbook of psychiatry* (2nd ed., vol. I, pp. 632–637). Oxford: Oxford University Press.

Beck, A. T. (Ed.). (1979). *Cognitive therapy of depression*. New York, NY: Guilford Press.

Beck, A. T., Davis, D. D., & Freeman, A. (Eds.). (2015). *Cognitive therapy of personality disorders*. New York, NY: Guilford Press.

Beck, A. T., & Emery, G. (1985). *Anxiety disorders and phobias: A cognitive perspective*. New York, NY: Basic Books.

Beck, A. T., Rush, A. J., Shaw, B. F., & Emery, G. (1987). *Cognitive therapy of depression*. New York, NY: Guilford Press.

Beck, A. T., Steer, R. A., & Brown, G. K. (1996). Beck depression inventory-II. *San Antonio, 78*(2), 490–498.

Beck, A. T., Ward, C. H., Mendelson, M., Mock, J. E., & Erbaugh, J. (1962). Reliability of psychiatric diagnosis: 2. A study of consistency of clinical judgements and ratings. *The American Journal of Psychiatry, 119*, 351–357.

Beck, A. T., & Weishaar, M. E. (2019). Cognitive therapy. In D. Wedding & R. J. Corsini (Eds.), *Current psychotherapies* (11th ed., pp. 237–272). Independence, KY: Cengage Publications.

Becker, C. B., Zayfert, C., & Anderson, E. (2004). A survey of psychologists' attitudes towards and utilization of exposure therapy for PTSD. *Behaviour Research and Therapy, 42*(3), 277–292.

Behrman, A. (2002). *Electroboy: A Memoir of Mania*. New York, NY: Random House.

Bello, N. T., & Hajnal, A. (2010). Dopamine and binge eating behaviors. *Pharmacology Biochemistry and Behavior, 97*(1), 25–33.

Belmaker, R. H. (2004). Bipolar disorder. *New England Journal of Medicine, 351*(5), 476–486.

Beltrán, S., Sit, L., & Ginsburg, K. R. (2021). A call to revise the diagnosis of oppositional defiant disorder: Diagnoses are for helping, not harming. *JAMA Psychiatry, 78*(11), 1181–1182.

Beltrani, A., & Zapf, P. A. (2020). Competence to stand trial and criminalization: An overview of the research. *CNS Spectrums, 25*(2), 161–172. https://doi.org/10.1017/S1092852919001597

Bem, S. L. (1981). *Bem sex role inventory*. Palo Alto, CA: Consulting Psychologists Press.

Benham, G. (2020, August 19). Sleep paralysis in college students. *Journal of American College Health*, 1–6. doi:10.1080/07448481.2020.1799807

Benjet, C., Bromet, E., Karam, E. G., Kessler, R. C., McLaughlin, K. A., Ruscio, A. M., . . . Alonso, J. (2016). The epidemiology of traumatic event exposure worldwide: Results from the World Mental Health Survey Consortium. *Psychological Medicine, 46*(2), 327–343.

Benuto, L. T., Casas, J. B., Bennett, N. M., & Leany, B. D. (2020). The MMPI-2-RF: A pilot study of Latinx vs. non-Latinx Whites profiles. *Professional Psychology: Research and Practice, 51*(5), 496–506. https://doi.org/10.1037/pro0000359

Bergeron, S., Reed, B. D., Wesselmann, U., & Bohm-Starke, N. (2020). Vulvodynia. *Nature Reviews Disease Primers, 6*(1), 1–21.

Berghuis, H., Bandell, C. C., & Krueger, R. F. (2021). Predicting dropout using DSM–5 Section II personality disorders, and DSM–5 Section III personality traits, in a (day) clinical sample of personality disorders. *Personality Disorders: Theory, Research, and Treatment, 12*(4), 331–338.

Bergner, R. M., & Bunford, N. (2017). Mental disorder is a disability concept, not a behavioral one. *Philosophy, Psychiatry, & Psychology, 24*(1), 25–40.

Bernal-Manrique, K. N., García-Martín, M. B., & Ruiz, F. J. (2020). Effect of acceptance and commitment therapy in improving interpersonal skills in adolescents: A randomized waitlist control trial. *Journal of Contextual Behavioral Science, 17*, 86–94.

Bernard, J. L. (1977). The significance for psychology of O'Connor v. Donaldson. *American Psychologist, 32*(12), 1085–1088.

Berrettini, W. (2017). A brief review of the genetics and pharmacogenetics of opioid use disorders. *Dialogues in Clinical Neuroscience, 19*(3), 229–236. https://doi.org/10.31887/DCNS.2017.19.3/wberrettini

Berry, S. M., Broglio, K., Bunker, M., Jayewardene, A., Olin, B., & Rush, A. J. (2013). A patient-level meta-analysis of studies evaluating vagus nerve stimulation therapy for treatment-resistant depression. *Medical Devices* (Auckland, NZ), *6*, 17.

Bertsch, K., Krauch, M., Roelofs, K., Cackowski, S., Herpertz, S. C., & Volman, I. (2019). Out of control? Acting out anger is associated with deficient prefrontal emotional action control in male patients with borderline personality disorder. *Neuropharmacology, 156*, 107463.

Bhat, V., & Kennedy, S. H. (2018). Vagus nerve stimulation: A treatment in evolution. *Cognitive and Behavioral Neurology, 31*(2), 99–100.

Bhukhari, S. R., Saba, F., & Fatima, S. I. (2018). The efficacy of cognitive behavior therapy for obsessive compulsive personality disorder. *Pakistan Journal of Clinical Psychology, 17*(1).

Bhutta, M. R., Hong, M. J., Kim, Y., & Hong, K. (2015). Single-trial lie detection using a combined fNIRS-polygraph system. *Frontiers in Psychology, 6*, 709.

Biederman, J., Mick, E., Faraone, S. V., Braaten, E., Doyle, A., Spencer, T., Wilens, T. E., Frazier, E., & Johnson, M. A. (2002). Influence of gender on attention deficit hyperactivity disorder in children referred to a psychiatric clinic. *The American Journal of Psychiatry, 159*(1), 36–42. https://doi.org/10.1176/appi.ajp.159.1.36

Billard, T. J. (2018). Attitudes toward transgender men and women: Development and validation of a new measure. *Frontiers in Psychology, 9*, 387.

Biondich, A. S., & Joslin, J. D. (2016). Coca: The history and medical significance of an ancient Andean tradition. *Emergency Medicine International, 2016*, 4048764. https://doi.org/10.1155/2016/4048764

Black, D. W. (2019). *Antisocial personality disorder: Epidemiology, clinical manifestations, course and diagnosis. UpToDate.* www.uptodate.com/contents/

antisocial-personality-disorder-epidemiology-clinical-manifestations-course-and-diagnosis

Black, D. W., & Shaw, M. (2019). The epidemiology of gambling disorder. In A. Heinz, N. Romanczuk-Seiferth, & M. Potenza (Eds.), *Gambling disorder* (pp. 29–48). Cham: Springer. https://doi.org/10.1007/978-3-030-03060-5_3

Blair, J., Mitchell, D., & Blair, K. (2005). *The psychopath: Emotion and the brain.* Malden, MA: Blackwell Publishing.

Blihar, D., Delgado, E., Buryak, M., Gonzalez, M., & Waechter, R. (2020). A systematic review of the neuroanatomy of dissociative identity disorder. *European Journal of Trauma & Dissociation, 4*(3), 100148.

Bloch, M. H., Landeros-Weisenberger, A., Rosario, M. C., Pittenger, C., & Leckman, J. F. (2008). Meta analysis of the symptom structure of obsessive-compulsive disorder. *The American Journal of Psychiatry, 165*(12), 1532–1542. doi:10.1176/appi.ajp.2008.08020320

Bloch, S., & Green, S. A. (Eds.). (2021). *Psychiatric ethics.* New York, NY: Oxford University Press.

Blythin, S. P., Nicholson, H. L., Macintyre, V. G., Dickson, J. M., Fox, J. R., & Taylor, P. J. (2020). Experiences of shame and guilt in anorexia and bulimia nervosa: A systematic review. *Psychology and Psychotherapy: Theory, Research and Practice, 93*(1), 134–159.

Bodryzlova, Y., Audet, J. S., Bergeron, K., & O'Connor, K. (2019). Group cognitive-behavioural therapy for hoarding disorder: Systematic review and meta-analysis. *Health & Social Care in the Community, 27*(3), 517–530.

Bodur, O. C., Özkan, E. H., Çolak, Ö., Arslan, H., Sarı, N., Dişli, A., & Arslan, F. (2021). Preparation of acetylcholine biosensor for the diagnosis of Alzheimer's disease. *Journal of Molecular Structure, 1223*, 129168.

Boelen, P. A., & Lenferink, L. I. (2020). Comparison of six proposed diagnostic criteria sets for disturbed grief. *Psychiatry Research, 285*, 112786.

Bogels, S. M., Alden, L., Beidel, D. C., Clark, L. A., Pine, D. S., Stein, M. B., & Voncken, M. (2010). Social anxiety disorder: Questions and answers for the DSM-V. *Depression and Anxiety, 27*, 168–189.

Boinstein, R. F. (2007). Might the Rorschach be a projective test after all? Social projection of an undesired trait alters Rorschach oral dependency scores. *Journal of Personality Assessment, 88*(3), 324–367.

Boness, C. L., Hershenberg, R., Kaye, J., Mackintosh, M. A., Grasso, D. J., Noser, A., & Raffa, S. D. (2020). An evaluation of cognitive behavioral therapy for insomnia: A systematic review and application of Tolin's criteria for

empirically supported treatments. *Clinical Psychology: Science and Practice, 27*(4). https://doi.org/10.1111/cpsp.12348

Bonfils, K. A., Lysaker, P. H., Yanos, P. T., Siegel, A., Leonhardt, B. L., James, A. V., ... Davis, L. W. (2018). Self-stigma in PTSD: Prevalence and correlates. *Psychiatry Research, 265*, 7–12.

Bonnet, L., Comte, A., Tatu, L., Millot, J. L., Moulin, T., & Medeiros de Bustos, E. (2015). The role of the amygdala in the perception of positive emotions: An "intensity detector." *Frontiers in Behavioral Neuroscience, 9*, 178.

Borkovec, T. D., Newman, M. G., & Castonguay, L. G. (2003). Cognitive-behavioral therapy for generalized anxiety disorder with integrations from interpersonal and experiential therapies. *CNS Spectrums, 8*, 382–389.

Bornstein, R. F. (2012). Dependent personality disorder. In T. A. Widiger (Ed.), *The Oxford handbook of personality disorders* (pp. 505–526). New York, NY: Oxford University Press. https://doi.org/10.1093/oxfordhb/9780199735013.013.0023

Botticelli, M. P., & Koh, H. K. (2016). Changing the language of addiction. *JAMA, 316*(13), 1361. https://doi.org/10.1001/jama.2016.11874

Bourgin, J., Tebeka, S., Mallet, J., Mazer, N., Dubertret, C., & Le Strat, Y. (2020). Prevalence and correlates of psychotic-like experiences in the general population. *Schizophrenia Research, 215*, 371–377.

Bowrey, G. D., & Smark, C. J. (2010). Measurement and the decline of moral therapy. In H. Yeatman (Ed.), *The Sinet 2010 eBook* (pp. 168–176). Wollongong, Australia: Sinet UOW.

Bradford, A. (2017). Treatment of female orgasmic disorder. *UpToDate.* www.uptodate.com/contents/treatment-of-female-orgasmic-disorder

Bradley, R., Conklin, C. Z., & Westen, D. (2007). Borderline personality disorder. In W. O'Donohue, K. A. Fowler, & S. O. Lilienfeld (Eds.), *Personality disorders: Toward the DSM-V* (pp. 167–201). London: Sage Publications.

Brady, K. T., Levin, F. R., Galanter, M., & Kleber, H. D. (2021). *The American Psychiatric Association Publishing textbook of substance use disorder treatment* (6th ed.). *Washington, DC:* American Psychiatric Association Publishing.

Braham, M. Y., Jedidi, M., Chkirbene, Y., Hmila, I., ElKhal, M. C., Souguir, M. K., & Ben Dhiab, M. (2017). Caregiver-fabricated illness in a child: A case report of three siblings. *Journal of Forensic Nursing, 13*(1), 39–42. https://doi.org/10.1097/JFN.0000000000000141

Brand, B. L., Sar, V., Stavropoulos, P., Krüger, C., Korzekwa, M., Martínez-Taboas, A., & Middleton, W. (2016). Separating fact from fiction: An empirical examination of six myths about dissociative identity disorder. *Harvard Review of Psychiatry, 24*(4), 257–270.

Braxton, L. E., Calhoun, P. S., William, J. E., & Boggs, C. D. (2007). Validity rates of the Personality Assessment Inventory and the Minnesota Multiphasic Personality Inventory-2 in a VA medical center setting. *Journal of Personality Assessment, 88*(1), 5–15.

Brefczynski-Lewis, J. A. (2020). Human neuroimaging-based connections between stress, cardiovascular disease and depression. In P. D. Chantler & K. T. Larkin (Eds.), *Cardiovascular implications of stress and depression* (pp. 141–173). London: Academic Press.

Brennan, T. J., & O'Reilly, F. (2017). *Shooting ghosts: A U.S. Marine, a combat photographer, and their journey back from war.* New York, NY: Viking.

Bressert, S. (2017). Fetishistic disorder symptoms. *PsychCentral.* https://psychcentral.com/disorders/fetishism-symptoms.

Brewster, G., Riegel, B., & Gehrman, P. R. (2018). Insomnia in the older adult. *Sleep Medicine Clinics, 13*(1), 13.

Bridler, R., Häberle, A., Müller, S. T., Cattapan, K., Grohmann, R., Toto, S., ... Greil, W. (2015). Psychopharmacological treatment of 2195 in-patients with borderline personality disorder: A comparison with other psychiatric disorders. *European Neuropsychopharmacology, 25*(6), 763–772.

Briggs, S., Netuveli, G., Gould, N., Gkaravella, A., Gluckman, N., Kangogyere, P., ... Lindner, R. (2019). The effectiveness of psychoanalytic/psychodynamic psychotherapy for reducing suicide attempts and self-harm: Systematic review and meta-analysis. *The British Journal of Psychiatry, 214*(6), 320–328. doi:10.1192/bjp.2019.33

Britton, J. C., Grillon, C., Lissek, S., Norcross, M. A., Szuhany, K. L., Chen, G., ... Pine, D. S. (2013). Response to learned threat: An fMRI study in adolescent and adult anxiety. *The American Journal of Psychiatry, 170*(10), 1195–1204.

Britton, J. C., & Rauch, S. L. (2009). Neuroanatomy and neuroimaging of anxiety disorders. In M. M. Antony & M. B. Stein (Eds.), *The Oxford handbook of anxiety and related disorders* (pp. 97–110). New York, NY: Oxford University Press.

Broft, A., Shingleton, R., Kaufman, J., Liu, F., Kumar, D., Slifstein, M., ... Walsh, B. T. (2012). Striatal dopamine in

bulimia nervosa: A PET imaging study. *International Journal of Eating Disorders, 45*(5), 648–656.

Brooks, S. J., Rask-Andersen, M., Benedict, C., & Schiöth, H. B. (2012). A debate on current eating disorder diagnoses in light of neurobiological findings: Is it time for a spectrum model? *BMC Psychiatry, 12*(1), 76. https://doi.org/10.1186/1471-244x-12-76

Brosschot, J. F., Van Dijk, E., & Thayer, J. F. (2007). Daily worry is related to low heart rate variability during waking and the subsequent nocturnal sleep period. *International Journal of Psychophysiology, 63*, 39–47.

Brown, E., Gray, R., Monaco, S. L., O'Donoghue, B., Nelson, B., Thompson, A., ... McGorry, P. (2020). The potential impact of COVID-19 on psychosis: A rapid review of contemporary epidemic and pandemic research. *Schizophrenia Research, 222*, 79–87.

Brown, G. R. (2017, September). Exhibitionistic disorder (exhibitionism). *Merck Manual.*

Bryant, R. A., Friedman, M. J., Spiegel, D., Ursano, R., & Strain, J. (2011). A review of acute stress disorder in DSM-5. *Depression and Anxiety, 28*, 802–817.

Bulik, C. M., Blake, L., & Austin, J. (2019). Genetics of eating disorders: What the clinician needs to know. *Psychiatric Clinics, 42*(1), 59–73.

Burcusa, S. L., & Iacono, W. G. (2007). Risk for recurrence in depression. *Clinical Psychology Review, 27*(8), 959–985.

Burkauskas, J., & Fineberg, N. A. (2020). History and epidemiology of OCPD. In J. E. Grant, A. Pinto, & S. R. Chamberlain (Eds.), *Obsessive-compulsive personality disorder* (pp. 1–26). Washington, DC: American Psychiatric Association Publishing.

Burke, T. A., Jacobucci, R., Ammerman, B. A., Piccirillo, M., McCloskey, M. S., Heimberg, R. G., & Alloy, L. B. (2018). Identifying the relative importance of non-suicidal self-injury features in classifying suicidal ideation, plans, and behavior using exploratory data mining. *Psychiatry Research, 262*, 175–183.

Busch, F. N., Milrod, B. L., Singer, M. B., & Aronson, A. C. (2012). *Manual of panic focused psychodynamic psychotherapy – extended range.* New York, NY: Routledge.

Butler, A. C., Chapman, J. E., Forman, E. M., & Beck, A. T. (2006, January). The empirical status of cognitive-behavioral therapy: A review of meta-analyses. *Clinical Psychology Review, 26*(1), 17–31. http://doi.org/10.1016/j.cpr.2005.07.003

Butler, B. (2006). NGRI revisited: Venirepersons' attitudes toward the insanity defense. *Journal of Applied Social*

Psychology, *36*(8), 1833–1847. https://doi.org/10.1111/j
.0021-9029.2006.00084.x

Bylsma, L. M., Taylor-Clift, A., & Rottenberg, J. (2011).
Emotional reactivity to daily events in major and minor
depression. *Journal of Abnormal Psychology*, *120*(1),
155–167.

Cabrera, F. J., Herrera, A. D. R. C., Rubalcava, S. J., &
Martínez, K. I. (2017). Behavior patterns of antisocial
teenagers interacting with parents and peers:
A longitudinal study. *Frontiers in Psychology*, *8*, 757.

Cahalan, S. (2019). *The great pretender: The undercover
mission that changed our understanding of madness*.
London: Hachette.

Cain, S. (2013). *Quiet: The power of introverts in a world
that can't stop talking*. New York, NY: Crown.

Calamari, J. E., Chik, H. M., Pontarelli, N. K., & DeJong,
B. L. (2012). Phenomenology and epidemiology of
obsessive compulsive disorder. In G. Steketee (Ed.), *The
Oxford handbook of obsessive compulsive and spectrum
disorders* (pp. 11–47). New York, NY: Oxford University
Press.

Cale, E. M., & Lilienfeld, S. O. (2002). Sex differences in
psychopathy and antisocial personality disorder: A review
and integration. *Clinical Psychology Review*, *22*(8),
1179–1207.

Caligor, E., & Clarkin, J. F. (2010). An object relations model
of personality and personality pathology. In J. F. Clarkin,
P. Fonagy, & G. O. Gabbard (Eds.), *Psychodynamic
psychotherapy for personality disorders: A clinical
handbook* (pp. 3–35). Washington, DC: American
Psychiatric Publishing.

Callahan, L. A., McGreevy, M. A., Cirincione, C., &
Steadman, H. J. (1992). Measuring the effects of the
guilty but mentally ill (GBMI) verdict. *Law and Human
Behavior*, *16*(4), 447–462.

Calzada-Reyes, A., Alvarez-Amador, A., Galán-García, L., &
Valdés-Sosa, M. (2012). Electroencephalographic
abnormalities in antisocial personality disorder. *Journal of
Forensic and Legal Medicine*, *19*(1), 29–34.

Campbell, S. J. (2021). Telling their stories: Photo exhibit at
ValleyCAST Battles Stigma of Mental Illness. *Telegram
& Gazette*, September 15. www.telegram.com/story/
lifestyle/2021/09/15/yellow-tulip-project-photo-exhibit-
valleycast-mental-illness-stigma/5665500001/.

Campbell, W. K., & Miller, J. D. (Eds.). (2011). *The
handbook of narcissism and narcissistic personality
disorder*. Hoboken, NJ: John Wiley & Sons.

Campbell-Sills, L., & Barlow, D. H. (2007). Incorporating
emotion regulation into conceptualizations and treatments

of anxiety and mood disorders. In J. J. Gross (Ed.),
Handbook of emotion regulation (pp. 542–559). New
York, NY: Guilford Press.

Canady, V. A. (2021). New reports reveals billions in cost of
schizophrenia. *Mental Health Weekly*, *31*(28), 7–8.

Canino, G., Polanczyk, G., Bauermeister, J. J., Rohde, L. A.,
& Frick, P. J. (2010). Does the prevalence of CD and
ODD vary across cultures?. *Social Psychiatry and
Psychiatric Epidemiology*, *45*(7), 695–704.

Cao, J., Wei, J., Fritzsche, K., Toussaint, A. C., Li, T., Jiang,
Y., . . . Ma, X. (2020). Prevalence of DSM-5 somatic
symptom disorder in Chinese outpatients from general
hospital care. *General Hospital Psychiatry*, *62*, 63–71.

Cardinale, E. M., Ryan, R. M., & Marsh, A. A. (2021).
Maladaptive fearlessness: An examination of the
association between subjective fear experience and
antisocial behaviors linked with callous unemotional
traits. *Journal of Personality Disorders*, *35*(Supplement
A), 39–56.

Cardozo, B. L., Kaiser, R., Gotway, C. A., & Agani, F. (2003).
Mental health, social functioning, and feelings of hatred and
revenge in Kosovar Albanians one year after the war in
Kosovo. *Journal of Traumatic Stress*, *16*, 351–360.

Cariola, L. (2020). Psychodynamic processes. In C. Zeigler-
Hill & T. Shackelford, (Eds.), *Encyclopedia of personality
and individual differences* (pp. 4131–4136). Cham:
Springer.

Carpenter, K. M., Williams, K., & Worly, B. (2017). Treating
women's orgasmic difficulties. In Z. D. Peterson (Ed.),
The Wiley handbook of sex therapy (pp. 57–71).
Chichester: John Wiley & Sons.

Carr, S. N., & Francis, A. J. (2010). Do early maladaptive
schemas mediate the relationship between childhood
experiences and avoidant personality disorder features?
A preliminary investigation in a non-clinical
sample. *Cognitive Therapy and Research*, *34*(4), 343–358.

Carson, A. J., Brown, R., David, A. S., Duncan, R., Edwards,
M. J., Goldstein, L. H., . . . Voon, V. (2012). Functional
(conversion) neurological symptoms: Research since the
millennium. *Journal of Neurology, Neurosurgery &
Psychiatry*, *83*(8), 842–850.

Cartwright, S. (1851). Diseases and peculiarities of the Negro
race: Africans in America. *De Bow's Review Southern and
Western States*.

Cascade, E., Kalali, A. H., & Kennedy, S. H. (2009). Real-
world data on SSRI antidepressant side effects. *Psychiatry
(Edgmont)*, *6*(2), 16–18.

Caseras, X., Lawrence, N. S., Murphy, K., Wise, R. G., &
Phillips, M. L. (2013). Ventral striatum activity in

response to reward: Differences between bipolar I and II disorders. *The American Journal of Psychiatry, 170*(5), 533–541.

Cash, S. S., Halgren, E., Dehghani, N., Rossetti, A. O., Thesen, T., Wang, C., . . . Ulbert, I. (2009). The human K-complex represents an isolated cortical down-state. *Science (New York, N.Y.), 324*(5930), 1084–1087. https://doi.org/10.1126/science.1169626

Castellini, G., Rellini, A. H., Appignanesi, C., Pinucci, I., Fattorini, M., Grano, E., . . . Ricca, V. (2018). Deviance or normalcy? The relationship among paraphilic thoughts and behaviors, hypersexuality, and psychopathology in a sample of university students. *The Journal of Sexual Medicine, 15*(9), 1322–1335.

Catanesi, R., Martino, V., Candelli, C., Troccoli, G., Grattagliano, I., Vella, G. D., & Carabellese, F. (2013). Posttraumatic stress disorder: Protective and risk factors in 18 survivors of a plane crash. *Journal of Forensic Sciences, 58*(5), 1388–1392.

CDC (2021, May 21). *Basics about FASDs*. Centers for Disease Control and Prevention. www.cdc.gov/ncbddd/fasd/facts.html

Celentano, D. (2020). The worldwide opioid pandemic: Epidemiologic perspectives. *Epidemiologic Reviews, 42*(1), 1–3. https://doi.org/10.1093/epirev/mxaa012

Cerdá, M., Nandi, V., Frye, V., Egan, J. E., Rundle, A., Quinn, J. W., . . . Van Tieu, H. (2017). Neighborhood determinants of mood and anxiety disorders among men who have sex with men in New York City. *Social Psychiatry and Psychiatric Epidemiology, 52*(6), 749–760.

Cerniglia, L., Muratori, P., Milone, A., Paciello, M., Ruglioni, L., Cimino, S., . . . Tambelli, R. (2017). Paternal psychopathological risk and psychological functioning in children with eating disorders and disruptive behavior disorder. *Psychiatry Research, 254*, 60–66.

Chadwick, P. K. (2014). Peer-professional first person account: Before psychosis—schizoid personality from the inside. *Schizophrenia Bulletin, 40*(3), 483–486.

Challa, M., Scott, C., & Turban, J. L. (2020). Epidemiology of pediatric gender identity. In M. Forcier, G. Van Schalkwyk, & J. L. Turban (Eds.), *Pediatric gender identity: Gender-affirming care for transgender & gender diverse youth* (pp. 15–31). Cham: Springer International.

Chapman, A. L., Hope, N. H., & Turner, B. J. (2020). Borderline personality disorder. In C. W. Lejuez & K. L. Gratz (Eds.), *The Cambridge handbook of personality disorders* (pp. 223–241). New York, NY: Cambridge University Press.

Charney, D. S. (2004). Psychobiological mechanisms of resilience and vulnerability: Implications for successful adaptation to extreme stress. *The American Journal of Psychiatry, 161*, 195–216.

Cheli, S. (2020). Assessment and treatment planning for schizotypal personality disorder: A metacognitively oriented point of view. *Psychiatric Rehabilitation Journal, 43*(4), 335–343.

Chemerinski, E., Triebwasser, J., Roussos, P., & Siever, L. J. (2013). Schizotypal personality disorder. *Journal of Personality Disorders, 27*(5), 652–679.

Chen, E. H., Shofer, F. S., Dean, A. J., Hollander, J. E., Baxt, W. G., Robey, J. L., . . . Mills, A. M. (2008). Gender disparity in analgesic treatment of emergency department patients with acute abdominal pain. *Academic Emergency Medicine, 15*(5), 414–418.

Chen, H.-F., Rose, A. M., Waisbren, S., Ahmad, A., & Prosser, L. A. (2021). Newborn screening and treatment of phenylketonuria: Projected health outcomes and cost-effectiveness. *Children, 8*(5), 381.

Cherry, K. (2015). What is a projective test? *About Education*. Retrieved from About.com: http://psychology.about.com/od/personality-testing

Chiarotti, F., & Venerosi, A. (2020). Epidemiology of autism spectrum disorders: A review of worldwide prevalence estimates since 2014. *Brain Sciences, 10*(5), 274.

Choi, B., Kim, I., Lee, G. Y., Kim, S., Kim, S. H., Lee, J. G., & Lim, M. H. (2020). Estimated prevalence and impact of the experience of becoming a victim of exhibitionism and frotteurism in Korea: A general population based study. *Criminal Behaviour and Mental Health, 30*(2–3), 132–140. https://doi.org/10.1002/cbm.2153

Chokroverty, S. (2008). *Questions & answers about sleep apnea*. Sudbury, MA: Jones and Bartlett Publishers.

Chorpita, B. F., & Barlow, D. H. (1998). The development of anxiety: The role of control in the early environment. *Psychological Bulletin, 124*(1), 2–21.

Chow, J. C. C., Jaffee, K., & Snowden, L. (2003). Racial/ethnic disparities in the use of mental health services in poverty areas. *American Journal of Public Health, 93*(5), 792–797.

Chu, J. (2011). *Rebuilding shattered lives: Treating complex PTSD and dissociative disorders*. Hoboken, NJ: John Wiley & Sons.

Chung, K.-F., Yeung, W.-F., Ho, F. Y.-Y., Yung, K.-P., Yu, Y.-M., & Kwok, C.-W. (2015). Cross-cultural and comparative epidemiology of insomnia: The Diagnostic and Statistical Manual (DSM), International Classification of Diseases (ICD) and International Classification of Sleep Disorders (ICSD). *Sleep Medicine, 16*(4), 477–482.

Ciardha, C. Ó., Gannon, T. A., & Ward, T. (2016). The cognitive distortions of child sexual abusers: Evaluating key theories. In D. P. Boer (Ed.), *The Wiley handbook on the theories, assessment and treatment of sexual offending* (pp. 207–222). Hoboken, NJ: John Wiley & Sons.

Cipriani, A., Furukawa, T. A., Salanti, G., Chaimani, A., Atkinson, L. Z., Ogawa, Y., . . . Higgins, J. P. (2018). Comparative efficacy and acceptability of 21 antidepressant drugs for the acute treatment of adults with major depressive disorder: A systematic review and network meta-analysis. *Focus, 16*(4), 420–429.

Cirincione, C., Steadman, H., & McGreevy, M. (1995). Rates of insanity acquittals and the factors associated with successful insanity pleas. *Bulletin of the American Academy of Psychiatry and the Law, 23*, 3.

Clark, D. A., & Beck, A. T. (2010). Cognitive theory and therapy of anxiety and depression: Convergence with neurobiological findings. *Trends in Cognitive Sciences, 14*, 418–424.

Claudat, K., Brown, T. A., Anderson, L., Bongiorno, G., Berner, L. A., Reilly, E., . . . Kaye, W. H. (2020). Correlates of co-occurring eating disorders and substance use disorders: A case for dialectical behavior therapy. *Eating Disorders, 28*(2), 142–156.

Cleveland Clinic (n.d.). Delirium and mental confusion: Symptoms, causes, treatment & prevention. https://my.clevelandclinic.org/health/diseases/15252-delirium

Coccaro, E. F., Lee, R., McCloskey, M., Csernansky, J. G., & Wang, L. (2015). Morphometric analysis of amygdala and hippocampus shape in impulsively aggressive and healthy control subjects. *Journal of Psychiatric Research, 69*, 80–86.

Coelho, C. M., Suttiwan, P., Arato, N., & Zsido, A. N. (2020). On the nature of fear and anxiety triggered by COVID-19. *Frontiers in Psychology, 11*, 3109.

Coelho, G. A. (2022). Sleep and gender differences. In C. Frange & F. M. S. Coelho (Eds.), *Sleep medicine and physical therapy* (pp. 275–283). Cham: Springer.

Coldwell-Harris, C. L., & Ayçiçegi, A. (2006). When personality and culture clash: The psychological distress of allocentrics in an individualistic culture and idiocentrics in a collectivistic culture. *Transcultural Psychiatry, 43*(3), 331–361.

Colins, O. F., Fanti, K. A., & Andershed, H. (2021). The DSM-5 limited prosocial emotions specifier for conduct disorder: Comorbid problems, prognosis, and antecedents. *Journal of the American Academy of Child and Adolescent Psychiatry, 60*(8), 1020–1029. https://doi.org/10.1016/j.jaac.2020.09.022

Colli, A., Tanzilli, A., Dimaggio, G., & Lingiardi, V. (2014). Patient personality and therapist response: An empirical investigation. *The American Journal of Psychiatry, 171*(1), 102–108. https://doi.org/10.1176/appi.ajp.2013.13020224

Comas-Díaz, L. (2014). Multicultural theories of psychotherapy. In D. Wedding & R. J. Corsini (Eds.), *Current psychotherapies* (10th ed., pp. 533–568). Independence, KY: Cengage Publications.

Comas-Díaz, L. (2016). Racial trauma recovery: A race-informed therapeutic approach to racial wounds. In A. N. Alvarez, C. T. H. Liang, & H. A. Neville (Eds.), *The cost of racism for people of color: Contextualizing experiences of discrimination* (pp. 249–272). Washington, DC: American Psychological Association. https://doi.org/10.1037/14852-012

Conklin, H. M., & Iacono, W. G. (2002). Schizophrenia: A neurodevelopmental perspective. *Current Directions in Psychological Science, 11*(1), 33. https://doi.org/Article

Connor, J. L. (2009). The role of driver sleepiness in car crashes: A review of the epidemiological evidence. In J. C. Verster, S. R. Pandi-Perumal, & J. G. Ramaekers (Eds.), *Drugs, driving and traffic safety* (pp. 187–205). Basel: Birkhäuser Verlag.

Conseglieri, A., & Villasante, O. (2021). Shock therapies in Spain (1939–1952) after the Civil War: Santa Isabel National Mental Asylum in Leganés. *History of Psychiatry, 32*(4), 402–418. https://doi.org/10.1177/0957154X211030790

Conway, C. R., & Xiong, W. (2018). The mechanism of action of vagus nerve stimulation in treatment-resistant depression: Current conceptualizations. *Psychiatric Clinics, 41*(3), 395–407.

Coogan, P., Schon, K., Li, S., Cozier, Y., Bethea, T., & Rosenberg, L. (2020). Experiences of racism and subjective cognitive function in African American women. *Alzheimer's & Dementia (Amsterdam, Netherlands), 12*(1), e12067. https://doi.org/10.1002/dad2.12067

Cook, B. L., Zuvekas, S. H., Carson, N., Wayne, G. F., Vesper, A., & McGuire, T. G. (2014). Assessing racial/ethnic disparities in treatment across episodes of mental health care. *Health Services Research, 49*(1), 206–229.

Cook, S. C., Schwartz, A. C., & Kaslow, N. J. (2017). Evidence-based psychotherapy: Advantages and challenges. *Neurotherapeutics: The Journal of the American Society for Experimental Neurotherapeutics, 14*(3), 537–545. doi:10.1007/s13311-017-0549-4

Cooper, M., Reilly, E. E., Siegel, J. A., Coniglio, K., Sadeh-Sharvit, S., Pisetsky, E. M., & Anderson, L. M. (2022). Eating disorders during the COVID-19 pandemic and quarantine: An overview of risks and recommendations for treatment and early intervention. *Eating Disorders*, *30*(1), 54–76.

Corathers, S. D. (2018). Collaboration is key to developing effective hormonal treatment paradigms for transgender youth. *Journal of Adolescent Health*, *62*(4), 361–362.

Corrigan, P. (2004). How stigma interferes with mental health care. *American Psychologist*, *59*(7), 614–625.

Cortese, S., Adamo, N., Del Giovane, C., Mohr-Jensen, C., Hayes, A. J., Carucci, S., ... Cipriani, A. (2018). Comparative efficacy and tolerability of medications for attention-deficit hyperactivity disorder in children, adolescents, and adults: A systematic review and network meta-analysis. *The Lancet Psychiatry*, *5*(9), 727–738. https://doi.org/10.1016/s2215–0366(18)30269-4

Cosgrove, L., & Riddle, B. (2003). Constructions of femininity and experiences of menstrual distress. *Women & Health*, *38*(3), 37–58.

Coskuner, E. R., & Ozkan, B. (2022). Premature ejaculation and endocrine disorders: A literature review. *The World Journal of Men's Health*, *40*(1), 38–51.

Courtois, C. A., Brown, L. S., Cook, J., Fairbank, J. A., Friedman, M., Gone, J. P., ... Kurtzman, H. (2017). *Clinical practice guideline for the treatment of posttraumatic stress disorder (PTSD) in adults*. American Psychological Association Guideline Development Panel for the Treatment of PTSD in Adults Adopted as APA Policy February 24, 2017.

Cox, J., Kopkin, M. R., Rankin, J. A., Tomeny, T. S., & Coffey, C. A. (2018). The relationship between parental psychopathic traits and parenting style. *Journal of Child and Family Studies*, *27*(7), 2305–2314.

Coyne, J. C. (1976). Toward an interactional description of depression. *Psychiatry*, *39*(1), 28–40.

Coyne, J. C., Thompson, R., & Palmer, S. C. (2002). Marital quality, coping with conflict, marital complaints, and affection in couples with a depressed wife. *Journal of Family Psychology*, *16*(1), 26–37.

Coyne, S. M., & Stockdale, L. (2021). Growing up with Grand Theft Auto: A 10-year study of longitudinal growth of violent video game play in adolescents. *Cyberpsychology, Behavior, and Social Networking*, *24*(1), 11–16.

Craddock, N., & Jones, I. (1999). Genetics of bipolar disorder. *Journal of Medical Genetics*, *36*(8), 585–594.

Craddock, N., & Mynors-Wallis, L. (2014). Psychiatric diagnosis: Impersonal, imperfect and important. *The British Journal of Psychiatry*, *204*(2), 93–95.

Craske, M. G., DeCola, J. P., Sachs, A. D., & Pontillo, D. C. (2003). Panic control treatment for agoraphobia. *Journal of Anxiety Disorders*, *17*(3), 321–333.

Crerand, C., Sarwer, D., Magee, L., Gibbons, L., Lowe, M., Bartlett, S., & Whitaker, L. A. (2004). Rate of body dysmorphic disorder among patients seeking facial plastic surgery. *Psychiatric Annals*, *34*, 958–965.

Crisp, H., & Gabbard, G. O. (2020). Principles of psychodynamic treatment for patients with narcissistic personality disorder. *Journal of Personality Disorders*, *34*(Supplement), 143–158.

Cristea, I. A., Gentili, C., Cotet, C. D., Palomba, D., Barbui, C., & Cuijpers, P. (2017). Efficacy of psychotherapies for borderline personality disorder: A systematic review and meta-analysis. *JAMA Psychiatry*, *74*(4), 319–328.

Crosson, F. J., Covinsky, K., & Redberg, R. F. (2021). Medicare and the shocking US Food and Drug Administration approval of aducanumab: Crisis or opportunity? *JAMA Internal Medicine*, *181*(10), 1278–1280.

Crow, S. J. (2017, July 17). Bulimia nervosa in adults: Pharmacotherapy. *UpToDate*. www.uptodate.com/contents/bulimia-nervosa-in-adults-pharmacotherapy

Crow, S. J., & Mitchell, J. E. (2019). Bulimia nervosa: Methods of treatment. In L. A. Mott & B. D. Lumsden (Eds.), *Understanding eating disorders* (pp. 203–218). New York, NY: Routledge.

Cruz-Sáez, S., Pascual, A., Wlodarczyk, A., & Echeburúa, E. (2020). The effect of body dissatisfaction on disordered eating: The mediating role of self-esteem and negative affect in male and female adolescents. *Journal of Health Psychology*, *25*(8), 1098–1108. https://doi.org/10.1177/1359105317748734

Cuijpers, P., & Gentili, C. (2017) Psychological treatments are as effective as pharmacotherapies in the treatment of adult depression: A summary from randomized clinical trials and neuroscience evidence. *Research in Psychotherapy: Psychopathology, Process and Outcome*, *20*, 147–152.

Cuijpers, P., Geraedts, A. S., van Oppen, P., Andersson, G., Markowitz, J. C., & van Straten, A. (2011). Interpersonal psychotherapy for depression: A meta-analysis. *The American Journal of Psychiatry*, *168*(6), 581–592. http://doi.org/10.1176/appi.ajp.2010.10101411

Cuijpers, P., Karyotaki, E., de Wit, L., & Ebert, D. D. (2020). The effects of fifteen evidence-supported therapies for adult depression: A meta-analytic review. *Psychotherapy Research*, *30*(3), 279–293.

Cuijpers, P., Reijnders, M., & Huibers, M. J. H. (2019). The role of common factors in psychotherapy outcomes. *Annual Review of Clinical Psychology*, *15*, 207–231. https://doi.org/10.1146/annurev-clinpsy-050718-095424

Cuijpers, P., Veen, S. C. V., Sijbrandij, M., Yoder, W., & Cristea, I. A. (2020). Eye movement desensitization and reprocessing for mental health problems: A systematic review and meta-analysis. *Cognitive Behaviour Therapy*, *49*(3), 165–180.

Cunningham, G. R., & Khera, M. (2018, January 31). Evaluation of male sexual dysfunction. *UpToDate*. www.uptodate.com/contents/evaluation-of-male-sexual-dysfunction

Cunningham, G. R., & Rosen, R. C. (2018, April 18). Overview of male sexual dysfunction. *UpToDate*. http://updodate.com

Curtis, D. A., Nicks, K. L., & Huang, H.-H. (2021). Patient deception in healthcare: Longitudinal effects of different educational interventions. *North American Journal of Psychology*, *23*(1), 77–94.

Czeisler, M. É., Lane, R. I., Petrosky, E., Wiley, J. F., Christensen, A., Njai, R., . . . Rajaratnam, S. M. W.(2020). Mental health, substance use, and suicidal ideation during the COVID-19 pandemic—United States, June 24–30, 2020. *Morbidity and Mortality Weekly Report*, *69*(32), 1049–1057.

Dafauce, L., Romero, D., Carpio, C., Barga, P., Quirce, S., Villasante, C., . . . Álvarez-Sala, R. (2021). Psycho-demographic profile in severe asthma and effect of emotional mood disorders and hyperventilation syndrome on quality of life. *BMC Psychology*, *9*(1), 1–15.

Dahlen, H. (2019). Female sexual dysfunction: Assessment and treatment. *Urologic Nursing*, *39*(1). doi:10.7257/1053-816X.2019.39.1.39

Daker, R. J., Cortes, R. A., Lyons, I. M., & Green, A. E. (2019). Creativity anxiety: Evidence for anxiety that is specific to creative thinking, from STEM to the arts. *Journal of Experimental Psychology: General*, *149*(1), 42–57.

Daley, T. (2021). *Coming Up for Air: What I Learned from Sport, Fame and Fatherhood*. London: Mira.

Dalle Grave, R., Sartirana, M., & Calugi, S. (2021). Eating disorder psychopathology and its consequences. In R. D. Grave, M. Sartirana, & S. Calugi (Eds.), *Complex cases and comorbidity in eating disorders* (pp. 15–27). Cham: Springer.

Dalvie, S., Koen, N., & Stein, D. J. (2020). Genomic contributions to anxiety disorders. In B. T. Baune (Ed.), *Personalized psychiatry* (pp. 297–306). London: Academic Press.

Daly, M., Baumeister, R.F., Delaney, L., & MacLachlan, M. (2014). Self-control and its relation to emotions and psychobiology: Evidence from a Day Reconstruction Method study. *Journal of Behavioral Medicine*, *37*(1), 81–93.

Dana, R. H. (2005). *Multicultural assessment: Principles, applications, and examples*. Mahwah, NJ: Lawrence Erlbaum.

Das-Munshi, J., Ford, T., Hotopf, M., Prince, M., & Stewart, R. (2020). *Practical psychiatric epidemiology*. New York, NY: Oxford University Press.

Dattilo, N. (2018) La belle indifférence. In J. S. Kreutzer, J. DeLuca, & B. Caplan (Eds.), *Encyclopedia of clinical neuropsychology*. Cham: Springer. https://doi.org/10.1007/978-3-319-57111-9_2080

Daud, N. M., Isa, F. S. M., Ismail, J., Nor, N. A. K., Yahya, A., & Ishak, B. (2021). Down syndrome: What are the possible risk factors of ocular anomalies? *International Journal of Allied Health Sciences*, *5*(3), 2251.

Davis, C., Levitan, R. D., Yilmaz, Z., Kaplan, A. S., Carter, J. C., & Kennedy, J. L. (2012). Binge eating disorder and the dopamine D2 receptor: Genotypes and sub-phenotypes. *Progress in Neuro-Psychopharmacology and Biological Psychiatry*, *38*(2), 328–335.

Dawood, S., Wu, L. Z., Bliton, C. F., & Pincus, A. L. (2020). Narcissistic and histrionic personality disorders. In C. W. Lejuez & K. L. Gratz (Eds.), *The Cambridge handbook of personality disorders* (pp. 277–291). New York, NY: Cambridge University Press.

de Giambattista, C., Ventura, P., Trerotoli, P., Margari, F., & Margari, L. (2021). Sex differences in autism spectrum disorder: Focus on high functioning children and adolescents. *Frontiers in Psychiatry*, *12*, 1063.

De Sousa, A. (2019) Disulfiram in the management of alcohol dependence. In A. De Sousa, *Disulfiram: Its use in alcohol dependence and other disorders* (pp. 21–30). Singapore: Springer. https://doi.org/10.1007/978-981-32-9876-7_3

de Vries, G. J., & Olff, M. (2009). The lifetime prevalence of traumatic events and posttraumatic stress disorder in the Netherlands. *Journal of Traumatic Stress: Official Publication of the International Society for Traumatic Stress Studies*, *22*(4), 259–267.

de Zwart, P. L., Jeronimus, B. F., & de Jonge, P. (2019). Empirical evidence for definitions of episode, remission, recovery, relapse and recurrence in depression: A systematic review. *Epidemiology and Psychiatric Sciences, 28*(5), 544–562.

Deacon, B. J., & Abramowitz, J. S. (2004). Cognitive and behavioral treatments for anxiety disorders: A review of meta-analytic findings. *Journal of Clinical Psychology, 60*(4), 429–441. http://onlinelibrary.wiley.com/doi/10.1002/jclp.10255/abstract

Dębiec, J., Díaz-Mataix, L., Bush, D. E., Doyère, V., & LeDoux, J. E. (2010). The amygdala encodes specific sensory features of an aversive reinforcer. *Nature Neuroscience, 13*(5), 536–537.

Dement, W. C., & Vaughan, C. (2000). *The promise of sleep: A pioneer in sleep medicine explores the vital connection between health, happiness, and a good night's sleep.* New York, NY: Dell.

Demi Lovato—Dancing with the devil (Official video). (n.d.). Retrieved from www.youtube.com/watch?v=EAg69LaLlS0

Desaulniers, J., Desjardins, S., Lapierre, S., & Desgagné, A. (2018). Sleep environment and insomnia in elderly persons living at home. *Journal of Aging Research, 2018.* https://doi.org/10.1155/2018/8053696

DiCarlo, F., Sociali, A., Picutti, E., Pettorruso, M., Vellante, F., Verrastro, V., . . . di Giannantonio, M. (2021). Telepsychiatry and other cutting-edge technologies in COVID-19 pandemic: Bridging the distance in mental health assistance. *International Journal of Clinical Practice, 75*(1). doi:10.1111/ijcp.13716

Diedrich, A., & Voderholzer, U. (2015). Obsessive-compulsive personality disorder: A current review. *Current Psychiatry Reports, 17*(2), 2.

Ding, J. M., & Kanaan, R. A. A. (2017). Conversion disorder: A systematic review of current terminology. *General Hospital Psychiatry, 45*, 51–55.

Dirks-Linhorst, P. A., Linhorst, D. M., & Loux, T. M. (2019). Criminal court-ordered psychiatric evaluations: Does gender play a role? *Women and Criminal Justice, 29*(6), 303–322. https://doi.org/10.1080/08974454.2018.1520673

Donders, J. (2020). The incremental value of neuropsychological assessment: A critical review. *The Clinical Neuropsychologist, 34*(1), 56–87.

Donelli, D., Antonelli, M., Bellinazzi, C., Gensini, G. F., & Firenzuoli, F. (2019). Effects of lavender on anxiety: A systematic review and meta-analysis. *Phytomedicine, 65.* doi:10.1016/j.phymed.2019.153099

Donovan, L. M., & Kapur, V. K. (2016). Prevalence and characteristics of central compared to obstructive sleep apnea: Analyses from the Sleep Heart Health Study cohort. *Sleep, 39*(7), 1353–1359.

Dorahy, M. J., Brand, B. L., Şar, V., Krüger, C., Stavropoulos, P., Martínez-Taboas, A., . . . Middleton, W. (2014). Dissociative identity disorder: An empirical overview. *Australian & New Zealand Journal of Psychiatry, 48*(5), 402–417. https://doi.org/10.1177/0004867414527523

Dow, C., & Siniscarco, M. (2021). Culture, mental health, and stigma. *Journal of Psychosocial Nursing and Mental Health Services, 59*(2), 5.

Dowd, E. T. (1989). Stasis and change in cognitive psychotherapy: Client resistance and reactance as mediating variables. In W. Dryden & P. Trower (Eds.), *Cognitive therapy: Stasis and change* (pp. 139–158). New York, NY: Springer.

Dowling, N. A., Ewin, C., Youssef, G. J., Merkouris, S. S., Suomi, A., Thomas, S. A., & Jackson, A. C. (2018). Problem gambling and family violence: Findings from a population-representative study. *Journal of Behavioral Addictions, 7*(3), 806–813.

Dozier, M. E., Porter, B., & Ayers, C. R. (2016). Age of onset and progression of hoarding symptoms in older adults with hoarding disorder. *Aging & Mental Health, 20*(7), 736–742.

Drake, R. E., Xie, H., & McHugo, G. J. (2020). A 16-year follow-up of patients with serious mental illness and co-occurring substance use disorder. *World Psychiatry, 19*(3), 397–398.

Drescher, J. (2015). Out of DSM: Depathologizing homosexuality. *Behavioral Sciences (Basel, Switzerland), 5*(4), 565–575. https://doi.org/10.3390/bs5040565

Dukakis, K., & Tye, L. (2007). *Shock: The healing power of electroconvulsive therapy.* New York, NY: Penguin.

Dunner, D. L., Aaronson, S. T., Sackeim, H. A., Janicak, P. G., Carpenter, L. L., Boyadjis, T., . . . Lanocha, K. (2014). A multisite, naturalistic, observational study of transcranial magnetic stimulation for patients with pharmacoresistant major depressive disorder: Durability of benefit over a 1-year follow-up period. *The Journal of Clinical Psychiatry, 75*(12), 1394–1401.

Dvoskin, J. A., Knoll, J. L., & Silva, M. (2020). A brief history of the criminalization of mental illness. *CNS Spectrums, 25*(5), 638–650.

Dygdon, J. A., & Dienes, K. A. (2013). Behavioral excesses in depression: A learning theory hypothesis. *Depression and Anxiety, 30*(6), 598–605. http://doi.org/10.1002/da.22111

Ebner-Priemer, U. W., Houben, M., Santangelo, P., Kleindienst, N., Tuerlinckx, F., Oravecz, Z., . . . Kuppens,

P. (2015). Unraveling affective dysregulation in borderline personality disorder: A theoretical model and empirical evidence. *Journal of Abnormal Psychology, 124*(1), 186–198.

Eftekhari, A., Crowley, J. J., & Rosen, C. S. (2020). *Predicting treatment dropout among veterans receiving prolonged exposure therapy. Psychological Trauma: Theory, Research, Practice, and Policy, 12*(4), 405–412.

Eggertson, L. (2010). Lancet retracts 12-year-old article linking autism to MMR vaccines. *Canadian Medical Association Journal, 182*(4), E199–E200. https://doi.org/10.1503/cmaj.109-3179

Eikenaes, I., Egeland, J., Hummelen, B., & Wilberg, T. (2015). Avoidant personality disorder versus social phobia: The significance of childhood neglect. *PLoS One, 10*(3), e0122846.

Eisenlohr-Moul, T. A., Kaiser, G., Weise, C., Schmalenberger, K. M., Kiesner, J., Ditzen, B., & Kleinstäuber, M. (2020). Are there temporal subtypes of premenstrual dysphoric disorder? Using group-based trajectory modeling to identify individual differences in symptom change. *Psychological Medicine, 50*(6), 964–972.

Elbogen, E. B., & Johnson, S. C. (2009). The intricate link between violence and mental disorder: Results from the National Epidemiologic Survey on Alcohol and Related Conditions. *Archives of General Psychiatry, 66*(2), 152–161.

Elhai, J. D., Gallinari, E. F., Rozgonjuk, D., & Yang, H. (2020). Depression, anxiety and fear of missing out as correlates of social, non-social and problematic smartphone use. *Addictive Behaviors, 105*, 106335.

Elias, G. J., Giacobbe, P., Boutet, A., Germann, J., Beyn, M. E., Gramer, R. M., . . . Lozano, A. M. (2020). Probing the circuitry of panic with deep brain stimulation: Connectomic analysis and review of the literature. *Brain Stimulation, 13*(1), 10–14.

Ellason, J. W., & Ross, C. A. (1997). Two-year follow-up of inpatients with dissociative disorder. *The American Journal of Psychiatry, 154*(6), 832–839. https://doi.org/10.1176/ajp.154.6.832

Ellicott, A., Hammen, C., Gitlin, M., Brown, G., & Jamison, K. (2019). Life events and the course of bipolar disorder. In S. Hyman (Ed.), *The science of mental health* (pp. 78–82). New York, NY: Routledge.

Elliott, R., Watson, J. C., Timulak, L., & Sharbanee, J. (2020). Research on humanistic-experiential psychotherapies: Updated review. In M. Barkham, W. Lutz, & L. G. Castonguay (Eds.), *Bergin and Garfield's handbook of psychotherapy and behavior change* (pp. 421–468). Hoboken, NJ: John Wiley & Sons.

Ellis, A. (1980). Rational-emotive therapy and cognitive behavior therapy: Similarities and differences. *Cognitive Therapy and Research, 4*(4), 325–340.

Ellison, J. W., Rosenfeld, J. A., & Shaffer, L. G. (2013). Genetic basis of intellectual disability. *Annual Review of Medicine, 64*, 441–450.

Emerson, E., Shahtahmasebi, S., Lancaster, G., & Berridge, D. (2010). Poverty transitions among families supporting a child with intellectual disability. *Journal of Intellectual and Developmental Disability, 35*(4), 224–234.

Emerson, N. D., & Bursch, B. (2020). Munchausen by proxy and pediatric factitious disorder imposed on self. In B. D. Carter & K. A. Kullgren (Eds.), *Clinical handbook of psychological consultation in pediatric medical settings* (pp. 463–474). Cham: Springer.

Emsley, R., Rabinowitz, J., & Medori, R. (2006). Time course for antipsychotic treatment response in first-episode schizophrenia. *The American Journal of Psychiatry, 163*(4), 743–745. https://doi.org/10.1176/appi.ajp.163.4.743

Enander, J., Ivanov, V. Z., Mataix-Cols, D., Kuja-Halkola, R., Ljótsson, B., Lundström, S., . . . Rück, C. (2018). Prevalence and heritability of body dysmorphic symptoms in adolescents and young adults: A population-based nationwide twin study. *Psychological Medicine, 48*(16), 2740–2747.

Engel, S., Steffen, K., & Mitchell, J. (2017). *Bulimia nervosa in adults: Clinical features, course of illness, assessment and diagnosis. UpToDate.* www.uptodate.com/contents/bulimia-nervosa-in-adults-clinical-features-course-of-illness-assessment-and-diagnosis

Erland, L. A. E., & Saxena, P. K. (2017). Melatonin natural health products and supplements: Presence of serotonin and significant variability of melatonin content. *Journal of Clinical Sleep Medicine, 13*(2), 275–281. https://doi.org/10.5664/jcsm.6462

Erlich, M. D., Smith, T. E., Horwath, E., & Cournos, F. (2014). Schizophrenia and other psychotic disorders. In J. Cutler (Ed.), *Psychiatry* (3rd ed., pp. 97–128). New York, NY: Oxford University Press.

Eschweiler, G. W., Vonthein, R., Bode, R., Huell, M., Conca, A., Peters, O., . . . Schlotter, W. (2007). Clinical efficacy and cognitive side effects of bifrontal versus right unilateral electroconvulsive therapy (ECT): A short-term randomised controlled trial in pharmaco-resistant major depression. *Journal of Affective Disorders, 101*(1–3), 149–157.

Eusei, D., & Delcea, C. (2020). Fetishistic disorder. In C. Delcea (Ed.), *Theoretical-Experimental Models in Sexual and Paraphilic Dysfunctions* (pp. 67–71). IJASS, International Journal of Advanced Studies in Sexology Monograph. Bologna: Filodiritto.

Evans, S. C., Reed, G. M., Roberts, M. C., Esparza, P., Watts, A. D., Ritchie, P. L. J., . . . Saxena, S., (2013). Psychologists' perspectives on the diagnostic classification of mental disorders: Results from the WHO-IUpsyS Global Survey. *International Journal of Psychology, 48*, 177–193. http://dx.doi.org/10.1080/00207594.2013.804189.

Exline, J. J., Pargament, K. I., Wilt, J. A., & Harriott, V. A. (2021). Mental illness, normal psychological processes, or attacks by the devil? Three lenses to frame demonic struggles in therapy. *Spirituality in Clinical Practice, 8*(3), 215–228.

Exner, J. E. (2003). *The Rorschach: A comprehensive system. Basic foundations and principles of interpretation* (4th ed.) New York, NY: John Wiley & Sons.

Eynan, R., Shah, R., & Links, P. (2016). Comorbid clinical and personality disorders: The risk of suicide. *Psychiatric Times, 33*(2).

Eysenck, M. W., Mogg, K., May, J., Richards, A, & Matthews, A. (1991). Bias in interpretation of ambiguous sentences related to threat in anxiety. *Journal of Abnormal Psychology, 100*(2), 144–150. doi:10.1037/002-843X.100.2.144

Fadus, M. C., Odunsi, O. T., & Squeglia, L. M. (2019). Race, ethnicity, and culture in the medical record: Implicit bias or patient advocacy? *Academic Psychiatry, 43*(5), 532–536.

Fairburn, C. G., Bailey-Straebler, S., Basden, S., Doll, H. A., Jones, R., Murphy, R., O'Connor, M. E., & Cooper, Z. (2015). A transdiagnostic comparison of enhanced cognitive behaviour therapy (CBT-E) and interpersonal psychotherapy in the treatment of eating disorders. *Behaviour Research and Therapy, 70*, 64–71.

Fallon, J. H. (2006). Neuroanatomical background to understanding the brain of the young psychopath. *Ohio State Journal of Criminal Law, 3*(34), 341–367.

Fallon, J. H. (2014). *The psychopath inside: A neuroscientist's personal journey into the dark side of the brain*. New York, NY: Penguin.

Faravelli, C., Guigni, A., Salvatori, S., & Ricca, V. (2004). Psychopathology after rape. *The American Journal of Psychiatry, 161*, 1483–1485.

Fariba, K., & Gokarakonda, S. B. (2021). Impulse control disorders. *StatPearls* [Internet]. Treasure Island (FL): StatPearls Publishing. www.ncbi.nlm.nih.gov/books/nbk562279/

Fatemi, S. H., & Folsom, T. D. (2009). The neurodevelopmental hypothesis of schizophrenia, revisited. *Schizophrenia Bulletin, 35*(3), 528–548. https://doi.org/10.1093/schbul/sbn187

Fatimah, H., Wiernik, B. M., Gorey, C., McGue, M., Iacono, W. G., & Bornovalova, M. A. (2020). Familial factors and the risk of borderline personality pathology: Genetic and environmental transmission. *Psychological Medicine, 50*(8), 1327–1337.

Fayyad, J., Sampson, N. A., Hwang, I., Adamowski, T., Aguilar-Gaxiola, S., Al-Hamzawi, A., . . . WHO World Mental Health Survey Collaborators (2017). The descriptive epidemiology of DSM-IV Adult ADHD in the World Health Organization World Mental Health Surveys. *Attention Deficit and Hyperactivity Disorders, 9*(1), 47–65. https://doi.org/10.1007/s12402–016-0208-3

Fedoroff, J. P. (2020). The pedophilia and orientation debate and its implications for forensic psychiatry. *The Journal of the American Academy of Psychiatry and the Law, 48*(2), 146–150. https://doi.org/10.29158/JAAPL.200011-20

Feldman, E., & Gitu, A. C. (2021). Recognizing personality disorders in patients presenting to the primary care provider. *Primary Care Reports, 27*(9).

Felthous, A. R., O'Shaughnessy, R., Kuten, J., François-Purssell, I., Medrano, J., & Carabellese, F. (2020). The clinician's duty to warn or protect: In the United States, England, Canada, New Zealand, France, Spain, and Italy. In A. R. Felthous & Henning Saß (Eds.), *The Wiley international handbook on psychopathic disorders and the law* (pp. 121–153). Hoboken, NJ: John Wiley & Sons.

Fentiman, L. C. (2020). Book review of P. Ash (Ed.), *From courtroom to clinic: Legal cases that changed mental health treatment. Journal of Legal Medicine, 40*(1), 131–133.

Ferber, A. L., Holcomb, K., & Wentling, T. (Eds.). (2016). *Sex, gender, and sexuality: The new basics – An anthology* (3rd ed.). New York, NY: Oxford University Press.

Ferguson, C. J., & Wang, C. J. (2021). Aggressive video games are not a risk factor for mental health problems in youth: A longitudinal study. *Cyberpsychology, Behavior, and Social Networking, 24*(1), 70–73.

Ferland, J.-M. N., & Hurd, Y. L. (2020). Deconstructing the neurobiology of cannabis use disorder. *Nature Neuroscience, 23*(5), 600–610. https://doi.org/10.1038/s41593–020-0611-0

Ferracioli-Oda, E., Qawasmi, A., & Bloch, M. H. (2013). Meta-analysis: Melatonin for the treatment of primary sleep disorders. *PLoS One, 8*(5). https://doi.org/10.1371/journal.pone.0063773

Ferrando, C., & Thomas, T. N. (2018). Transgender surgery: Male to female. *UpToDate.* www.uptodate.com/contents/transgender-surgery-male-to-female

Ferrão, Y. A. (2019). Other obsessive-compulsive related disorders. In L. F. Fontenelle & M. Yücel (Eds.), *A transdiagnostic approach to obsessions, compulsions and related phenomena* (pp. 413–423). New York, NY: Cambridge University Press.

Fettes, P., Schulze, L., & Downar, J. (2017). Cortico-striatal-thalamic loop circuits of the orbitofrontal cortex: Promising therapeutic targets in psychiatric illness. *Frontiers in Systems Neuroscience, 11*, 25.

Fichter, M. M., Naab, S., Voderholzer, U., & Quadflieg, N. (2021). Mortality in males as compared to females treated for an eating disorder: A large prospective controlled study. *Eating and Weight Disorders: Studies on Anorexia, Bulimia and Obesity, 26*(5), 1627–1637.

Finger, E. C. (2016). Frontotemporal dementias. *Continuum: Lifelong Learning in Neurology, 22*(2), 464–489.

Fink, M., Kellner, C. H., & McCall, W. V. (2014). The role of ECT in suicide prevention. *The Journal of ECT, 30*(1), 5–9.

Fink, P. (2004). The prevalence of somatoform disorders among internal medical inpatients. *Journal of Psychosomatic Research, 56*(4), 413–418. https://doi.org/10.1016/S0022–3999(03)00624-X

Fino, E., & Mazzetti, M. (2019). Monitoring healthy and disturbed sleep through smartphone applications: A review of experimental evidence. *Sleep and Breathing, 23*(1), 13–24.

First, M. B., Williams, J. B., Karg, R. S., & Spitzer, R. L. (2016). *User's guide for the SCID-5-CV Structured Clinical Interview for DSM-5® disorders: Clinical version.* Washington, DC: American Psychiatric Publishing.

Fisher, C. A., Skocic, S., Rutherford, K. A., & Hetrick, S. E. (2019). Family therapy approaches for anorexia nervosa. *Cochrane Database of Systematic Reviews, 5*. doi:10.1002/14651858.CD004780.pub4

Fisher, K. A., & Marwaha, R. (2020). Paraphilia. *StatPearls* [Internet]. Treasure Island (FL): StatPearls Publishing. www.ncbi.nlm.nih.gov/books/NBK554425/

Fitch, W. L. (2014). *White Paper: Forensic mental health services in the United States.* National Association of State Mental Health Program Directors. www.nasmhpd.org/sites/default/files/Assessment%203%20-%20Updated%20Forensic%20Mental%20Health%20Services.pdf

Fitzgerald, P. B. (2020). An update on the clinical use of repetitive transcranial magnetic stimulation in the treatment of depression. *Journal of Affective Disorders, 276*, 90–103.

Flessner, C. A., Lochner, C., Stein, D. J., Woods, D. W., Franklin, M. E., & Keuthen, N. J. (2010). Age of onset of trichotillomania symptoms: Investigating clinical correlates. *The Journal of Nervous and Mental Disease, 198*(12), 896–900.

Flynn-Evans, E. E., Shekleton, J. A., Miller, B., Epstein, L. J., Kirsch, D., Brogna, L. A., . . . Gehrman, P. (2017). Circadian phase and phase angle disorders in primary insomnia. *Sleep, 40*(12). doi:10.1093/sleep/zsx163

Fogelkvist, M., Gustafsson, S. A., Kjellin, L., & Parling, T. (2020). Acceptance and commitment therapy to reduce eating disorder symptoms and body image problems in patients with residual eating disorder symptoms: A randomized controlled trial. *Body Image, 32*, 155–166.

Foote, B., Smolin, Y., Kaplan, M., Legatt, M.E., & Lipschitz, D. (2006). Prevalence of dissociative disorders in psychiatric outpatients. *The American Journal of Psychiatry, 163*, 623–629.

Forman, S., Yager, J., & Solomon, D. (2016). Eating disorders: Overview of epidemiology, clinical features and diagnosis. *UpToDate.* www.uptodate.com/contents/eating-disorders-overview-of-epidemiology-clinical-features-and-diagnosis

Foster, J. D., Keith Campbell, W., & Twenge, J. M. (2003). Individual differences in narcissism: Inflated self-views across the lifespan and around the world. *Journal of Research in Personality, 37*(6), 469–486. https://doi.org/https://doi.org/10.1016/S0092–6566(03)00026-6

Frances, A. J., & Nardo, J. M. (2013). ICD-11 should not repeat the mistakes made by DSM-5. *British Journal of Psychiatry, 203*(1), 1–2. http://doi.org/10.1192/bjp.bp.113.127647

Frank, E., Kupfer, D. J., Thase, M. E., Mallinger, A. G., Swartz, H. A., Fagiolini, A. M., . . . Monk, T. (2005). Two-year outcomes for interpersonal and social rhythm therapy in individuals with bipolar I disorder. *Archives of General Psychiatry, 62*(9), 996–1004.

Franz, L., Chambers, N., von Isenburg, M., & de Vries, P. J. (2017). Autism spectrum disorder in sub-Saharan Africa: A comprehensive scoping review. *Autism Research, 10*(5), 723–749.

Frederick, D. A., John, H. K. S., Garcia, J. R., & Lloyd, E. A. (2018). Differences in orgasm frequency among gay, lesbian, bisexual, and heterosexual men and women in a US national sample. *Archives of Sexual Behavior, 47*(1), 273–288.

Freedman, J., Hage, S., & Quatromoni, P. A. (2021). Eating disorders in male athletes: Factors associated with onset and maintenance. *Journal of Clinical Sport Psychology, 1*, 1–22.

Freis, D. (2019). The rise and fall of mental hygiene. In D. Freis, *Psycho-politics between the World Wars* (pp. 239–330). Cham: Palgrave Macmillan.

French, J. H., & Hameed, S. (2021). Illness anxiety disorder. *StatPearls* [Internet]. Treasure Island (FL): StatPearls Publishing. www.ncbi.nlm.nih.gov/books/NBK554399/

French, J. H., & Shrestha, S. (2020). Histrionic personality disorder. *StatPearls* [Internet]. Treasure Island (FL): StatPearls Publishing. https://www.ncbi.nlm.nih.gov/books/NBK542325/

Freud, S. (1933). *New introductory lectures on psychoanalysis*. New York, NY: Norton.

Frías, Á., González, L., Palma, C., & Farriols, N. (2017). Is there a relationship between borderline personality disorder and sexual masochism in women? *Archives of Sexual Behavior, 46*(3), 747–754.

Frick, P. J., & Matlasz, T. M. (2018). Disruptive, impulse-control, and conduct disorders. In M. M. Martel (Ed.), *Developmental pathways to disruptive, impulse-control and conduct disorders* (pp. 3–20). London: Academic Press.

Friedman, M., & Rosenman, R. H. (1974). *Type A behavior and your heart*. New York, NY: Knopf.

Friedman, M. J., Resik, P. A., Bryant, R. A., Strain, J., Horowitz, M., & Spiegel, D. (2011). *Classification of trauma and stressor-related disorders in DSM-5. Depression and Anxiety, 28*, 737–749.

Friedrich, M. J. (2017). Depression is the leading cause of disability around the world. *JAMA, 317*(15), 1517.

Frost, R. O., Steketee, G., & Tolin, D. F. (2011). Comorbidity in hoarding disorder. *Depression and Anxiety, 28*, 876–884.

Frost, R. O., Steketee, G., & Tolin, D. F. (2012). Diagnosis and assessment of hoarding disorder. *Annual Review of Clinical Psychology, 8*, 219–242.

Fusar-Poli, P., Salazar de Pablo, G., Rajkumar, R. P., López-Díaz, Á., Malhotra, S., Heckers, S., Lawrie, S. M., & Pillmann, F. (2022). Diagnosis, prognosis, and treatment of brief psychotic episodes: a review and research agenda. *The Lancet Psychiatry, 9*(1), 72–83. https://doi.org/https://doi.org/10.1016/S2215-0366(21)00121-8

Galderisi, S. (2000). Qualitative MRI findings in patients with schizophrenia: A controlled study. *Psychiatry Research: Neuroimaging, 98*(2), 117–126. https://doi.org/10.1016/S0925-4927(00)00047-0

Galling, B., Garcia, M. A., Osuchukwu, U., Hagi, K., & Correll, C. U. (2015). Safety and tolerability of antipsychotic-mood stabilizer co-treatment in the management of acute bipolar disorder: Results from a systematic review and exploratory meta-analysis. *Expert Opinion on Drug Safety, 14*(8), 1181–1199.

Gallo, A. (2020). Treatment for non-contact sexual offenders: What we know and what we need. *Sexual Addiction & Compulsivity, 27*, 149–163.

Galmiche, M., Déchelotte, P., Lambert, G., & Tavolacci, M. P. (2019). Prevalence of eating disorders over the 2000–2018 period: A systematic literature review. *The American Journal of Clinical Nutrition, 109*, 1402–1413. https://doi.org/10.1093/ajcn/nqy342

Gamache, K., Platania, J., & Zaitchik, M. (2021). Perceptions of criminal responsibility through the lens of race. *Applied Psychology in Criminal Justice, 16*(1), 52–64.

Gandhi, S., Padmavathi, N., Raveendran, R., Jadhav, P., Sahu, M., Gurusamy, J., & Muliyala, K. P. (2020). Perception of expressed emotion among persons with mental illness. *Journal of Psychosocial Rehabilitation and Mental Health, 7*(2), 121–130.

Gannon, T. A., Tyler, N., Ciardha, C. Ó., & Alleyne, E. (2022). *Adult deliberate firesetting: Theory, assessment, and treatment*. Hoboken, NJ: John Wiley & Sons.

Gaudiano, B. A. (2013, October 9). Psychotherapy's image problem. *The New York Times*.

Gautam, M., Tripathi, A., Deshmukh, D., & Gaur, M. (2020). Cognitive behavioral therapy for depression. *Indian Journal of Psychiatry, 62*(Supplement 2), S223–S229.

Geller, J. (2012). Advocacy: The push and pull of psychiatrists. In J. M. Ranz & J. M. Feldman (Eds.), *Handbook of community psychiatry* (pp. 61–78). New York, NY: Springer.

Genovese, A., & Butler, M. G. (2020). Clinical assessment, genetics, and treatment approaches in autism spectrum disorder (ASD). *International Journal of Molecular Sciences, 21*(13), 4726.

Geradt, M., Jahnke, S., Heinz, J., & Hoyer, J. (2018). Is contact with children related to legitimizing beliefs toward sex with children among men with pedophilia? *Archives of Sexual Behavior, 47*(2), 375–387.

Geyer, N. K. (2021). Beyond accommodations: Considerations for supporting and improving academic outcomes for neurodivergent students in post-secondary education. Seminar paper. https://minds.wisconsin.edu/bitstream/handle/1793/81778/Geyer,%20Natasha.pdf?sequence=1

Gillan, C. M., & Rutledge, R. B. (2021). Smartphones and the neuroscience of mental health. *Annual Review of Neuroscience, 44*, 129–151.

Gim, C. S.., Lillystone, D., & Caldwell, P. H.. (2009). Efficacy of the bell and pad alarm therapy for nocturnal enuresis. *Journal of Paediatrics and Child Health, 45*, 405–408.

Gitlin, M. J. (2002). Pharmacological treatment of depression. In I. H. Gotlib & C. L. Hammen (Eds.), *Handbook of depression* (pp. 360–382). New York, NY: Guilford Press.

Givler, A., & Maani-Fogelman, P. A. (2020). The importance of cultural competence in pain and palliative care. *StatPearls* [Internet]. Treasure Island (FL): StatPearls Publishing. www.ncbi.nlm.nih.gov/books/NBK493154/

Glantz, M. D., Bharat, C., Degenhardt, L., Sampson, N. A., Scott, K. M., Lim, C., ... Kessler, R. C. (2020). The epidemiology of alcohol use disorders cross-nationally: Findings from the World Mental Health Surveys. *Addictive Behaviors, 102*, 106128. https://doi.org/10.1016/j.addbeh.2019.106128

Glaser, R., Rice, J., Sheridan, J., & Fertel, R. (1987). Stress-related immune suppression: Health implications. *Brain, Behavior, and Immunity, 1*(1), 7–20. https://doi.org/10.1016/0889-1591(87)90002-X

Glass, R. M. (2001). Electroconvulsive therapy. *JAMA, 285*(10), 1346–1348. http://doi.org/10.1001/jama.285.10.1346

Glenn, A. L., Johnson, A. K., & Raine, A. (2013). Antisocial personality disorder: A current review. *Current Psychiatry Reports, 15*(12), 427.

Glick, R. L. (2021). Malingering and factitious disorder in the emergency department. In L. S. Zun, K. Nordstrom, & M. P. Wilson (Eds.), *Behavioral emergencies for healthcare providers* (pp. 151–155). Cham: Springer.

Glied, S., & Frank, R. G. (2014). Mental illness and violence: Lessons from the evidence. *American Journal of Public Health, 104*(2), e5–e6. https://doi.org/10.2105/AJPH.2013.301710

Goff, P. A., Jackson, M. C., Di Leone, B. A. L., Culotta, C. M., & DiTomasso, N. A. (2014). The essence of innocence: Consequences of dehumanizing Black children. *Journal of Personality and Social Psychology, 106*(4), 526–545.

Golden, C. J., & Freshwater, S. M. (2001). Luria-Nebraska Neuropsychological Battery. In W. I. Dorfman & S. M. Freshwater (Eds.), *Understanding psychological assessment* (pp. 59–75). Dordrecht: Kluwer Academic.

Goldenberg, I., Goldenberg, H., & Goldenberg Pelavin, E. (2014). Family therapy. In D. Wedding & R. J. Corsini (Eds.), *Current psychotherapies* (10th ed., pp. 373–410). Independence, KY: Cengage Publications.

Goldstein, A. N., & Walker, M. P. (2014). The role of sleep in emotional brain function. *Annual Review of Clinical Psychology, 10*, 679–708.

Goldstein, I., Clayton, A. H., Goldstein, A. T., Kim, N. N., & Kingsberg, S. A. (Eds.). (2018). *Textbook of female sexual function and dysfunction: Diagnosis and treatment*. Hoboken, NJ: John Wiley & Sons.

Gómez-Gil, E., Esteva, I., Almaraz, M. C., Pasaro, E., Segovia, S., & Guillamon, A. (2010). Familiality of gender identity disorder in non-twin siblings. *Archives of Sexual Behavior, 39*(2), 546–552.

González, H. M., Tarraf, W., Whitfield, K. E., & Vega, W. A. (2010). The epidemiology of major depression and ethnicity in the United States. *Journal of Psychiatric Research, 44*(15), 1043–1051. http://doi.org/10.1016/j.jpsychires.2010.03.017

Goode, R. W., Cowell, M. M., Mazzeo, S. E., Cooper-Lewter, C., Forte, A., Olayia, O. I., & Bulik, C. M. (2020). Binge eating and binge-eating disorder in Black women: A systematic review. *International Journal of Eating Disorders, 53*(4), 491–507. https://doi.org/10.1002/eat.23217

Goodman, M. (2013). Patient highlights: Female genital plastic/cosmetic surgery. *Journal of Sexual Medicine, 10*(8), 2125–2126.

Goossen, B., van der Starre, J., & van der Heiden, C. (2019). A review of neuroimaging studies in generalized anxiety disorder: "So where do we stand?" *Journal of Neural Transmission, 126*(9), 1203–1216. http://dx.doi.org.ezaccess.libraries.psu.edu/10.1007/s00702-019-02024-w

Gordovez, F. J. A., & McMahon, F. J. (2020). The genetics of bipolar disorder. *Molecular Psychiatry, 25*(3), 544–559.

Gorman, J. M. (2003). Treating generalized anxiety disorder. *Journal of Clinical Psychiatry, 64*(Supplement 2), 24–29.

Gotlib, I. H., Lewinsohn, P. M., & Seeley, J. R. (1995). Symptoms versus a diagnosis of depression: Differences in psychosocial functioning. *Journal of Consulting and Clinical Psychology, 63*(1), 90–100.

Gottesman, I. I. (1991). *Schizophrenia genesis: The origins of madness*. New York, NY: Henry Holt & Co.

Graham, J. R. (2014). *MMPI-2: Assessing personality and psychopathology* (5th ed.). New York, NY: Oxford University Press.

Granic, I., & Patterson, G. R. (2006). Toward a comprehensive model of antisocial development: A dynamic systems approach. *Psychological Review, 113*(1), 101–131. https://doi.org/10.1037/0033-295X.113.1.101

Grant, B. F., Hasin, D. S., Stinson, F. S., Dawson, D. A., Chou, S. P., Ruan, W. J., & Pickering, R. P. (2004). Prevalence, correlates, and disability of personality disorders in the United States: Results from the national epidemiologic survey on alcohol and related conditions. *The Journal of Clinical Psychiatry, 65*(7), 948–958.

Grant, I., Gonzalez, R., Carey, C. L., Natarajan, L., & Wolfson, T. (2003). Non-acute (residual) neurocognitive effects of cannabis use: A meta-analytic study. *Journal of the International Neuropsychological Society: JINS, 9*(5), 679–689. https://doi.org/10.1017/S1355617703950016

Grant, J. E., & Chamberlain, S. R. (2018). Symptom severity and its clinical correlates in kleptomania. *Annals of Clinical Psychiatry, 30*(2), 97–101.

Grant, J. E., Donahue, C. B., & Odlaug, B. L. (2011). *Treating impulse control disorders: A cognitive-behavioral therapy program, therapist guide.* New York, NY: Oxford University Press.

Grant, J. E., Stein, D. J., Woods, D. W., & Keuthen, N. J. (Eds.). (2012). *Trichotillomania, skin picking, and other body-focused repetitive behaviors.* Arlington, VA: American Psychiatric Publishing.

Gravitz, M. A., & Page, R. A. (2019). Hypnosis in the management of stress reactions. In G. S. Everly, Jr. & J. M. Lating, *A clinical guide to the treatment of the human stress response* (4th ed., pp. 353–366). New York, NY: Springer.

Greenberg, P. E., Pike, C. T., & Kessler, R. C. (2015). The economic burden of adults with major depressive disorder in the United States (2005 and 2010). *Journal of Clinical Psychiatry, 76*(2), 155–162. http://doi.org/10.4088/JCP.14m09298

Greengard, P. (2001). The neurobiology of slow synaptic transmission. *Science, 294*(5544), 1024–1030.

Gregory, B., & Peters, L. (2017). Changes in the self during cognitive behavioural therapy for social anxiety disorder: A systematic review. *Clinical Psychology Review, 52,* 1–18. https://doi.org/https://doi.org/10.1016/j.cpr.2016.11.008

Greiner, T., Haack, B., Toto, S., Bleich, S., Grohmann, R., Faltraco, F., ... Schneider, M. (2020). Pharmacotherapy of psychiatric inpatients with adjustment disorder: Current status and changes between 2000 and 2016. *European Archives of Psychiatry and Clinical Neuroscience, 270*(1), 107–117. doi:http://dx.doi.org.ezaccess.libraries.psu.edu/10.1007/s00406-019-01058-1

Grier, B. C., Wilkins, M. L., & Jeffords, E. H. (2010). Diagnosis and treatment of pediatric bipolar disorder. In P. C. McCabe & S. R. Shaw (Eds.), *Psychiatric disorders:* *Current topics and interventions for educators* (pp. 17–27). Thousand Oaks, CA: Corwin Press.

Griner, D., & Smith, T. B. (2006). Culturally adapted mental health intervention: A meta-analytic review. *Psychotherapy: Theory, Research, Practice, Training, 43*(4), 531–548. http://doi.org/10.1037/0033-3204.43.4.531

Grisham, J. R., Norberg, M. M., & Certoma, S. P. (2012). Treatment of compulsive hoarding. In G. Steketee (Ed.), *The Oxford handbook of obsessive compulsive and spectrum disorders* (pp. 422–435). New York, NY: Oxford University Press.

Grisso, T., & Appelbaum, P. S. (1995). Comparison of standards for assessing patients' capacities to make treatment decisions. *The American Journal of Psychiatry, 152*(7), 1033–1037.

Gual, N., García-Salmones, M., Brítez, L., Crespo, N., Udina, C., Pérez, L. M., & Inzitari, M. (2020). The role of physical exercise and rehabilitation in delirium. *European Geriatric Medicine, 11*(1), 83–93. https://doi.org/10.1007/s41999-020-00290-6

Gunderson, J. G., Stout, R. L., McGlashan, T. H., Shea, M. T., Morey, L. C., Grilo, C. M., ... Skodol, A. E. (2011). Ten-year course of borderline personality disorder: Psychopathology and function from the Collaborative Longitudinal Personality Disorders study. *Archives of General Psychiatry, 68*(8), 827–837. https://doi.org/10.1001/archgenpsychiatry.2011.37

Gustafson, P. E., Larson, I., Nelson, N., & Gustafson, P. A. (2009). Sociocultural disadvantage, traumatic life events, and psychiatric symptoms in preadolescent children. *American Journal of Orthopsychiatry, 79,* 387–397.

Guterman, J. T., Martin, C. V., & Rudes, J. (2011). A solution-focused approach to frotteurism. *Journal of Systemic Therapies, 30*(1), 59–72.

Gutman, D. A., & Nemeroff, C. B. (2011). Stress and depression. In R. Contrada & A. Baum (Eds.), *The handbook of stress science: Biology, psychology, and health* (pp. 345–357). New York, NY: Springer.

Gyawali, S., & Patra, B. N. (2019). Trends in concept and nosology of autism spectrum disorder: A review. *Asian Journal of Psychiatry, 40,* 92–99.

Haddad, P. M., Al Abdulla, M., Latoo, J., & Iqbal, Y. (2020). Brief psychotic disorder associated with quarantine and mild COVID-19. *BMJ Case Reports, 13*(12), e240088.

Hadley, S., Kim, S., Priday, L., & Hollander, E. (2006). Pharmacologic treatment of body dysmorphic disorder. *Primary Psychiatry, 13,* 61–69.

Haedt-Matt, A. A., & Keel, P. K. (2011). Revisiting the affect regulation model of binge eating: A meta-analysis of studies using ecological momentary assessment. *Psychological Bulletin, 137*(4), 660–681.

Hammen, C. (2005). Stress and depression. *Annual Review of Clinical Psychology, 1*, 293–319.

Hardaker, M., & Tsakanikos, E. (2021). Early information processing in narcissism: Heightened sensitivity to negative but not positive evaluative attributes. *Personality and Individual Differences, 168*, 110386.

Hare, R. D., McPherson, L. M., & Forth, A. E. (1988). Male psychopaths and their criminal careers. *Journal of Consulting and Clinical Psychology, 56*(5), 710–714. https://doi.org/10.1037//0022-006x.56.5.710

Haroz, E. E., Ritchey, M., Bass, J. K., Kohrt, B. A., Augustinavicius, J., Michalopoulos, L., ... Bolton, P. (2017). How is depression experienced around the world? A systematic review of qualitative literature. *Social Science & Medicine, 183*, 151–162.

Harris, B. (2017). Bedlam: The asylum and beyond. *Bulletin of the History of Medicine, 91*(2), 434–435.

Harris, L., Gilmore, D., Longo, A., & Hand, B. N. (2021). Patterns of US federal autism research funding during 2017–2019. *Autism, 25*(7), 2135–2139.

Hartung, C. M., & Lefler, E. K. (2019). Sex and gender in psychopathology: DSM-5 and beyond. *Psychological Bulletin, 145*(4), 390–409.

Harvey, A. G. (2008). Sleep and circadian rhythms in bipolar disorder: Seeking synchrony, harmony, and regulation. *The American Journal of Psychiatry, 165*(7), 820–829.

Hashmi, A., Shad, M., Rhoades, H. M., & Parsaik, A. K. (2014). Involuntary detention: Do psychiatrists clinically justify continuing involuntary hospitalization? *Psychiatric Quarterly, 85*(3), 285–293.

Hasin, D. S., Sarvet, A. L., Meyers, J. L., Saha, T. D., Ruan, W. J., Stohl, M., & Grant, B. F. (2018). Epidemiology of adult DSM-5 major depressive disorder and its specifiers in the United States. *JAMA Psychiatry, 75*(4), 336–346.

Hastings, M. H., Maywood, E. S., & Brancaccio, M. (2019). The mammalian circadian timing system and the suprachiasmatic nucleus as its pacemaker. *Biology, 8*(1), 13.

Hauser, S. R., Katner, S. N., Waeiss, R. A., Truitt, W. A., Bell, R. L., McBride, W. J., & Rodd, Z. A. (2020). Selective breeding for high alcohol preference is associated with increased sensitivity to cannabinoid reward within the nucleus accumbens shell. *Pharmacology Biochemistry and Behavior, 197*, 173002.

Hay, P. (2020). Current approach to eating disorders: A clinical update. *Internal Medicine Journal, 50*(1), 24–29. https://doi.org/10.1111/imj.14691

Hayes, S. C. (2019). Acceptance and commitment therapy: Towards a unified model of behavior change. *World Psychiatry, 18*(2), 226–227.

Hayley, A. C., Williams, L. J., Kennedy, G. A., Holloway, K. L., Berk, M., Brennan-Olsen, S. L., & Pasco, J. A. (2015). Excessive daytime sleepiness and falls among older men and women: Cross-sectional examination of a population-based sample. *BMC Geriatrics, 15*(1), 1–11.

Haynes, S. N., O'Brien, W., & Kaholokula, J. (2011). *Behavioral assessment and case formulation.* New York, NY: John Wiley & Sons.

Heishman, S. J., Kleykamp, B. A., & Singleton, E. G. (2010). Meta-analysis of the acute effects of nicotine and smoking on human performance. *Psychopharmacology, 210*(4), 453–469. https://doi.org/10.1007/s00213-010-1848-1

Henningsen, P. (2018). Management of somatic symptom disorder. *Dialogues in Clinical Neuroscience, 20*(1), 23–31.

Henriksen, M. G., Nordgaard, J., & Jansson, L. B. (2017). Genetics of schizophrenia: Overview of methods, findings and limitations. *Frontiers in Human Neuroscience, 11*, 332.

Herane-Vives, A., Fischer, S., De Angel, V., Wise, T., Papadopoulos, A., Arnone, D., ... Cleare, A. (2016). Cortisol levels in major depressive episode using fingernail specimens. *Psychoneuroendocrinology, 71*, 21. http://doi.org/10.1016/j.psyneuen.2016.07.062

Hermes, E. D., Hoff, R., & Rosenheck, R. A. (2014). Sources of the increasing number of Vietnam era veterans with a diagnosis of PTSD using VHA services. *Psychiatric Services, 65*(6), 830–832.

Herrmann, E. S., Johnson, P. S., Johnson, M. W., & Vandrey, R. (2016). Novel drugs of abuse. In V. R. Preedy (Ed.), *Neuropathology of drug addictions and substance misuse* (vol. 3, pp. 893–902). Amsterdam: Elsevier. https://doi.org/10.1016/b978-0-12-800634-4.00088-3

Hertenstein, E., Feige, B., Gmeiner, T., Kienzler, C., Spiegelhalder, K., Johann, A., ... Baglioni, C. (2019). Insomnia as a predictor of mental disorders: A systematic review and meta-analysis. *Sleep Medicine Reviews, 43*, 96–105. https://doi.org/10.1016/j.smrv.2018.10.006

Heylens, G., De Cuyper, G., Zucker, J.J. Schelfaut, C., Elaut, E., Vanden Bossche, H., ... T'Sjoen, G. (2012). Gender identity disorder in twins: A review of the case report literature. *Journal of Sexual Medicine, 9*(3), 751–757.

Hilbert, A., Hoek, H. W., & Schmidt, R. (2017). Evidence-based clinical guidelines for eating disorders. *Current Opinion in Psychiatry, 30*(6), 423–437. doi:10.1097/YCO.0000000000000360.

Hilbert, A., Petroff, D., Herpertz, S., Pietrowsky, R., Tuschen-Caffier, B., Vocks, S., & Schmidt, R. (2020). Meta-analysis on the long-term effectiveness of psychological and medical treatments for binge-eating disorder. *International Journal of Eating Disorders, 53*(9), 1353–1376.

Hinshaw, S. P. (2018). Attention deficit hyperactivity disorder (ADHD): Controversy, developmental mechanisms, and multiple levels of analysis. *Annual Review of Clinical Psychology, 14*, 291–316. https://doi.org/10.1146/annurev-clinpsy-050817-084917

Hinshaw, S. P., & Stier, A., (2008). Stigma as related to mental disorders. *Annual Review of Clinical Psychology, 4*, 367–393.

Hirsch, M., & Birnbaum, R. J. (2019). *Tricyclic and tetracyclic drugs: Pharmacology, administration, and side effects. UpToDate.* www.uptodate.com/contents/tricyclic-and-tetracyclic-drugs-pharmacology-administration-and-side-effects

Hirschtritt, M. E., Olfson, M., & Kroenke, K. (2021). Balancing the risks and benefits of benzodiazepines. *JAMA, 325*(4), 347–348.

Hjorthøj, C., Albert, N., & Nordentoft, M. (2018). Association of substance use disorders with conversion from schizotypal disorder to schizophrenia. *JAMA Psychiatry, 75*(7), 733–739.

Hock, L. E., & Karnik, N. S. (2017). Should clinicians medicate against structural violence? Potential iatrogenic risks and the need for social interventions. *AMA Journal of Ethics, 19*(8), 753–761.

Hodder, S. L., Feinberg, J., Strathdee, S. A., Shoptaw, S., Altice, F. L., Ortenzio, L., & Beyrer, C. (2021). The opioid crisis and HIV in the USA: Deadly synergies. *The Lancet, 397*(10279), 1139–1150. https://doi.org/10.1016/s0140-6736(21)00391-3

Hoffman, K. M., Trawalter, S., Axt, J. R., & Oliver, M. N. (2016). Racial bias in pain assessment and treatment recommendations, and false beliefs about biological differences between blacks and whites. *Proceedings of the National Academy of Sciences, 113*(16), 4296–4301.

Hoffman, L. W. (1991). The influence of the family environment on personality: Accounting for sibling differences. *Psychological Bulletin, 110*(2), 187–203.

Holoyda, B. J., & Kellaher, D. C. (2016). The biological treatment of paraphilic disorders: An updated review. *Current Psychiatry Reports, 18*(2), 19.

Holtzheimer, P. E., Kelley, M. E., Gross, R. E., Filkowski, M. M., Garlow, S. J., Barrocas, A., ... Mayberg, H. S. (2012). Subcallosal cingulate deep brain stimulation for treatment-resistant unipolar and bipolar depression. *Archives of General Psychiatry, 69*(2), 150. http://doi.org/10.1001/archgenpsychiatry.2011.1456

Holzer, K. J., & Vaughn, M. G. (2017). Antisocial personality disorder in older adults: A critical review. *Journal of Geriatric Psychiatry and Neurology, 30*(6), 291–302.

Holzer, K. J., Vaughn, M. G., Fearn, N. E., Loux, T. M., & Mancini, M. A. (2021). Age bias in the criteria for antisocial personality disorder. *Journal of Psychiatric Research, 137*, 444–451.

Honberg, R. S. (2020). Mental illness and gun violence: Research and policy options. *The Journal of Law, Medicine & Ethics, 48*(Supplement), 137–141. https://doi.org/10.1177/1073110520979414

Hong, V. (2016). Borderline personality disorder in the emergency department: Good psychiatric management. *Harvard Review of Psychiatry, 24*(5), 357–366.

Hoogman, M., Bralten, J., Hibar, D. P., Mennes, M., Zwiers, M. P., Schweren, L. S. J., ... Franke, B. (2017). Subcortical brain volume differences in participants with attention deficit hyperactivity disorder in children and adults: A cross-sectional mega-analysis. *The Lancet Psychiatry, 4*(4), 310–319. https://doi.org/10.1016/s2215-0366(17)30049-4

Hoppenbrouwers, S. S., Neumann, C. S., Lewis, J., & Johansson, P. (2015). A latent variable analysis of the Psychopathy Checklist–Revised and behavioral inhibition system/behavioral activation system factors in North American and Swedish offenders. *Personality Disorders: Theory, Research, and Treatment, 6*(3), 251–260. https://doi.org/10.1037/per0000115

Hopwood, C. J., Kotov, R., Krueger, R. F., Watson, D., Widiger, T. A., Althoff, R. R., ... Zimmermann, J. (2018). The time has come for dimensional personality disorder diagnosis. *Personality and Mental Health, 12*(1), 82–86. https://doi.org/10.1002/pmh.1408

Hopwood, C. J., & Thomas, K. M. (2012). Paranoid and schizoid personality disorders. In T. A. Widiger (Ed.), *The Oxford handbook of personality disorders* (pp. 582–602). New York, NY: Oxford University Press. https://doi.org/10.1093/oxfordhb/9780199735013.013.0027

Horigome, T., Kurokawa, S., Sawada, K., Kudo, S., Shiga, K., Mimura, M., & Kishimoto, T. (2020). Virtual reality exposure therapy for social anxiety disorder: A systematic review and meta-analysis. *Psychological Medicine*, *50*(15), 2487–2497.

Hosie, R. (2021, October 14). Tom Daley says he had an eating disorder due to weight pressure from his former coach. *Insider*. www.insider.com/tom-daley-had-eating-disorder-weight-pressure-from-former-coach-2021-10

Hossack, M. R., Reid, M. W., Aden, J. K., Gibbons, T., Noe, J. C., & Willis, A. M. (2020). Adverse childhood experience, genes, and PTSD risk in soldiers: A methylation study. *Military Medicine*, *185*(3–4), 377–384.

Houben, M., Mestdagh, M., Dejonckheere, E., Obbels, J., Sienaert, P., van Roy, J., & Kuppens, P. (2021). The statistical specificity of emotion dynamics in borderline personality disorder. *Journal of Personality Disorders*, *35*(6), 819–840.

Howard, R. M., Potter, S. J., Guedj, C. E., & Moynihan, M. M. (2019). Sexual violence victimization among community college students. *Journal of American College Health*, *67*(7), 674–687.

Howell, M. J., & Schenck, C. H. (2009). Treatment of nocturnal eating disorders. *Current Treatment Options in Neurology*, *11*(5), 333–339.

Howes, O. D., Rogdaki, M., Findon, J. L., Wichers, R. H., Charman, T., King, B. H., ... Murphy, D. G. (2018). Autism spectrum disorder: Consensus guidelines on assessment, treatment and research from the British Association for Psychopharmacology. *Journal of Psychopharmacology*, *32*(1), 3–29.

Hróbjartsson, A., & Norup, M. (2003). The use of placebo interventions in medical practice: A national questionnaire survey of Danish clinicians. *Evaluation & the Health Professions*, *26*(2), 153–165. https://doi.org/10.1177/0163278703026002002

Huang, C. Y., Fang, S. C., & Shao, Y. H. J. (2021). Comparison of long-acting injectable antipsychotics with oral antipsychotics and suicide and all-cause mortality in patients with newly diagnosed schizophrenia. *JAMA Network Open*, *4*(5), e218810.

Huang, W. L., Liao, S. C., & Gau, S. S. F. (2021). Association between Stroop tasks and heart rate variability features in patients with somatic symptom disorder. *Journal of Psychiatric Research*, *136*, 246–255.

Huang, Y., Kotov, R., De Girolamo, G., Preti, A., Angermeyer, M., Benjet, C., ... Kessler, R. (2009). DSM–IV personality disorders in the WHO World Mental Health Surveys. *British Journal of Psychiatry*, *195*(1), 46–53. doi:10.1192/bjp.bp.108.058552

Hughto, J. M. W., Clark, K. A., Altice, F. L., Reisner, S. L., Kershaw, T. S., & Pachankis, J. E. (2018). Creating, reinforcing, and resisting the gender binary: A qualitative study of transgender women's healthcare experiences in sex-segregated jails and prisons. *International Journal of Prisoner Health*, *14*(2), 69–88.

Huh, J., Le, T., Reeder, B., Thompson, H. J., & Demiris, G. (2013). Perspectives on wellness self-monitoring tools for older adults. *International Journal of Medical Information*, *82*(11), 1092–1103.

Huhn, M., Nikolakopoulou, A., Schneider-Thoma, J., Krause, M., Samara, M., Peter, N., ... Cipriani, A. (2019). Comparative efficacy and tolerability of 32 oral antipsychotics for the acute treatment of adults with multi-episode schizophrenia: A systematic review and network meta-analysis. *The Lancet*, *394*(10202), 939–951.

Hui, T. P., Kandola, A., Shen, L., Lewis, G., Osborn, D. P. J., Geddes, J. R., & Hayes, J. F. (2019). A systematic review and meta-analysis of clinical predictors of lithium response in bipolar disorder. *Acta Psychiatrica Scandinavica*, *140*(2), 94–115. https://doi.org/10.1111/acps.13062

Hyde, J. S., & Mezulis, A. H. (2020). Gender differences in depression: Biological, affective, cognitive, and sociocultural factors. *Harvard Review of Psychiatry*, *28*(1), 4–13.

Hyland, P., Murphy, J., Shevlin, M., Vallières, F., McElroy, E., Elklit, A., ... Cloitre, M. (2017). Variation in post-traumatic response: The role of trauma type in predicting ICD-11 PTSD and CPTSD symptoms. *Social Psychiatry and Psychiatric Epidemiology*, *52*(6), 727–736.

Iacovino, J. M., Jackson, J. J., & Oltmanns, T. F. (2014). The relative impact of socioeconomic status and childhood trauma on Black-White differences in paranoid personality disorder symptoms. *Journal of Abnormal Psychology*, *123*(1), 225–230. https://doi.org/10.1037/a0035258

Ibrahim, K., Eilbott, J. A., Ventola, P., He, G., Pelphrey, K. A., Mccarthy, G., & Sukhodolsky, D. G. (2019). Reduced amygdala–prefrontal functional connectivity in children with autism spectrum disorder and co-occurring disruptive behavior. *Biological Psychiatry: Cognitive Neuroscience and Neuroimaging*, *4*(12), 1031–1041. https://doi.org/10.1016/j.bpsc.2019.01.009

Inder, M. L., Crowe, M. T., Luty, S. E., Carter, J. D., Moor, S., Frampton, C. M., & Joyce, P. R. (2015). Randomized, controlled trial of interpersonal and social rhythm therapy for young people with bipolar disorder. *Bipolar Disorders*, *17*(2), 128–138.

Inouye, S. K., Westendorp, R. G., & Saczynski, J. S. (2014). Delirium in elderly people. *The Lancet, 383*(9920), 911–922.

Irwin, M. R., & Opp, M. R. (2017). Sleep health: Reciprocal regulation of sleep and innate immunity. *Neuropsychopharmacology, 42*(1), 129–155.

Izon, E., Berry, K., Wearden, A., Carter, L.-A., Law, H., & French, P. (2021). Investigating expressed emotion in individuals at-risk of developing psychosis and their families over 12 months. *Clinical Psychology & Psychotherapy, 28*(5), 1285–1296. https://doi.org/10.1002/cpp.2576

Jacobs, A. (1997, September 28). Shoplifting: The life style; when having enough is not enough. Why people with money raid the aisles. *The New York Times.* www.nytimes.com/1997/09/28/nyregion/shoplifting-life-style-when-having-enough-not-enough-why-people-with-money-raid.html

Jacobs, G. D. (2009). *Say goodnight to insomnia: A drug-free programme developed at Harvard Medical School.* New York, NY: Holt.

Jacobson, R. (2018). College students and eating disorders. *Child Mind Institute.* https://childmind.org/article/eating-disorders-and-college/

Jaffe, J. H. (1990). *Drug addiction and drug abuse* (8th ed.). Oxford: Pergamon.

Jafferany, M., Khalid, Z., McDonald, K. A., & Shelley, A. J. (2018). Psychological aspects of factitious disorder. *The Primary Care Companion for CNS Disorders, 20*(1). https://doi.org/10.4088/PCC.17nr02229

Jakubovski, E., Johnson, J. A., Nasir, M., Müller-Vahl, K., & Bloch, M. H. (2019). Systematic review and meta-analysis: Dose–response curve of SSRIs and SNRIs in anxiety disorders. *Depression and Anxiety, 36*(3), 198–212.

Jalnapurkar, I., Allen, M., & Pigott, T. (2018). Sex differences in anxiety disorders: A review. *Journal of Psychiatry, Depression & Anxiety, 4*(12), 3–16.

Jenkins, A. J., & Gates, M. J. (2020). Hallucinogens and psychedelics. In B. S. Levine & S. Kerrigan (Eds.), *Principles of forensic toxicology* (pp. 467–489). Cham: Springer.

Jennings, J. (2017). *Being jazz: My life as a (transgender) teen.* New York, NY: Random House.

Johns, M. M., Beltran, O., Armstrong, H. L., Jayne, P. E., & Barrios, L. C. (2018). Protective factors among transgender and gender variant youth: A systematic review by socioecological level. *The Journal of Primary Prevention, 39*(3), 263–301. https://doi.org/10.1007/s10935-018-0508-9

Johnson, J. G., Cohen, P., Chen, H., Kasen, S., & Brook, J. S. (2006). Parenting behaviors associated with risk for offspring personality disorder during adulthood. *Archives of General Psychiatry, 63*(5), 579–587. https://doi.org/10.1001/archpsyc.63.5.579

Johnson, M. W., Hendricks, P. S., Barrett, F. S., & Griffiths, R. R. (2019). Classic psychedelics: An integrative review of epidemiology, therapeutics, mystical experience, and brain network function. *Pharmacology & Therapeutics, 197*, 83–102. https://doi.org/10.1016/j.pharmthera.2018.11.010

Johnson, R. S., & Netherton, E. (2016). Fire setting and the impulse-control disorder of pyromania. *American Journal of Psychiatry: Residents' Journal, 11*(7), 14–16. https://doi.org/10.1176/appi.ajp-rj.2016.110707

Johnson, R. S., Ostermeyer, B., Sikes, K. A., Nelsen, A. J., & Coverdale, J. H. (2014). Prevalence and treatment of frotteurism in the community: A systematic review. *Journal of the American Academy of Psychiatry and the Law, 42*(4), 478–483.

Jonas, D. E., Cusack, K., Forneris, C. A., Wilkins, T. M., Sonis, J., Middleton, J. C., ... Olmsted, K. R. (2013). Psychological and pharmacological treatments for adults with posttraumatic stress disorder (PTSD). Rockville, MD: Agency for Healthcare Research and Quality (US); 2013 Apr. Report No. 13-EHC011-EF.

Jones, K. C. (2021). Update on major neurocognitive disorders. *Focus, 19*(3), 271–281.

Jones, M. C. (1924). A laboratory study of fear: The case of Peter. *The Pedagogical Seminary and Journal of Genetic Psychology, 31*(4), 308–315. https://doi.org/10.1080/08856559.1924.9944851

Jorge, J. C., Valerio-Pérez, L., Esteban, C., & Rivera-Lassen, A. I. (2021). Intersex care in the United States and international standards of human rights. *Global Public Health, 16*(5), 679–691.

Joseph, S., & Linley, P. A. (2006). *Positive therapy: A meta-theory for positive psychological practice.* London: Routledge.

Joseph, S. M., & Siddiqui, W. (2020). Delusional disorder. *StatPearls* [Internet]. Treasure Island (FL): StatPearls Publishing. www.ncbi.nlm.nih.gov/books/NBK539855/

Joyal, C. C. (2017). Linking crime to paraphilia: Be careful with label. *Archives of Sexual Behavior, 46*(4), 865–866.

Joyal, C. C., & Carpentier, J. (2017). The prevalence of paraphilic interests and behaviors in the general population: A provincial survey. *The Journal of Sex Research, 54*(2), 161–171.

Juhasz, G., Eszlari, N., Pap, D., & Gonda, X. (2012). Cultural differences in the development and characteristics of depression. *Neuropsychopharmacologia Hungarica,* *14*(4), 259–265.

Juvonen, J., & Ho, A. Y. (2008). Social motives underlying antisocial behavior across middle school grades. *Journal of Youth and Adolescence, 37*(6), 747–756.

Kagan, J. (2007). The limitations of concepts in developmental psychology. In G. W. Ladd (Ed.), *Appraising the human developmental sciences: Essays in honor of Merrill-Palmer Quarterly* (pp. 30–37). Detroit, MI: Wayne State University Press.

Kahn, J. (2012, May 11). Can you call a 9-year-old a psychopath? *The New York Times.* www.nytimes.com/ 2012/05/13/magazine/can-you-call-a-9-year-old-a-psychopath.html

Kallweit, U., & Bassetti, C. L. (2017). Pharmacological management of narcolepsy with and without cataplexy. *Expert Opinion on Pharmacotherapy, 18*(8), 809–817.

Kamenskov, M. Y., & Gurina, O. (2019). Neurotransmitter mechanisms of paraphilic disorders. *Zhurnal nevrologii i psikhiatrii imeni SS Korsakova, 119*(8), 61–67.

Kaminen-Ahola, N. (2020). Fetal alcohol spectrum disorders: Genetic and epigenetic mechanisms. *Prenatal Diagnosis, 40*(9), 1185–1192.

Kaminski, J. W., Valle, L. A., Filene, J. H., & Boyle, C. L. (2008). A meta-analytic review of components associated with parent training program effectiveness. *Journal of Abnormal Child Psychology, 36*(4), 567–589. https://doi .org/10.1007/s10802–007-9201-9

Kanayama, G., & Pope, H. G. (2021). Anabolic steroid use disorders: Diagnosis and treatment. In N. El-Guebaly, G. Carrà, & M. Galanter (Eds.), *Textbook of addiction treatment* (pp. 307–323). Cham: Springer.

Kanter, J. W., Rosen, D. C., Manbeck, K. E., Branstetter, H. M., Kuczynski, A. M., Corey, M. D., ... Williams, M. T. (2020). Addressing microaggressions in racially charged patient-provider interactions: A pilot randomized trial. *BMC Medical Education, 20*(1), 1–14.

Kaplan, M. (2016). Clinical considerations regarding regression in psychotherapy with patients with conversion disorder. *Psychodynamic Psychiatry, 44*(3), 367–384.

Kaplan, M. S., & Krueger, R. B. (2012). Cognitive-behavioral treatment of the paraphilias. *Israel Journal of Psychiatry and Related Sciences, 49*(4), 291–296.

Kapoor, R., Wasser, T. D., Funaro, M. C., & Norko, M. A. (2020). Hospital treatment of persons found not guilty by reason of insanity. *Behavioral Sciences & the Law, 38*(5), 426–440.

Kashima, Y. (2019). A history of cultural psychology: Cultural psychology as a tradition and a movement. In D.

Cohen & S. Kitayama (Eds.), *Handbook of cultural psychology* (pp. 53–78). New York, NY: Guilford Press.

Kato, K., Jevas, S., & Culpepper, D. (2011). Body image disturbances in NCAA Division I and III female athletes. *Sport Journal, 14*(1), 1–2.

Kaufman, A. R., Way, B. B., & Suardi, E. (2012). Forty years after Jackson v. Indiana: States' compliance with "reasonable period of time" ruling. *Journal of the American Academy of Psychiatry and the Law, 40*(2), 261–265.

Kaussner, Y., Kuraszkiewicz, A. M., Schoch, S., Markel, P., Hoffmann, S., Baur-Streubel, R., ... Pauli, P. (2020). Treating patients with driving phobia by virtual reality exposure therapy: A pilot study. *PLoS One, 15*(1), 1–14.

Kaye, W. H., Bulik, C. M., Thornton, L., Barbarich, N., Masters, K., & Price Foundation Collaborative Group (2004). Comorbidity of anxiety disorders with anorexia and bulimia nervosa. *The American Journal of Psychiatry, 161*(12), 2215–2221.

Kaye, W. H., Wagner, A., Frank, G., & Bailer, U. F. (2018). Review of brain imaging in anorexia and bulimia nervosa. *Annual Review of Eating Disorders Part 2–2006,* 113–130.

Keefe, J. R., McMain, S. F., McCarthy, K. S., Zilcha-Mano, S., Dinger, U., Sahin, Z., ... Barber, J. P. (2020). A meta-analysis of psychodynamic treatments for borderline and cluster C personality disorders. *Personality Disorders: Theory, Research, and Treatment, 11*(3), 157–169. https:// doi.org/10.1037/per0000382

Keenan, L., & Van Gundy, K. (2021). The neurological consequences of sleep deprivation. In L. M. DelRosso & R. Ferri (Eds.), *Sleep neurology* (pp. 45–55). Cham: Springer.

Keene, C. D., Montine, T. J., & Kuller, L. H. (2017). *Epidemiology, pathology, and pathogenesis of Alzheimer disease. UpToDate.* www.uptodate.com/contents/ epidemiology-pathology-and-pathogenesis-of-alzheimer-disease

Keightley, A. (2017). *Ian Brady: The untold story of the Moors murders.* New York, NY: HarperCollins.

Keller, N. E., Hennings, A. C., & Dunsmoor, J. E. (2020). Behavioral and neural processes in counterconditioning: Past and future directions. *Behaviour Research and Therapy, 125,* 103532.

Kellett, S., & Hardy, G. (2014). Treatment of paranoid personality disorder with cognitive analytic therapy: A mixed methods single case experimental design. *Clinical Psychology & Psychotherapy, 21*(5), 452–464.

Kelley, E., Bastow, B., Lakshmin, P., & Kingsberg, S. A. (2021). Female sexual dysfunctions and reproductive psychiatry. In L. A. Hutner, L. A. Catapano, S. M. Nagle-Yang, K. E. Williams, & L. M. Osborne (Eds.), *Textbook of women's reproductive mental health* (pp. 67–92). Washington, DC: American Psychiatric Association Publishing.

Kelly, J. F., Abry, A., Ferri, M., & Humphreys, K. (2020). Alcoholics Anonymous and 12-step facilitation treatments for alcohol use disorder: A distillation of a 2020 Cochrane Review for clinicians and policy makers. *Alcohol and Alcoholism*, *55*(6), 641–651. https://doi.org/10.1093/alcalc/agaa050

Kendall, P. C., Hollon, S. D., Beck, A. T., Hammen, C. L., & Ingram, R. E. (1987). Issues and recommendations regarding use of the Beck Depression Inventory. *Cognitive Therapy & Research*, *11*, 289–299.

Kendler, K. S., & Walsh, D. (1995). Schizotypal personality disorder in parents and the risk for schizophrenia in siblings. *Schizophrenia Bulletin*, *21*(1), 47–52.

Kerns, J. G. (2020). Cluster A personality disorders. In C. W. Lejuez & K. L. Gratz (Eds.), *The Cambridge handbook of personality disorders* (pp. 195–211). New York, NY: Cambridge University Press. https://doi.org/10.1017/9781108333931.037

Keski-Rahkonen, A. (2021). Epidemiology of binge eating disorder: Prevalence, course, comorbidity, and risk factors. *Current Opinion in Psychiatry*, *34*(6), 525–531.

Kessler, R. C., Berglund, P., Demler, O., Jin, R., & Walters, E. E. (2005). Trends in suicide ideation, plans, gestures, and attempts in the United States, 1990–1992 to 2001–2003. *JAMA*, *293*, 2487–2495.

Kessler, R. C., Chiu, W. T., Jin, R., Ruscio, A. M., Shear, K., & Walters, E. E. (2006). The epidemiology of panic attacks, panic disorder, and agoraphobia in the National Comorbidity Survey Replication. *Archives of General Psychiatry*, *63*, 415–424.

Kessler, R. C., Hudson, J. I., Shahly, V., Kiejna, A., & Cardoso, G. (2018). Bulimia nervosa and binge-eating disorder. In K. M. Scott, P. de Jonge, D. J. Stein, & R. C. Kessler (Eds.), *Mental disorders around the world: Facts and figures from the WHO World Mental Health Surveys* (pp. 263–285). New York, NY: Cambridge University Press. https://doi.org/10.1017/9781316336168.018

Kessler, R. C., McGonagle, K. A., Zhao, S., Nelson, C. B., Hughes, M., Eshleman, S., ... Kendler, K. S. (1994). Lifetime and 12-month prevalence of DSM-III-R psychiatric disorders in the United States: Results from the National Comorbidity Survey. *Archives of General Psychiatry*, *51*(1), 8–19.

Kessler, R. C., & Wang, P. S. (2008). The descriptive epidemiology of commonly occurring mental disorders in the United States. *Annual Review of Public Health*, *29*, 115–129.

Khera, M., & Cunningham, G. R. (2018). Treatment of male sexual dysfunction. *UpToDate*. www.uptodate.com/contents/treatment-of-male-sexual-dysfunction

Khoury, J. M., Roque, M. A. V., & Garcia, F. D. (2016). Pedophilic disorder. In R. Balon (Ed.), *Practical guide to paraphilia and paraphilic disorders* (pp. 141–154). Cham: Springer.

Kibria, A. A., & Metcalfe, N. H. (2016). A biography of William Tuke (1732–1822): Founder of the modern mental asylum. *Journal of Medical Biography*, *24*(3), 384–388.

Kiedis, A., & Sloman, L. (2004). *Scar tissue*. New York, NY: Hyperion.

Kihlstrom, J. F., Glisky, M. L., & Angiulo, M. J. (1994). Dissociative tendencies and dissociative disorders. *Journal of Abnormal Psychology*, *103*(1), 117–124.

Kikkert, M. J., Driessen, E., Peen, J., Barber, J. P., Bockting, C., Schalkwijk, F., ... Dekker, J. J. (2016). The role of avoidant and obsessive-compulsive personality disorder traits in matching patients with major depression to cognitive behavioral and psychodynamic therapy: A replication study. *Journal of Affective Disorders*, *205*, 400–405.

Killion, B., Hai, A. H., Alsolami, A., Vaughn, M. G., Sehun Oh, P., & Salas-Wright, C. P. (2021). LSD use in the United States: Trends, correlates, and a typology of use. *Drug and Alcohol Dependence*, *223*, 108715. https://doi.org/10.1016/j.drugalcdep.2021.108715

Kim, K. M. (2021). What makes adolescents psychologically distressed? Life events as risk factors for depression and suicide. *European Child & Adolescent Psychiatry*, *30*(3), 359–367.

King, R. M., Grenyer, B. F., Gurtman, C. G., & Younan, R. (2020). A clinician's quick guide to evidence-based approaches: Narcissistic personality disorder. *Clinical Psychologist*, *24*(1), 91–95.

Kingsberg, S. A., Althof, S., Simon, J. A., Bradford, A., Bitzer, J., Carvalho, J., ... Rezaee, R. L. (2017). Female sexual dysfunction: Medical and psychological treatments, committee 14. *The Journal of Sexual Medicine*, *14*(12), 1463–1491.

Kingsberg, S. A., & Simon, J. A. (2020). Female hypoactive sexual desire disorder: A practical guide to causes, clinical diagnosis, and treatment. *Journal of Women's Health, 29*(8), 1101–1112. https://doi.org/10.1089/jwh.2019.7865

Kirchebner, J., Günther, M. P., Sonnweber, M., King, A., & Lau, S. (2020). Factors and predictors of length of stay in offenders diagnosed with schizophrenia – a machine-learning-based approach. *BMC Psychiatry, 20*, 1–12.

Kirmayer, L. J., & Ryder, A. G. (2016). Culture and psychopathology. *Current Opinion in Psychology, 8*, 143–148. https://doi.org/10.1016/j.copsyc.2015.10.020

Kirsch, D. B. (2020). Obstructive sleep apnea. *Continuum: Lifelong Learning in Neurology, 26*(4), 908–928. https://doi.org/10.1212/CON.0000000000000885

Klein, D., & Attia, E. (2017). Anorexia nervosa in adults: Clinical features, course of illness, assessment, and diagnosis. *UpToDate.* www.uptodate.com/contents/anorexia-nervosa-in-adults-clinical-features-course-of-illness-assessment-and-diagnosis

Klein, D. N. (2010). Chronic depression: Diagnosis and classification. *Current Directions in Psychological Science, 19*(2), 96–100.

Knapp, M., Mangalore, R., & Simon, J. (2004). The global costs of schizophrenia. *Schizophrenia Bulletin, 30*, 279–293.

Knekt, P., Lindfors, O., Harkanen, T., Valikoski, M., Virtala, E., Laaksonen, M. A., … Renlund, C. (2008). Randomized trial on the effectiveness of long- and short-term psychodynamic psychotherapy and solution-focused therapy on psychiatric symptoms during a 3-year follow-up. *Psychological Medicine, 38*(5), 689–703. https://doi.org/10.1017/S003329170700164X

Knopf, A. (2021). Update on new boxed warning for benzodiazepines. *Alcoholism & Drug Abuse Weekly, 33*(8), 6–7.

Koenen, K. C., Ratanatharathorn, A., Ng, L., McLaughlin, K. A., Bromet, E. J., Stein, D. J., … Atwoli, L. (2017). Posttraumatic stress disorder in the World Mental Health Surveys. *Psychological Medicine, 47*(13), 2260–2274.

Koenigsberg, H. W., Harvey, P. D., Mitropoulou, V., New, A. S., Goodman, M., Silverman, J., … Siever, L. J. (2001). Are the interpersonal and identity disturbances in the borderline personality disorder criteria linked to the traits of affective instability and impulsivity? *Journal of Personality Disorders, 15*(4), 358–370. https://doi.org/10.1521/pedi.15.4.358.19181

Kollins, S. H., DeLoss, D. J., Cañadas, E., Lutz, J., Findling, R. L., Keefe, R. S., … Faraone, S. V. (2020). A novel digital intervention for actively reducing severity of paediatric ADHD (STARS-ADHD): A randomised

controlled trial. *The Lancet Digital Health, 2*(4), e168–e178.

Konarski, J. Z., McIntyre, R. S., Kennedy, S. H., Rafi-Tari, S., Soczynska, J. K., & Ketter, T. A. (2008). Volumetric neuroimaging investigations in mood disorders: Bipolar disorder versus major depressive disorder. *Bipolar Disorders, 10*(1), 1–37. http://doi.org/10.1111/j.1399-5618.2008.00435.x

Kondo, K., Noonan, K. M., Freeman, M., Ayers, C., Morasco, B. J., & Kansagara, D. (2019). Efficacy of biofeedback for medical conditions: An evidence map. *Journal of General Internal Medicine, 34*(12), 2883–2893.

Kontis, D., & Theochari, E. (2012). Dopamine in anorexia nervosa: A systematic review. *Behavioural Pharmacology, 23*(5–6), 496–515. https://doi.org/10.1097/FBP.0b013e328357e115

Kothgassner, O. D., Goreis, A., Robinson, K., Huscsava, M. M., Schmahl, C., & Plener, P. L. (2021). Efficacy of dialectical behavior therapy for adolescent self-harm and suicidal ideation: A systematic review and meta-analysis. *Psychological Medicine, 51*(7), 1–11.

Kraaijenvanger, E. J., Pollok, T. M., Monninger, M., Kaiser, A., Brandeis, D., Banaschewski, T., & Holz, N. E. (2020). Impact of early life adversities on human brain functioning: A coordinate-based meta-analysis. *Neuroscience & Biobehavioral Reviews, 113*, 62–76.

Krieg, A., & Xu, Y. (2018). From self-construal to threat appraisal: Understanding cultural differences in social anxiety between Asian Americans and European Americans. *Cultural Diversity and Ethnic Minority Psychology, 24*(4), 477–488.

Krijn, M., Emmelkamp, P. M. G., Olafsson, R. P., & Biemond, R. (2004). Virtual reality exposure therapy for anxiety disorders: A review. *Clinical Psychology Review, 24*(3), 259–281. doi:10.1017/S003329170700164X

Kring, A. M., & Sloan, D. M. (Eds.). (2009). *Emotion regulation and psychopathology: A transdiagnostic approach to etiology and treatment.* New York, NY: Guilford Press.

Kritsotaki, D. (2019). Social and mental hygiene: Models of mental illness prevention in twentieth-century Greece (1900–1980). In D. Kritsotaki, V. Long, & M. Smith (Eds.), *Preventing mental illness* (pp. 111–130). Cham: Palgrave Macmillan.

Krizan, Z., Miller, A., & Hisler, G. (2020). Does losing sleep unleash anger? *Sleep, 43*, A105.

Kroll, J. (1973). A reappraisal of psychiatry in the middle ages. *Archives of General Psychiatry, 29*(2), 276–283.

Kunst, M. J. J., Winkel, F. W., & Bogaerts, S. (2011). Posttraumatic anger, recalled peritraumatic emotions, and PTSD in victims of violent crime. *Journal of Interpersonal Violence, 26*(17), 3561–3579.

Kuperman, S., Chan, G., Kramer, J. R., Wetherill, L., Bucholz, K. K., Dick, D., ... Schuckit, M. (2013). A model to determine the likely age of an adolescent's first drink of alcohol. *Pediatrics, 131*(2), 242–248.

Kurlansik, S. L., & Maffei, M. S. (2016). Somatic symptom disorder. *American Family Physician, 93*(1), 49–54. https://pubmed.ncbi.nlm.nih.gov/26760840/

Kvarstein, E. H., Antonsen, B. T., Klungsøyr, O., Pedersen, G., & Wilberg, T. (2021). Avoidant personality disorder and social functioning: A longitudinal, observational study investigating predictors of change in a clinical sample. *Personality Disorders: Theory, Research, and Treatment, 12*(6), 594–605. http://dx.doi.org/10.1037/per0000471

Kwapil, T. R., & Barrantes-Vidal, N. (2012). Schizotypal personality disorder: An integrative review. In T. A. Widiger (Ed.), *The Oxford handbook of personality disorders* (pp. 437–477). New York, NY: Oxford University Press. https://doi.org/10.1093/oxfordhb/9780199735013.013.0021

Labrecque, F., Potz, A., Larouche, É., & Joyal, C. C. (2021). What is so appealing about being spanked, flogged, dominated, or restrained? Answers from practitioners of sexual masochism/submission. *The Journal of Sex Research, 58*(4), 409–423. https://doi.org/10.1080/00224499.2020.1767025

LaFortune, K. A. (2018). Eliminating offensive legal language. *Monitor on Psychology, 49*(5). www.apa.org/monitor/2018/05/jn

LaFrance, W. C., Baird, G. L., Barry, J. J., Blum, A. S., Webb, A. F., Keitner, G. I., ... Szaflarski, J. P. (2014). Multicenter pilot treatment trial for psychogenic nonepileptic seizures: A randomized clinical trial. *JAMA Psychiatry, 71*(9), 997–1005.

LaFreniere, L. S., & Newman, M. G. (2020). Exposing worry's deceit: Percentage of untrue worries in generalized anxiety disorder treatment. *Behavior Therapy, 51*(3), 413–423.

Lai, C. H. (2019). Fear network model in panic disorder: The past and the future. *Psychiatry Investigation, 16*(1), 16–26.

Lalonde, J. K., Hudson, J. I., Gigante, R. A., & Pope Jr., H. G. (2001). Canadian and American psychiatrists' attitudes toward dissociative disorders diagnoses. *The Canadian Journal of Psychiatry, 46*(5), 407–412.

Lamb, H. R., & Weinberger, L. E. (2020). Deinstitutionalization and other factors in the criminalization of persons with serious mental illness and how it is being addressed. *CNS Spectrums, 25*(2), 173–180. https://doi.org/10.1017/s1092852919001524

Lambert, M. J. (2010). Using outcome data to improve the effects of psychotherapy: Some illustrations. In M. J. Lambert, *Prevention of treatment failure: The use of measuring, monitoring, and feedback in clinical practice* (pp. 203–242). Washington, DC: American Psychological Association.

Lamm, C., & Singer, T. (2010). The role of anterior insular cortex in social emotions. *Brain Structure and Function, 214*(5–6), 579–591. http://doi.org/10.1007/s00429–010-0251-3

Lampe, L., & Malhi, G. (2018). Avoidant personality disorder: Current insights. *Psychology Research and Behavior Management, 11*, 55–66. https://doi.org/10.2147/prbm.s121073

Lan, M. J., & Mann, J. J. (2016). Serotonergic dysfunction in bipolar disorder. In J. C. Soares & A. H. Young (Eds.), *Bipolar disorders: Basic mechanisms and therapeutic implications* (pp. 43–48). New York, NY: Cambridge University Press.

Langberg, J. M., & Becker, S. P. (2012). Does long-term medication use improve the academic outcomes of youth with attention-deficit/hyperactivity disorder? *Clinical Child and Family Psychology Review, 15*(3), 215–233.

Latreille, V., von Ellenrieder, N., Peter-Derex, L., Dubeau, F., Gotman, J., & Frauscher, B. (2020). The human K-complex: Insights from combined scalp-intracranial EEG recordings. *NeuroImage, 213*, 116748. https://doi.org/10.1016/j.neuroimage.2020.116748

Laursen, T. M. (2019). Causes of premature mortality in schizophrenia: A review of literature published in 2018. *Current Opinion in Psychiatry, 32*(5), 388–393.

Lavender, J. M., Brown, T. A., & Murray, S. B. (2017). Men, muscles, and eating disorders: An overview of traditional and muscularity-oriented disordered eating. *Current Psychiatry Reports, 19*(6), 1–7.

Lazarus, R. S., & Folkman, S. (1984). *Stress, appraisal, and coping*. New York, NY: Springer.

Lazarus, S. A., Cheavens, J. S., Festa, F., & Zachary Rosenthal, M. (2014). Interpersonal functioning in borderline personality disorder: A systematic review of behavioral and laboratory-based assessments. *Clinical Psychology Review, 34*(3), 193–205. https://doi.org/10.1016/j.cpr.2014.01.007

Le, J., Feygin, Y., Creel, L., Lohr, W. D., Jones, V. F., Williams, P. G., . . . Davis, D. W. (2020). Trends in diagnosis of bipolar and disruptive mood dysregulation disorders in children and youth. *Journal of Affective Disorders, 264,* 242–248.

Leavitt, C. E., Leonhardt, N. D., & Busby, D. M. (2019). Different ways to get there: Evidence of a variable female sexual response cycle. *The Journal of Sex Research, 56*(7), 899–912. https://doi.org/10.1080/00224499.2019 .1616278

LeBeau, R. T., Glenn, D., Liao, B., Wittchen, H.-U., Beesdo-Baum, K., Ollendick, T., & Craske, M. G. (2010). Specific phobia: A review of DSM-IV specific phobia and preliminary recommendations for DSM-V. *Depression and Anxiety, 27*(2), 148–167.

Lebow, J. L., Chambers, A. L., Christensen, A., & Johnson, S. M. (2012). Research on the treatment of couple distress. *Journal of Marital and Family Therapy, 38*(1), 145–168.

Leclerc, J., Lesage, A., Rochette, L., Huỳnh, C., Pelletier, É., & Sampalis, J. (2020). Prevalence of depressive, bipolar and adjustment disorders, in Quebec, Canada. *Journal of Affective Disorders, 263,* 54–59.

Lee, C. D., Chippendale, T. L., & McLeaming, L. (2020). Postoperative delirium prevention as standard practice in occupational therapy in acute care. *Physical & Occupational Therapy in Geriatrics, 38*(3), 264–270.

Leeuwerik, T., Cavanagh, K., & Strauss, C. (2019). Patient adherence to cognitive behavioural therapy for obsessive-compulsive disorder: A systematic review and meta-analysis. *Journal of Anxiety Disorders, 68,* 102135. doi:10.1016/j.janxdis.2019.102135

Leichsenring, F., & Klein, S. (2020). Evidence for psychodynamic psychotherapy in specific mental disorders. In M. Leuzinger-Bohleber, M. Solms, & S. E. Arnold (Eds.), *Outcome research and the future of psychoanalysis: Clinicians and researchers in dialogue* (pp. 99–127). New York, NY: Routledge.

Leichsenring, F., Salzer, S., Beutel, M. E., Herpertz, S., Hiller, W., Hoyer, J., . . . Leibing, E. (2014). Long-term outcome of psychodynamic therapy and cognitive-behavioral therapy in social anxiety disorder. *The American Journal of Psychiatry, 171*(10), 1074–1082.

Leisman, G., Machado, C., Melillo, R., & Mualem, R. (2012). Intentionality and 'free-will' from a neurodevelopmental perspective. *Frontiers in Integrative Neuroscience, 6,* 1–12. doi:10.3389/fnint.2012.00036

Lejoyeux, M., & Germain, C. (2011). Pyromania: Phenomenology and epidemiology. In J. E. Grant & M. N. Potenza (Eds.), *The Oxford handbook of impulse control disorders* (pp. 135–148). New York, NY: Oxford University Press.

Lentz, A. M., & Zaikman, Y. (2021). The big "O": Sociocultural influences on orgasm frequency and sexual satisfaction in women. *Sexuality & Culture, 25*(3), 1096–1123. https://doi.org/10.1007/s12119–020-09811-8

Lescai, E. F. (2020). The transvestic disorder. *International Journal of Advanced Studies in Sexology, 2*(1), 25–31.

Lessard, L. M., Watson, R. J., & Puhl, R. M. (2020). Bias-based bullying and school adjustment among sexual and gender minority adolescents: The role of gay-straight alliances. *Journal of Youth and Adolescence, 49*(5), 1094–1109.

Levenson, J. (2018). Somatic symptom disorder: Epidemiology and clinical presentation. *UpToDate.* www .medilib.ir/uptodate/show/109552

Levine, S. B. (2021). Reflections on the clinician's role with individuals who self-identify as transgender. *Archives of Sexual Behavior, 50,* 3527–3536.

Levinson, D. F. (2006). The genetics of depression: A review. *Biological Psychiatry, 60*(2), 84–92. http://doi.org/10 .1016/j.biopsych.2005.08.024

Levy, J. J., Lebeaux, R. M., Hoen, A. G., Christensen, B. C., Vaickus, L. J., & MacKenzie, T. A. (2020). Longevity associated geometry identified in satellite images: Sidewalks, driveways and hiking trails. *arXiv preprint.* arXiv:2003.08750

Lévy, P., Kohler, M., McNicholas, W., Barbé, F., McEvoy, R., Somers, V., . . . Pepin, J. (2015). Obstructive sleep apnoea syndrome. *Nature Reviews Disease Primers, 1,* 15015.

Lewis, K. C., & Ridenour, J. M. (2020). Paranoid personality disorder. In C. Zeigler-Hill & T. Shackelford, (Eds.), *Encyclopedia of personality and individual differences* (pp. 3413–3421). Cham: Springer.

Lewis-Fernández, R., Guarnaccia, P. J., Martínez, I. E., Salmán, E., Schmidt, A. B., & Liebowitz, M. (2020). Comparative phenomenology of 'ataques de nervios,' panic attacks, and panic disorder. In D. E. Hinton & B. J. Good (Eds.), *Culture and panic disorder* (pp. 135–156). Stanford, CA: Stanford University Press.

Lewis-Fernández, R., Hinton, D. E., Laria, A. J., Patterson, E. H., Hofmann, S. G., Craske, M. G., . . . Liao, B. (2010). Culture and the anxiety disorders: Recommendations for the *DSM-V. Depression and Anxiety, 27,* 212–229.

Li, C. Y., Larsen, S., & Yap, T. (2017). Nocturnal penile tumescence study. In S. Minhas & J. Mulhall (Eds.), *Male sexual dysfunction: A clinical guide* (pp. 129–132). Chichester: John Wiley & Sons.

Li, M., Yao, X., Sun, L., Zhao, L., Xu, W., Zhao, H., . . . Yang, W. (2020). Effects of electroconvulsive therapy on depression and its potential mechanism. *Frontiers in Psychology, 11*. doi:10.3389/fpsyg.2020.00080

Li, Z., & Arthur, D. (2005). Family education for people with schizophrenia in Beijing, China: Randomised controlled trial. *The British Journal of Psychiatry, 187*(4), 339–345.

Lilienfeld, S. O. (2014). DSM-5: Centripetal scientific and centrifugal antiscientific forces. *Clinical Psychology: Science and Practice, 21*(3), 269–279.

Lilienfeld, S. O., & Arkowitz, H. (2010). *Living with schizophrenia. Scientific American.* https://doi.org/10.1038/scientificamericanmind0310-66

Lilienfeld, S. O., Wood, J. M., & Garb, H. N. (2000). The scientific status of projective techniques. *Psychological Science in the Public Interest, 1*(2), 27–66.

Lind, M. J., Aggen, S. H., Kirkpatrick, R. M., Kendler, K. S., & Amstadter, A. B. (2015). A longitudinal twin study of insomnia symptoms in adults. *Sleep, 38*(9), 1423–1430.

Linden, S. C., & Jones, E. (2014). 'Shell shock' revisited: An examination of the case records of the National Hospital in London. *Medical History, 58*(4), 519–545.

Lindner, P., Savic, I., Sitnikov, R., Budhiraja, M., Liu, Y., Jokinen, J., . . . Hodgins, S. (2016). Conduct disorder in females is associated with reduced corpus callosum structural integrity independent of comorbid disorders and exposure to maltreatment. *Translational Psychiatry, 6*(1), e714–e714.

Lindsey, M. A., Joe, S., Muroff, J., & Ford, B. E. (2010). Social and clinical factors associated with psychiatric emergency service use and civil commitment among African American youth. *General Hospital Psychiatry, 32*(3), 300–309.

Linehan, M. M. (1993). *Skills training manual for treating borderline personality disorder.* New York, NY: Guilford Press.

Linehan, M. M. (1999). Standard protocol for assessing and treating suicidal behaviors for patients in treatment. In D. G. Jacobs (Ed.), *The Harvard Medical School guide to suicide assessment and intervention* (pp. 146–187). San Francisco, CA: Jossey-Bass.

Linehan, M. M. (2020). *Building a life worth living: A memoir.* New York, NY: Random House.

Linehan, M. M., Korslund, K. E., Harned, M. S., Gallop, R. J., Lungu, A., Neacsiu, A. D., . . . Murray-Gregory, A. M. (2015). Dialectical behavior therapy for high suicide risk in individuals with borderline personality disorder: A randomized clinical trial and component analysis. *JAMA Psychiatry, 72*(5), 475–482.

Liu, A. (2007). *Gaining: The truth about life after eating disorders.* New York, NY: Warner Books.

Lobbestael, J., & Arntz, A. (2012). Cognitive contributions to personality disorders. In T. A. Widiger (Ed.), *The Oxford handbook of personality disorders* (pp. 325–344). New York, NY: Oxford University Press.

Lochner, C., Grant, J. E., Odlaug, B. L., Woods, D. W., Keuthen, N. J., & Stein, D. J. (2012). DSM-5 field survey: Hair-pulling disorder (trichotillomania). *Depression and Anxiety, 29*, 1025–1031. doi:10.1002/da.22011

Loewenstein, R. J. (2018). Dissociation debates: Everything you know is wrong. *Dialogues in Clinical Neuroscience, 20*(3), 229–242.

Loftus, T. J., Filiberto, A. C., Rosenthal, M. D., Arnaoutakis, G. J., Sarosi Jr., G. A., Dimick, J. B., & Upchurch Jr., G. R. (2020). Performance advantages for grit and optimism. *The American Journal of Surgery, 220*(1), 10–18.

López-López, J. A., Davies, S. R., Caldwell, D. M., Churchill, R., Peters, T. J., Tallon, D., . . . Lewis, G. (2019). The process and delivery of CBT for depression in adults: A systematic review and network meta-analysis. *Psychological Medicine, 49*(12), 1937–1947.

López-Muñoz, F., & Alamo, C. (2009). Monoaminergic neurotransmission: The history of the discovery of antidepressants from 1950s until today. *Current Pharmaceutical Design, 15*(14), 1563–1586.

Loria, K. (2019, January 23). Does melatonin really help you sleep? *Consumer Reports.* www.consumerreports.org/vitamins-supplements/does-melatonin-really-help-you-sleep/

Lovato, N., & Lack, L. (2019). Insomnia and mortality: A meta-analysis. *Sleep Medicine Reviews, 43*, 71–83.

Löwe, B., Levenson, J., Depping, M., Hüsing, P., Kohlmann, S., Lehmann, M., . . . Weigel, A. (2021). Somatic symptom disorder: A scoping review on the empirical evidence of a new diagnosis. *Psychological Medicine, 52*(4), 1–17. doi:10.1017/S0033291721004177

Luca, M., Bellia, S., Bellia, M., Luca, A., & Calandra, C. (2014). Prevalence of depression and its relationship with work characteristics in a sample of public workers. *Neuropsychiatric Disease and Treatment, 10*, 519–525.

Lui, S., Deng, W., Huang, X., Jiang, L., Ma, X., Chen, H., . . . Zou, L. (2009). Association of cerebral deficits with clinical symptoms in antipsychotic-naive first-episode schizophrenia: An optimized voxel-based morphometry and resting state functional connectivity study. *The American Journal of Psychiatry, 166*(2), 196–205.

Lyng, J., Swales, M. A., Hastings, R. P., Millar, T., Duffy, D. J., & Booth, R. (2020). Standalone DBT group skills training versus standard (i.e. all modes) DBT for borderline personality disorder: A natural quasi-experiment in routine clinical practice. *Community Mental Health Journal, 56*(2), 238–250.

Lynn, S. J., Maxwell, R., Merckelbach, H., Lilienfeld, S. O., van Heugten-van der Kloet, D., & Miskovic, V. (2019). Dissociation and its disorders: Competing models, future directions, and a way forward. *Clinical Psychology Review, 73*, 101755.

Macdonald, P., Hibbs, R., Corfield, F., & Treasure, J. (2012). The use of motivational interviewing in eating disorders: A systematic review. *Psychiatry Research, 200*(1), 1–11.

MacLennan, S. (2020). Down's syndrome. *InnovAiT, 13*(1), 47–52.

MacPherson, H. A. (2020). More than medication: The importance of family treatments for pediatric bipolar disorder. *The Brown University Child and Adolescent Behavior Letter, 36*(1), 1–6.

Madden, J. M., Lakoma, M. D., Lynch, F. L., Rusinak, D., Owen-Smith, A. A., Coleman, K. J., ... Croen, L. A. (2017). Psychotropic medication use among insured children with autism spectrum disorder. *Journal of Autism and Developmental Disorders, 47*(1), 144–154.

Maeder, E. M., Yamamoto, S., & McLaughlin, K. J. (2020). The influence of defendant race and mental disorder type on mock juror decision-making in insanity trials. *International Journal of Law and Psychiatry, 68*, 101536.

Maenner, M. J., Shaw, K. A., & Baio, J. (2020). Prevalence of autism spectrum disorder among children aged 8 years: Autism and developmental disabilities monitoring network, 11 sites, United States, 2016. *MMWR Surveillance Summaries, 69*(4), 1–12.

Maercker, A., & Lorenz, L. (2018). Adjustment disorder diagnosis: Improving clinical utility. *The World Journal of Biological Psychiatry, 19*(Supplement 1), S3–S13.

Magon, N., Chauhan, M., Malik, S., & Shah, D. (2012). Sexuality in midlife: Where the passion goes? *Journal of Mid-Life Health, 3*(2), 61–65. https://doi.org/10.4103/0976-7800.104452

Maher, B. A., & Maher, W. B. (1994). Personality and psychopathology: A historical perspective. *Journal of Abnormal Psychology, 103*(1), 72–77.

Maietta, J. E., Paul, N. B., & Allen, D. N. (2020). Cultural considerations for schizophrenia spectrum disorders part I: Symptoms, diagnosis, and prevalence. In L. T. Benuto, F. R. Gonzalez, & J. Singer (Eds.), *Handbook of cultural factors in behavioral health* (pp. 363–380). Cham: Springer.

Malcolm, A., Pikoos, T. D., Castle, D. J., & Rossell, S. L. (2021). An update on gender differences in major symptom phenomenology among adults with body dysmorphic disorder. *Psychiatry Research, 295*, 113619. https://doi.org/https://doi.org/10.1016/j.psychres.2020.113619

Malhi, G. S., Tanious, M., Das, P., Coulston, C. M., & Berk, M. (2013). Potential mechanisms of action of lithium in bipolar disorder. *CNS Drugs, 27*(2), 135–153.

Maller, J. J., Thaveenthiran, P., Thomson, R. H., McQueen, S., & Fitzgerald, P. B. (2014). Volumetric, cortical thickness and white matter integrity alterations in bipolar disorder type I and II. *Journal of Affective Disorders, 169*, 118–127.

Manahan, V. J. (2004). When our system of involuntary civil commitment fails individuals with mental illness: Russell Weston and the case for effective monitoring and medication delivery mechanisms. *Law & Psychology Review, 28*, 1–33.

Marder, S. R. (2021). Changing the face of schizophrenia. *The American Journal of Psychiatry, 178*(7), 584–585. https://doi.org/10.1176/appi.ajp.2021.21050480

Maree, D. J. (2020). The applicative split: The science-practitioner model of training and practice. In D. J. Maree, *Realism and Psychological Science* (pp. 43–53). Cham: Springer.

Marrus, N., & Hall, L. (2017). Intellectual disability and language disorder. *Child and Adolescent Psychiatric Clinics of North America, 26*(3), 539–554. https://doi.org/10.1016/j.chc.2017.03.001

Marshall, W. L., Serran, G. A., Marshall, L. E., & O'Brien, M. D. (2008). Sexual deviation. In M. Hersen & J. Rosqvist (Eds.), *Handbook of psychological assessment, case conceptualization and treatment, Vol. 1: Adults* (pp. 590–615). Hoboken, NJ: John Wiley & Sons.

Martell, C. R., Dimidjian, S., & Herman-Dunn, R. (2010). *Behavioral activation for depression: A clinician's guide.* New York, NY: Guilford Press.

Martin, A., & Rief, W. (2011). Relevance of cognitive and behavioral factors in medically unexplained syndromes and somatoform disorders. *Psychiatric Clinics, 34*(3), 565–578.

Martin, P. R., Lae, L., & Reece, J. (2007). Stress as a trigger for headaches: Relationship between exposure and sensitivity. *Anxiety, Stress & Coping: An International Journal, 20*(4), 393–407. https://doi.org/10.1080/10615800701628843

Martin, S. F., & Levine, S. B. (2018). Fetishistic disorder. *UpToDate.* www.uptodate.com/contents/fetishistic-disorder/print

Martín-Blanco, A., Soler, J., Villalta, L., Feliu-Soler, A., Elices, M., Pérez, V., ... Pascual, J. C. (2014). Exploring the interaction between childhood maltreatment and temperamental traits on the severity of borderline personality disorder. *Comprehensive Psychiatry, 55*(2), 311–318. https://doi.org/10.1016/j.comppsych.2013.08.026

Martínez-Monteagudo, M. C., Delgado, B., Inglés, C. J., & Escortell, R. (2020). Cyberbullying and social anxiety: A latent class analysis among Spanish adolescents. *International Journal of Environmental Research and Public Health, 17*(2), 406. https://doi.org/10.3390/ijerph17020406

Masheb, R. M., Grilo, C. M., & White, M. A. (2011). An examination of eating patterns in community women with bulimia nervosa and binge eating disorder. *International Journal of Eating Disorders, 44*(7), 618–624.

Mason, N. L., Theunissen, E. L., Hutten, N. R., Tse, D. H., Toennes, S. W., Jansen, J. F., ... Ramaekers, J. G. (2021). Reduced responsiveness of the reward system is associated with tolerance to cannabis impairment in chronic users. *Addiction Biology, 26*(1), e12870.

Massau, C., Kärgel, C., Weiß, S., Walter, M., Ponseti, J., HC Krueger, T., ... Schiffer, B. (2017). Neural correlates of moral judgment in pedophilia. *Social Cognitive and Affective Neuroscience, 12*(9), 1490–1499.

Masters, W. H., & Johnson, V. E. (1966). *Human sexual response.* Boston, MA: Little, Brown.

Masters, W. H., & Johnson, V. J. (1980). *Human sexual inadequacy.* New York, NY: Bantam Books.

Masuda, A., Qinaʻau, J., Juberg, M., & Martin, T. (2020). Bias in the Diagnostic and Statistical Manual 5 and psychopathology. In L. T. Benuto, M. P. Duckworth, & A. Masuda (Eds.), *Prejudice, Stigma, Privilege, and Oppression* (pp. 215–234). Cham: Springer.

Mataix-Cols, D., Frost, R. O., Pertusa, A., Clark, L. A., Saxena, S., Leckman, J. F., ... Wilhelm, S. (2010). Hoarding disorder: A new diagnosis for DSM-V? *Depression and Anxiety, 27*, 556–572.

Mattina, G. F., & Steiner, M. (2020). Premenstrual dysphoric disorder. In J. Rennó Jr., G. Valadares, A. Cantilino, J. Mendes-Ribeiro, R. Rocha, & A. Geraldo da Silva (Eds.), *Women's mental health* (pp. 73–93). Cham: Springer.

Matusiewicz, A. K., Hopwood, C. J., Banducci, A. N., & Lejuez, C. (2010). The effectiveness of cognitive behavioral therapy for personality disorders. *Psychiatric Clinics, 33*(3), 657–685.

May, P. A., Hasken, J. M., Hooper, S. R., Hedrick, D. M., Jackson-Newsom, J., Mullis, C. E., ... Hoyme, H. E. (2021). Estimating the community prevalence, child traits, and maternal risk factors of fetal alcohol spectrum disorders (FASD) from a random sample of school children. *Drug and Alcohol Dependence, 227*, 108918. https://doi.org/10.1016/j.drugalcdep.2021.108918

Mayes, S. D., Mathiowetz, C., Kokotovich, C., Waxmonsky, J., Baweja, R., Calhoun, S. L., & Bixler, E. O. (2015). Stability of disruptive mood dysregulation disorder symptoms (irritable-angry mood and temper outbursts) throughout childhood and adolescence in a general population sample. *Journal of Abnormal Child Psychology, 43*(8), 1543–1549.

Maymone, M. B., Neamah, H. H., Secemsky, E. A., Kundu, R. V., Saade, D., & Vashi, N. A. (2017). The most beautiful people: Evolving standards of beauty. *JAMA Dermatology, 153*(12), 1327–1329.

Mayo, C., & George, V. (2014). Eating disorder risk and body dissatisfaction based on muscularity and body fat in male university students. *Journal of American College Health, 62*(6), 407–415.

Mazure, C. M. (1998). Life stressors as risk factors in depression. *Clinical Psychology: Science and Practice, 5*(3), 291–313. https://doi.org/10.1111/j.1468-2850.1998.tb00151.x

McCabe, R. (2018). Specific phobia in adults: Epidemiology, clinical manifestations, course and diagnosis. *UpToDate.* www.uptodate.com/contents/specific-phobia-in-adults-epidemiology-clinical-manifestations-course-and-diagnosis

McDermott, B. E., Leamon, M. H., Feldman, M. D., & Scott, C. L. (2012). Factitious disorder and malingering. In J. A. Bourgeois, U. Parthasarathi, & A. Hategan (Eds.), *Psychiatry review and Canadian certification exam preparation guide* (pp. 267–276). Arlington, VA: American Psychiatric Publishing.

McDermott, B. E., Ventura, M. I., Juranek, I. D., & Scott, C. L. (2020). Role of mandated community treatment for justice-involved individuals with serious mental illness. *Psychiatric Services, 71*(7), 656–662.

McDermott, B. E., Warburton, K., & Auletta-Young, C. (2020). A longitudinal description of incompetent to stand trial admissions to a state hospital. *CNS Spectrums, 25*(2), 223–236.

McDonald, W. M. (2017). Overview of neurocognitive disorders. *Focus, 15*(1), 4–12.

McGoldrick, M., Loonan, R., & Wohlsifer, D. (2007). Sexuality and culture. In S. R. Leiblum (Ed.), *Principles and practice of sex therapy* (4th ed., pp. 416–441). New York, NY: Guilford Press.

McGrath, J. J., Féron, F. P., Burne, T. H. J., Mackay-Sim, A., & Eyles, D. W. (2003). The neurodevelopmental hypothesis of schizophrenia: A review of recent developments. *Annals of Medicine, 35*(2), 86–93. www.ncbi.nlm.nih.gov/pubmed/12795338

McGrath, J. J., Saha, S., Al-Hamzawi, A., Alonso, J., Bromet, E. J., Bruffaerts, R., . . . Kessler, R. C. (2015). Psychotic experiences in the general population: A cross-national analysis based on 31,261 respondents from 18 countries. *JAMA Psychiatry, 72*(7), 697–705.

McGrath, R. E., & Carroll, E. J. (2012). The current status of "projective" "tests". In H. Cooper, P.M. Camic, D.L. Long, A.T. Panter, D. Rindskopf, & K.J. Sher (Eds.), *APA handbook of research methods in psychology, vol. 1: Foundations, planning, measures, and psychometrics* (pp. 329–348). Washington, DC: American Psychological Association.

McGuffin, P., Rijsdijk, F., Andrew, M., Sham, P., Katz, R., & Cardno, A. (2003). The heritability of bipolar affective disorder and the genetic relationship to unipolar depression. *Archives of General Psychiatry, 60*(5), 497–502.

McIntosh, A. M., Sullivan, P. F., & Lewis, C. M. (2019). Uncovering the genetic architecture of major depression. *Neuron, 102*(1), 91–103.

McKenzie, K. C., & Gross, J. J. (2014). Nonsuicidal self-injury: An emotion regulation perspective. *Psychopathology, 47*(4), 207–219.

McLemore, K. A. (2018). A minority stress perspective on transgender individuals' experiences with misgendering. *Stigma and Health, 3*(1), 53–64.

McManus, M. A., Hargreaves, P., Rainbow, L., & Alison, L. J. (2013). Paraphilias: Definition, diagnosis and treatment. *F1000Prime Reports, 5*, 36. http://f1000.com/prime/reports/m/5/36

McSweeney, S. (2004). Depression in women. In P. J. Caplan & L. Cosgrove (Eds.), *Bias in psychiatric diagnosis* (pp. 183–188). Lanham, MD: Jason Aronson.

Meana, M., Fertel, E., & Maykut, C. (2017). Treating genital pain associated with sexual intercourse. In Z. D. Peterson (Ed.), *The Wiley handbook of sex therapy* (pp. 98–11). Chichester: John Wiley & Sons.

Mechler, K., Banaschewski, T., Hohmann, S., & Häge, A. (2021). Evidence-based pharmacological treatment options for ADHD in children and adolescents. *Pharmacology & Therapeutics, 230*, 107940. https://doi.org/10.1016/j.pharmthera.2021.107940

Medda, P., Toni, C., Mariani, M. G., De, L. S., Mauri, M., & Perugi, G. (2015). Electroconvulsive therapy in 197 patients with a severe, drug-resistant bipolar mixed state: Treatment outcome and predictors of response. *The Journal of Clinical Psychiatry, 76*(9), 1168–1173.

Meersand, P. (2011) Psychological testing and the analytically trained child psychologist. *Psychoanalytic Psychology, 28*(1), 117–131.

Mei, S., Hu, Y., Sun, M., Fei, J., Li, C., Liang, L., & Hu, Y. (2021). Association between bullying victimization and symptoms of depression among adolescents: A moderated mediation analysis. *International Journal of Environmental Research and Public Health, 18*(6), 3316. https://doi.org/10.3390/ijerph18063316

Meloy, J. R., & Yakeley, J. (2010). *Psychodynamic treatment of antisocial personality disorder.* In J. F. Clarkin, P. Fonagy, & G. O. Gabbard (Eds.), *Psychodynamic Psychotherapy for Personality Disorders: A Clinical Handbook* (pp. 311–336). Arlington, VA: American Psychiatric Publishing.

Mendoza, M. D., & Russell, H. A. (2020). Epidemiology and public health implications of the opioid crisis. In R. D. Shah & S. Suresh (Eds.), *Opioid therapy in infants, children, and adolescents* (pp. 3–15). Cham: Springer.

Merikangas, K. R., He, J. P., Burstein, M., Swendsen, J., Avenevoli, S., Case, B., . . . Olfson, M. (2011). Service utilization for lifetime mental disorders in US adolescents: Results of the National Comorbidity Survey–Adolescent Supplement (NCS-A). *Journal of the American Academy of Child & Adolescent Psychiatry, 50*(1), 32–45.

Merrill, L. L., Thomsen, C. J., Sinclair, B. B., Gold, S. R., & Milner, J. S. (2001). Predicting the impact of child sexual abuse on women: The role of abuse severity, parental support, and coping strategies. *Journal of Consulting & Clinical Psychology, 69*, 992–1006.

Metz, M. E., Epstein, N. B., & McCarthy, B. (2017). *Cognitive-behavioral therapy for sexual dysfunction.* New York, NY: Routledge.

Meyer, R. G., & Weaver, C. M. (2006). *The clinician's handbook: Integrated diagnostics, assessment, and intervention in adult and adolescent psychopathology.* Long Grove, IL: Waveland Press.

Micallef-Trigona, B. (2014). Comparing the effects of repetitive transcranial magnetic stimulation and electroconvulsive therapy in the treatment of depression: A systematic review and meta-analysis. *Depression Research and Treatment, 2014*, 135049. https://doi.org/10.1155/2014/135049

Miklowitz, D. J., & Chung, B. (2016). Family-focused therapy for bipolar disorder: Reflections on 30 years of research. *Family Process, 55*(3), 483–499. http://doi.org/10.1111/famp.12237

Miller, I. W., Uebelacker, L. A., Keitner, G. I., Ryan, C. E., & Solomon, D. A. (2004). Longitudinal course of bipolar I disorder. *Comprehensive Psychiatry, 45*(6), 431–440.

Miller, J. D., Lynam, D. R., Hyatt, C. S., & Campbell, W. K. (2017). Controversies in narcissism. *Annual Review of Clinical Psychology, 13*, 291–315.

Miller, J. N., & Black, D. W. (2020). Bipolar disorder and suicide: A review. *Current Psychiatry Reports, 22*(2), 1–10.

Miller, K., & Nied, J. (2020, February 5). *Jazz Jennings just posted a hospital photo after her 3rd gender confirmation surgery. Women's Health.* www.womenshealthmag.com/health/a23828566/jazz-jennings-gender-confirmation-surgery-complication/

Mindell, J. A., & Owens, J. A. (2015). *A clinical guide to pediatric sleep: Diagnosis and management of sleep problems.* Philadelphia, PA: Lippincott Williams & Wilkins.

Mineka, S., & Zinbarg, R. (2006). A contemporary learning theory perspective on the etiology of anxiety disorders: It's not what you thought it was. *The American Psychologist, 61*(1), 10–26. doi:10.1037/0003-066X.61.1.10

Mishra, P., & Srivastava, A. K. (2018). The association of impatience, hostility and hypertension: A review. *IAHRW International Journal of Social Sciences Review, 6*(4), 721–723.

Miyamoto, S., Lieberman, J., Fleishhacker, W., Aoba, A., & Marder, S. (2003). Antipsychotic drugs. In J. Tasman, J. Kay, & J. Lieberman (Eds.), *Psychiatry* (2nd ed., pp. 1928–1964). New York, NY: John Wiley & Sons.

Mizuki, Y., Sakamoto, S., Okahisa, Y., Yada, Y., Hashimoto, N., Takaki, M., & Yamada, N. (2021). Mechanisms underlying the comorbidity of schizophrenia and type 2 diabetes mellitus. *International Journal of Neuropsychopharmacology, 24*(5), 367–382. https://doi.org/10.1093/ijnp/pyaa097

Modak, A., & Fitzgerald, P. B. (2021). Personalising transcranial magnetic stimulation for depression using neuroimaging: A systematic review. *The World Journal of Biological Psychiatry, 22*(9), 647–669.

Mojibi, N., Ghazanfari-Sarabi, S., & Hashemi-Soteh, S. M. B. (2021). The prevalence and incidence of congenital phenylketonuria in 59 countries: A systematic review. *Journal of Pediatrics Review, 9*(2), 83–96.

Möllmann, A., Hunger, A., Schulz, C., Wilhelm, S., & Buhlmann, U. (2020). Gazing rituals in body dysmorphic disorder. *Journal of Behavior Therapy and Experimental Psychiatry, 68*, 101522. doi:10.1016/j.jbtep.2019.101522

Monahan, J. (2018). Predictions of violence. In T. Grisso & S. L. Brodsky (Eds.), *The roots of modern psychology and law: A narrative history* (pp. 143–157). New York, NY: Oxford University Press.

Montgomery, A., Ventriglio, A., & Bhugra, D. (2020). Standards in intercultural psychotherapy. In M. Schouler-Ocak & M. C. Kastrup (Eds.), *Intercultural psychotherapy* (pp. 29–46). Cham: Springer.

Montlahuc, C., Curis, E., Laroche, D. G., Bagoe, G., Etain, B., Bellivier, F., & Chevret, S. (2019). Response to lithium in patients with bipolar disorder: What are psychiatrists' experiences and practices compared to literature review? *Pharmacopsychiatry, 52*(2), 70–77.

Moore, A. A., Silberg, J. L., Roberson-Nay, R., & Mezuk, B. (2017). Life course persistent and adolescence limited conduct disorder in a nationally representative US sample: prevalence, predictors, and outcomes. *Social Psychiatry and Psychiatric Epidemiology, 52*(4), 435–443.

Mora, G. (2008). Renaissance conceptions and treatments of madness. In E. R. Wallace & J. Gach (Eds.), *History of psychiatry and medical psychology* (pp. 227–254). New York, NY: Springer.

Morandi, A., Zambon, A., Di Santo, S. G., Mazzone, A., Cherubini, A., Mossello, E., . . . Rispoli, V. (2020). Understanding factors associated with psychomotor subtypes of delirium in older inpatients with dementia. *Journal of the American Medical Directors Association, 21*(4), 486–492.

Morgentaler, A., Polzer, P., Althof, S., Bolyakov, A., Donatucci, C., Ni, X., . . . Basaria, S. (2017). Delayed ejaculation and associated complaints: Relationship to ejaculation times and serum testosterone levels. *The Journal of Sexual Medicine, 14*(9), 1116–1124.

Morrison, A. S., & Heimberg, R. G. (2013). Social anxiety and social anxiety disorder. *Annual Review of Clinical Psychology, 9*, 249–274.

Moser, C., & Kleinplatz, P. J. (2020). Conceptualization, history, and future of the paraphilias. *Annual Review of Clinical Psychology, 16*, 379–399.

Mourilhe, C., Moraes, C. E. de, Veiga, G. de, da Luz, F. Q., Pompeu, A., Nazar, B. P., . . . Appolinario, J. C. (2021). An evaluation of binge eating characteristics in individuals with eating disorders: A systematic review and meta-analysis. *Appetite, 162*, 105176. https://doi.org/https://doi.org/10.1016/j.appet.2021.105176

Mueller, S. C., De Cuypere, G., & T'Sjoen, G. (2017). Transgender research in the 21st century: A selective critical review from a neurocognitive perspective. *The American Journal of Psychiatry, 174*(12), 1155–1162.

Munder, T., Flückiger, C., Leichsenring, F., Abbass, A. A., Hilsenroth, M. J., Luyten, P., . . . Wampold, B. E. (2019). Is psychotherapy effective? A re-analysis of treatments for depression. *Epidemiology and Psychiatric Sciences*, *28*(3), 268–274.

Munsch, S., Meyer, A. H., Quartier, V., & Wilhelm, F. H. (2012). Binge eating in binge eating disorder: A breakdown of emotion regulatory process? *Psychiatry Research*, *195*(3), 118–124. https://doi.org/10.1016/j.psychres.2011.07.016

Murad, M. H., Elamin, M. B., Garcia, M. Z., Mullan, R. J., Murad, A., Erwin, P. J., & Montori, V. M. (2010). Hormonal therapy and sex reassignment: A systematic review and meta-analysis of quality of life and psychosocial outcomes. *Clinical Endocrinology*, *72*(2), 214–231. https://doi.org/10.1111/j.1365-2265.2009.03625.x

Murphy, M. J., & Peterson, M. J. (2015). Sleep disturbances in depression. *Sleep Medicine Clinics*, *10*(1), 17–23.

Murray, R. M., Quattrone, D., Natesan, S., van Os, J., Nordentoft, M., Howes, O., . . . Taylor, D. (2016). Should psychiatrists be more cautious about the long-term prophylactic use of antipsychotics?. *The British Journal of Psychiatry*, *209*(5), 361–365.

Murrie, D. C., Gardner, B. O., & Torres, A. N. (2020). Competency to stand trial evaluations: A state-wide review of court-ordered reports. *Behavioral Sciences & the Law*, *38*(1), 32–50.

Nahata, L., Quinn, G. P., Caltabellotta, N. M., & Tishelman, A. C. (2017). Mental health concerns and insurance denials among transgender adolescents. *LGBT Health*, *4*(3), 188–193.

Narr, R. K., Allen, J. P., Tan, J. S., & Loeb, E. L. (2019). Close friendship strength and broader peer group desirability as differential predictors of adult mental health. *Child Development*, *90*(1), 298–313.

Narrow, W. E., Regier, D. A., Rae, D. S., Manderscheid, R. W., & Locke, B. Z. (1993). Use of services by persons with mental and addictive disorders: Findings from the National Institute of Mental Health Epidemiologic Catchment Area Program. *Archives of General Psychiatry*, *50*(2), 95–107.

Neugebauer, R. (1979). Medieval and early modern theories of mental illness. *Archives of General Psychiatry*, *36*(4), 477–483.

Newcomb, M. E., & Mustanski, B. (2014). Diaries for observation or intervention of health behaviors: Factors that predict reactivity in a sexual diary study of men who have sex with men. *Annals of Behavioral Medicine*, *47*(3), 325–334.

Newman, W. C., Chivukula, S., & Grandhi, R. (2016). From mystics to modern times: A history of craniotomy & religion. *World Neurosurgery*, *92*, 148–150.

NFPA report—Fire loss in the United States (2021). www.nfpa.org/News-and-Research/Data-research-and-tools/US-Fire-Problem/Fire-loss-in-the-United-States

Nichtová, A., Volavka, J., Vevera, J., Příhodová, K., Juríčková, V., Klemsová, A., . . . Papoušková, E. (2020). Deconstructing violence in acutely exacerbating psychotic patients. *CNS Spectrums*, *26*(6), 643–647.

Nicolini, H., Salin-Pascual, R., Cabrera, B., & Lanzagorta, N. (2017). Influence of culture in obsessive-compulsive disorder and its treatment. *Current Psychiatry Reviews*, *13*(4), 285–292.

NIMH (National Institute of Mental Health) (2019) *Mental health services.* www.nimh.nih.gov/health/statistics/mental-illness

Nippert, K. E., Tomiyama, A. J., Smieszek, S. M., & Incollingo Rodriguez, A. C. (2021). The media as a source of weight stigma for pregnant and postpartum women. *Obesity*, *29*(1), 226–232.

Nobler, M. S., Oquendo, M. A., Kegeles, L. S., Malone, K. M., Campbell, C., Sackeim, H. A., & Mann, J. J. (2001). Decreased regional brain metabolism after ECT. *The American Journal of Psychiatry*, *158*(2), 305–308.

Nolan, R. P., Feldman, R., Dawes, M., Kaczorowski, J., Lynn, H., Barr, S. I., . . . Surikova, J. (2018). Randomized controlled trial of e-counseling for hypertension: REACH. *Circulation: Cardiovascular Quality and Outcomes*, *11*(7), e004420.

Nolen-Hoeksema, S., & Hilt, L. M. (2013). The emergence of gender differences in depression in adolescence. In S. Nolen-Hoeksema & L. M. Hilt (Eds.), *Handbook of depression in adolescents* (pp. 111–136). New York, NY: Routledge.

Norcross, J. C., & Goldfried, M. R. (Eds.). (2005). *Handbook of psychotherapy integration* (2nd ed.). New York, NY: Oxford University Press.

Novais, F., Araújo, A. M., & Godinho, P. (2015). Historical roots of histrionic personality disorder. *Frontiers in Psychology*, *6*, 1463.

Novosad, D., Banfe, S., Britton, J., & Bloom, J. D. (2016). Conditional release placements of insanity acquittees in Oregon: 2012–2014. *Behavioral Sciences & the Law*, *34*(2–3), 366–377.

Novotney, A. (2014, September). Students under pressure: College and university counseling centers are examining how best to serve the growing number of students seeking their services. *Monitor on Psychology*, *36*.

Noyes, D. (2016). *Ten days a madwoman: The daring life and turbulent times of the original "girl" reporter, Nellie Bly.* New York, NY: Penguin.

Nusslock, R., Abramson, L. Y., Harmon-Jones, E., Alloy, L. B., & Hogan, M. E. (2007). A goal-striving life event and the onset of bipolar episodes: Perspective from the Behavioral Approach System (BAS) dysregulation theory. *Journal of Abnormal Psychology, 116,* 105–115.

Nutt, D. (2019). Psychedelic drugs: A new era in psychiatry? *Dialogues in Clinical Neuroscience, 21*(2), 139–147.

O'Connor, D. B., Thayer, J. F., & Vedhara, K. (2021). Stress and health: A review of psychobiological processes. *Annual Review of Psychology, 72,* 663–688.

O'Donnell, E. (2020). *Examining the impact of competency to stand trial and judicial instructions on NGRI verdicts.* New York, NY: City University of New York John Jay College of Criminal Justice.

O'Donnell, M. L., Agathos, J. A., Metcalf, O., Gibson, K., & Lau, W. (2019). Adjustment disorder: Current developments and future directions. *International Journal of Environmental Research and Public Health, 16*(14), 2537.

O'Hara, M., & Howard, C. (2021). Does CBT decrease physical symptoms in somatic symptom disorder in adults? *Evidence-Based Practice, 24*(9), 30–31.

Ohikuare, J. (2014, January 21). Life as a nonviolent psychopath. *The Atlantic.* www.theatlantic.com/health/archive/2014/01/life-as-a-nonviolent-psychopath/282271/

Olaya, B., Moneta, M. V., Miret, M., Ayuso-Mateos, J. L., & Haro, J. M. (2018). Epidemiology of panic attacks, panic disorder and the moderating role of age: Results from a population-based study. *Journal of Affective Disorders, 241,* 627–633.

Olsen, S., Smith, S., Oei, T. P. S., & Douglas, J. (2010). Cues to starting CPAP in obstructive sleep apnea: Development and validation of the cues to CPAP use questionnaire. *Journal of Clinical Sleep Medicine, 6*(3), 229–237. www.ncbi.nlm.nih.gov/pmc/articles/PMC2883033/

Olson, B. D., Emshoff, J., & Rivera, R. (2017). Substance use and misuse: The community psychology of prevention, intervention, and policy. In M. A. Bond, I. Serrano-García, C. B. Keys, & M. Shinn (Eds.), *APA handbook of community psychology: Methods for community research and action for diverse groups and issues* (pp. 393–407). Washington, DC: American Psychological Association. https://doi.org/10.1037/14954-023

Olson-Kennedy, J., Forcier, M., Geffner, M. E., & Blake, D. (2018). Management of transgender and gender-diverse children and adolescents. *UpToDate.* www.uptodate.com/contents/management-of-transgender-and-gender-diverse-children-and-adolescents

Olver, M. E., Lewis, K., & Wong, S. (2013). Risk reduction treatment of high-risk psychopathic offenders: The relationship of psychopathy and treatment change to violent recidivism. *Personality Disorders, 4*(2), 160–167. https://doi.org/10.1037/a0029769

Osaji, J., Ojimba, C., & Ahmed, S. (2020). The use of acceptance and commitment therapy in substance use disorders: A review of literature. *Journal of Clinical Medicine Research, 12*(10), 629–633.

Ospina, J. P., King IV, F., Madva, E., & Celano, C. M. (2018). Epidemiology, mechanisms, diagnosis, and treatment of delirium: A narrative review. *Clinical Medicine and Therapeutics, 1*(1), 3. doi:10.24983/scitemed.cmt.2018.00085

Otto, M. W., & Applebaum, A. J. (2011). The nature and treatment of bipolar disorder and the bipolar spectrum. In D. H. Barlow (Ed.), *The Oxford handbook of clinical psychology* (pp. 294–310). New York, NY: Oxford University Press

Owen, M. J., Cardno, A. G., & O'Donovan, M. C. (2000). Psychiatric genetics: Back to the future. *Molecular Psychiatry, 5*(1), 22–31.

Paintain, E., & Cassidy, S. (2018). First-line therapy for post-traumatic stress disorder: A systematic review of cognitive behavioural therapy and psychodynamic approaches. *Counselling and Psychotherapy Research, 18*(3), 237–250.

Palma-Gudiel, H., Córdova-Palomera, A., Navarro, V., & Fañanás, L. (2020). Twin study designs as a tool to identify new candidate genes for depression: A systematic review of DNA methylation studies. *Neuroscience & Biobehavioral Reviews, 112,* 345–352. https://doi.org/10.1016/j.neubiorev.2020.02.017

Pandya, N. H., Mevada, A., Patel, V., & Surthar, M. (2013). Study of effects of advanced maternal age related risks for Down syndrome & other trisomies. *International Journal of Biomedical and Advance Research, 4*(2), 123–127.

Parcesepe, A. M., & Cabassa, L. J. (2013). Public stigma of mental illness in the United States: A systematic literature review. *Administration and Policy in Mental Health and Mental Health Services Research, 40*(5), 384–399.

Paris, J. (2013). *The intelligent clinician's guide to the DSM-5®.* New York, NY: Oxford University Press.

Paris, J. (2018). Childhood adversities and personality disorders. In W. J. Livesley & R. Larstone (Eds.), *Handbook of personality disorders: Theory, research, and treatment* (pp. 301–308). New York, NY: Guilford Press.

Park, M., & Unützer, J. (2014). Hundred forty eight more days with depression: The association between marital conflict and depression-free days. *International Journal of Geriatric Psychiatry, 29*(12), 1271–1277. http://doi.org/10.1002/gps.4107

Patel, A., & Hinton, D. (2020). Two peas in a pod? Understanding cross-cultural similarities and differences in anxiety disorders. In E. Bui, M. E. Charney, & A. W. Baker (Eds.), *Clinical handbook of anxiety disorders* (pp. 59–75). Cham: Springer.

Patel, D. R., Cabral, M. D., Ho, A., & Merrick, J. (2020). A clinical primer on intellectual disability. *Translational Pediatrics, 9*(Supplement 1), S23–S35.

Patel, S. Y., Mehrotra, A., Huskamp, H. A., Uscher-Pines, L., Ganguli, I., & Barnett, M. L. (2021). Trends in outpatient care delivery and telemedicine during the COVID-19 pandemic in the US. *JAMA Internal Medicine, 181*(3), 388–391.

Peckmezian, T., & Paxton, S. J. (2020). A systematic review of outcomes following residential treatment for eating disorders. *European Eating Disorders Review, 28*(3), 246–259.

Peebles, R., Lesser, A., Park, C. C., Heckert, K., Timko, C. A., Lantzouni, E., . . . Weaver, L. (2017). Outcomes of an inpatient medical nutritional rehabilitation protocol in children and adolescents with eating disorders. *Journal of Eating Disorders, 5*(1), 1–14.

Pereira-Lourenço, M., e Brito, D. V., & Pereira, B. J. (2019). Premature ejaculation: From physiology to treatment. *Journal of Family & Reproductive Health, 13*(3), 120–131.

Perlick, D. A., Berk, L., Kaczynski, R., Gonzalez, J., Link, B., Dixon, L., . . . Miklowitz, D. J. (2016). Caregiver burden as a predictor of depression among family and friends who provide care for persons with bipolar disorder. *Bipolar Disorders, 18*(2), 183–191. http://doi.org/10.1111/bdi.12379

Perlin, M. L. (2000). *The hidden prejudice: Mental disability on trial*. Washington, DC: American Psychological Association. https://doi.org/10.1037/10379-000

Perrotta, G. (2019). Panic disorder: Definitions, contexts, neural correlates and clinical strategies. *Current Trends in Clinical & Medical Sciences, 1*. doi:10.33552/CTCMS.2019.01.000508

Persico, A. M., Ricciardello, A., Lamberti, M., Turriziani, L., Cucinotta, F., Brogna, C., . . . Arango, C. (2021). The pediatric psychopharmacology of autism spectrum disorder: A systematic review, part I – the past and the present. *Progress in Neuropsychopharmacology and Biological Psychiatry*. doi:10.1016/j.pnpbp.2021.110326

Peterson, C., Maier, S. F., & Seligman, M. E. (1993). *Learned helplessness: A theory for the age of personal control*. New York, NY: Oxford University Press.

Peterson, C., Semmel, A., Baeyer, C. Abramson. L. Y., Metalsky, G. I., & Seligman, M. E. P. (1982). The attributional style questionnaire. *Cognitive Therapy and Research, 6*(3), 287–300. https://doi.org/10.1007/BF01173577

Peterson, Z. D. (Ed.). (2017). *The Wiley handbook of sex therapy*. Chichester: John Wiley & Sons.

Pew Charitable Trusts (2009). *States cope with rising homelessness*. www.pewtrusts.org/en/research-and-analysis/blogs/stateline/2009/03/18/states-cope-with-rising-homelessness

Phillips, K. A., Dufresne, R. G., Wilkel, C. S., & Vittorio, C. C. (2000). Rate of body dysmorphic disorder in dermatology patients. *Journal of the American Academy of Dermatology, 42*, 436–441.

Phillips, K. A., Grant, J., Siniscalchi, J., & Albertini, R. S. (2001). Surgical and nonpsychiatric medical treatment of patients with body dysmorphic disorder. *Psychosomatics, 42*, 504–510.

Phillips, K. A., Menard, W., Fay, C., & Weisberg, R. (2005). Demographic characteristics, phenomenology, comorbidity, and family history in 200 individuals with body dysmorphic disorder. *The American Journal of Psychiatry, 163*, 907–912.

Phillips, K. A., Wilhelm, S., Koran, L. M., Didie, E. R., Fallon, B. A., Feusner, J., & Stein, D. J. (2010). Body dysmorphic disorder: Some key issues for DSM-V. *Depression and Anxiety, 27*, 573–591.

Pike, K., Yager, J., & Solomon, D. Anorexia nervosa in adults: Cognitive-behavioral therapy (CBT). *Cochrane Database* 2017.

Pinna, M., Manchia, M., Visioli, C., & Tondo, L. (2020). Clinical response and metabolic effects of lithium in 323 mood disorder patients. *Journal of Affective Disorders, 270*, 9–14.

Piper, A., & Mersky, H. (2004). The persistence of folly: A critical examination of dissociative identity disorder, part I: The excesses of an improbable concept. *Canadian Journal of Psychiatry, 49*, 592–600.

Plomin, R., Asbury, K., & Dunn, J. (2001). Why are children in the same family so different? Nonshared environment a decade later. *The Canadian Journal of Psychiatry, 46*(3), 225–233.

Plomin, R., DeFries, J. C., McClearn, G. E., & McGuffin, P. (2000). *Behavioral genetics*. New York, NY: Worth.

Polanczyk, G. V., Salum, G. A., Sugaya, L. S., Caye, A., & Rohde, L. A. (2015). Annual research review: A meta-analysis of the worldwide prevalence of mental disorders in children and adolescents. *Journal of Child Psychology and Psychiatry, 56*(3), 345–365.

Pollklas, M., Widemann, L., Lochschmidt, M., Plakhuta, A., & Gerlach, A. L. (2020). Cyberchondriasis: The effect of searching the internet on health concerns. *Zeitschrift für Psychologie, 228*(2), 110–118.

Pons, E. V., Salvador-Carulla, L., Calcedo-Barba, A., Paz, S., Messer, T., Paccardi, B., & Zeller, S. L. (2020). The capacity of schizophrenia and bipolar disorder individuals to make autonomous decisions about pharmacological treatments for their illness in real life: A scoping review. *Health Science Reports, 3*(3), e179.

Possin, K. L., Tsoy, E., & Windon, C. C. (2021). Perils of race-based norms in cognitive testing: The case of former NFL players. *JAMA Neurology, 78*(4), 377–378.

Postlethwaite, A., Kellett, S., & Mataix-Cols, D. (2019). Prevalence of hoarding disorder: A systematic review and meta-analysis. *Journal of Affective Disorders, 256,* 309–316.

Potter, N. N., Kincaid, H., & Sullivan, J. A. (2014). Oppositional defiant disorder: Cultural factors that influence interpretations of defiant behavior and their social and scientific consequences. In H. Kincaid & J. A. Sullivan (Eds.), *Classifying psychopathology: Mental kinds and natural kinds* (pp. 175–194). Cambridge, MA: MIT Press.

Pozzi, E., Capogrosso, P., Boeri, L., Cazzaniga, W., Matloob, R., Ventimiglia, E., ... Salonia, A. (2021). Trends in reported male sexual dysfunction over the past decade: An evolving landscape. *International Journal of Impotence Research, 33,* 596–602. https://doi.org/10.1038/s41443-020-0324-7

Preston, J. D., O'Neal, J. H., Talaga, M. C., & Moore, B. A. (2021). *Handbook of clinical psychopharmacology for therapists.* Oakland, CA: New Harbinger Publications.

Preti, E., Di Pierro, R., Fanti, E., Madeddu, F., & Calati, R. (2020). Personality disorders in time of pandemic. *Current Psychiatry Reports, 22*(12). https://doi.org/10.1007/s11920–020-01204-w

Pretsky, J. (2020). Teaching empirical research in psychodynamic psychotherapy: How to make research really matter. In M. Leuzinger-Bohleber, M. Solms, & S. E. Arnold (Eds.), *Outcome research and the future of psychoanalysis* (pp. 238–248). New York, NY: Routledge.

Probst, T., Kleinstäuber, M., Lambert, M. J., Tritt, K., Pieh, C., Loew, T. H., ... Delgadillo, J. (2020). Why are some cases not on track? An item analysis of the Assessment for Signal Cases during inpatient psychotherapy. *Clinical Psychology & Psychotherapy, 27*(4), 559–566.

Prochaska, J. O., & Norcross, J.C. (2018). *Systems of psychotherapy: A transtheoretical analysis* (9th ed.). New York, NY: Oxford University Press.

Przybylski, A. K., & Weinstein, N. (2019). Violent video game engagement is not associated with adolescents' aggressive behaviour: Evidence from a registered report. *Royal Society Open Science, 6*(2), 171474. https://doi.org/doi:10.1098/rsos.171474

Puckett, J. A., Maroney, M. R., Wadsworth, L. P., Mustanski, B., & Newcomb, M. E. (2020). Coping with discrimination: The insidious effects of gender minority stigma on depression and anxiety in transgender individuals. *Journal of Clinical Psychology, 76*(1), 176–194. http://dx.doi.org.ezaccess.libraries.psu.edu/10.1002/jclp.22865

Pueschel, S. M., & Goldstein, A. (1991). Genetic counseling. In J. L. Matson & J. A. Mulick (Eds.), *Handbook of mental retardation* (pp. 279–291). New York, NY: Pergamon.

Puhl, R. M., & Heuer, C. A. (2009). The stigma of obesity: A review and update. *Obesity, 17*(5), 941–964.

Pyke, R. E. (2020). Sexual performance anxiety. *Sexual Medicine Reviews, 8*(2), 183–190.

Quinsey, V. L. (2003). The etiology of anomalous sexual preferences in men. *Annals of the New York Academy of Sciences, 989*(1), 105–117.

Raihani, N. J., & Bell, V. (2019). An evolutionary perspective on paranoia. *Nature Human Behaviour, 3*(2), 114–121. https://doi.org/10.1038/s41562–018-0495-0

Raj, V., Rowe, A. A., Fleisch, S. B., Paranjape, S. Y., Arain, A. M., & Nicolson, S. E. (2014). Psychogenic pseudosyncope: Diagnosis and management. *Autonomic Neuroscience: Basic and Clinical, 184,* 66–72.

Rao, S. (2020). Treatment of personality disorders. In R. Sagar & S. Sarkar (Eds.), *Drug therapy for psychiatric disorders* (pp. 110–118). New Delhi: JP Medical Publishers.

Rathee, S. (2020). Dissociative disorders: Phenomenology and management. *Delhi Psychiatry Journal, 23*(1), 138–144.

Reddy, Y. J., Sudhir, P. M., Manjula, M., Arumugham, S. S., & Narayanaswamy, J. C. (2020). Clinical practice guidelines for cognitive-behavioral therapies in anxiety disorders and obsessive-compulsive and related disorders. *Indian Journal of Psychiatry, 62*(Supplement 2), S230–S250.

Rees, S., Silove, D., Verdial, T., Tam, N., Savio, E., Fonseca, Z., . . . Steel, Z. (2013). Intermittent explosive disorder amongst women in conflict affected Timor-Leste: Associations with human rights trauma, ongoing violence, poverty, and injustice. *PLoS One, 8*(8), e69207.

Reinares, M., Bonnín, C. M., Hidalgo-Mazzei, D., Sánchez-Moreno, J., Colom, F., & Vieta, E. (2016). The role of family interventions in bipolar disorder: A systematic review. *Clinical Psychology Review, 43*, 47–57. http://doi.org/10.1016/j.cpr.2015.11.010

Reinders, A. S., Willemsen, A. T., Vos, H. P., den Boer, J. A., & Nijenhuis, E. R. (2012). Fact or factitious? A psychobiological study of authentic and simulated dissociative identity states. *PloS One, 7*(6), e39279.

Ren, J., Li, H., Palaniyappan, L., Liu, H., Wang, J., Li, C., & Rossini, P. M. (2014). Repetitive transcranial magnetic stimulation versus electroconvulsive therapy for major depression: A systematic review and meta-analysis. *Progress in Neuro-Psychopharmacology and Biological Psychiatry, 51*, 181–189.

Resick, P. A., & Calhoun, K. S. (2001). Posttraumatic stress disorder. In D. H. Barlow (Ed.), *Clinical handbook of psychological disorders: A step-by-step treatment manual* (3rd ed., pp. 60–113). New York, NY: Guilford Press.

Reynolds, C. R., Altmann, R. A., & Allen, D. N. (2021). The problem of bias in psychological assessment. In C. R. Reynolds & R. B. Livingston (Eds.), *Mastering modern psychological testing* (pp. 573–613). Harlow: Pearson.

Ribeiro, R. V. E. (2017). Prevalence of body dysmorphic disorder in plastic surgery and dermatology patients: A systematic review with meta-analysis. *Aesthetic Plastic Surgery, 41*(4), 964–970.

Richey, L. N., Krieg, A., & Rao, V. (2019). *Johns Hopkins psychiatry guide: Culture-bound syndromes.* www.hopkinsguides.com/hopkins/view/Johns_Hopkins_Psychiatry_Guide/787377/all/Culture_bound_Syndromes

Rief, W., Mewes, R., Martin, A., Glaesmer, H., & Braehler, E. (2010). Are psychological features useful in classifying patients with somatic symptoms? *Psychosomatic Medicine, 72*(7), 648–655.

Ritchie, H. (2019, May 29). Does the news reflect what we die from? *Our World in Data.* https://ourworldindata.org/does-the-news-reflect-what-we-die-from

Roaiah, M., Elkhayat, Y., Rashed, L., GamalEl Din, S., El Guindi, A., & Abd El Salam, M. (2018). Study of the prevalence of 5 HT-2C receptor gene polymorphisms in Egyptian patients with lifelong premature ejaculation. *Andrologia, 50*(2), e12855.

Roberts, A. L., Gilman, S. E., Brelau, J., & Koenen, K. C. (2011). Race/ethnic differences in exposure to traumatic events, development of post-traumatic stress disorder, and treatment-seeking for post-traumatic stress disorder in the United States. *Psychological Medicine, 41*, 71–83.

Robins, C. J., Schmidt, H. III, & Linehan, M. M. (2004). Dialectical behavior therapy: Synthesizing radical acceptance with skillful means. In S. C. Hayes, V. M. Follette, & M. M. Linehan (Eds.), *Mindfulness and acceptance: Expanding the cognitive-behavioral tradition* (pp. 30–44). New York, NY: Guilford Press.

Robles, R., Fresán, A., Vega-Ramírez, H., Cruz-Islas, J., Rodríguez-Pérez, V., Domínguez-Martínez, T., & Reed, G. M. (2016). Removing transgender identity from the classification of mental disorders: A Mexican field study for ICD-11. *The Lancet Psychiatry, 3*(9), 850–859.

Rodewald, F., Wilhelm-Gosling, C., Emrich, H.M., Reddemann, L., & Gast, U. (2011). Axis-I comorbidity in female patients with dissociative identity disorder not otherwise specified. *Journal of Nervous and Mental Disease, 199*, 122–131.

Rodgers, N., McDonald, S., & Wootton, B. M. (2021). Cognitive behavioral therapy for hoarding disorder: An updated meta-analysis. *Journal of Affective Disorders, 290*, 128–135. https://doi.org/10.1016/j.jad.2021.04.067

Rodgers, R. F., Berry, R., & Fischer, L. E. (2020). Anxiety disorders: A feminist ecological approach. In E. Bui, M. E. Charney, & A. W. Baker (Eds.), *Clinical handbook of anxiety disorders* (pp. 43–58). Cham: Springer.

Rogers, C. (1989). *The Carl Rogers reader.* New York, NY: Mariner Books.

Rogers, J. C., & De Brito, S. A. (2016). Cortical and subcortical gray matter volume in youths with conduct problems: A meta-analysis. *JAMA Psychiatry, 73*(1), 64–72.

Rolls, E. T., Cheng, W., Gong, W., Qiu, J., Zhou, C., Zhang, J., . . . Feng, J. (2019). Functional connectivity of the anterior cingulate cortex in depression and in health. *Cerebral Cortex, 29*(8), 3617–3630. https://doi.org/10.1093/cercor/bhy236

Ronningstam, E. (2013). An update on narcissistic personality disorder. *Current Opinion in Psychiatry, 26*(1), 102–106. https://doi.org/10.1097/YCO.0b013e328359979c

Roscoe, R. A. (2021). The battle against mental health stigma: Examining how veterans with PTSD communicatively manage stigma. *Health Communication, 36*(11), 1378–1387.

Rosell, D. R. (2017). Schizotypal personality disorder: Epidemiology, pathogenesis, clinical manifestations, course, and diagnosis. *UpToDate.* www.uptodate.com/contents/schizotypal-personality-disorder-epidemiology-pathogenesis-clinical-manifestations-course-and-diagnosis

Rosell, D. R., Futterman, S. E., McMaster, A., & Siever, L. J. (2014). Schizotypal personality disorder: A current review. *Current Psychiatry Reports, 16*(7), 452. https://doi.org/10.1007/s11920–014-0452-1

Rosen, E., Bakshi, N., Watters, A., Rosen, H. R., & Mehler, P. S. (2017). Hepatic complications of anorexia nervosa. *Digestive Diseases and Sciences, 62*(11), 2977–2981. https://doi.org/10.1007/s10620–017-4766-9

Rosen, T. E., Mazefsky, C. A., Vasa, R. A., & Lerner, M. D. (2018). Co-occurring psychiatric conditions in autism spectrum disorder. *International Review of Psychiatry, 30*(1), 40–61.

Rosenberg, E. (2018, November 14). The CIA explored using a 'truth-serum' on terrorism detainees after 9/11, newly released report shows. *The Washington Post.* www.washingtonpost.com/nation/2018/11/14/cia-explored-using-truth-serum-terror-detainees-after-newly-released-report-shows/

Ross, C. A., & Ness, L. (2010). Symptom patterns in dissociative identity disorder patients and the general population. *Journal of Trauma and Dissociation, 11*, 458–468.

Ross, D. A., Arbuckle, M. R., Travis, M. J., Dwyer, J. B., van Schalkwyk, G. I., & Ressler, K. J. (2017). An integrated neuroscience perspective on formulation and treatment planning for posttraumatic stress disorder: An educational review. *JAMA Psychiatry, 74*(4), 407–415.

Roth, G. A. (2018). Global Burden of Disease Collaborative Network. Global Burden of Disease Study 2017 (GBD 2017) Results. Seattle, United States: Institute for Health Metrics and Evaluation (IHME), 2018. *The Lancet, 392*, 1736–1788.

Roth, T., Coulouvrat, C., Hajak, G., Lakoma, M. D., Sampson, N. A., Shahly, V., . . . Kessler, R. C. (2011). Prevalence and perceived health associated with insomnia based on DSM-IV-TR; international statistical classification of diseases and related health problems, tenth revision; and research diagnostic criteria/international classification of sleep disorders, criteria: results from the America insomnia survey. *Biological Psychiatry, 69*(6), 592–600.

Rowe, R., Costello, E. J., Angold, A., Copeland, W. E., & Maughan, B. (2010). Developmental pathways in oppositional defiant disorder and conduct disorder. *Journal of Abnormal Psychology, 119*(4), 726–773.

Rowland, D. L., & Cooper, S. E. (2017). Treating men's orgasmic difficulties. In Z. D. Peterson (Ed.), *The Wiley handbook of sex therapy* (pp. 72–97). Chichester: John Wiley & Sons.

Roytman, E. (2020). Kahler v. Kansas: The end of the insanity defense. *Duke Journal of Constitutional Law & Public Policy Sidebar, 15*, 43–58.

Rucker, J. J. H., Iliff, J., & Nutt, D. J. (2018). Psychiatry & the psychedelic drugs: Past, present & future. *Neuropharmacology, 142*, 200–218. https://doi.org/10.1016/j.neuropharm.2017.12.040

Rueger, S. Y., Malecki, C. K., Pyun, Y., Aycock, C., & Coyle, S. (2016). A meta-analytic review of the association between perceived social support and depression in childhood and adolescence. *Psychological Bulletin, 142*(10), 1017–1067. http://doi.org/10.1037/bul0000058

Russo, F. (2017, January 6). Where transgender is no longer a diagnosis. *Scientific American.* www.scientificamerican.com/article/where-transgender-is-no-longer-a-diagnosis/

Sadeh, N., Londahl-Shaller, E. A., Piatigorsky, A., Fordwood, S., Stuart, B. K., McNiel, D. E., . . . Yaeger, A. M. (2014). Functions of non-suicidal self-injury in adolescents and young adults with borderline personality disorder symptoms. *Psychiatry Research, 216*(2), 217–222.

Sadock, B. J., & Sadock, V. A. (Eds.). (2010). *Kaplan and Sadock's pocket handbook of clinical psychiatry.* Philadelphia, PA: Lippincott Williams & Wilkins.

Safer, J. D., & Tangpricha, V. (2019). Care of the transgender patient. *Annals of Internal Medicine, 171*(1), ITC1–ITC16.

Saitz, R., Miller, S. C., Fiellin, D. A., & Rosenthal, R. N. (2021). Recommended use of terminology in addiction medicine. *Journal of Addiction Medicine, 15*(1), 3–7. doi:10.1097/ADM.0000000000000673

Saks, E. R. (2007). *The center cannot hold: My journey through madness.* New York, NY: Hyperion.

Samulowitz, A., Gremyr, I., Eriksson, E., & Hensing, G. (2018). "Brave men" and "emotional women": A theory-guided literature review on gender bias in health care and gendered norms towards patients with chronic pain. *Pain Research and Management, 2018*, 6358624. doi:10.1155/2018/6358624

Samura, O. (2020). Update on noninvasive prenatal testing: A review based on current worldwide research. *Journal of Obstetrics and Gynaecology Research, 46*(8), 1246–1254.

Sansone, R. A., & Sansone, L. A. (2011). Personality disorders: A nation-based perspective on prevalence. *Innovations in Clinical Neuroscience, 8*(4), 13–18.

Sar, V. (2011). Epidemiology of dissociative disorders: An overview. *Epidemiology Research International, 2011.* https://doi.org/10.1155/2011/404538

Sarbin, T. R., & Juhasz, J. B. (1967). The historical background of the concept of hallucination. *Journal of the History of the Behavioral Sciences, 3*(4), 339–358.

Sareen, J. (2014). Posttraumatic stress disorder in adults: Impact, comorbidity, risk factors, and treatment. *The Canadian Journal of Psychiatry, 59*(9), 460–467. https://doi.org/10.1177/070674371405900902

Sareen, J., Stein, M., & Hermann, R. (2018). Posttraumatic stress disorder in adults: Epidemiology, pathophysiology, clinical manifestations, course, assessment, and diagnosis. *UpToDate.* www.uptodate.com/contents/posttraumatic-stress-disorder-in-adults-epidemiology-pathophysiology-clinical-manifestations-course-assessment-and-diagnosis

Savage, J. (Ed.). (2009). *The development of persistent criminality.* New York, NY: Oxford University Press. https://doi.org/10.1093/acprof:oso/9780195310313.001.0001

Saveanu, R. V., & Nemeroff, C. B. (2012). Etiology of depression: Genetic and environmental factors. *The Psychiatric Clinics of North America, 35*(1), 51–71. http://doi.org/10.1016/j.psc.2011.12.001

Scaramutti, C., Salas-Wright, C. P., Vos, S. R., & Schwartz, S. J. (2019). The mental health impact of Hurricane Maria on Puerto Ricans in Puerto Rico and Florida. *Disaster Medicine and Public Health Preparedness, 13*(1), 24–27.

Scarella, T., Boland, R., & Barsky, A. (2019). Illness anxiety disorder: Psychopathology, epidemiology, clinical characteristics, and treatment. *Psychosomatic Medicine, 81*(5), 398–407. doi:10.1097/PSY.0000000000000691

Scher, C. D., Suvak, M. K., & Resick, P. A. (2017). Trauma cognitions are related to symptoms up to 10 years after cognitive behavioral treatment for posttraumatic stress disorder. *Psychological Trauma: Theory, Research, Practice, and Policy, 9*(6), 750–757.

Schifano, F., Chiappini, S., Corkery, J. M., Scherbaum, N., & Guirguis, A. (2021). The e-psychonaut drugs' psychopharmacology. *Current Opinion in Pharmacology, 57*, 165–174.

Schiller, L., & Bennett, A. (2008). *The quiet room: A journey out of the torment of madness.* London: Hachette.

Schmidt, A. (2019). Comparison of Kernberg's and Kohut's theory of narcissistic personality disorder. *Turkish Journal of Psychiatry, 30*(2), 137–141.

Schmidt, N. B., Lerew, D. R., & Jackson, R. J. (1997). The role of anxiety sensitivity in the pathogenesis of panic: Prospective evaluation of spontaneous panic attacks during acute stress. *Journal of Abnormal Psychology, 106*(3), 355–364.

Schneider, S. C., Mond, J., Turner, C. M., & Hudson, J. L. (2019). Sex differences in the presentation of body dysmorphic disorder in a community sample of adolescents. *Journal of Clinical Child and Adolescent Psychology, 48*(3), 516–528. http://dx.doi.org.ezaccess.libraries.psu.edu/10.1080/15374416.2017.1321

Schulman, J. K., & Erickson-Schroth, L. (2017). Mental health in sexual minority and transgender women. *Psychiatric Clinics, 40*(2), 309–319.

Schultz, S. K. (2007). Depression in the older adult: The challenge of medical comorbidity. *The American Journal of Psychiatry, 164*(6), 847–848.

Schutter, D. J. L. G. (2009). Antidepressant efficacy of high-frequency transcranial magnetic stimulation over the left dorsolateral prefrontal cortex in double-blind sham-controlled designs: A meta-analysis. *Psychological Medicine, 39*(1), 65–75. http://doi.org/10.1017/S0033291708003462

Scott, C. L., Hilty, D. M., & Brook, M. (2003). Impulse-control disorders not elsewhere classified. In R. E. Hales & S. C. Yudofsky (Eds.), *Textbook of clinical psychiatry* (4th ed., pp. 781–802). Washington, DC: American Psychiatric Publishing.

Scott, H. R., Pitman, A., Kozhuharova, P., & Lloyd-Evans, B. (2020). A systematic review of studies describing the influence of informal social support on psychological wellbeing in people bereaved by sudden or violent causes of death. *BMC Psychiatry, 20*(1). https://doi.org/10.1186/s12888-020-02639-4

Scott, K. M., De Jonge, P., Stein, D. J., & Kessler, R. C. (eds.) (2018). *Mental Disorders Around the World: Facts and Figures from the WHO World Mental Health Surveys.* Cambridge University Press.

Scott, K. M., De Vries, Y. A., Aguilar-Gaxiola, S., Al-Hamzawi, A., Alonso, J., Bromet, E. J., ... De Jonge, P. (2020). Intermittent explosive disorder subtypes in the general population: Association with comorbidity, impairment and suicidality. *Epidemiology and Psychiatric Sciences, 29*, e138. https://doi.org/10.1017/S2045796020000517

Scott, K. M., Lim, C. C. W., Al-Hamzawi, A., & Alonso, J. (2018). Intermittent explosive disorder. In K. M. Scott, P. de Jonge, D. J. Stein, & R. C. Kessler (Eds.), *Mental Disorders Around the World: Facts and Figures from the*

WHO World Mental Health Surveys (pp. 182–194). New York, NY: Cambridge University Press. https://doi.org/10 .1017/9781316336168.013

Scott, S., Briskman, J., & O'Connor, T. G. (2014). Early prevention of antisocial personality: Long-term follow-up of two randomized controlled trials comparing indicated and selective approaches. *The American Journal of Psychiatry, 171*(6), 649–657. https://doi.org/10.1176/appi .ajp.2014.13050697

Seibel, B. L., de Brito Silva, B., Fontanari, A., Catelan, R. F., Bercht, A. M., Stucky, J. L., . . . Koller, S. H. (2018). The impact of the parental support on risk factors in the process of gender affirmation of transgender and gender diverse people. *Frontiers in Psychology, 9*, 399. https:// doi.org/10.3389/fpsyg.2018.00399

Seiler, A., Fagundes, C. P., & Christian, L. M. (2020). The impact of everyday stressors on the immune system and health. In A. Choukèr (Ed.), *Stress challenges and immunity in space* (pp. 71–92). New York, NY: Springer.

Sekuła, M., Boniecka, I., & Paśnik, K. (2019). Bulimia nervosa in obese patients qualified for bariatric surgery: Clinical picture, background and treatment. *Wideochirurgia I Inne Techniki Maloinwazyjne, 14*(3). https://doi.org/10.5114/wiitm.2019.81312

Selby, E. A., Anestis, M. D., Bender, T. W., & Joiner Jr., T. E. (2009). An exploration of the emotional cascade model in borderline personality disorder. *Journal of Abnormal Psychology, 118*(2), 375–387.

Seligman, M. E. (1975). *Helplessness: On depression, development, and death*. New York, NY: W. H. Freeman.

Seligman, M. E., & Maier, S. F. (1967). Failure to escape traumatic shock. *Journal of Experimental Psychology, 74*(1), 1–9.

Senaratna, C. V., Perret, J. L., Lodge, C. J., Lowe, A. J., Campbell, B. E., Matheson, M. C., Hamilton, G. S., & Dharmage, S. C. (2017). Prevalence of obstructive sleep apnea in the general population: A systematic review. *Sleep Medicine Reviews, 34*, 70–81. https://doi .org/10.1016/j.smrv.2016.07.002

Setlack, J., Brais, N., Keough, M., & Johnson, E. A. (2020). Workplace violence and psychopathology in paramedics and firefighters: Mediated by posttraumatic cognitions. *Canadian Journal of Behavioural Science/Revue canadienne des sciences du comportement, 53*(3), 211–220.

Severus, E., Taylor, M. J., Sauer, C., Pfennig, A., Ritter, P., Bauer, M., & Geddes, J. R. (2014). Lithium for prevention of mood episodes in bipolar disorders: Systematic review and meta-analysis. *International Journal of Bipolar Disorders, 2*(1), 15.

Shapiro, F. (2001). *EMDR: Eye movement desensitization and reprocessing*. New York, NY: Guilford Press.

Sharf, R.S. (2015). *Theories of psychotherapy and counseling: Concepts and cases*. Belmont, CA: Brooks/ Cole.

Sharma, A., & Brody, A. L. (2009). In vivo brain imaging of human exposure to nicotine and tobacco. In J. E. Henningfield, E. D. London, & S. Pogun (Eds.), *Handbook of experimental pharmacology* (pp. 145–171). New York, NY: Springer.

Sharma, S., Ghosh, S. N., & Sharma, M. (2004). Life events stress, emotional vital signs and peptic ulcer. *Psychological Studies, 49*(2–3), 167–176.

Shattuck, E. C., Perrotte, J. K., Daniels, C. L., Xu, X., & Sunil, T. S. (2020). The contribution of sociocultural factors in shaping self-reported sickness behavior. *Frontiers in Behavioral Neuroscience, 14*, 4. https://doi .org/10.3389/fnbeh.2020.00004

Shear, M. K., Wang, Y., Skritskaya, N., Duan, N., Mauro, C., & Ghesquiere, A. (2014). Treatment of complicated grief in elderly persons: A randomized clinical trial. *JAMA Psychiatry, 71*(11), 1287–1295.

Sheerin, C. M., Lind, M. J., Bountress, K. E., Nugent, N. R., & Amstadter, A. B. (2017). The genetics and epigenetics of PTSD: Overview, recent advances, and future directions. *Current Opinion in Psychology, 14*, 5–11.

Shell shock (1922). *The British Medical Journal, 2*(3216), 322–323. www.jstor.org/stable/20420866

Shen, O., Al-Jamaly, H., Siemers, M., & Stone, N. (2018). Death: Reality vs reported. https://twistedsifter.com/2018/ 04/causes-of-death-google-media-reality/

Sherin, J. E., & Nemeroff, C. B. (2011). Overview of psychological trauma, post-traumatic stress disorder, and biological markers. *Dialogues in Clinical Neuroscience, 13*, 263–278.

Shifren, J. L. (2018) *Sexual dysfunction in women: Epidemiology, risk factors, and evaluation*. UpToDate. www.uptodate.com/contents/overview-of-sexual- dysfunction-in-females-epidemiology-risk-factors-and- evaluation

Shin, J. C., Parab, K. V., An, R., & Grigsby-Toussaint, D. S. (2020). Greenspace exposure and sleep: A systematic review. *Environmental Research, 182*, 109081.

Shin, L. M., Bush, G., Milad, M. R., Lasko, N. B., Brohawn, K. H., Hughes, K. C., . . . Pitman, R. K. (2011). Exaggerated activation of dorsal anterior cingulate cortex during cognitive interference: A monozygotic twin study of posttraumatic stress disorder. *The American Journal of Psychiatry, 168,* 979–985.

Shindel, A. W., Althof, S. E., Carrier, S., Chou, R., McMahon, C. G., Mulhall, J. P., . . . Sharlip, I. D. (2020). *Home guidelines clinical guidelines disorders of ejaculation disorders of ejaculation: An AUA/SMSNA guideline panel members guideline statements premature ejaculation.* www.auanet.org/guidelines/disorders-of-ejaculation

Shostrom, E. L. (Producer). (1965). *Three approaches to psychotherapy [Film]. Orange Country,* CA: Psychological Films.

Sicile-Kira, C. (2014). *Autism spectrum disorder: The complete guide to understanding autism.* New York, NY: Penguin.

Siegel, J. M., & Boehmer, L. N. (2006). Narcolepsy and the hypocretin system: Where motion meets emotion. *Nature Clinical Practice Neurology, 2*(10), 548–556. https://doi.org/10.1038/ncpneuro0300

Siever, L. J., & Davis, K. L. (2004). The pathophysiology of schizophrenia disorders: Perspectives from the spectrum. *The American Journal of Psychiatry, 161*(3), 398–413.

Sigman, M., Spence, S. J., & Wang, A. T. (2006). Autism from developmental and neuropsychological perspectives. *Annual Review of Clinical Psychology, 2,* 327–355.

Silva, B., Canas-Simião, H., & Cavanna, A. E. (2020). Neuropsychiatric aspects of impulse control disorders. *Psychiatric Clinics of North America, 43*(2), 249–262. https://doi.org/10.1016/j.psc.2020.02.001

Silver, E., Cirincione, C., & Steadman, H. J. (1994). Demythologizing inaccurate perceptions of the insanity defense. *Law and Human Behavior, 18*(1), 63–70.

Silverman, J. A. (1997). Sir William Gull (1819–1890): Limner of anorexia nervosa and myxoedema. *Eating and Weight Disorders: Studies on Anorexia, Bulimia and Obesity, 2*(3), 111–116.

Simonsson, P., Farwell, M. M., & Solomon, P. L. (2020). Judges' perceptions of violence risk among defendants with mental illness. *The Journal of Forensic Psychiatry & Psychology, 31*(3), 385–390.

Sinclair, B. (2019). Early teens gaming online more—study. *GamesIndustry.Biz.* www.gamesindustry.biz/articles/2019-01-31-early-teens-gaming-online-more-study

Singer, J. (2017). *NeuroDiversity: The birth of an idea.* Lexington, KY: n.p.

Sipahi, L., Wildman, D. E., Aiello, A. E., Koenen, K. C., Galea, S., Abbas, A., & Uddin, M. (2014). Longitudinal epigenetic variation of DNA methyltransferase genes is associated with vulnerability to post-traumatic stress disorder. *Psychological Medicine, 44*(15), 3165–3179.

Skewes, M. C., & Gonzalez, V. M. (2013). The biopsychosocial model of addiction. *Principles of Addiction, 1,* 61–70.

Skodol, A. (2017). Borderline personality disorder: Epidemiology, clinical features, course, assessment, and diagnosis. *UpToDate.* www.uptodate.com/contents/borderline-personality-disorder-epidemiology-pathogenesis-clinical-features-course-assessment-and-diagnosis

Slobodin, O., & Masalha, R. (2020). Challenges in ADHD care for ethnic minority children: A review of the current literature. *Transcultural Psychiatry, 57*(3), 468–483. https://doi.org/10.1177/1363461520902885

Smith, B., Gasby, D., & Shnayerson, M. (2016). *Before I forget: Love, hope, help, and acceptance in our fight against Alzheimer's.* New York, NY: Harmony.

Smith, D. J., Langan, J., McLean, G., Guthrie, B., & Mercer, S. W. (2013). Schizophrenia is associated with excess multiple physical-health comorbidities but low levels of recorded cardiovascular disease in primary care: cross-sectional study. *BMJ Open, 3*(4), e002808. https://doi.org/10.1136/bmjopen-2013-002808

Smith, M. L., Glass, G. V., & Miller, T. I. (1980). *The benefits of psychotherapy.* Baltimore, MD: Johns Hopkins University Press.

Smith, R., Shepard, C., Wiltgen, A., Rufino, K., & Fowler, J. C. (2017). Treatment outcomes for inpatients with obsessive-compulsive personality disorder: An open comparison trial. *Journal of Affective Disorders, 209,* 273–278.

Smithson, S., & Pignone, M. P. (2017). Screening adults for depression in primary care. *Medical Clinics of North America, 101*(4), 807–821. http://doi.org/10.1016/j.mcna.2017.03.010

Sohn, E. (2021, July 16). Righting the gender imbalance in autism studies. *Spectrum.* www.spectrumnews.org/features/deep-dive/righting-gender-imbalance-autism-studies/

Solmi, M., Radua, J., Olivola, M., Croce, E., Soardo, L., de Pablo, G. S., . . . Kim, J. H. (2021). Age at onset of mental disorders worldwide: Large-scale meta-analysis of 192 epidemiological studies. *Molecular Psychiatry, 27,* 281–295.

Somer, E., Amos-Williams, T., & Stein, D. J. (2013). Evidence-based treatment for depersonalisation-derealisation disorder (DPRD). *BMC Psychology, 1*(1), 1–13.

Sommers-Flanagan, J., & Sommers-Flanagan, R. (2013). *Clinical interviewing* (5th ed.). Hoboken, NJ: John Wiley & Sons.

Sorensen, J., Bautista, K. E., Lamvu, G., & Feranec, J. (2018). Evaluation and treatment of female sexual pain: A clinical review. *Cureus, 10*(3), e2379. doi:10.7759/cureus.2379

Speyer, R., Chen, Y. W., Kim, J. H., Wilkes-Gillan, S., Nordahl-Hansen, A. J., Wu, H. C., & Cordier, R. (2021). Non-pharmacological interventions for adults with autism: A systematic review of randomised controlled trials. *Review Journal of Autism and Developmental Disorders*, 1–31. https://doi.org/10.1007/s40489-021-00250-1

Spiegel, D., Lowenstein, R.J., Lewis-Fernández, R., Sar, V., & Simeon, D. (2011). Dissociative disorders in DSM-5. *Depression and Anxiety, 28*, 824–852.

Spires-Jones, T. L., & Hyman, B. T. (2014). The intersection of amyloid beta and tau at synapses in Alzheimer's disease. *Neuron, 82*(4), 756–771.

Spoont, M. R., Nelson, D. B., Murdoch, M., Rector, T., Sayer, N. A., Nugent, S., & Westermeyer, J. (2014). Impact of treatment beliefs and social network encouragement on initiation of care by VA service users with PTSD. *Psychiatric Services, 65*(5), 654-662. https://doi.org/10.1176/appi.ps.201200324

Srivastava, P., Lampe, E. W., Michael, M. L., Manasse, S., & Juarascio, A. S. (2021). Stress appraisal prospectively predicts binge eating through increases in negative affect. *Eating and Weight Disorders, 26*(7), 2413–2420.

Stahl, S. M. (2017). *Prescriber's guide: Stahl's essential psychopharmacology.* (6th ed.). New York, NY: Cambridge University Press.

Stahl, S. M. (2021). *Stahl's essential psychopharmacology: Neuroscientific basis and practical applications* (5th ed.). New York, NY: Cambridge University Press.

Starr, L. R., & Davila, J. (2008). Excessive reassurance seeking, depression, and interpersonal rejection: A meta-analytic review. *Journal of Abnormal Psychology, 117*(4), 762–775. http://doi.org/10.1037/a0013866

Steardo, L., Luciano, M., Sampogna, G., Zinno, F., Saviano, P., Staltari, F., ... Fiorillo, A. (2020). Efficacy of the interpersonal and social rhythm therapy (IPSRT) in patients with bipolar disorder: Results from a real-world, controlled trial. *Annals of General Psychiatry, 19*(1), 1–7.

Stefan, S., Cristea, I. A., Szentagotai Tatar, A., & David, D. (2019). Cognitive-behavioral therapy (CBT) for generalized anxiety disorder: Contrasting various CBT

approaches in a randomized clinical trial. *Journal of Clinical Psychology, 75*(7), 1188–1202.

Stein, D. J., Chiu, W. T., Hwang, I., Kessler, R. C., Sampson, N., Alonso, J., ... Nock, M. K. (2010). Cross-national analysis of the associations between traumatic events and suicidal behavior: Findings from the WHO World Mental Health Surveys. *PLoS One, 5*, e10574.

Stein, D. J., Kupfer, D. J., & Schatzberg, A. F. (2005). *The American Psychiatric Publishing textbook of mood disorders.* Washington, DC: American Psychiatric Publishing.

Steinglass, J. E., & Devlin, M. J. (2017). Finding the disorder in binge eating disorder. *Acta Psychiatrica Scandinavica, 136*(2), 145–146. https://doi.org/10.1111/acps.12766

Stewart, D., Goodwin, S. R., & Karagiannis, N. (2021). Does the United States need a comprehensive national health system? A discussion of views, facts, challenges, and potential benefits. www.global-isp.org/wp-content/uploads/WP-129.pdf

Stewart, T. M., & Williamson, D. A. (2008). Bulimia nervosa. In M. Hersen & J. Rosqvist (Eds.), *Handbook of psychological assessment, case conceptualization and treatment, vol. 1: Adults* (pp. 463–497). Hoboken, NJ: John Wiley & Sons.

Stice, E., & Shaw, H. (2017). Eating disorders: Insights from imagining and behavioral approaches to treatment. *Journal of Psychopharmacology, 31*(11), 11485–11495.

Stone, J., & Sharpe, M. (2018). *Conversion disorder in adults: Terminology, diagnosis, and differential diagnosis. UpToDate.* www.uptodate.com/contents/conversion-disorder-in-adults-terminology-diagnosis-and-differential-diagnosis

Strain, E. (2021, April 17). *Medication for opioid use disorder. UpToDate.* www.uptodate.com/contents/medication-for-opioid-use-disorder

Strakowski, S. M., Adler, C. M., Almeida, J., Altshuler, L. L., Blumberg, H. P., Chang, K. D., ... Townsend, J. D. (2012). The functional neuroanatomy of bipolar disorder: A consensus model. *Bipolar Disorders, 14*(4), 313–325. http://doi.org/10.1111/j.1399-5618.2012.01022.x

Studer, L. H., & Aylwin, A. S. (2006). Pedophilia: The problem with diagnosis and limitations of CBT in treatment. *Medical Hypotheses, 67*(4), 774–781.

Subramanyam, A. A., Somaiya, M., Shankar, S., Nasirabadi, M., Shah, H. R., Paul, I., & Ghildiyal, R. (2020). Psychological interventions for dissociative disorders. *Indian Journal of Psychiatry, 62*(Supplement 2), S280–S289.

Sullivan, P. F., Neale, M. C., & Kendler, K. S. (2000). Genetic epidemiology of major depression: Review and meta-analysis. *American Journal of Psychiatry, 157*(10), 1552–1562. http://doi.org/10.1176/appi.ajp.157.10.1552

Suor, J. H., Jimmy, J., Monk, C. S., Phan, K. L., & Burkhouse, K. L. (2020). Parsing differences in amygdala volume among individuals with and without social and generalized anxiety disorders across the lifespan. *Journal of Psychiatric Research, 128*, 83–89.

Suppes, T., Baldessarini, R. J., Faedda, G. L., & Tohen, M. (1991). Risk of recurrence following discontinuation of lithium treatment in bipolar disorder. *Archives of General Psychiatry, 48*(12), 1082–1088.

Sutar, R., & Sahu, S. (2019). Pharmacotherapy for dissociative disorders: A systematic review. *Psychiatry Research, 281*, 112529.

Swann, A. C. (2009). Impulsivity in mania. *Current Psychiatry Reports, 11*(6), 481–487. http://doi.org/10.1007/s11920–009-0073-2

Swift, J. K., & Greenberg, R. P. (2014). A treatment by disorder meta-analysis of dropout from psychotherapy. *Journal of Psychotherapy Integration, 24*(3), 193–207.

Swinnen, N., Vandenbulcke, M., & Vancampfort, D. (2020). Exergames in people with major neurocognitive disorder: A systematic review. *Disability and Rehabilitation: Assistive Technology*, 1–14. https://doi.org/10.1080/17483107.2020.1785566

Szasz, T. S. (1971). The sane slave: An historical note on the use of medical diagnosis as justificatory rhetoric. *American Journal of Psychotherapy, 25*(2), 228–239.

Szechtman, H., & Woody, E. (2004). Obsessive-compulsive disorder as a disturbance of security motivation. *Psychological Review, 111*(1), 111–127. doi:10.1037/0033-295X.111.1.111

Szumski, F., & Kasparek, K. (2020). Encountering an exhibitionist: The female victim's perspective. *The Journal of Sex Research, 57*(5), 610–623. https://doi.org/10.1080/00224499.2019.1669523

Tan, P. Z., Forbes, E. E., Dahl, R. E., Ryan, N. D., Siegle, G. J., Ladouceur, C. D., & Silk, J. S. (2012). Emotional reactivity and regulation in anxious and nonanxious youth: A cell-phone ecological momentary assessment study. *Journal of Child Psychology & Psychiatry, 53*, 197–206.

Tasca, C., Rapetti, M., Carta, M. G., & Fadda, B. (2012). Women and hysteria in the history of mental health. *Clinical Practice and Epidemiology in Mental Health, 8*, 110–119.

Tatu, L., Aybek, S., & Bogousslavsky, J. (2018). Munchausen syndrome and the wide spectrum of factitious disorders. *Neurologic-Psychiatric Syndromes in Focus – Part II, 42*, 81–86.

Tavares, I. M., Laan, E. T., & Nobre, P. J. (2018). Sexual inhibition is a vulnerability factor for orgasm problems in women. *The Journal of Sexual Medicine, 15*(3), 361–372.

Taylor, D., Gehrman, P., Dautovich, N. D., Lichstein, K. L., & McCrae, C. S. (2014). Causes of insomnia. In D. Taylor, P. Gehrman, & N. D. Dautovich (Eds.), *Handbook of insomnia* (pp. 11–27). New York, NY: Springer.

Taylor, L. E., Swerdfeger, A. L., & Eslick, G. D. (2014). Vaccines are not associated with autism: An evidence-based meta-analysis of case-control and cohort studies. *Vaccine, 32*(29), 3623–3629. https://doi.org/10.1016/j.vaccine.2014.04.085

Tefft, B. C. (2018). Acute sleep deprivation and culpable motor vehicle crash involvement. *Sleep, 41*(10). doi:10.1093/sleep/zsy144

Ten Have, M., Nuyen, J., Beekman, A., & De Graaf, R. (2013). Common mental disorder severity and its association with treatment contact and treatment intensity for mental health problems. *Psychological Medicine, 43*(10), 2203–2213. doi:10.1017/S0033291713000135

Thackray, A. E., Deighton, K., King, J. A., & Stensel, D. J. (2016). Exercise, appetite and weight control: Are there differences between men and women? *Nutrients, 8*(9), 583. doi:10.3390/nu8090583

Thase, M. E., & Denko, T. (2008). Pharmacotherapy of mood disorders. *Annual Review of Clinical Psychology, 4*, 53–91. http://doi.org/10.1146/annurev.clinpsy.2.022305.095301

Thibaut, F., Bradford, J. M., Briken, P., De La Barra, F., Häßler, F., Cosyns, P., & Disorders, W. T. F. o. S. (2016). The World Federation of Societies of Biological Psychiatry (WFSBP) guidelines for the treatment of adolescent sexual offenders with paraphilic disorders. *The World Journal of Biological Psychiatry, 17*(1), 2–38.

Thom, R. P., Levy-Carrick, N. C., Bui, M., & Silbersweig, D. (2019). Delirium. *The American Journal of Psychiatry, 176*(10), 785–793. https://doi.org/10.1176/appi.ajp.2018.18070893

Thompson, D., Ramos, C., & Willett, J. (2014). Psychopathy: Clinical features, developmental basis and therapeutic challenges. *Journal of Clinical Pharmacy and Therapeutics, 39*(5), 485–495.

Tick, B., Bolton, P., Happé, F., Rutter, M., & Rijsdijk, F. (2016). Heritability of autism spectrum disorders: A meta-analysis of twin studies. *Journal of Child Psychology and Psychiatry, 57*(5), 585–595.

Tohver, G. C., & Feher, A. (2020). Health and personality. In B. J. Carducci, C. S. Nave, A. Di Fabio, D. H. Saklofske, & C. Stough (Eds.), *The Wiley encyclopedia of personality and individual differences, vol. 3: Personality processes and individual differences* (pp. 221–226). Hoboken, NJ: John Wiley & Sons.

Torales, J., González, I., Castaldelli-Maia, J. M., & Ventriglio, A. (2020). Kleptomania as a neglected disorder in psychiatry. *International Review of Psychiatry, 32*(5–6), 451–454.

Torgersen, S., Myers, J., Reichborn-Kjennerud, T., Røysamb, E., Kubarych, T. S., & Kendler, K. S. (2012). The heritability of Cluster B personality disorders assessed both by personal interview and questionnaire. *Journal of Personality Disorders, 26*(6), 848–866.

Toro, P. A. (2007). Toward an international understanding of homelessness. *Journal of Social Issues, 63*(3), 461-481.

Tozdan, S., & Briken, P. (2021). *Paraphilias: Diagnostics, comorbidities, and treatment*. In M. Lew-Starowicz, A. Giraldi, & T. Krüger (Eds.), *Psychiatry and sexual medicine* (pp. 407–416). Cham: Springer.

Traig, J. (2008). *Well enough alone: A cultural history of my hypochondria*. New York, NY: Riverhead Books.

Treadway, M. T., Pizzagalli, D. A., Schkade, D., Schwarz, N., Stone, A., Hevenor, S., . . . Greenberg, B. (2014). Imaging the pathophysiology of major depressive disorder: From localist models to circuit-based analysis. *Biology of Mood & Anxiety Disorders, 4*(1), 5. http://doi.org/10.1186/2045-5380-4-5

Treasure, J., Duarte, T. A., & Schmidt, U. (2020, March 14). Eating disorders. *The Lancet.* https://doi.org/10.1016/S0140–6736(20)30059-3

Triebwasser, J., Chemerinski, E., Roussos, P., & Siever, L. J. (2013). Paranoid personality disorder. *Journal of Personality Disorders, 27*(6), 795–805.

Tseng, W.-S., & Hsu, J. (1970). Chinese culture, personality formation and mental illness. *International Journal of Social Psychiatry, 16*(1), 5–14.

Tsui, P., Deptula, A., & Yuan, D. Y. (2017). Conversion disorder, functional neurological symptom disorder, and chronic pain: Comorbidity, assessment, and treatment. *Current Pain and Headache Reports, 21*(6), 1–10.

Turner, B. J., Hu, C., Posada Villa, J., & Nock, M. K. (2018). Oppositional defiant disorder and conduct disorder. In K. M. Scott, P. de Jonge, D. J. Stein, & R. C. Kessler (Eds.), *Mental disorders around the world: Facts and figures from the WHO World Mental Health Surveys* (pp. 209–222). New York, NY: Cambridge University Press. https://doi.org/10.1017/9781316336168.015

Turner, B. J., Prud'homme, J., & Legg, N. (2020). Environmental and sociocultural influences on personality disorders. In C. W. Lejuez & K. L. Gratz (Eds.), *The Cambridge handbook of personality disorders* (pp. 50–64). New York, NY: Cambridge University Press. https://doi.org/10.1017/9781108333931.011

Turner, D., Petermann, J., Harrison, K., Krueger, R., & Briken, P. (2019). Pharmacological treatment of patients with paraphilic disorders and risk of sexual offending: An international perspective. *The World Journal of Biological Psychiatry, 20*(8), 616–625. https://doi.org/10.1080/15622975.2017.1395069

Uddin, M., Amstadter, A. B., Nugent, N. R., & Koenen, K. C. (2012). Genetics and genomics of posttraumatic stress disorder. In J. G. Beck & D. M. Sloan (Eds.), *The Oxford handbook of traumatic stress disorders* (pp. 143–158). New York, NY: Oxford University Press.

Uher, R., & Treasure, J. (2003). Neuroimaging and eating disorders. In C. H. Y. Fu, C. Senior, T. Russell, D. R. Weinberger, & R. Murray (Eds.), *Neuroimaging in psychiatry* (pp. 171–191). New York, NY: Routledge.

Ulualp, S. O. (2010). Snoring and obstructive sleep apnea. *Medical Clinics of North America, 94*(5), 1047–1055. http://linkinghub.elsevier.com/retrieve/pii/S0025712510000763

Unger, W. J., Mirabelli, C., Cousins, M., & Boydell, K. M. (2006). A qualitative analysis of a dyad approach to health-related quality of life measurement in children with asthma. *Social Science & Medicine, 63*(9), 2354–2366.

Unwin, G. L., & Deb, S. (2011). Efficacy of atypical antipsychotic medication in the management of behaviour problems in children with intellectual disabilities and borderline intelligence: A systematic review. *Research in Developmental Disabilities, 32*(6), 2121–2133.

Ursu, S., Stenger, V. A., Shear, M. K., Jones, M. R., & Carter, C. S. (2003). Overactive action monitoring in obsessive-compulsive disorder: Evidence from functional magnetic resonance imaging. *Psychological Science, 14*(4), 347–353.

US Census Bureau (2016, May 19). *U.S. Census Bureau projections show a slower growing, older, more diverse nation a half century from now – population – newsroom – U.S. Census Bureau.* www.census.gov/newsroom/releases/archives/population/cb12-243.html

US Department of Health and Human Services, Substance Abuse and Mental Health Services Administration, Center for Behavioral Health Statistics and Quality (SAMHSA) (2013). *National Survey on Drug Use and Health 2013* (NSDUH-2016-DS0001). https://datafiles.samhsa.gov/

US Department of Health and Human Services, Substance Abuse and Mental Health Services Administration, Center for Behavioral Health Statistics and Quality (SAMHSA) (2017). *National Survey on Drug Use and Health 2017* (NSDUH-2016-DS0001). https://datafiles.samhsa.gov/

US Department of Health and Human Services, Substance Abuse and Mental Health Services Administration, Center for Behavioral Health Statistics and Quality (SAMHSA) (2018). *National Survey on Drug Use and Health 2018* (NSDUH-2016-DS0001). https://datafiles.samhsa.gov/

Vaccarino, S. R., Adamsahib, F., Milev, R. V., Parikh, S. V., Lam, R. W., Blier, P., . . . Bhat, V. (2022). The effects of ketamine on cognition in unipolar and bipolar depression: A systematic review. *The Journal of Clinical Psychiatry*, *83*(1), 38984.

Vall, E., & Wade, T. D. (2015). Predictors of treatment outcome in individuals with eating disorders: A systematic review and meta-analysis. *International Journal of Eating Disorders*, *48*(7), 946–971.

Van Baak, T. E., Coarfa, C., Dugué, P. A., Fiorito, G., Laritsky, E., Baker, M. S., . . . Waterland, R. A. (2018). Epigenetic supersimilarity of monozygotic twin pairs. *Genome Biology*, *19*(1), 1–20.

van der Velden, P. G., van Loon, P., Benight, C. C., & Eckardt, T. (2012). Mental health problems among search and rescue workers deployed in the Haiti earthquake 2010: A pre-post comparison. *Psychiatry Research*, *198*, 100–105.

van Es, R. M. S., Kunst, M. J. J., & De Keijser, J. W. (2020). Forensic mental health expert testimony and judicial decision-making: A systematic literature review. *Aggression and Violent Behavior*, *51*, 101387.

Van Laar, M., Volkerts, E., & Verbaten, M. (2001). Subchronic effects of the GABA-agonist lorazepam and the 5-HT2A/2C antagonist ritanserin on driving performance, slow wave sleep and daytime sleepiness in healthy volunteers. *Psychopharmacology (Berlin)*, *154*, 189–197.

van Minnen, A., Hendriks, L., & Olff, M. (2010). When do trauma experts choose exposure therapy for PTSD patients? A controlled study of therapist and patient factors. *Behaviour Research and Therapy*, *48*(4), 312–320. https://doi.org/10.1016/j.brat.2009.12.003

Van Ryzin, M. J., Fosco, G. M., & Dishion, T. J. (2012). Family and peer predictors of substance use from early adolescence to early adulthood: An 11-year prospective analysis. *Addictive Behaviors*, *37*(12), 1314–1324.

Vander Wal, J. S., Gibbons, J. L., & Grazioso, M. (2008). The sociocultural model of eating disorder development: Application to a Guatemalan sample. *Eating Behaviors*, *9*(3), 277–284. https://doi.org/10.1016/j.eatbeh.2007.10.002

Vargas, J. M., & Adesso, V. J. (1976). A comparison of aversion therapies for nailbiting behavior. *Behavior Therapy*, *7*(3), 322–329. https://doi.org/10.1016/S0005-7894(76)80058-5

VentureBeat (2020). SuperData: Games hit $120.1 billion in 2019, with Fortnite topping $1.8 billion. *VentureBeat*. https://venturebeat.com/2020/01/02/superdata-games-hit-120-1-billion-in-2019-with-fortnite-topping-1-8-billion/

Vermeiden, M., Janssens, M., Thewissen, V., Akinsola, E., Peeters, S., Reijnders, J., . . . Lataster, J. (2019). Cultural differences in positive psychotic experiences assessed with the Community Assessment of Psychic Experiences-42 (CAPE-42): A comparison of student populations in the Netherlands, Nigeria and Norway. *BMC Psychiatry*, *19*(1). https://doi.org/10.1186/s12888-019-2210-8

Villemagne, V. L., Doré, V., Burnham, S. C., Masters, C. L., & Rowe, C. C. (2018). Imaging tau and amyloid-β proteinopathies in Alzheimer disease and other conditions. *Nature Reviews Neurology*, *14*(4), 225–236. https://doi.org/10.1038/nrneurol.2018.9

Vogel, L. (2019). Fat shaming is making people sicker and heavier. *Canadian Medical Association Journal*, *191*(23), E649–E649. https://doi.org/10.1503/cmaj.109-5758

Voigt, K., Nagel, A., Meyer, B., Langs, G., Braukhaus, C., & Loewe, B. (2010). Towards positive diagnostic criteria: A systematic review of somatoform disorder diagnosis and suggestions for future classification. *Journal of Psychosomatic Research*, *68*, 403–414.

Volkert, J., Gablonski, T.-C., & Rabung, S. (2018). Prevalence of personality disorders in the general adult population in Western countries: Systematic review and meta-analysis. *The British Journal of Psychiatry*, *213*(6), 709–715. https://doi.org/10.1192/bjp.2018.202

Volkow, N. D., Jones, E. B., Einstein, E. B., & Wargo, E. M. (2019). Prevention and treatment of opioid misuse and addiction: A review. *JAMA Psychiatry*, *76*(2), 208–216. https://doi.org/10.1001/jamapsychiatry.2018.3126

Voss, M., & Brust, A. (2020). Bulimia nervosa. In Y. N. Evans & A. D. Docter (Eds.), *Adolescent nutrition* (pp. 427–469). Cham: Springer.

Voth, E. A., & Schwartz, R. H. (1997). Medicinal applications of delta-9-tetrahydrocannabinol and marijuana. *Annals of Internal Medicine*, *126*(10), 791–798. www.ncbi.nlm.nih.gov/pubmed/9148653

Wade, T. D. (2019). Recent research on bulimia nervosa. *Psychiatric Clinics of North America*, *42*(1), 21–32. https://doi.org/10.1016/j.psc.2018.10.002

Wagner, A. F., Bennett, B. L., Stefano, E. C., & Latner, J. D. (2020). Thin, muscular, and fit-ideals: Prevalence and correlates in undergraduate women. *Journal of American College Health*, 1–7. https://doi.org/10.1080/07448481.2020.1865981

Wakefield, J. C. (2009). Mental disorder and moral responsibility: Disorders of personhood as harmful dysfunctions, with special reference to alcoholism. *Philosophy, Psychiatry, & Psychology*, *16*(1), 91–99.

Walentynowicz, M., Raes, F., Van Diest, I., & Van den Bergh, O. (2017). The specificity of health-related autobiographical memories in patients with somatic symptom disorder. *Psychosomatic Medicine*, *79*(1), 43–49.

Walker, H. (2008). *Breaking free: My life with dissociative identity disorder*. New York, NY: Simon & Schuster.

Walker, L. E., Shapiro, D., & Akl, S. (2020). Criminal responsibility. In C. R. Bartol & A. M. Bartol (Eds.), *Introduction to Forensic Psychology* (pp. 37–51). Cham: Springer.

Wallace, E. R., & Gach, J. (Eds.). (2010). *History of psychiatry and medical psychology: With an epilogue on psychiatry and the mind-body relation*. New York, NY: Springer.

Wampold, B. E., & Imel, Z. E. (2015). *The great psychotherapy debate: The evidence for what makes psychotherapy work*. New York, NY: Routledge.

Wang, J., Liu, P., Zhang, A., Yang, C., Liu, S., Wang, J., ... Sun, N. (2021). Specific gray matter volume changes of the brain in unipolar and bipolar depression. *Frontiers in Human Neuroscience*, *14*, 591. https://doi.org/10.3389/fnhum.2020.592419

Wang, P. S., Berglund, P., Olfson, M., Pincus, H. A., Wells, K. B., & Kessler, R. C. (2005). Failure and delay in initial treatment contact after first onset of mental disorders in the National Comorbidity Survey Replication. *Archives of General Psychiatry*, *62*(6), 603–613. http://doi.org/10.1001/archpsyc.62.6.603

Warburton, K., McDermott, B. E., Gale, A., & Stahl, S. M. (2020). A survey of national trends in psychiatric patients found incompetent to stand trial: Reasons for the reinstitutionalization of people with serious mental illness in the United States. *CNS Spectrums*, *25*(2), 245–251.

Wardenaar, K. J., Lim, C. C., Al-Hamzawi, A. O., Alonso, J., Andrade, L. H., Benjet, C., ... De Jonge, P. (2017). The cross-national epidemiology of specific phobia in the World Mental Health Surveys. *Psychological Medicine*, *47*(10), 1744–1760.

Wassenaar, E., Friedman, J., & Mehler, P. S. (2019). Medical complications of binge eating disorder. *Psychiatric Clinics*, *42*(2), 275–286.

Watkins, L. E., Sprang, K. R., & Rothbaum, B. O. (2018). Treating PTSD: A review of evidence-based psychotherapy interventions. *Frontiers in Behavioral Neuroscience*, *12*, 258. https://doi.org/10.3389/fnbeh.2018.00258

Watson, H. J., Yilmaz, Z., Thornton, L. M., Hubel, C., & Coleman, J. R., Gaspar, H. A., ... Bulik, C. M. (2019). Genome-wide association study identifies eight risk loci and implicates metabo-psychiatric origins for anorexia nervosa. *Nature Genetics*, *51*(8), 1207–1214.

Weinbrecht, A., Schulze, L., Boettcher, J., & Renneberg, B. (2016). Avoidant personality disorder: A current review. *Current Psychiatry Reports*, *18*(3), 29.

Wendzel, B. (2020). Not guilty, yet continuously confined: Reforming the insanity defense. *American Criminal Law Review*, *57*, 391–411.

West, S. (2020). Does your patient have the right to refuse medications? *Current Psychiatry*, *19*(4), 22–30.

Weston, C. S. E. (2019). Four social brain regions, their dysfunctions, and sequelae, extensively explain autism spectrum disorder symptomatology. *Brain Sciences*, *9*(6), 130. https://doi.org/10.3390/brainsci9060130

Wheeler, L. J., & Guntupalli, S. R. (2020). Female sexual dysfunction: Pharmacologic and therapeutic interventions. *Obstetrics & Gynecology*, *136*(1), 174–186.

Whisman, M. A. (2017). Interpersonal perspectives on depression. In R. J. DeRubeis & D. R. Strunk (Eds.), *The Oxford handbook of mood disorders* (pp. 167–178). New York, NY: Oxford University Press.

Whitman, M. R., Tylicki, J. L., Mascioli, R., Pickle, J., & Ben-Porath, Y. S. (2020). Psychometric properties of the Minnesota Multiphasic Personality Inventory-3 (MMPI-3) in a clinical neuropsychology setting. *Psychological Assessment*, *33*(2), 142–155.

WHO (2017). Depression fact sheet. www.who.int/mediacentre/factsheets/fs369/en/

Wick, M. R., & Keel, P. K. (2020). Posting edited photos of the self: Increasing eating disorder risk or harmless behavior? *International Journal of Eating Disorders*, *53*(6), 864–872.

Wilksch, S. M., O'Shea, A., Ho, P., Byrne, S., & Wade, T. D. (2020). The relationship between social media use and disordered eating in young adolescents. *International Journal of Eating Disorders*, *53*(1), 96–106. https://doi.org/10.1002/eat.23198

Williams, M. T., Metzger, I. W., Leins, C., & DeLapp, C. (2018). Assessing racial trauma within a DSM-5 framework: The UConn Racial/Ethnic Stress & Trauma Survey. *Practice Innovations*, *3*(4), 242–260. https://doi.org/10.1037/pri0000076

Wilson, G. T. (2018). Cognitive-behavioral therapy for eating disorders. In W. S. Agras & A. Robinson (Eds.), *The Oxford handbook of eating disorders* (pp. 271–286). New York, NY: Oxford University Press.

Winarick, D. J. (2020). Schizoid personality disorder. In B. J. Carducci, C. S. Nave, A. Di Fabio, D. H. Saklofske, & C. Stough (Eds.), *The Wiley encyclopedia of personality and individual differences, vol. 4: Clinical, applied, and cross-cultural research* (pp. 181–185). Hoboken, NJ: John Wiley & Sons.

Wirtz, A. L., Poteat, T. C., Malik, M., & Glass, N. (2020). Gender-based violence against transgender people in the United States: A call for research and programming. *Trauma, Violence, & Abuse*, *21*(2), 227–241.

Witchel, S. F. (2018). Disorders of sex development. *Best Practice & Research Clinical Obstetrics & Gynaecology*, *48*, 90–102.

Wittchen, H. U., Gloster, A. T., Beesdo-Baum, K., Fava, G. A., & Craske, M. G. (2010). Agoraphobia: A review of the diagnostic classificatory position and criteria. *Depression and Anxiety*, *27*(2), 113–133.

Witte, T. H., Wright, A., & Stinson, E. A. (2019). Factors influencing stigma toward individuals who have substance use disorders. *Substance Use & Misuse*, *54*(7), 1115–1124.

Witthöft, M., Gropalis, M., & Weck, F. (2018). Somatic symptom and related disorders. In J. N. Butcher & J. M. Hooley (Eds.), *APA handbook of psychopathology: Psychopathology. Understanding, assessing, and treating adult mental disorders* (pp. 531–556). Washington, DC: American Psychological Association. https://doi.org/10.1037/0000064-022

Wittkowski, H., Hinze, C., Häfner-Harms, S., Oji, V., Masjosthusmann, K., Monninger, M., ... Foell, D. (2017). Munchausen by proxy syndrome mimicking systemic autoinflammatory disease: Case report and review of the literature. *Pediatric Rheumatology*, *15*(1), 19.

Wonderlich, S. A., Bulik, C. M., Schmidt, U., Steiger, H., & Hoek, H. W. (2020). Severe and enduring anorexia nervosa: Update and observations about the current clinical reality. *International Journal of Eating Disorders*, *53*(8), 1303–1312.

Wood, J. J., Kendall, P. C., Wood, K. S., Kerns, C. M., Seltzer, M., Small, B. J., ... Storch, E. A. (2020). Cognitive behavioral treatments for anxiety in children with autism spectrum disorder: A randomized clinical trial. *JAMA Psychiatry*, *77*(5), 474–483.

Woolfolk, R. L., & Allen, L. A. (2011). Somatoform and physical disorders. In D. H. Barlow (Ed.), *The Oxford handbook of clinical psychology* (pp. 334–358). New York, NY: Oxford University Press.

Wortmann, F. (2012). *Triggered: A memoir of obsessive-compulsive disorder*. New York, NY: St. Martin's Press.

Wortzel, H. S., Borges, L. M., Barnes, S. M., Nazem, S., McGarity, S., Clark, K., ... Matarazzo, B. B. (2020). Therapeutic risk management for violence: Clinical risk assessment. *Journal of Psychiatric Practice*, *26*(4), 313–319.

Wright, K. D., Lebell, M. A. A., & Carleton, R. N. (2016). Intolerance of uncertainty, anxiety sensitivity, health anxiety, and anxiety disorder symptoms in youth. *Journal of Anxiety Disorders*, *41*, 35–42.

Wu, G., & Shi. J. (2005). The problem of AIM and countermeasure for improvement in interviews. *Psychological Science (China)*, *28*(4), 952–955.

Wu, M., Mennin, D. S., Ly, M., Karim, H. T., Banihashemi, L., Tudorascu, D. L., ... Andreescu, C. (2019). When worry may be good for you: Worry severity and limbic-prefrontal functional connectivity in late-life generalized anxiety disorder. *Journal of Affective Disorders*, *257*, 650–657. doi:http://dx.doi.org.ezaccess.libraries.psu.edu/10.1016/j.jad.2019.07.022

Wyatt, G. W., & Parham, W. D. (2007). The inclusion of culturally sensitive course materials in graduate school and training programs. *Psychotherapy: Theory, Research, Practice, Training*, *22*(2), 461–468.

Yakeley, J., & Wood, H. (2014). Paraphilias and paraphilic disorders: Diagnosis, assessment and management. *Advances in Psychiatric Treatment*, *20*(3), 202–213. doi:10.1192/apt.bp.113.011197

Yakobov, E., Jurcik, T., & Sullivan, M. J. (2017). Conversion disorder. In M. A. Budd, S. Hough, S. T. Wegener, & W. Stiers (Eds.), *Practical psychology in medical rehabilitation* (pp. 277–285). Cham: Springer.

Yakushev, I., & Sidorov, P. (2013). Philippe Pinel and the psychiatry of late XVII – early XIX centuries. *Problemy sotsial'noi gigieny, zdravookhraneniia i istorii meditsiny*, *1*, 57–59.

Yang, Y., Li, W., Lok, K. I., Zhang, Q., Hong, L., Ungvari, G. S., ... Xiang, Y. T. (2020). Voluntary admissions for patients with schizophrenia: A systematic review and meta-analysis. *Asian Journal of Psychiatry*, *48*, 101902. https://doi.org/10.1016/j.ajp.2019.101902

Yap, W. S., Dolzhenko, A. V., Jalal, Z., Hadi, M. A., & Khan, T. M. (2019). Efficacy and safety of lavender essential oil

(Silexan) capsules among patients suffering from anxiety disorders: A network meta-analysis. *Scientific Reports, 9*(1), 1–11.

Yates, G. P., & Feldman, M. D. (2016). Factitious disorder: A systematic review of 455 cases in the professional literature. *General Hospital Psychiatry, 41*, 20–28.

Yatham, S., Sivathasan, S., Yoon, R., da Silva, T. L., & Ravindran, A. V. (2018). Depression, anxiety, and post-traumatic stress disorder among youth in low and middle income countries: A review of prevalence and treatment interventions. *Asian Journal of Psychiatry, 38*, 78–91.

Ye, M., Du, K., Zhou, J., Zhou, Q., Shou, M., Hu, B., . . . Liu, Z. (2018). A meta-analysis of the efficacy of cognitive behavior therapy on quality of life and psychological health of breast cancer survivors and patients. *Psycho-oncology, 27*(7), 1695–1703.

Yealland, L. R. (1918). *Hysterical disorders of warfare.* London: Macmillan.

Yehuda, R. (2002). Post-traumatic stress disorder. *New England Journal of Medicine, 346*(2), 108–114.

Yehuda, R., Teicher, M. H., Seckl, J. R., Grossman, R. A., Morris, A., & Bierer, L. M. (2007). Parental posttraumatic stress disorder as a vulnerability factor for low cortisol trait in offspring of holocaust survivors. *Archives of General Psychiatry, 64*(9), 1040–1048. https://doi.org/10.1001/archpsyc.64.9.1040

Yockey, R. A., King, K. A., & Vidourek, R. A. (2019). "Go ask Alice, when she's 10-feet tall": Psychosocial correlates to lifetime LSD use among a national sample of US adults. *Journal of Psychedelic Studies, 3*(3), 308–314. https://doi.org/10.1556/2054.2019.014

Young, K., Fine, N., & Hendler, T. (2021). fMRI neurofeedback for disorders of emotion regulation. In M. Hampson (Ed.), *fMRI Neurofeedback* (pp. 187–205). London: Academic Press.

Yourstone, J., Lindholm, T., Grann, M., & Svenson, O. (2008). Evidence of gender bias in legal insanity evaluations: A case vignette study of clinicians, judges and students. *Nordic Journal of Psychiatry, 62*(4), 273–278. https://doi.org/10.1080/08039480801963135

Yuni, I. G. A. A. P., Aryani, L. N. A., & Lesmana, C. B. J. (2020). Correlation of family expressed emotion and frequency of relapse schizophrenia patients. *Journal of Clinical and Cultural Psychiatry, 1*(2), 35–37.

Zaki, J., & Ochsner, K. (2012). The neuroscience of empathy: Progress, pitfalls and promise. *Nature Neuroscience, 15*(5), 675–680.

Zanarini, M. C. (2000). Childhood experiences associated with the development of borderline personality disorder.

Psychiatric Clinics of North America, 23(1), 89–101. https://doi.org/10.1016/S0193–953X(05)70145-3

Zanarini, M. C., Frankenburg, F. R., Reich, D. B., & Fitzmaurice, G. M. (2016). Fluidity of the subsyndromal phenomenology of borderline personality disorder over 16 years of prospective follow-up. *The American Journal of Psychiatry, 173*(7), 688–694.

Zelkowitz, P., Paris, J., Guzder, J., & Feldman, R. (2001). Borderline pathology. *Journal of the American Academy of Child & Adolescent Psychiatry, 40*(10), 1124–1125.

Zerbe, K. J. (2010). Psychodynamic therapy for eating disorders. In C. M. Zilo & J. E. Mitchell (Eds.), *The treatment of eating disorders: A clinical handbook* (pp. 339–358). New York, NY: Guilford Press.

Zhou, D.-D., Zhou, X.-X., Li, Y., Zhang, K.-F., Lv, Z., Chen, X.-R., . . . Kuang, L. (2019). Augmentation agents to serotonin reuptake inhibitors for treatment-resistant obsessive-compulsive disorder: A network meta-analysis. *Progress in Neuropsychopharmacology and Biological Psychiatry, 90*, 277–287. https://doi.org/10.1016/j.pnpbp.2018.12.009

Zilboorg, G., & Henry, G. W. (1941). *A history of medical psychology.* New York, NY: W. W. Norton.

Zimring, F. E. (2020). Firearms and violence in American life—50 years later. *Criminology & Public Policy, 19*(4), 1359–1369.

Zinzaw, H. M., Resnick, H. S., McCauley, J. L., Amstadter, A. B., Ruggiero, K. J., & Kilpatrick, D. G. (2012). Prevalence and risk of psychiatric disorders as a function of variant rape histories: Results from a national survey of women. *Social Psychiatry and Psychiatric Epidemiology, 47*, 893–902.

Zoellner, L. A., Ojalehto, H. J., Rosencrans, P., Walker, R. W., Garcia, N. M., Sheikh, I. S., & Bedard-Gilligan, M. A. (2020). Anxiety and fear in PTSD. In M. T. Tull & N. A. Kimbrel (Eds.), *Emotion in posttraumatic stress disorder* (pp. 43–63). London: Academic Press.

Zucker, K. J. (2017). Epidemiology of gender dysphoria and transgender identity. *Sexual Health, 14*(5), 404–411.

Zuckerman, K. E., & Pachter, L. M. (2019). Race, ethnicity, socioeconomic factors, and attention-deficit hyperactivity disorder. *Journal of Developmental and Behavioral Pediatrics, 40*(2), 150–151. https://doi.org/10.1097/dbp.0000000000000645

Zvolensky, M. J., Rogers, A. H., Bakhshaie, J., Viana, A. G., Walker, R., Mayorga, N. A., . . . Ruiz, A. C. (2019). Perceived racial discrimination, anxiety sensitivity, and mental health among Latinos in a federally qualified health center. *Stigma and Health, 4*(4), 473–479.

Index

Note: Page numbers in bold refer to Glossary items

exposure therapy, 55–56
external locus of control, 58
extroversion, 390–91
eye movement desensitization and
        reprocessing (EMDR)
        therapy, 158–59

face validity, 72
factitious disorder, 216–17, **513**
factitious disorder imposed on another,
        217
Fallon, James, 397
Falret, Jean-Pierre, 187
family
        influence on eating disorders, 309–10
family-focused therapy, 206–7
family studies, 39–40
family systems therapy, 206
family therapy, 62–63, 206–7, 309–10
fat shaming, 292–93
fear, 98
fear response, 39
female orgasmic disorder, 266, 267, 272,
        513
female sexual interest/arousal disorder,
        264, **514**
Feminist Ecological model, 120
fetal alcohol spectrum disorder,
        463–64
fetishistic disorder, 274–75, **514**
        models and treatments, 281–83
Fetzima, 196
fight, flee, or freeze response, 37, 99
        generalized anxiety disorder and,
                117–18
        symptoms of, 132
fight or flight response, 34, 99
        See also fight, flee, or freeze response
fixation (Freud), 47
flat or restricted affect, 418
flibanserin, 271
fluoxetine, 44, 114, 130, 152, 308, 325
fluvoxamine, 130
Food and Drug Administration (FDA), 42
forebrain, 33–35
Foster, Jodie, 497
Fragile X syndrome, 462, **514**
free association, 48
Freud, Sigmund, 15–16, 119, 221
        assessment of the psychodynamic
                perspective, 49–50
        defense mechanisms, 47
        personality theory, 45–46

psychodynamic therapies, 47–49,
        517
psychosexual stages of development,
        46–47
theory of personality development,
        46–47
views of women, 49
frontal lobes, 35
frontotemporal neurocognitive disorder,
        475, **514**
frotteuristic disorder, 277–79, **514**
        models and treatments, 281–83
functional magnetic resonance imaging
        (fMRI), 78, **514**
functional neurological symptom
        disorder, 219–21

GABA (gamma-aminobutyric acid), 36
GABA neurotransmitter system, 118
gambling disorder, 365–67, **514**
        diagnostic overview, 366
        prevalence of, 367
        symptoms and description, 351–66
        trajectory, 367
gamma hydroxybutyrate (GHB), 365
gay panic defense, 496
gender
        distinction from sex, 255–56
        social construction of, 283–84
gender confirmation surgery, 259–60
gender diversity
        case study (Jazz Jennings), 253–54,
                259
gender dysphoria, 254, 256–57, **514**
        biological models and treatments,
                259–60
        models and treatments, 259–62
        prevalence, 257–58
        psychological models and treatments,
                260–62
        symptoms and clinical description,
                257
        trajectory, 257–58
gender expression, 255, **514**
gender identity, 254–55, **514**
        misgendering, 258–59
gender pronouns, 258–59
gender reveal parties, 255–56
Gender Unicorn, 74
gender variations, 256–57
gene expression
        effects of trauma, 150–51
        role of methylation, 150–51

generalized anxiety disorder, 116–21
        biological models and treatment,
                117–19
        cognitive and behavioral models and
                treatment, 119–20
        diagnostic overview, 117
        Feminist Ecological model, 120
        fight, flee, or freeze response, 117–18
        heritability of, 117
        hypervigilance, 121
        medications for, 118–19
        models, 117–21
        multiperspective models and
                treatment, 121
        predisposing factors, 121
        prevalence, 117
        protective behaviors, 121
        psychodynamic models and
                treatment, 119
        sociocultural models and treatment,
                120–21
        symptoms and description, 116–17
        trajectory, 117
        treatments, 117–21
genetic model of PTSD, 150–51
genetics
        chromosomes, 38–39
        dominant genes, 39
        environmental influences on
                populations, 39
        influence on psychopathology, 37–39
        nature-nurture debate, 37
        polygenic traits, 39
        principles of genetic inheritance,
                38–39
        recessive genes, 39
        role of DNA, 38–39
genetics research
        adoption studies, 40
        family studies, 39–40
        heritability estimate, 40
        methods, 39–41
        Minnesota Study of Twins Reared
                Apart (MISTRA), 40–41
        twin studies, 40–41
genito-pelvic pain/penetration disorder,
        267–69, **514**
genograms, 73–74
genuineness
        in client-centered therapy, 52
Geodon, 43
George III, King
        madness of, 1–2, 71

For EU product safety concerns, contact us at Calle de José Abascal, 56–1°, 28003 Madrid, Spain or eugpsr@cambridge.org.

www.ingramcontent.com/pod-product-compliance
Ingram Content Group UK Ltd.
Pitfield, Milton Keynes, MK11 3LW, UK
UKHW051048150625
459647UK00016B/1816